P9-CRG-966

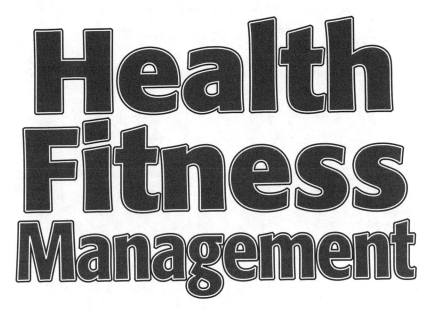

Health Fitness Management

A Comprehensive Resource for Managing and Operating Programs and Facilities

William C. Grantham, MS

General Manager of Little Rock Athletic Club
Little Rock, Arkansas

Robert W. Patton, PhD

Regents Professor
Department of Kinesiology, Health Promotion, and Recreation
University of North Texas

Tracy D. York, MS

Director of Operations, Lake Austin Spa Resort
Austin, Texas

Mitchel L. Winick, JD

Management Consultant
Dallas, Texas

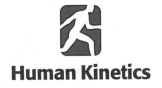

Human Kinetics

Library of Congress Cataloging-in-Publication Data

Health fitness management : a comprehensive resource for managing and operating programs and
  facilities / William C. Grantham . . . [et al.].
      p.   cm.
    Includes bibliographical references and index.
    ISBN 0-88011-559-9
    1. Physical fitness centers--United States--Management.
  2. Physical fitness--Study and teaching--United States.
I. Grantham, William C., 1950-
  GV428.5.H43   1997
  613.7'068--dc21   97-26549
                                                                               CIP

ISBN-10: 0-88011-559-9
ISBN-13: 978-0-88011-559-9

Copyright © 1998 by William C. Grantham, Robert W. Patton, Tracy D. York, and Mitchel L. Winick

All rights reserved. Except for use in a review, the reproduction or utilization of this work in any form or by any
electronic, mechanical, or other means, now known or hereafter invented, including xerography, photocopying, and
recording, and in any information storage and retrieval system, is forbidden without the written permission of the
publisher.

Notice: Permission to reproduce the following material is granted to instructors and agencies who have purchased
Health Fitness Management: pp. 119, 122, 123, 124, 128, 129-130, 132, 134, 148, 155, 156, 159, 176, 180, 184, 185, 230-232,
255, 259, 260, 265-271, 288, 290, 304, 305, 306-307, 310, 311-312, 313-314, 316, 317-318, 320, 323, 332, 340, 341, 342, 343,
351, 422, 424, 440, 444, 459, 460, 461, 465, 478. The reproduction of other parts of this book is expressly forbidden by
the above copyright notice. Persons or agencies who have not purchased *Health Fitness Management* may not
reproduce any material.

Acquisitions Editor: Scott Wikgren; **Developmental Editor:** Julie Rhoda; **Assistant Editor:** Sandra Merz Bott;
Editorial Assistants: Jennifer Jeanne Hemphill and Laura T. Seversen; **Copyeditor:** Denelle Eknes; **Proofreader:**
Pam Johnson; **Indexer:** Craig Brown; **Graphic Designer:** Stuart Cartwright; **Graphic Artist:** Kim Maxey;
Photographer: Tom Roberts; **Photo Editor:** Boyd LaFoon; **Cover Designer:** Jack Davis; **Illustrator:** Chuck Nivens;
Printer: Braun-Brumfield, Inc.; **Cover Photo:** Courtesy of Four Seasons Resort and Clubs at Las Colinas, Irving,
Texas

Printed in the United States of America   10   9   8

Human Kinetics
Web site: www.HumanKinetics.com

United States: Human Kinetics
P.O. Box 5076
Champaign, IL 61825-5076
800-747-4457
e-mail: humank@hkusa.com

Canada: Human Kinetics
475 Devonshire Road Unit 100
Windsor, ON N8Y 2L5
800-465-7301 (in Canada only)
e-mail: orders@hkcanada.com

Europe: Human Kinetics
107 Bradford Road
Stanningley
Leeds LS28 6AT, United Kingdom
+44 (0) 113 255 5665
e-mail: hk@hkeurope.com

Australia: Human Kinetics
57A Price Avenue
Lower Mitcham, South Australia 5062
08 8277 1555
e-mail: liaw@hkaustralia.com

New Zealand: Human Kinetics
Division of Sports Distributors NZ Ltd.
P.O. Box 300 226 Albany
North Shore City
Auckland
0064 9 448 1207
e-mail: info@humankinetics.co.nz

To my lovely and very understanding wife, Jamie; and to my mother and father, Barbara and J.O. Grantham, without their continued encouragement and inspiration this book would still be a dream.

W.C.G.

To my mother, Ruth Patton, for her nurturing and unconditional love; to my wife, Elisa, for her unending support, love, and wonderful companionship; and, to my children, Laura and Scott, for enriching my life and giving me hope for the future.

R.W.P.

To Lucille York. Thanks for your unwavering support, example of integrity, and unconditional love. I am the luckiest kid in the world. I love you, Mom.

T.D.Y.

To my wife, Debbie, for taking more than her share of the parenting responsibilities while I realized my dream of writing; to our children, Tyler and Lezah, for providing inspiration for the future; to my parents, Veta and Darvin, for providing inspiration—past and present; and to my sister Mara Beth and brother Seth for their high expectations for big brother.

M.L.W.

CONTENTS

PREFACE

Health Fitness Management—A Comprehensive Resource for Managing and Operating Programs and Facilities is the third in a trilogy of books designed to assist students and active professionals in the health fitness field. *Implementing Health/Fitness Programs* (1986), the first book in the series, developed a model for successful delivery of wellness programs in varied settings. The explosive growth of health fitness programs designed to promote high-level wellness began during the early and mid-1980s. This growth appeared in diverse settings, such as shopping centers, corporations, and hospitals, and the industry needed a resource for a generic program delivery model. Moreover, colleges and universities were initiating professional preparation programs for students interested in the health fitness industry. This first book galvanized the delivery concepts in disparate settings and was timely in meeting the book market needs. *Developing and Managing Health/Fitness Facilities* (1989), the second book, provided a model for planning, designing, constructing, equipping, and staffing health fitness facilities. The timely introduction of this book was in the late 1980s, the height of the construction boom in which the number of health fitness facilities increased more than 120 percent during an eight-year period (International Health, Racquet and Sportsclub Association [IHRSA] 1995). Moreover, professional preparation programs were expanding and needing a text for facility development courses they were adopting. *Health Fitness Management—A Comprehensive Resource for Managing and Operating Programs and Facilities* completes the trilogy by presenting a set of management theories and operational models for health fitness programs.

According to the International Health, Racquet and Sportsclub Association (IHRSA 1995), during the mid-1990s there has been a 16 percent decline, followed by a recent slow reversal in the number of health fitness facilities across the United States while membership has continued to increase. Owners and operators of single- or multiple-site facilities have adopted their own management and operational

guidelines. Management practices in this industry are varied and without consensus. Individuals with diverse backgrounds, often with no formal training, manage and operate facilities. Marginally operated facilities failing to make profits or achieve program objectives are closing their doors. In short, the industry is maturing and competition is vigorous. Poorly managed programs are perishing at record rates and well-run programs are flourishing. Unfortunately, there is no industry-wide reference to guide managers and operators of these programs. There is also no reference text for the colleges and universities providing students information on health fitness management. We have designed this book to meet these needs and are confident that it provides a valuable resource both for readers' current needs and for future reference.

Health Fitness Management—A Comprehensive Resource for Managing and Operating Programs and Facilities brings conventional business management principles and operational guidelines to the unconventional business of health and fitness. The book introduces the reader to the health fitness industry and its members before addressing management practices and operational issues. The book finally provides a means of evaluating existing programs and strategically planning for the future.

Part I sets the stage for managing and operating facilities. Following an introduction to the field and the type of member frequenting the various program settings, we address some management concepts. Through this process, we review the nature of managing facilities from a contemporary approach. We then present organizational considerations to provide you with alternative viewpoints toward organizational structure. We discuss organizational leadership, emphasizing the importance of dynamic leadership and personal communications for successful program operation.

We make a distinction between *front-of-the-house* and *back-of-the-house* management and operations. The former relates to those activities that directly impact member and guest service, such as member name recognition, staff attitude, and member service. The latter relates to those operations that are not as apparent in their impact on member service but must be accomplished effectively if programs are to run smoothly and efficiently. Examples of these operations include facility and equipment maintenance, business office management, financial management, legal issues, and insurance matters.

Part II deals with front-of-the-house management issues, which directly impact the member or participant's experience. We discuss topics such as sales and marketing, member management, service desk management, program management, profit centers, as well as personnel management and equipment issues. This section reinforces the importance of member relations and illustrates methods of ensuring quality control in this vital area of running a successful operation.

Part III addresses back-of-the-house management issues, which are less visible to the member but critically important to the successful management of a program: health and safety standards, maintenance, finance, compensation, legal, insurance, and computer issues. This section underscores that no number of smiling faces or name recognitions can overcome member discontent associated with such things as dirty locker rooms or constant billing problems. We present practical information and tactics to minimize these back-of-the-house problems.

Part IV presents the evaluation and planning processes and includes areas such as facility, personnel, program, marketing, and financial evaluation. We provide an easy-to-use instrument to facilitate program evaluation. By focusing on strategic planning and issues for the future we hope to ensure that the ongoing evaluation of programs can forecast change for optimal development.

The book uses many examples from for-profit commercial environments because this is the largest sector of health fitness settings in the industry. Moreover, for-profit environments address both revenue production and expense management issues. Most nonprofit programs, on the other hand, primarily deal with expense management regarding financial issues. Thus, considerations surrounding sales and marketing, membership dues, and other revenue issues may not seem as relevant to readers interested in nonprofit health fitness settings. Keep in mind, though, that both for-profit and nonprofit institutions need to hire and train quality staff; keep facilities clean, safe, and operational; and service members with good programs. These topics dominate the content of the book.

We have also introduced a management model for the health fitness industry. In addition to the traditional scheme of planning, organizing, leading, and controlling functions of management, we have included the thought that this core of management theory must include the concepts of information gathering, innovative thinking, and implementation that we have identified as the I-formation management model. A thorough discussion of this model is presented in chapter 4 and will clarify our thinking on the subject. Throughout the book we have included the icons to reinforce the I-formation management model.

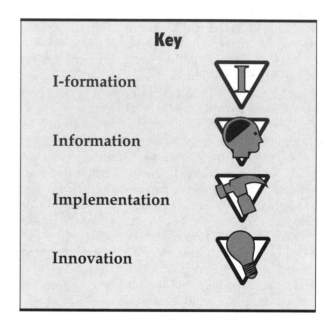

We have highlighted key points throughout the chapters to focus attention on main issues. These key points are set off by the I-formation icons mentioned above and presented in detail in chapter 4. Each chapter also highlights and discusses key terms and lists them at the end. We designed these key points and key terms to help the student quickly recall new terminology and important concepts presented on the chapter topics. The book includes sample forms and checklists that you can adapt to site-specific requirements for a cross section of health fitness facilities. These ready references should prove helpful to the practitioner seeking quick solutions to ongoing management and operational problems.

We have designed this book for you to use both as a reference tool and as a classroom textbook. The professional health fitness facility owner or manager will be able to use the checklists, forms, illustrations, and graphs to develop or improve specific operational guidelines. In fact, we recommend that practitioners start using the book with an evaluation of their programs. Chapter 20 provides an instrument for this purpose. The practitioner can then clarify any deficits observed from this evaluation and make improvements using the book. The college instructor of an organizational or an administration course in health fitness management can use this book as a primary text. We have organized the content logically and designed it for the teacher to present following the order of the book. This book should also be a helpful reference to those seeking professional certifications. Some certifications are now expecting that candidates have a working knowledge of managing and operating facilities. Certainly, the material in this book should prove helpful for those seeking such health fitness management information.

RECOMMENDED READINGS

International Health, Racquet and Sportsclub Association (IHRSA). 1995. *The 1995 IHRSA report on the state of the health club industry.* Boston: IHRSA

International Health, Racquet and Sportsclub Association (IHRSA). 1997. *1997 IHRSA report on the state of the health club industry.* Boston: IHRSA.

Patton, R.W., J.M. Corry, L.R. Gettman, and J.S. Graf. 1986. *Implementing health/fitness programs.* Champaign, IL: Human Kinetics.

Patton, R.W., W.C. Grantham, R.F. Gerson, and L.R. Gettman. 1989. *Developing and managing health/fitness facilities.* Champaign, IL: Human Kinetics.

ACKNOWLEDGMENTS

We would like to thank everyone who taught us what we know about the health fitness industry. Without their help this book would not have been possible. We would also like to thank Human Kinetics for undertaking this project. Rainer Martens endorsed the book project without hesitation. Julie Rhoda, our developmental editor, was terrific and provided endless support throughout the book's development.

Two other individuals were instrumental in the development of this book: Mary Olson for editing, copying, and providing helpful feedback, and Pat M. Riley, Jr., for lending support and feedback and assisting in general manager duties of the Little Rock Athletic Club, which provided me the time to complete the book.

W.C.G.

I would like to thank all my students who went on to work in the health fitness industry—and then taught me how things really work in the trenches. Aside from my coauthors, Bill Baun is most noteworthy, who provided critical reviews of the book and suggested the framework for the evaluation model we adopted. I would also like to thank Cindy Ford for helping with the manuscript development and my wife, Elisa, for enduring unintended neglect during the book's development, which took longer than we all expected.

R.W.P.

There are no words to express my gratitude to so many for their support and encouragement throughout this project. Without the understanding of those close to me and the time and talents of many skilled professionals, this book would never have become a reality. A huge thank you to Lydia for her constant support and understanding, to my coauthors from whom I have learned so much, and to my family and friends for putting up with two years of unintended absence and neglect. I also thank my past and present coworkers and associates from whom I learned so much and made so many lifelong friendships. Thanks.

T.D.Y.

First and foremost I thank my personal friend, mentor, and coauthor Bob Patton. His contributions to the growth of the health fitness industry, the success of numerous health fitness organizations, and the education and career development of hundreds (if not thousands) of young professionals, is represented in one small way by this book. As his peers, students, and former students would undoubtedly agree, it would take an encyclopedia rather than a single volume to capture the full range of Dr. Bob's knowledge. I also thank my coauthors Bill Grantham and Tracy York: they have brought valuable, hands-on experience and insight to the book and exhibited more than a full measure of patience and professionalism toward an often-delinquent coauthor.

M.L.W.

INTRODUCTION TO HEALTH FITNESS MANAGEMENT

The Health Fitness Industry

The *fitness boom* arising during the last half of the 20th century has created an explosive growth in the health fitness industry. For decades participation in physical activity, membership in health clubs, and expansion of fitness facilities increased exponentially. The result has been that more than 20 million Americans frequent health clubs plus a 82 percent increase in home exercisers from 1987 through 1996. Even with this explosive growth, nearly 80 percent of Americans fail to get enough exercise to enhance quality and quantity of life. It is this sedentary group that represents a tremendous market potential for the health fitness industry.

The explosive growth in facilities and memberships in the health fitness industry has abated. This slowing growth gives us pause to examine the industry, define some of its essential characteristics, and position ourselves for the new marketplace. Currently, the health fitness industry can be divided into four distinct segments, described as commercial, corporate, clinical, and community settings. Although each setting is distinct, there are many similarities in operational functions and management concepts.

This chapter explores trends in the industry and the status of settings in which health fitness services are conducted. The chapter also contrasts these settings in terms of program functions, practitioner roles, and facility design. This information provides the aspiring health fitness professional with insight into functional differences existing in the various settings. It is helpful for the health fitness student or entry-level professional planning and directing a career path. The settings also serve as a platform for the remainder of the book, as we apply fundamental business practices to them and give a model for managing and operating programs in this diverse industry.

THE HEALTH FITNESS MOVEMENT

The health fitness movement in the United States has unclear origins. Some might argue that the roots of our current health and fitness consciousness began before the 20th century with physical education programs developing in the schools and YMCAs. Others might argue that the health fitness movement is a more recent phenomenon related to the aerobics movement in the 1970s, the explosive construction of commercial fitness facilities in the 1980s, or some other concurrent trend. Regardless of the origin of the so-called fitness boom, the greatest of health and fitness growth has been during the last half of this century. Participation by Americans in fitness activities, for example, has increased expo-

nentially since 1960. Figure 1.1 illustrates this explosive growth pattern. Only recently has the growth in participation begun to slow. However, according to American Sports Data, Inc. (1994), the growth in participation resumed during 1994 with an 11 percent surge. It is uncertain what lies ahead, but we have enjoyed great progress thus far and there is little to prevent continued growth. We are forecasting modest, but not explosive, growth in fitness participation in the coming decade and into the 21st century.

During 1996, there were approximately 20 million Americans participating in some type of health fitness club or facility away from the home. This represents a compound growth of 10 percent during each of the preceding two years. Figure 1.2 illustrates participation levels in a variety of health club settings during 1996. The commercial sector, or the for-profit environment, is currently capturing the largest number of users. The Y programs rank second in market penetration, with the category of single-purpose facilities, such as aerobic studios, tennis centers, aquatic clubs, bodybuilding gyms, and racquetball centers, ranking third. Corporate fitness centers come in a distant fourth as the most popular setting for those who exercise outside the home. No single-purpose facility approaches the annual usage of the corporate fitness center category. Many individuals use more than one type of facility during a year and would contribute to some estimate inflation in these categories. Nonetheless, from 1987 to 1996 health fitness membership in the health club environment has grown by 51 percent and currently shows no sign of letting up.

Yet, with all the growth in activity participation, we are not making a large enough improvement in our exercise behaviors.

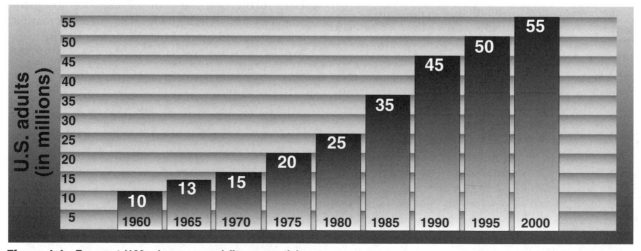

Figure 1.1   Frequent (100+ days per year) fitness participants.

Adapted, by permission, from IHRSA, 1997, *Profiles of Success* (Boston: IHRSA).

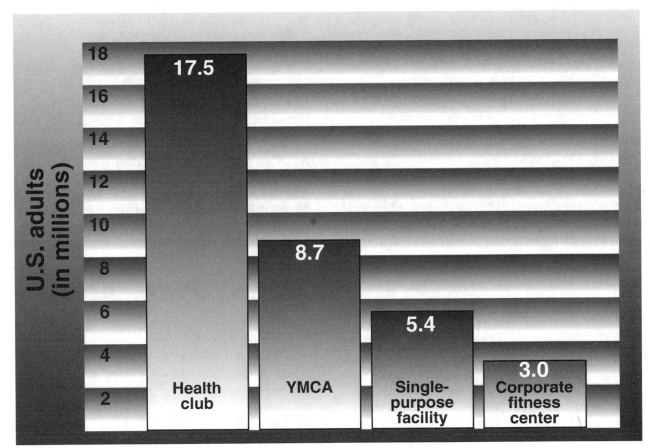

Figure 1.2 Usage of health fitness facilities in 1996.

Adapted, by permission, from IHRSA, 1997, *Profiles of success* (Boston: IHRSA).

> *Only 22 percent of Americans partici-
> pate in physical activity enough to enjoy the
> protective effects of exercise from such diseases
> as coronary heart disease, hypertension, diabe-
> tes, osteoporosis, anxiety, and depression.*

Figure 1.3 shows that four out of five Americans are inactive, that is, not exercising at home or at a club enough to ward off hypokinetic disease, which accounts for as much as 80 percent of the death, disease, and disability in our culture, according to the Centers for Disease Control and Prevention (U.S. Department of Health and Human Services 1996). Despite efforts by many professional organizations and legions of fitness professionals, little headway is occurring in the nationwide campaign toward the goal set by the federally-supported project Healthy People 2000 of getting 30 percent of our population regularly physically active by the turn of the century. Demographic data show that, on average, men are more active than women and that regular physical activity declines with age. Furthermore, ethnic minorities, especially minority women, are less active than Caucasian Americans. Ethnic differences in physical activity can be attributed to differences in education and socioeconomic status. Data further indicate that participation in leisure time physical activity increases with an increase in education and annual income level. The primary explanations for low participation among all adult Americans include lack of sufficient time for participation, lack of confidence in the ability to be physically active, perceived barriers to activity, and lack of enjoyment derived from physical activity. There is a huge and untapped market represented by the underactive and underfit people in America. Most fitness conscious Americans have bought into the fitness movement, joined clubs, or initiated a home exercise program. We have gathered the low-hanging fruit. The sedentary market will be the next and greatest challenge we face as health fitness professionals because of resistance among these underactive individuals to include exercise in their lifestyles. However, there is reason for hope. According to a national study conducted in 1993 for the President's Council on Physical Fitness and Sports and the Sporting Goods Manufacturers Association, 59 percent of the inactive Americans surveyed desire to become more physically active. Apparently, they are just having some difficulty getting started.

> *According to a national study conducted in 1993 for the President's Council on Physical Fitness and Sports and the Sporting Goods Manufacturers Association, 59 percent of the inactive Americans surveyed desire to become more physically active.*

Some headway is occurring in making exercise more appealing to the currently inactive. The Surgeon General's 1996 report on physical activity will help immensely in promoting exercise to our population of inactive Americans (U.S. Department of Health and Human Services 1996). Prestigious organizations such as the American College of Sports Medicine and the Centers for Disease Control and Prevention have endorsed what some have labeled *Exercise Lite,* suggesting that extremely vigorous activity is not the only way to get significant and lasting benefits from exercise (Pate et al. 1995). Although vigorous activity, such as running, is necessary to achieve high levels of fitness, moderate activity, such as walking, gardening, and taking the stairs instead of elevators, can achieve health benefits if undertaken for a total of 30 minutes most days of the week. Individuals don't need to accomplish this 30 minutes per day during continuous movement. They can accumulate it with intermittent trips during the workday to the next floor in an office building or walking from a distantly parked car to their work site. The health fitness industry has yet to incorporate this Exercise Lite approach into their system of program delivery. It will be interesting to see how this concept unfolds and is incorporated into health fitness programs in the coming years.

Home exercise presents another great opportunity for increasing physical activity levels in Americans. Between 1987 and 1996, frequent home exercise participation skyrocketed by 82 percent according to American Sports Data, Inc. (IHRSA 1997). Perhaps we are doing a better job at promoting exercise participation in our schools and health fitness centers than we

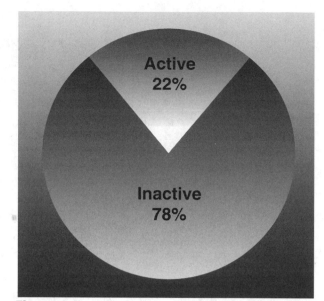

Figure 1.3   Active versus chronically inactive adult Americans in 1994.

think. Several barriers for belonging to a club are not present in the home setting for some individuals. In any event, this explosive growth is not occurring at the expense of health fitness club memberships. As mentioned previously, a 82 percent increase in home participation occurred during the same nine-year period as a 51 percent increase in club memberships. The focus for this book, however, is not on home exercise programs; it is with managing and operating health fitness facilities and programs. Let's examine the various settings in which this membership growth has occurred during recent years.

CONTRASTING THE HEALTH FITNESS SETTINGS

Perhaps the best way to understand health fitness management is to examine the various settings in which programs are managed and operated. We devote the remainder of this chapter to examining the *commercial, corporate, clinical,* and *community settings.* First, we look at the growth patterns and functional differences in managing various programs. Next, we explore the roles that professionals exhibit in different settings. We also mention other contrasts, such as facility differences. Finally, we identify factors, such as the program's objectives and type of participants, that tend to define the program and render each setting unique. Throughout the book we will illustrate different approaches each setting takes in managing and operating programs.

Table 1.1 The Type, Number, and Membership of Health Fitness Facilities in the United States		
Type	Number	Membership based
Commercial centers		
Health clubs/fitness facilities	13,000	100%
Corporate fitness centers	2,000	25%
Clinical hospital-based wellness centers	1,000	25%
Community centers		
Recreation fitness facilities	8,000	15%
Hotel fitness facilities	3,000	25%
Country club fitness facilities	4,000	100%
YMCAs, JCCs, Boys Clubs	3,000	100%
Residential developments	4,000	25%
Schools and universities	4,000	15%
	Total 42,000	

Adapted, by permission, from IHRSA, 1997, Profiles of success (Boston: IHRSA).

The commercial, corporate, clinical, and community settings each play an important, but different, role in the health fitness industry. Management processes, although using fundamental business principles, are emphasized differently in each setting. It is important that health fitness professionals recognize these differences because many of our career paths take us into diverse settings when we least expect it. Each setting has unique approaches to problem solving and programming, and it behooves us to know about this industry's diversity to prepare for unexpected opportunities for advancement and challenge.

Growth Patterns and Trends

According to the International Health, Racquet and Sportsclub Association (IHRSA) (1994, 1997), there are currently more than 40 thousand health fitness facilities in the United States delivering programs in different settings with varied membership structures. Table 1.1 illustrates the breakdown of facilities in these settings.

Commercial Programs

The commercial setting has grown in both memberships and facilities during the past two decades; however, membership growth has far exceeded facility development in recent times. Figure 1.4 shows how memberships in health fitness programs have risen from a market penetration of 7.6 percent of the U.S. population (12.8 million) in 1987 to more than

8.0 percent of the population in 1995 (19.1 million), according to the IHRSA (1995, 1997). Facility development of the 1980s resulted in a net growth of more than 120 percent but has declined more than 15 percent in the early to mid-1990s. According to IHRSA, the decline in facilities indicates a shakeout of marginally operated facilities and programs. Many believe this to be a positive trend for the surviving clubs embracing sound operational and management practices. This consolidation of the industry has resulted in fewer and larger players. Table 1.2 represents the industry's current major players in the commercial sector.

There are several major trends occurring in the commercial setting, including:

- continued movement away from single-purpose clubs, such as racquetball centers, which have lost 50 percent in membership over the past 10 years, to a multipurpose athletic, fitness, and social club, which has gained almost 50 percent in membership over the past 10 years;

- movement from indoor-only to four-season indoor and outdoor clubs;

- greater emphasis on personalized programming using a value-added basis, as seen in the rapid growth of personal training offered in clubs;

- movement from an annual dues plus pay-as-you-play pricing system to an initiation fee plus monthly dues payment system, which holds clubs more accountable to members on a regular basis and encourages increased service levels;

Table 1.2	The Industry's Big Players in the Commercial Sector							
Number of clubs	1989	1990	1991	1992	1993	1994	1995	1996
Gold's Gym franchises	296	330	350	375	400	420	---	503
Bally Fitness Center divisions*	---	---	307	310	336	339	---	320
Club Corporation of America*, **	---	---	200	230	231	231	---	250
World Gym franchises	68	88	120	145	175	194	---	255
Family Fitness*, **	33	48	54	60	65	72	---	---
American Club Systems, Inc.**	---	---	---	15	15	42	---	661
*Owned clubs ** Managed clubs								

Adapted by permission, from IHRSA, 1997, *Profiles of success* (Boston: IHRSA).

- focus on more comprehensive wellness programs addressing increased health concerns of members; and
- shift of commercial health fitness program development to focus on mid- to small-sized companies seeking a cost-effective environment for their employee health promotion activities.

Commercial organizations are increasingly forming joint ventures with hospitals and other health care providers seeking venues for cost-effective delivery sites for preventive managed care. Table 1.3 presents some of the popular programs for 1997 in the commercial setting and reflects some trends just mentioned.

The financial incentives for the commercial sector continue to be a challenge because growth is barely keeping pace with current inflation. Price competition abounds in the commercial sector because fewer facilities are chasing the increasingly sophisticated and demanding consumer. Moreover, nonprofit facilities, such as YMCAs and other community facilities, offer lower prices because they benefit from United Way subsidies and federal tax relief.

The industry's dollar volume is astounding. According to 1993 estimates of the National Sporting Goods Association, the retail fitness equipment industry generated over $2 billion—much of which was targeted for the burgeoning home fitness market. Institutional fitness equipment sales accounted for another $120 million. The total estimated revenue for the health fitness industry was $7.4 billion. These figures continue to grow regardless of fluctuations in the economy. We are forecasting more than $10 billion revenue in the health fitness industry by the 21st century.

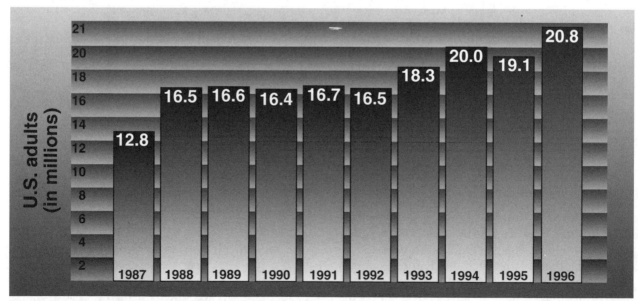

Figure 1.4 Health club membership growth in America.

Adapted, by permission, from IHRSA, 1997, *Profiles of success* (Boston: IHRSA).

Table 1.3	Top Ten Hot Programs for 1997 in the Commercial Setting

1. Personal training
2. Nutritional programs
3. Senior's fitness
4. Children's fitness
5. Mind-body programs
6. Physical therapy
7. Spinning
8. Wellness education
9. Massage
10. Adventure fitness

Adapted, by permission, from IHRSA, 1997, *Profiles of success* (Boston: IHRSA).

The health fitness boom is alive and well in America, and it shows no sign of letting up any time soon. Memberships are growing. Fitness equipment sales are explosive, and home exercise participation is increasing exponentially.

Corporate Programs

There has been good growth in the number of corporate health fitness program participants in recent years. As figure 1.5 illustrates, participation had increased more than 50 percent from 1989 to 1994.

It is difficult to explain the marked increase in participation rates for corporate health fitness programs from 1993 to 1994—especially when this increase came on the heels of successive years of declining participation. Regardless of aberrations in measures of participation rates, the corporate health fitness setting is alive and well at the moment. We should note, however, that corporate programs are dependent on the size of the workforce. The vast majority of companies in America have fewer than 100 employees. Table 1.4 reveals that companies with fewer than 100 employees are significantly less likely to have health fitness programs than companies with more than 750 employees. Moreover, the variety of program offerings is less in the smaller companies when compared with the larger companies. The logical assumption from these data would be that smaller companies do not have the resources to offer the breadth of programs seen in the larger companies. However, many smaller companies unable to develop in-house facilities for health promotion programs frequently contract these activities to other providers or fitness facilities in local commercial, clinical, or community settings where there is greater economy of scale. As mentioned earlier, many commercial programs offer financial incentives and specialized programming for such associations.

There is no data giving reliable information on the number of facilities being developed in the corporate setting at the moment. One might speculate that parallel patterns exist between corporate and commercial settings in facilities and programs developed. Speculating further, one might conclude that large corporations made a commitment to developing health fitness facilities during the boom years of the 1980s when all their corporate colleagues were

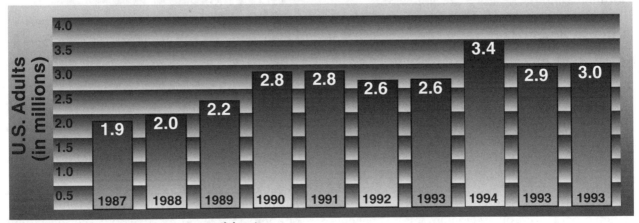

Figure 1.5 Corporate fitness center participants.

Adapted, by permission, from IHRSA, 1997, *Profiles of success* (Boston: IHRSA).

Table 1.4   Percent of Worksites Offering Specific Health Promotion Activities

Type of activity	Worksite size (number of employees)			
	50–99	100–249	250–749	750+
Health risk appraisal	18.4%	34.0%	41.8%	66.2%
Exercise/fitness	14.5	22.7	32.4	33.7
Back care	19.5	34.8	41.4	47.4
Smoking cessation	30.1	37.5	39.5	57.9
Weight control	8.1	13.5	22.9	48.8
Nutrition education	8.6	19.8	21.9	48.0
Stress management	14.5	32.7	37.5	60.8

Reprinted from National survey of worksite health promotion activities (p. 10) by U.S. Department of Health and Human Services, Public Health Service, Office of Disease Prevention and Health Promotion, 1987, Silver Spring, MD: ODPHP National Health Information Center.

undergoing wellness center construction. Perhaps the health care and insurance industries also had something to do with this wellness center development. However, the role of the health care industry as an incentive for corporate program development is clouded now by the polarized influences of private health insurance companies and managed care providers. We will discuss the role of managed care later in this chapter and further in chapter 21.

The types of programs in the corporate setting differ from those in other environments. We can presume corporate programs pay dividends to the company by increased employee health and a better bottom line through greater productivity, lower health care costs, and fewer absences, to mention a few outcomes. Commercial programs, however, reflect a more physical performance and appearance focus in delivering services. The professional association for corporate health fitness centers has recently undergone a name change from the Association for Fitness in Business to the Association for Worksite Health Promotion, reflecting this broadening concern in the corporate setting. Corporate programs are now addressing many health issues in addition to fitness program development.

Clinical Programs

There are approximately 1,000 hospital-based health fitness facilities in the country, accounting for only 5 percent of the fitness centers available to consumers. Roughly one out of four hospitals now has a health fitness facility providing community outreach programs. Most of these facilities are closely associated with outpatient services, such as physical therapy, sports medicine, and cardiac rehabilitation and frequently provide both types of programs in the same facility. This is especially true where cardiac rehabilitation programs are offered to unmonitored patients not requiring direct physician supervision.

One might question the wisdom of according an entire category in this book to such a sparsely represented segment of the industry. The reason for giving such emphasis to hospital-based fitness programs is more because of their potential impact than present representation in the health fitness industry. Managed care is taking on a greater role in American health care delivery; the focus in managed care is to empty rather than fill hospital beds and to reduce rather than increase patient care. The only way this can be effectively accomplished is through prevention, which diminishes health care volume and thus reduces costs. We know that health fitness programs are cost beneficial and cost effective. White papers abound explaining the financial merits of preventive health care services and health promotion programs. Health care administrators are only now recognizing the importance of prevention. Either that or the reimbursement system is now being capitated at a fixed annual rate for a subscriber, and managed care is using prevention as a tool for conserving revenues.

Many managed care organizations are now beginning to allocate resources to health fitness services. This trend can only continue and grow in an increasingly capitated cost environment.

At this writing, there are over 4,000 hospitals and only 25 percent have health fitness centers. It is conceivable that the future hospital or comprehensive health care complex, having a market service radius of approximately 30 miles, would align itself with several health fitness centers, each with a market service radius of approximately 10 miles. Such an alliance could provide comprehensive health care, including prevention, to an entire community. It is also conceivable that a joint venture, or even a merger, between major players in the health care industry and the health fitness industry could occur in the future. This would be most likely between managed care entities and larger commercial fitness players mentioned in table 1.2. Community recreation centers supported by tax dollars and hotels with fitness centers designed to maximize guest registrations have different missions than commercial programs and are unlikely candidates for takeovers by the health care industry. We are forecasting a rich future for the clinical health fitness arena.

Community Programs

The community setting consists of many outlets for health fitness services. Some outlets, such as hotels, we have arbitrarily placed in this grouping. Parks and recreation departments offer fitness programs in many of their community recreation centers. Hotels are increasingly attractive to guests because of newly developed fitness complexes complete with exercise equipment, spas, and other amenities. This is especially true in the larger hotels catering to the corporate guests or convention business. The YMCAs, YWCAs, Jewish Community Centers (JCC), and other nonprofit organizations have a major presence in the health fitness services offered in the community. Urban-centered Y programs are so focused on health fitness services in the downtown business districts that it is difficult to distinguish these facilities from commercial fitness facilities. Schools and universities are offering services to their enrolled students and local citizens through

community outreach programs. Apartment complexes, responding in a similar fashion to hotels, are also building fitness complexes to accommodate fitness-conscious residents. The magnitude of the community setting in providing health fitness services is enormous. Figure 1.6 illustrates the incredible impact Ys and other nonprofit programs are making in exercise participation.

Management Functions

The major functional aspects of running health fitness programs, regardless of the type of setting, fall under the activity categories of (a) promotion, (b) program, and (c) management (Patton et al. 1986; Patton et al. 1989). *Promotional activities* include advertising, marketing, public relations, membership drives, and other activities that create an attractive image for the program. *Programming activities* include fitness and nutrition testing and prescription, exercise classes, seminars, and workshops. *Management activities* include supervision, budgeting, office operations, insurance, payroll, scheduling, and maintenance. A good health fitness manager must be skilled in all three functions or have staff well trained in these areas. However, the relative emphasis of each function will differ according to the setting (see figure 1.7).

Commercial Programs

Commercial health clubs promote their facilities by making year-round marketing efforts, launching membership drives, and selling memberships. The membership sales function, even in mature clubs, is a vital aspect of the business. It is not uncommon for the annual attrition in a mature commercial health

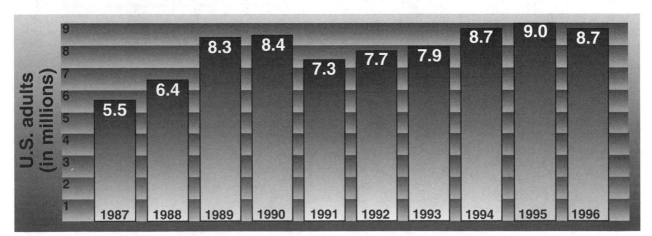

Figure 1.6 **Nonprofit facility participants.**
Adapted, by permission, from IHRSA, 1997, *Profiles of success* (Boston: IHRSA).

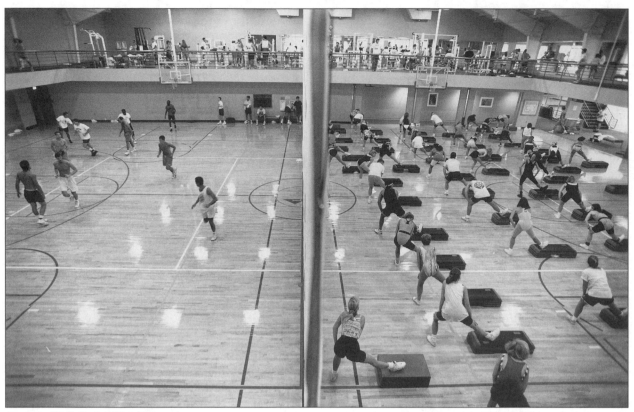

Courtesy of Little Rock Athletic Club

club membership to approach or even exceed 50 percent. Because of this attrition, the sales staff must constantly promote and sell new memberships. Consider that for membership to grow by 10 percent annually, with a 50 percent annual attrition, the club must make new sales of 60 percent during the year. Approximately 20 percent of Americans move annually. This accounts for a significant portion of a club's attrition; however, we can associate most of the remainder with participant dissatisfaction in facilities, staff, and programs.

Commercial clubs have been criticized for focusing on sales and neglecting quality indicators, such as well-trained professional personnel and highly organized, informative, and exciting programs for the members. Fortunately, there is a trend toward

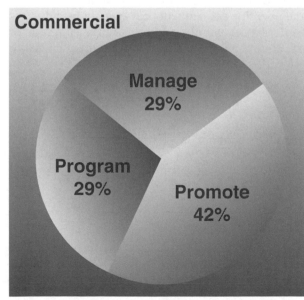

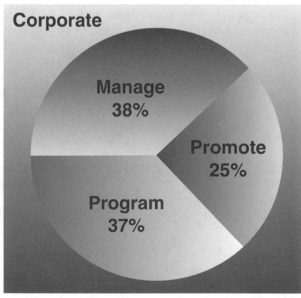

Figure 1.7   Emphasis of functional areas in the various settings.

(continued)

more qualified personnel and enriching the programming in the commercial sector. It seems that new and bright, shiny equipment is no longer a distinguishing factor among commercial clubs—they now all have this feature. Quality programs and professionally trained personnel are necessary to attract the increasingly knowledgeable and demanding consumer. Indeed, some of the more popular programs being offered now include nutrition, physical therapy, personal training, and stress management—these programs require well-trained staff to implement.

> ▽ *The commitment to improved quality in personnel is reflected in the industry standard of payroll costs growing from 30 percent a decade ago to approximately 40 percent of current annual expenses.*

Management activities, on the other hand, are the benchmark of the commercial setting. The effective health fitness manager must maximize revenues and minimize expenses while maintaining positive cash flow and desirable balance sheets. To accomplish this, management activities must be foremost in the minds of decision makers and action takers in the commercial sector, weighing in balance the cost effectiveness of their decisions.

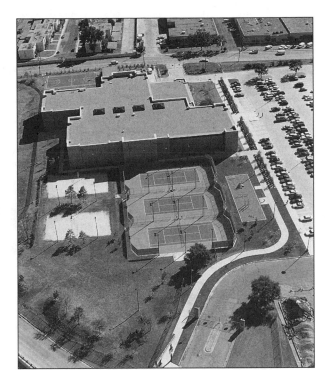

Courtesy of Dallas Texins Association

Corporate Programs

Corporate health fitness programs, in contrast to commercial programs, have not been concerned with external promotion of their programs but have focused their promotional energies on programming for their employees. Usually, their prospective consumers reside within the corporate complex during the center's operating hours. Internal marketing, therefore, prevails in this setting. Everyone coming through the fitness center's doors is precious and

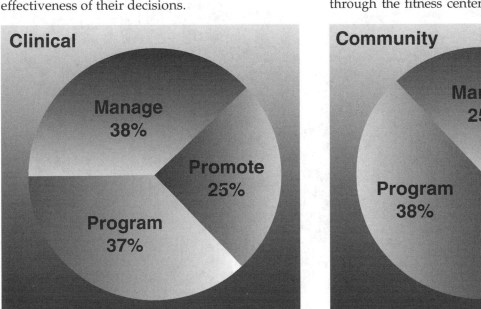

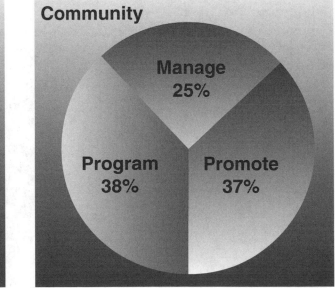

Clinical
Manage 38%
Promote 25%
Program 37%

Community
Manage 25%
Program 38%
Promote 37%

Figure 1.7 a-d adapted, with permission, from R.W. Patton, W.C. Grantham, R.F. Gerson, and L.R. Gettman, 1989, *Developing and managing health/fitness facilities* (Champaign, IL: Human Kinetics), 7.

must receive a positive experience. This is true more in the corporate setting than others because of the finite number of employees from which it draws members. It must be a lasting impression, or it may be their last impression. Corporate programs are, therefore, characterized by facility- and personnel-intensive features, providing the most effective programming experiences possible for the employees to optimize their adherence to the program. Management functions in the corporate setting are restricted because other corporate departments accomplish many functions. For example, there is little to concern the manager from a financial point of view beyond expense management—revenue production is typically not an issue. Financial management is relegated to managing the allocated budget. Likewise, facility management is often another corporate manager's concern. Another department frequently handles maintenance and cleaning, and the corporation might contract an outside vendor as a night cleaning service to supplement the routine cleaning by the maintenance staff.

The corporate health fitness manager is largely concerned with personnel and program management. The corporate fitness center manager must also continually evaluate programs to demonstrate participation levels, corporate impact, and cost ef-

fectiveness. These programs either flourish or perish, depending on the corporation's quarterly or annual performance. Surviving during the inevitable down cycles of a company requires a persuasive manager capable of considerable number crunching and compelling presentations.

Clinical Programs

The marketing and promotion activities for cardiac rehabilitation, physical therapy, and other clinical services revolve around physicians serving as gatekeepers for referring patients. Without a physician referral, no clinical services can be performed in the United States. This is not true worldwide. For example, in some countries physical therapists do not require physician referrals. The marketing for employee wellness services in the hospital setting, on the other hand, is similar to a corporate fitness program. Internal marketing activities must be employed in this context. If the program has a community outreach dimension and a fitness complex, then the marketing takes on a commercial setting focus. Marketing activities for a broad-based health fitness program in a hospital need to be quite sophisticated to be effective. Usually, a marketing department within the clinical organization assists in the promotional activities.

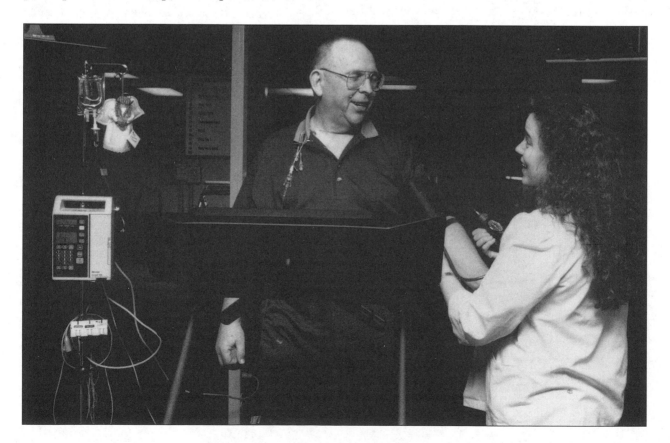

The programming area is extremely labor, equipment, and facility intensive. Unquestionably, the programming in a clinical setting is the most rigorous of all settings. Frequently in the clinical service areas, the outcomes of programming, such as cardiac rehabilitation, are a life or death matter and cannot be taken lightly. Besides the seriousness of the services, there are many accreditation constraints (e.g., Joint Commission on Accreditation of Healthcare Organizations and Occupational Safety and Health Administration) regulating the type and amount of programming activities. Licensure of staff, continuing education requirements, quality assurance of services, and compliance to environmental standards are ever-present reminders of these constraints. Delivering programs concurrently for employee populations and community members can be accomplished without a hitch, but these programs cannot impede or restrict the clinical programs. For example, a cardiac rehabilitation class with monitored patients will frequently have a priority for facilities and equipment over the regular adult fitness activities going on in the center.

Community Programs

Community health fitness programs describe the remainder of the programs within the health fitness industry. These would include the YMCA, YWCA, JCC programs, parks and recreation centers, college and university programs, country clubs, and residential fitness centers. These programs, as a whole, tend to emphasize promotion, program, and management with nearly equal weight. For example, the well-established Y programs are based on a formula that has worked for them for more than a century. Y administrators have come to

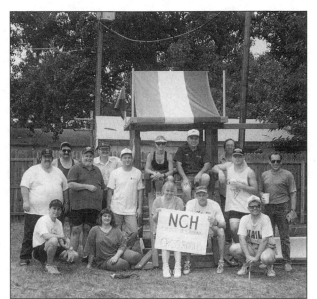

Courtesy of NCH Corporation, Dallas, Texas.

recognize that, although marketing is important, it should never outweigh the importance of the program they are delivering or the management system supporting that program. The Y system has a long and rich history of providing health fitness services; many of our industry leaders, such as health fitness organizational presidents, have their roots in these programs.

Community parks and recreation departments have also become active in the health fitness industry recently. Many suburban recreation centers have established dedicated space within a center to provide fitness programs and services on a value-added basis. In essence, these programs function as a commercial environment in a profit center housed within a nonprofit entity.

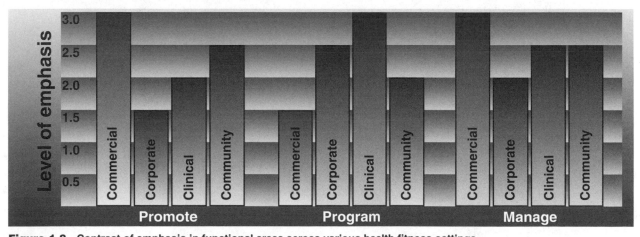

Figure 1.8 Contrast of emphasis in functional areas across various health fitness settings.

Adapted, by permission, from R.W. Patton, W.C. Grantham, R.F. Gerson, and L.R. Gettman, 1989, *Developing and managing health/fitness facilities* (Champaign, IL: Human Kinetics), 7.

As these discussions about promotion, programming, and management show, each area has a different emphasis in the various settings in the health fitness industry. Professionals in this industry need to be aware of these changing emphases as career paths in this profession are subject to change with little notice. It behooves us to prepare and be able to respond to these challenges.

If you are a student trying to chart a course for your career path in this profession, examine figure 1.8, which illustrates the relative emphasis of each functional area in the commercial, corporate, clinical, and community settings. Notice the commercial environment is rich in opportunity for someone interested in marketing and sales. This setting places a heavy emphasis on sales because the loss rate of members is inevitable and their replacement is necessary. The commercial setting is also a good place to get a broad exposure to all the management areas within the industry, unlike other settings that inherently limit exposure to some aspects of management. The career path in this area is extensive if one is fortunate enough to achieve an ownership position.

If your passion for entering this profession revolves around the scientific aspects of fitness and being directly involved in the program delivery of fitness services, you might want to explore the clinical or corporate settings, which provide rich opportunities in programming. As opportunities in the health care industry unfold for health fitness professionals, we may become viewed as paramedical professionals and may even acquire licensure status at some point, creating some parity with other therapists. Some community settings afford good exposure to programming. Many community

---

Table 1.5   Some Characteristic Duties of the Health Fitness Practitioner

Manager
- Administer daily operation
- Design program activities
- Control program
- Guide and direct staff
- Purchase equipment
- Maintain facilities
- Regulate budget
- Schedule activities
- Communicate with staff
- Cooperate with other departments

Supervisor
- Hire and dismiss staff
- Oversee program and staff
- Motivate staff
- Evaluate staff

Exercise leader
- Guide participants
- Conduct classes
- Create safe environment
- Be a role model

Counselor
- Advise participants
- Suggest changes
- Express opinions
- Recommend action
- Consult with participants

Assessor
- Conduct participant tests
- Interpret test results
- Follow safe procedures
- Follow up on results
- Encourage retests

Planner
- Assess organizational needs
- Establish goals for program
- Design program
- Organize resources
- Arrange schedule

Educator
- Train staff
- Instruct members
- Evaluate learning
- Develop curricula

Motivator
- Give impetus to program
- Persuade participants
- Influence participants
- Incite action

Promoter
- Design marketing technique
- Encourage participation
- Use sales techniques
- Promote program
- Be an ambassador of health

Evaluator
- Design program evaluation procedures
- Perform statistical analyses
- Interpret results
- Analyze program trends
- Convey reports to management

Adapted, by permission, from R.W. Patton, J.M. Corry, L.R. Gettman, and J.S. Graf, 1986, Implementing health/fitness programs (Champaign, IL: Human Kinetics), 74.

Table 1.6   Relative Emphasis of Practitioner Roles in Health Fitness Settings

Role	Commercial	Corporate	Clinical	Community
Manager	5	4	5	5
Planner	5	5	5	4
Supervisor	4	4	5	3
Educator	2	4	5	3
Exercise leader	3	4	5	3
Motivator	3	4	4	3
Counselor	4	4	4	3
Promoter	5	3	2	4
Assessor	3	5	5	3
Evaluator	4	5	4	4

Note: 1 = lowest; 5 = highest

Adapted, by permission, from R.W. Patton, W.C. Grantham, R.F. Gerson, and L.R. Gettman, 1989, *Developing and managing health/fitness facilities* (Champaign, IL: Human Kinetics), 16.

programs also have a social and recreational focus.

For students interested in management aspects of this industry, any setting will present opportunities; however, inherent within the commercial setting lies a broad spectrum of management areas that are minimized or missing in some other settings.

Practitioner's Roles

The health fitness practitioner takes on roles at many levels within the organization—ranging from the entry level to upper management. Two major factors generally influence these roles. First, the level of responsibility within the organization influences the role the practitioner will play. The entry-level professional, for example, has far more direct contact with members than someone in upper management. The senior staff person might spend more time with the overall management process than with direct member contact. We provide more discussion of the roles and tasks of the various professionals in chapter 4.

The setting also influences the role that the practitioner plays in the organization. Previously, we explained that program emphasis in the clinical setting is probably more intense than in the commercial setting. In an earlier book (Patton et al. 1989) the authors developed some generic practitioner roles that remain well accepted in the health fitness industry. These roles are delineated in table 1.5.

Certainly all these roles will not be performed in each setting, and it is unlikely that one person would perform all these tasks in a professional lifetime. However, this list describes the tasks commonly viewed as essential by practitioners in our profession. Table 1.6 places these roles in the context of emphasis exhibited by the various health fitness settings. This table reveals the roles that appeal to practitioners and provides some assistance in career path planning.

Table 1.7   Space Allocations in Health Fitness Settings (Square Feet / Percent of Total)

Area	Commercial	Corporate	Clinical	Community
Administrative	3,095 / 8%	2,109 / 5%	1,758 / 5%	1,695 / 4%
Exercise areas	16,419 / 42%	18,050 / 49%	16,688 / 49%	16,806 / 43%
Warm-up areas	3,895 / 10%	4,050 / 11%	4,895 / 13%	3,450 / 9%
Multipurpose	1,375 / 4%	2,461 / 7%	3,403 / 9%	2,475 / 6%
Locker rooms	6,450 / 17%	6,466 / 18%	4,950 / 13%	7,087 / 18%
Storage space	1,027 / 3%	963 / 3%	1,631 / 4%	858 / 2%
Laundry	422 / 1%	422 / 1%	675 / 2%	450 / 1%
Nursery	774 / 2%	----	----	900 / 2%
Snack bar	844 / 2%	----	----	675 / 2%
Circulation	4,458 / 11%	2,350 / 6%	1,800 / 5%	4,061 / 13%
Total sq. ft.	38,729	36,871	37,800	38,421

Adapted, by permission, from R.W. Patton, W.C. Grantham, R.F. Gerson, and L.R. Gettman, 1989, *Developing and managing health/fitness facilities* (Champaign, IL: Human Kinetics), 17.

Facilities

The final contrast among health fitness settings is in the facilities. Because the programs often have functional differences, they need various facility layouts to serve their needs. The facilities developed in various settings are slightly different, always reflecting the nuances from other sectors of the industry. Table 1.7 reflects these differences by illustrating the space allocations of commonly needed areas in the various settings. We can see, for example, that the commercial facility requires almost twice the space for administrative purposes as the other settings. This reflects the need for sales office space to accommodate the membership sales staff and marketing areas not required in other settings. The multipurpose space allocation in the clinical setting has about twice the relative space dedication as in the commercial setting because of the need for patient education that is so critical in rehabilitation.

The examples used in table 1.7 are based on large facilities. The average commercial health fitness center in the United States is larger than the average facilities in other settings. The average commercial health fitness center is about 25,000 square feet—considerably smaller than the illustrations used for comparison. So, the illustration is hypothetical and serves simply to offer a contrast of facility function to reflect varying program needs.

PROGRAM MODIFIERS

Many factors influence the nature and scope of a health fitness program. The cultural trends of a heightened health consciousness and a general concern for fitness have been a boost to programs. The baby boomers are now middle age, and their growing and changing demands for fitness programs have favorably positioned the industry.

> ▼I
> *The concern about reducing health care costs and taking more control of one's health has influenced a trend toward more alternative programming, such as nutrition, weight control, and stress management.*

The size of the industry itself has led to program specialization and diversification and to a consolida-

tion of the industry players. These are all examples of how cultural changes can influence the direction of program development. Two additional modifiers are *program objectives* and *target populations*. These two modifiers are extremely important in defining any program and serve as the underlying basis for the diversity of programs in this industry.

Program Objectives

The objectives of any program influence everything that goes on in a health fitness center. If profit is the main objective, every program and activity must be evaluated against its profitability. Various departments, such as pro shops and food bars, for example, may even be called profit centers, and their viability and longevity within the organization depend on a consistent and measurable profitability. Some programs have objectives that are less tangible—employee morale in the corporate setting, community visibility in the hospital-based environment, guest satisfaction in the hotel-based program, to mention a few. The list could continue for the different settings; programs are founded and uniquely manifested by these objectives. Because of this, no two programs are alike. This uniqueness is what makes the health fitness industry so exciting and challenging. Let's examine some primary and secondary objectives frequently found in each setting.

Commercial Programs

Commercial or for-profit health fitness enterprises have been around for many years. Earlier discussions have revealed an explosive growth of these programs now exceeding 13,000 in the United States. The common objective in these facilities is profit. They expect profit from all departments or program areas, such as fitness, racquet sports, food bar, retail outlets, and personal training. Profit is ex-

Table 1.8	Objectives for Commercial Health Fitness Centers	
Primary	**Secondary**
Obtain reasonable profit on capital growth invested.	Maintain sustained membership. Increase member satisfaction. Increase member retention. Increase program offerings. Improve quality of staff. Improve quality of facilities available.

Adapted from Patton, et al. 1989.

Table 1.9   Relationship Between Levels of Program Development and Program Objectives

Program objectives	Level I Awareness	Level II Assessment	Level III Education	Level IV Behavior change
Image enhancement				
General visibility	1	1	2	4
Employee recruiting	2	2	2	4
Productivity improvement				
Morale	3	3	3	4
Turnover	2	2	2	4
Absenteeism	2	2	2	4
Tardiness	1	1	2	2
Work ethic	1	2	2	3
Health related				
Health costs reduced	1	1	2	3-4
Disability costs reduced	1	1	2	2-3
Life insurance reduced	1	1	2	2-3

Note: 1 = impact unlikely; 2 = impact possible; 3 = impact probable; 4 = impact very probable

Adapted, by permission, from M. O'Donnell, 1986, "Design of workplace health promotion programs," *American Journal of Health Promotion* 1: 22.

pected from each department and ultimately the entire facility. Otherwise, the organization perishes—it cannot pay debts and bankruptcy follows.

Although profit is the primary objective, there are many secondary objectives for a commercial fitness center. We could consider high levels of membership service, staff development, program implementation, and similar topics as secondary objectives in the commercial setting. These are illustrated in table 1.8.

Corporate Programs

Corporate health fitness programs can have both tangible and intangible goals. The tangible goals relate to measurable changes in such things as reducing employee absenteeism, health care costs, and turnover rates. The intangible goals of a program might include improving employee morale, reducing employee tardiness, and increasing enthusiasm for the workplace. These goals are intimately related to the expectations of upper management of the company. If the champion of the program is the CEO, who is a fitness enthusiast, it is unlikely that the program will need hard data on tangible objectives to justify its progress and achievement. Tangible objectives are assumed. Programs of this type are based on the intangible objectives of a program, such as increased participation in fitness programs, special events, and improved employee morale. If, on the other hand, the decision makers are data based and there is no obvious champion at the upper management levels, detailed analyses must be performed to justify programs, and tangible objectives frequently become

necessary. These programs do a lot of testing and evaluating and interact frequently with medical and human resources departments gathering essential data for evaluation. Seasoned health fitness managers in the corporate environment are quick to point out that a sympathetic CEO today requiring little hard data to justify programs may be replaced tomorrow with a different approach to evaluating programs. Managers of corporate health fitness programs are well advised to constantly evaluate, carefully using as much data as possible.

Generally, programs have to reflect their mission, goals, and objectives. Regardless, the level of impact desired from the programs depends on the level of program development. Programs operated in the cafeteria before or after work by interested volunteers are generally not as effective as those conducted in well-equipped, dedicated facilities with professional staff. Table 1.9 illustrates the relationship between the level of program development and the expected impact that it can make on different program objectives. High levels of program development are necessary to effect significant behavior change that has lasting value.

Clinical Programs

It is difficult to identify clear objectives, in a generic fashion, for a clinical health fitness program. Some programs will operate in a nonprofit environment where the objective is increased community visibility for the hospital. Community outreach programs of this nature are presumed to enhance institutional loyalty and, thereby, increase patient volume.

Table 1.10   Objectives for a Clinical Health Fitness Program

Primary	Secondary
Improve compliance of patients with treatment regimens (for-profit and nonprofit, private and public community hospitals).	Create a marketing vehicle to develop goodwill within the community.
Gain reasonable profit for services rendered to community and corporate worlds (community and private, for-profit hospitals).	Recruit patients/clients for the hospital for both inpatient and outpatient services.
Render services to community on a cost-recovery basis (nonprofit community hospital).	Provide patient education materials for outpatient cardiac rehabilitation patients.
Meet accreditation standards for Joint Commission (all hospitals).	Improve general health of the community as a part of the hospital's overall mission.
Provide hospital employee health fitness programs to reduce health care costs and to increase productivity.	Increase health fitness levels of citizens in the countywide service area.

Adapted, by permission, from R.W. Patton, W.C. Grantham, R.F. Gerson, and L.R. Gettman, 1989, *Developing and managing health/fitness facilities* (Champaign, IL: Human Kinetics), 11.

Some programs are organizationally located in a for-profit environment in which the program will operate as if it were a commercial entity and a profit center for the hospital. The profit motive in this instance is foremost, and the programs compete in the same marketplace as other commercial facilities.

Other programs have objectives that seem like a combination of commercial and corporate facilities. The hospital employees may use the facility with membership fees paid by the employer and participate alongside the community member who may pay monthly membership fees. Patients may also use these facilities for outpatient health care, such as cardiac rehabilitation, where insurance or private payment may underwrite reimbursement. The objectives of such an environment are highly variable and complex. Nonetheless, the program will always function according to its expressed goals and objectives. In a multifocused environment, such as the clinical setting, it is essential that the relative importance of each objective is clearly established and understood by all concerned. Otherwise, chaos prevails. See table 1.10 for a generic statement of program objectives for a clinical health fitness program.

Community Programs

Many organizations and agencies serve clients in community settings, including voluntary health agencies (American Heart Association, American Cancer Society, YMCA, YWCA, JCC, American Red Cross, etc.), schools, churches, and private social service agencies. In each setting, the objectives depend on the expected goals of the particular

organization. For example, the goals of a health care organization, such as the American Heart Association, might revolve around collecting donations to support research and interventions for heart disease. The goals of a health fitness YMCA program might revolve around health promotion of its members and community service projects.

Target Population

The target population of a program has an immense impact on the direction a program takes in its development and operation.

> *One major issue to consider in developing any health fitness program is the size of the target population.*

A corporate employee fitness program, for example, has a finite number of individuals from which to draw. Due to this finite number, each participant becomes a precious commodity; failure to involve any person or to create a positive experience for this individual effectively reduces the population on which program impact can be made. The health fitness professional in the corporate setting is acutely aware that every experience for a prospective or existing member must be positive, thus creating a program-intensive environment.

The nearly infinite population from which

commercial fitness centers draw members places less burden on the health fitness professional to make a positive first impression (or subsequent impressions, for that matter). Because the target population normally lives or works within 10 minutes travel time of the facility, there is usually someone waiting in the wings to replace a disgruntled member in the commercial setting. In fact, a previously commonplace tactic was to lure a prospect to become a member through payment in advance of an annual fee, then to discourage continued attendance through inattention and indifference. This tactic provided a larger membership base for any size of facility. Moreover, the initiation fees facilitated the cash flow statement for the enterprise. Most of today's commercial fitness centers no longer use such marketing tactics and tend to follow the strategies of the other health fitness settings by promoting retention through quality programming. One major reason is that the increased density of facilities in any geographical area effectively reduces the once infinite target population to a more finite number of increasingly intelligent and discriminating consumers.

The more precious the prospective member becomes, the more program intensive the facility and staff must become.

The clinical health fitness program must also respond to the supply-demand equation for available patients and members. Competition is becoming intense in the hospital arena for the health care services of a community. The more comprehensive the range of services offered by the hospital, the better the image for delivering health care services. Therefore, health fitness services become an important dimension to the hospital community outreach marketing program. Stiff competition exists in communities for rehabilitation patient populations as well. Physicians frequently maintain privileges in more than one hospital. Vying for the referrals from physicians practicing in several hospitals becomes ferocious. Gaining allegiance from a physician who is better served by spreading referrals across all the hospitals in which he or she practices is extremely difficult. The health and fitness business is a market-driven enterprise, regardless of whether the patient or member is a rehabilitation patient in a clinic or a personal training client in a hospital-based fitness center.

Community health fitness facilities have a participant population consisting of diverse individuals seeking a variety of services. The size of the target population depends to a great extent on the size of each facility and its overall objectives. Larger communities can afford the luxury of having dedicated health fitness facilities in their community Ys and recreation centers. Smaller communities must have a multipurpose program designed to serve a host of consumer types. Some larger communities are developing residential spaces with a narrow market focus to better serve a particular market segment. A housing complex may, for example, cater to young singles seeking hard-core health fitness facilities, equipment, and programs. Others may focus on a seniors housing center or real estate development surrounding a golf and tennis complex. Again, the market drives the type of health fitness program and facility that develops. You can find more information on marketing and sales in chapter 5.

Those who are developing the health fitness projects need to heed the importance of market analysis. Define your target population early in the project development, and reexamine it periodically as the market area grows and changes. Facilities, personnel, and programs must be constantly fluctuating to remain viable in a changing marketplace. Otherwise, the program withers and dies.

IN CLOSING

This chapter segmented the health fitness industry into four settings: commercial, corporate, clinical, and community. Although each setting aspires to unique objectives, target markets, and practitioner roles and provides different facilities, they all must focus on three primary functions in differing degrees: promotion, programming, and management. Thus, despite some expectations of what health fitness programs should look and work like, there will never be two that are identical in how they are managed and operated. Because there are more than 40 thousand facilities currently serving more than 20 million members, there is considerable diversity. Yet, we can make some generalizations about the health fitness industry after 40 years of booming growth. This is especially true now that the growth seems to be slowing. We are in a position to apply some sound business principles and practices to this maturing industry. This is the mission of the remainder of the book.

KEY TERMS

Clinical setting

Commercial setting

Community setting

Corporate fitness

Exercise Lite

Fitness boom

Management activities

Programming activities

Program objectives

Promotional activities

Target population

RECOMMENDED READINGS

American Heart Association. 1992. Statement on exercise: Benefits and recommendations for physical activity programs for all Americans. *Circulation* 86: 340-344.

Association for Fitness in Business. 1992. *Guidelines for employee health promotion programs*. Champaign, IL: Human Kinetics.

Blair, S.N., H.W. Kohl, R.S. Paffenbarger, D.G. Clark, K.H. Cooper, and L.W. Gibbons. 1989. Physical fitness and all-cause mortality: A prospective study of healthy men and women. *Journal of the American Medical Association* 262: 2395-2401.

Howley, E.T., and B.D. Franks. 1992. *Health fitness instructor's handbook*. Champaign, IL: Human Kinetics.

International Health, Racquet and Sportsclub Association. 1994. *Profiles of success: The 1994 IHRSA/Gallup industry data survey of the health and fitness club industry*. Boston: IHRSA.

———. 1997. *Health club trend report*. Boston: IHRSA.

Markarian, M. 1993. How does your club compare to the typical club? *Club Industry* (February): 23-29.

Moffat, T. 1995. The home front. *Club Industry* (September): 25-31.

Pate, R.R., M. Pratt, S.N. Blair, W.L. Haskell, C.A. Macera, and C. Bouchard. 1995. Physical activity and public health: A recommendation from the Centers for Disease Control and Prevention and the American College of Sports Medicine. *Journal of the American Medical Association* 273: 402-407

Patton, R.W., J.M. Corry, L.F. Gettman, and J.S. Graf. 1986. *Implementing health/fitness programs*. Champaign, IL: Human Kinetics.

Patton, R.W., W.C. Grantham, R.F. Gerson, and L.R. Gettman. 1989. *Developing and managing health/fitness facilities*. Champaign, IL: Human Kinetics.

U.S. Department of Health and Human Services. 1996. *Physical activity and health: A report of the Surgeon General*. Atlanta, Georgia: U.S. Department of Health and Human Services, Centers for Disease Control and Prevention, National Center for Chronic Disease Prevention and Health Promotion.

Wilson, B.R.A., and T.E. Glaros. 1994. *Managing health promotion programs*. Champaign, IL: Human Kinetics.

Understanding Your Customer or Member

Understanding your customer or member is a key ingredient for learning how to better serve the client. Today's customers have more options than ever before. If your organization does not offer what the member wants or needs and if you do not provide a staff that interacts in a manner meeting or exceeding the members' expectations, then they will probably do business with a competitor. This option alone should motivate everyone involved in the health fitness industry to learn all they can about prospective customers and existing members.

In this chapter, we contrast the behaviors associated with a sedentary lifestyle with patterns of an active lifestyle. We examine the reasons people start an exercise program and what factors make them adhere or drop out of their program. We also explore member demographics and participation patterns and analyze data about trends on activities most preferred by Americans today. Finally, we discuss the importance of tracking member usage, adherence and attrition, and membership growth.

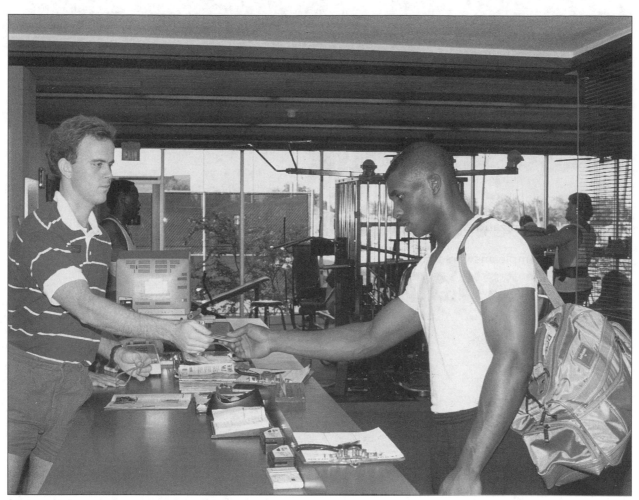

Courtesy of Dallas Texins Association

The health fitness industry is market driven. The need to know and understand the member is critical. Studies show that it costs five times as much to attract a new member as it does to retain an existing one. In today's competitive fitness market, most businesses continue to target prospective customers but concentrate on retaining existing members as well. Maintaining this delicate balance is the challenge for every owner or manager operating a health fitness facility.

Membership data in various health fitness settings indicate that there are distinguishing characteristics associated with members in the commercial, corporate, community, and clinical sectors. Although these findings are not representative of all patrons, they do provide an average member profile, which can assist management in solving marketing and operational issues.

For example, in 1996 the typical commercial club member was between 18 and 34 years old, was pursuing or had a college degree, and had a house-hold income over $75,000 annually. The average YMCA member was between 35 and 54 years old and earned $25,000 to $49,000 annually (IHRSA and American Sports Data, Inc. 1997). Corporate facilities are male dominated and tend to attract more white-collar employees than blue-collar. Members are more homogeneous because of the size and limitation of the corporate workforce as the target population. Clinical members often need a fitness program for special reasons, such as cardiac and injury rehabilitation or professional weight management classes. Physician referrals include workers' compensation, postrehabilitation patients, or members who are now crossing between the medical and fitness communities.

Because the commercial fitness market represents more than 13,350 clubs with a total membership of more than 11.3 million, compared with the 20.8 million who frequent all health clubs and recreational facilities (for-profit and nonprofit combined), we focus on the for-profit or commercial member to achieve the sense of a typical consumer (IHRSA and American Sports Data, Inc. 1997). When appropriate, we will present data for nonprofit entities to provide comparative values.

Achieving success in the health fitness business starts with understanding the members and knowing how to project and respond to their needs. Given equal facilities, staffing, and programs, why do some fitness centers succeed while others fail? What makes a member prefer one facility more than another? What does it take to meet the market's needs? How can the odds be increased to attract new customers while retaining existing members? Why does one organization outperform the competition?

There are no simple answers to these questions, but what successful organizations have in common is that they are able to anticipate members' needs and exceed their expectations. This emphasis is communicated to members through the actions of all employees. A well-trained staff responds appropriately at the point of encounter with the customer. Consequently, by meeting the needs and desires of the consumer, a one-time customer is transformed into a loyal member.

> *Successful organizations anticipate members' needs and exceed their expectations.*

CUSTOMER CHARACTERISTICS

To fully understand the customer, it's important to recognize two basic characteristics that affect actions: preconditioning and attitudes. Whether consciously or subconsciously, each of these characteristics influences how the consumers view the service they are considering purchasing.

Preconditioning

Today more than ever, customer's attitudes have been preconditioned. Many are cynical about the health fitness industry and its personnel. Inconsistent discounting practices, unkept promises, and encounters with untrained personnel have contributed to this *preconditioning*. Other factors play a role

in this cynicism as well. Attitudes and beliefs learned from parents and peers, societal events, and personal experiences precondition consumers' views.

The health fitness professional should ask, "How can I capitalize on this preconditioned customer and convert him or her to purchase my services?" or, "How can I train my staff to respond properly to the preconditioned customer?" The answers to these questions depend on what motivates customers to buy. Is the motivation pricing? Is it service? Is it the quality of personnel or the cleanliness of the facility? Regardless of the reason, the important thing to remember is that preconditioned views project themselves into customers' attitudes toward purchasing.

Attitudes

Determining individuals' attitudes is an acquired skill.

> *It does not take a professional psychologist to understand the signals being sent by consumers, but knowing human nature helps us recognize and respond to these signals.*

Consider those businesses that represent service excellence; the companies that excel are those sending a marketing message that meets a wide range of preconditioned consumer needs. For example, the McDonald's fast-food chain has achieved a level of service excellence by regularly incorporating its motto, "Quality, Service, Cleanliness, and Value." This motto has become the standard of comparison for the whole fast-food industry.

Attitudes can be influenced in a variety of ways. There are *internal attitudes*, which are those influenced by the quality of the service and the relationship between the buyer and the seller. Internal influences include everything from the initial marketing message to the services offered. The marketing message will shape an expectation. This expectation will be either raised or lowered by initial contact with the service or product. Take, for example, an advertisement promoting a weekend spa special. If the advertisement shows the spa positioned on a beautiful beach, the customer will

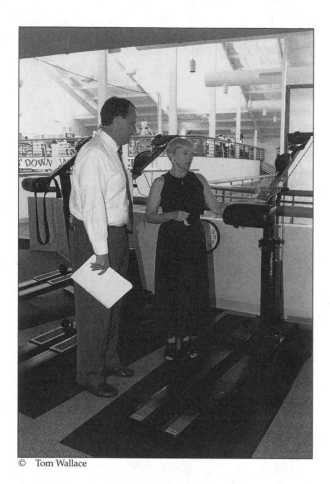

© Tom Wallace

not be fulfilled with anything less than an identical setting. The customer's expectation will be further reinforced upon arriving at the destination and seeing several beautiful beaches. Expectations continue to rise if the customer is promised a room overlooking a beach. If, for some reason, any of this scenario changes, expectations will be lowered and any cynical preconditioned attitude will be reinforced. The attitudes and expectations have already been shaped before the customer talks with any service personnel.

Another form of influence is *external attitudes*, which are factors less likely to be controlled by the business but are just as important in the successful service of the customers. External influences have nothing to do with the presell message or the service being provided. For example, a service desk attendant extends a pleasant greeting to a member but encounters an irate response such as, "Can't you move any faster with checking us in!" Unfortunately, the service desk attendant was not aware that the member was running four hours late due to flight delays at the airport. Personnel must be trained to respond to customers who have just gone through a severe attitude-changing experience.

The behavior of the customer is predetermined by the message being sent and the external influences received before the purchase experience. Knowing what to say in a message and how to handle the unexpected attitude are two factors in retaining customers.

How employees react to various customer characteristics is an important issue in retaining members. If service desk attendants react personally to an irate member who is unfairly attacking them because of an external influence, a lose-lose situation will likely result. However, if all employees are properly trained in customer relations, they will learn to react using a prepared response.

> *A good service employee is one who learns to act according to a prepared response script and, when necessary, assumes responsibility to resolve problems.*

With an understanding of customer reactions based on internal and external stimuli, let's apply these concepts to fitness behavior. Specifically, what are the factors that influence a sedentary lifestyle, and what are the reasons for beginning an active lifestyle? The prospective market is not individuals already participating in a fitness program but those who never or rarely exercise.

SEDENTARY LIFESTYLE

Despite common knowledge that exercise is helpful, the 1996 Surgeon General's report on *Physical Activity and Health* stated that more than 60 percent of American adults are not regularly active, and 25 percent of adults are not active at all. Also, many people who have embarked on an exercise program rarely sustain their participation. Clearly, the need to understand the reasons behind a sedentary lifestyle and develop interventions for changing this behavior are necessary.

In 1994, Dr. Christine Brooks conducted a study at the University of Michigan entitled *How Consumers View Health and Sports Clubs*. Although the research was deemed qualitative in nature, it was the first time in a study that participants were able to convey attitudes toward exercise and the health

Table 2.1 Sedentary Adults' Views on Health Fitness Facilities	
Impressions	**Desires**
Clientele	**Clientele**
People who frequented clubs were quite different from them.	Wide variety of fitness levels.
Members were described as young, fit, and unfriendly.	Friendly and accepting patrons.
Men ogled at women and displayed their vanity.	Wide variety of ages.
Women dressed up and applied makeup before working out.	
Facilities	**Facilities**
Liked the wide variety of equipment and facilities.	A wide variety of activities and equipment.
Weights and weight machines were difficult to use.	Easy to use equipment.
Neatness and cleanliness were important.	Clean and neat.
Personnel	**Personnel**
Concerned about personnel qualifications.	Skilled, qualified professionals.
Impression was that staff was unqualified.	Accepting and helpful to beginners.
Some staff portrayed an indifference to those who were not in shape.	Age ranges that match those of clients.
	Coaching and instruction ongoing.
Atmosphere	**Atmosphere**
Atmosphere at most facilities was too social.	Not a social, pickup atmosphere.
Some facility names gave an impression of intimidation and unwelcome.	Should feel welcome to all ages and fitness levels.
	Low emphasis on fashionable workout attire.
Programs	**Programs**
Many had a positive experience with aerobics classes.	Individual attention to develop and monitor progress.
Sometimes the pace of the class was too fast, and their lack of conditioning made it embarrassing.	Classes and workouts geared to a variety of fitness levels.
Positive, thoughtful instructors were a critical component.	
Costs	**Costs**
Negative comments regarding the hard sell approach for membership.	More trial memberships.
Some felt unethical business practices were being used.	Reasonably priced per visit passes.
Quoting a special price for one day was unfavorable.	No high-pressure sales tactics.
Advertising	**Advertising**
Models in ads were too thin and unhealthy looking.	Feature real people.
Models did not inspire them because they were too unrealistic.	Portray realistic results.

Reprinted, by permission, from C. Brooks, 1994, *How consumers view health and sports clubs* (The University of Michigan: IHRSA).

fitness industry (see table 2.1). The information gathered from this study is valuable in understanding consumer views on sedentary and active lifestyles.

A section of Dr. Brooks' study addressed the sedentary population and their reasons for leading an inactive lifestyle. As shown on the following page, six factors influenced this behavior.

Factors Influencing Sedentary Behavior

1. *Competing priorities.* Unlike active individuals who prioritize daily schedules to make time for workouts, sedentary individuals find other ways to fill their days. This attitude does not necessarily mean they don't understand the importance of physical activity; it only signifies that they place precedence on other interests. Often, these other interests serve as obstacles to finding time to exercise.

   In addition, sedentary individuals confess to not enjoying the process of working out: changing into exercise clothes, sweating, enduring the monotony of riding a stationary cycle, and even taking showers. As a result, individuals within this group will deliberately choose to do nothing rather than engage in an activity in which they have to experience the workout process.

2. *Lack of exposure.* Most individuals with sedentary lifestyles grow up in a household that places little emphasis on physical activity. Rarely do parents or siblings participate in exercise or sport programs. Developing motor skills and learning various sports did not occur unless it was part of a mandatory school physical education class. Personal experiences in these classes often result in a negative self-image, further reducing interest and desire in adopting an active lifestyle.

   The primary peer group among inactive individuals often consists of classmates and friends who are nonexercisers as well. A distinct feeling of separation, and sometimes even defiance, results between those who participate in school sport programs and those who do not. Interestingly enough, as adults, the same peer group distinction exists. Friends and colleagues who were sedentary during their adolescent years tend to remain inactive as adults.

3. *Lack of incentive.* Another factor influencing sedentary behavior is that some individuals are satisfied with their overall physical appearance. The aging process is not a big concern and they have no fear of potential health risks. As a result, many do not see the need to begin exercising. If they look good, feel good, and are healthy, why do they need to exercise?

   Many in this group never start an exercise program unless there is a specific reason to do so. For example, a doctor informs them of a life-threatening medical problem, or they notice increased weight gain, or they observe graying hair while looking in the mirror one day. One of these reasons could be enough to change a sedentary lifestyle into an active lifestyle. However, without stimulus, no action typically occurs.

4. *Lack of motivation.* Some individuals who lead a sedentary lifestyle know the benefits of regular exercise and the resulting health attributes. Unfortunately, in some cases, internal factors cause a reluctance to act on the desire to get fit. Various fears surface when exercise or health fitness facilities are discussed, for example, concerns about the lack of physical skills and embarrassment or fear of getting sore because of being so out of shape. Another concern is the negative image associated with some health fitness facilities, muscle head gyms, body beautiful clientele, and instructors who act the part but don't really assist patrons. Collectively, these views affect the decision-making process for beginning an exercise program.

   Often, a friend's or relative's persistence is necessary to motivate individuals in this category. Sometimes laziness or support factors contribute to the need for encouragement from friends and family. Without this assistance, many sedentary individuals would not have the willpower to choose an active lifestyle.

5. *Boredom.* Without quick, noticeable results, individuals in this group are prone to drop out. If changes in weight, strength, or body tone do not occur rapidly, many will give up and stop exercising. These people must experience some kind of reward in the early stages or they rarely give fitness a second chance. The lack of early results perpetuates frustration and apathy, generally resulting in terminating an exercise program. Without positive reinforcement, this cycle is likely to occur.

   Many of these individuals also seek out devices to assist in breaking the monotony associated with stationary exercise equipment. For example, televisions, reading racks, and headphones on cardiovascular equipment are preferences for individuals in this category. They find it necessary to be entertained while working out.

6. *Psychological barriers.* A number of internal, psychological concerns can prevent people from being active. These concerns include

- a high degree of self-consciousness about their body's appearance,
- a lack of skill or strength in using the equipment,
- the feeling of others watching and making negative appraisals, and

- a feeling of self-consciousness when compared with others who are younger and more fit.

Many of these barriers start in childhood and are perpetuated in adulthood. The lack of self-esteem discourages many individuals from even considering an active lifestyle. These individuals dismissed notions of becoming fit or improving their physical appearance due to these psychological obstacles.

Reasons for Becoming Active

Having discussed the reasons for assuming a sedentary lifestyle, the Brooks study also addresses the issue of what it would take for a sedentary individual to become more active. The study lists three reasons:

1. *Health risks.* The suggestion of their physician was key. The underlying motivation for most individuals to become more active is to live longer. Studies have indicated that for all demographic groups, the desire to live longer outweighs other reasons by a margin of 2:1. The diagnosis of a health problem by a personal physician is often enough impetus to change sedentary behavior, especially if fitness activity positively affects the problem.

2. *Appearance, either to lose weight or tone up.* How-

ever, when comparing the general U.S. population to fitness center patrons nearly half (48 percent) of the fitness center patrons surveyed listed factors relating to improving appearance as the number one reason for adopting an exercise program (see table 2.2). These findings were substantiated in a study conducted in 1995 by the International Health, Racquet and Sportsclub Association and American Sports Data, Inc., entitled *Why and Where People Exercise.* Eighty-five percent of all fitness center patrons listed weight control and muscle tone as the two biggest motivators to start an exercise program.

3. *The push of a friend or partner to motivate them to begin.* With encouragement from friends and relatives, many individuals in this category become motivated. However, without this support, many would not make the decision on their own.

Table 2.2   Reasons for Adopting a Fitness Program

Improving appearance		**48%**
Tone muscles	2%	
Build bulk	12%	
Reduce weight	34%	
Improving health		**26%**
Get into shape	17%	
Overcome a health problem	9%	
Feeling good		**16%**
Relieve stress	3%	
Strengthen self-image	3%	
Generally feel better	5%	
To do more things	5%	
Other reasons		**10%**
Continuation of active lifestyle	9%	
Function	1%	**Total 100%**

Reprinted from C. Brooks, 1994, *How consumers view health and sports clubs* (The University of Michigan: IHRSA). Copyright 1994 by IHRSA.

Consumers' Views of Fitness Centers

Understanding consumers' views in joining a health fitness center is a crucial element in determining the design of a facility, program offerings, and staffing options. Essentially, this means establishing the likes and dislikes associated with the fitness business through the eyes of the consumer.

Operators and fitness professionals need to address what consumers view as key elements for a successful fitness club. Understanding what the consumers need is the first step toward achieving their confidence. The second step is to constantly evaluate existing facilities with those elements in mind. Finally, for the benefit of the consumers, the facility management must not be afraid to change. When necessary, management must adopt new policies or procedures, expand facilities, or upgrade equipment to ensure that they are meeting consumers' needs.

In addition to understanding the likes and dislikes of the fitness industry through the eyes of the consumers, Brooks' study also provided a summary of the components that consumers wanted in a fitness center. These components are as follows:

- Neat, clean facilities
- A wide variety of activities and equipment
- Equipment that is easy to use
- Individual attention to develop a fitness program and monitor progress
- Classes and workouts geared to a variety of fitness levels
- An accepting and helpful approach to beginners
- Age ranges of staff matching those of members
- Ongoing instruction and coaching from staff
- A welcoming atmosphere to people of all ages and fitness levels
- Low emphasis on fashionable workout attire
- Members representing a wide variety of ages and fitness levels
- Friendly and accepting members

The U.S. Department of Health and Human Services 1995 report entitled *Healthy People 2000* found that only 20 percent of adults in the United States are active at the level recommended for health benefits. Twenty-six percent are completely sedentary, and the remaining 54 percent are inadequately active. Unfortunately, such sedentary lifestyles can have adverse consequences for the future.

Analyzing the sedentary population should be a high priority for today's fitness professionals. Identifying and understanding the perceptions of this group are the first steps toward reversing many misconceptions. Learning to dissolve psychological barriers, internal fears, excessively high expectations, and low self-esteem are all factors in changing sedentary lifestyles and improving the overall health and well-being of the U.S. public.

ATTITUDES TOWARD EXERCISE

Studies show a stark contrast between active behavior and sedentary lifestyles. *The American Health Club Experience*, a study conducted for IHRSA by American Sports Data, Inc. (1997) found that 55 percent of Americans are either very likely or certain to begin a program of regular exercise soon; an equal percentage stated they were more interested in fitness than they were two or three years ago. The study also revealed that Americans believe:

- Older people need to exercise just as often as younger ones (86 percent).
- People who exercise regularly will probably live longer than those who do not (85 percent).
- Regular exercisers are happier (73 percent).
- Regular exercisers are more productive on the job (70 percent).

The study also discovered four typologies which epitomized American attitudes toward exercise and fitness.

I. Non-Believers (2 percent): "I just don't think exercise is all that important."

II. Indifferent (17 percent): "Exercise may be important, but I just don't feel the need to get involved in fitness activities."

III. Uninitiated Believers (64 percent): "I know exercise is important, and I'd like to participate in fitness activities more than I do."

IV. Hard Core Fitness Enthusiasts (15 percent): "Exercise is very important to me, and I am a frequent participant in fitness activities."

Figure 2.1 summarizes these attitudes towards exercise and fitness.

Although exercise participation is at an all-time high (memberships in all health fitness facilities now exceed over 20 million, or 9 percent of the U.S. population), nonexercisers still make up a large

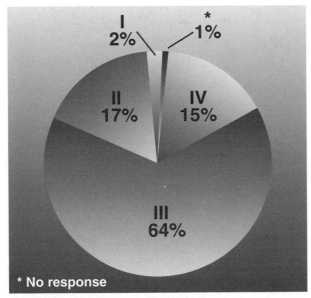

I
2%

*
1%

II
17%

IV
15%

III
64%

* No response

Figure 2.1   Four fitness typologies.

majority of the population (60 percent). It becomes apparent from the results of the IHRSA/ASD study that the uninitiated believers (64 percent), who are considered "fence sitters," is the group to pursue in the future. They realize exercise is important, but for some reason have not made the commitment to begin exercising. We hope the interest stimulated by the U.S. Surgeon General's report on *Physical Activity and Health* (1996) will reinforce the belief that regular exercise can add significantly to the quality of life. Unfortunately, this increased consciousness toward the fitness movement is slow moving and will continue to take time before noticeable behavior changes are initiated.

Despite the positive nature of the IHRSA/ASD study toward the benefits of exercise, other contrasting attitudes were also discovered:

- Nearly half the population (46 percent) admits that if they could take a "magic pill" that would prevent them from gaining weight, they would be less likely to exercise.

- While 65 percent of the population offer lack of time as an excuse for not exercising more, the more revealing statistic is the 68 percent majority who admit that the problem is a lack of self-discipline—especially among the overweight (77 percent).

Attitudes of this nature exhibit true societal views toward exercise and fitness. If a "magic pill" could be taken to enhance physical fitness or assist in losing weight, the majority of individuals will al-

ways opt for the quick and easy method. Over the years, excuses for not wanting to exercise have been plentiful, yet those who consider exercise as a priority in their lives always seem to find time for workouts.

Health fitness professionals should understand that these attitudes toward exercise and fitness are inherent and will probably never change. The challenge is to determine ways to continue motivating individuals to exercise despite the perception society has toward fitness.

MEMBER DEMOGRAPHICS

Having a good comprehension of target market information is another factor in understanding the customer or member. By definition, a *target market* consists of the individuals or groups for which a service or product is intended. Specifically, a target market refers to that group of prospective consumers or, in the case of a corporate fitness program, employees, who can be distinguished from other customers. The distinctions are made according to a set of characteristics possessed by one group but not by another. These characteristics refer to certain pertinent data on individuals' backgrounds and demographic information within a geographic service area.

Demographics are the most common characteristics used to segment a market. The primary demographics include age, gender, marital status, family size, personal and household income, people per household, education, and occupation. Geographic demographics refer to a region, city or county, population density, corporate density, and climate. Usually, these are classified where people live and work.

According to the 1996 IHRSA industry data survey, *Profiles of Success*, the tracking of member profiles includes three demographic categories: gender distribution, age distribution, and household income. Although demographic figures change annually, the responsibility of every health fitness operator is to regularly evaluate and determine the factors that make up the "average" member of a respective club setting.

Data collected from each category reflects a composite of the typical member in the for-profit commercial setting and the nonprofit YMCA or community market. Information derived from reports of this nature can assist owners, managers, and fitness professionals in preparing marketing strategies, programming mix, staffing philosophy, and facility design.

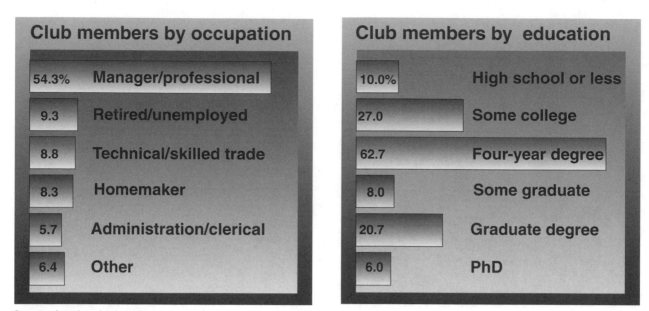

Club members by occupation

54.3%	Manager/professional
9.3	Retired/unemployed
8.8	Technical/skilled trade
8.3	Homemaker
5.7	Administration/clerical
6.4	Other

Club members by education

10.0%	High school or less
27.0	Some college
62.7	Four-year degree
8.0	Some graduate
20.7	Graduate degree
6.0	PhD

Occupational and educational demographics of for-profit clubs.

Gender Distribution

Of the 11.3 million commercial fitness center members in the United States today, 60 percent are women and 40 percent are men. In previous years, commercial fitness centers generally averaged a 1:1 ratio between male and female members. However, recent findings are now showing that women memberships are increasing annually at a higher percentage than their male counterparts (1.5:1 ratio). Additional data from the Universal Gym survey (Marketing Development Consultants 1993) discovered that, on average, more than two-thirds of these members were married, one-fifth were single, and about one-tenth were divorced.

Comparatively, in a nonprofit setting the ratio is still 1:1 (50.1 percent men versus 49.9 percent women). Yet, in this category, women memberships are increasing annually at a higher rate than men.

Regarding commercial facility usage, men continue to participate more frequently than women, averaging 88 days per year versus 82 days for women. This is also true for nonprofit organizations where men have an even higher frequency rate, averaging 111 days per year versus 89 days for females. Figure 2.2 reflects the gender summaries for men and women in the commercial and nonprofit settings.

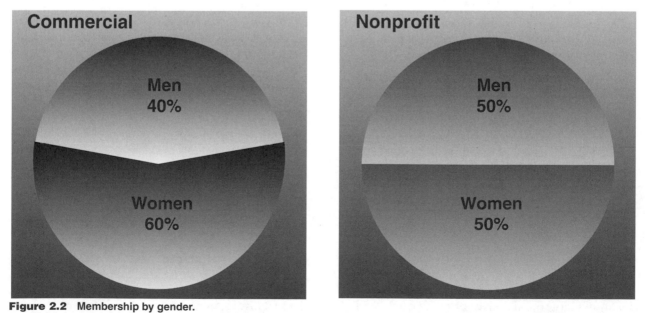

Commercial

Men 40%

Women 60%

Nonprofit

Men 50%

Women 50%

Figure 2.2   **Membership by gender.**
Reprinted, by permission, from American Sports Data, Inc., 1997, *Health Club Trend Report* (Hartsdale, NY: American Sports Data, Inc.).

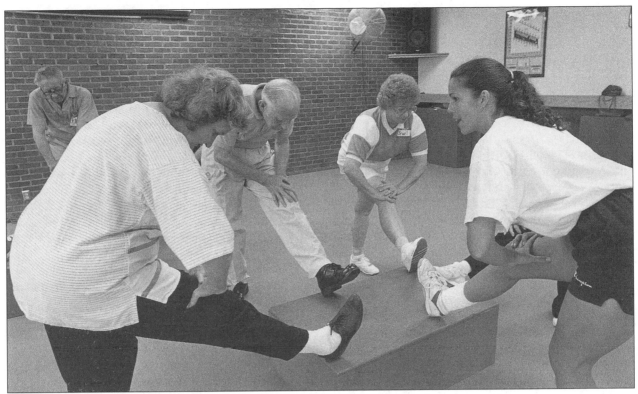

Courtesy of Dallas Texins Association

Age Distribution

As shown in figure 2.3, the largest age group of exercise participants in the for-profit commercial setting is the 18 to 34 year olds, who comprise 42 percent of the total health fitness population. The second largest age group is the 35- to 54-year-old category, which comprises 38 percent of the total population. Following this group are those 55 or older, who represent 12 percent of participants, and the under-18 age group comprising 8 percent of the total for-profit member population.

In the nonprofit fitness settings the findings are similar. Figure 2.3 shows that both the 18 to 34 year

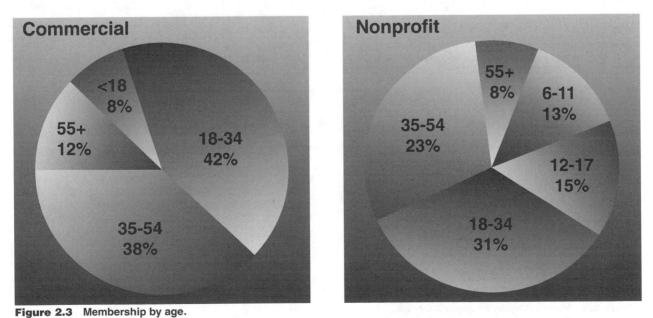

Figure 2.3 Membership by age.

Reprinted, by permission, from American Sports Data, Inc., 1997, *Health Club Trend Report* (Hartsdale, NY: American Sports Data, Inc.).

olds (31 percent) and the 35 to 54 year olds (33 percent) combine for 64 percent of the total population. However, one major difference is the percentage of young patrons from 6 to 11 years old (13 percent) and 12 to 17 years old (15 percent). The remaining 8 percent are members 55 or more years of age.

According to the 1997 *Health Club Trend Report* conducted by American Sports Data, Inc. (IHRSA 1997), fitness participation has increased in all age categories since 1987. The two groups showing the greatest potential for growth in the future are the under-18 year olds and the senior market (55 or more years). Between 1987 and 1995, growth in the under-18 age group increased 73 percent, and the 55 or more age group increased 70 percent. These findings hold true in both the for-profit and nonprofit settings. Professionals in the health fitness industry project that the growth in participation since 1987 for both the senior and youth market will continue increasing at the same rate or even accelerate through the year 2000.

Another category to become familiar with is the average number of days per year each age group participates in each facility setting. Senior members participate most frequently of all age segments in the commercial market. Of the 1.5 million members in this category, 37.2 percent use the club more than 100 days per year, compared with 37 percent for the 35 to 54 age group and 36.6 percent for the 18 to 34 age group. The increased usage demonstrated by the senior market is due primarily to two reasons: the amount of leisure time available to that age group and their perception that exercise is a necessity rather than a luxury.

When compared with the nonprofit sector, the difference is the facility patrons are much younger. Consequently, the under-18 age groups reflect a higher usage rate than adults. Respectively, the 6 to 11 year olds average 146 days per year, and the 12 to 17 year olds average 165 days per year.

As leisure time increases, as well as the awareness of the benefits derived from regular exercise, the senior market is positioned for major growth in the next 10 to 15 years. Although the senior population grew minimally between 1987 and 1996, it is projected to increase by 37 percent between 1997 and 2010. This compares with a projected 13 percent growth rate for the United States as a whole.

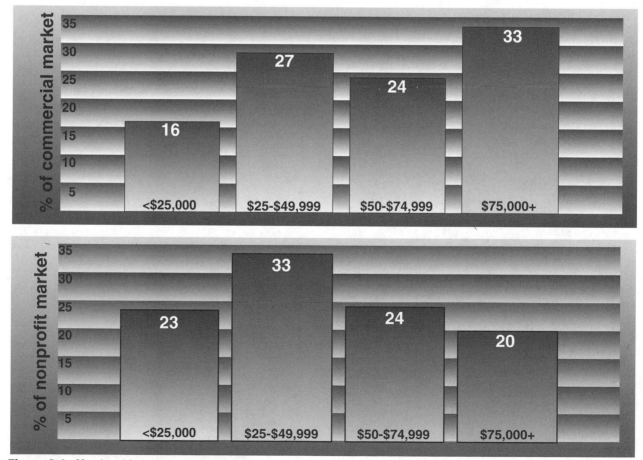

Figure 2.4 Membership by household income.

Reprinted, by permission, from American Sports Data, Inc., 1997, *Health Club Trend Report* (Hartsdale, NY: American Sports Data, Inc.).

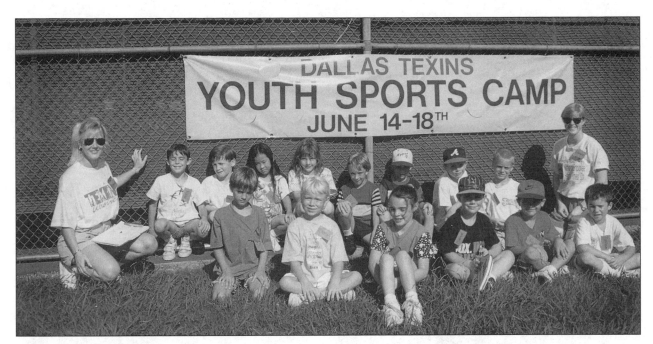

Courtesy of Dallas Texins Association

Household Incomes

As shown in figure 2.4, the average household income for the commercial fitness market is approximately $75,000+ (1996 dollars) This category represents 33 percent of the total commercial club membership. Of those earning $50,000 to $74,999, 24 percent are club members. Twenty-seven percent of households with incomes of $25,000 to $49,999 are commercial club members. Households with incomes of $25,000 or less comprise 16 percent of the market.

Figure 2.4 reflects 1996 nonprofit membership income levels. The largest membership income bracket (33 percent) is households earning between $25,000 and $49,999. Behind this category, however, are the categories $50,000 to $74,999, comprising 24 percent of the membership, and $75,000 and above, comprising 20 percent. In total 77 percent of members participating in nonprofit settings have incomes between $25,000 and $74,999.

There is a stark contrast between the household income levels of the profit and nonprofit settings compared with the U.S. population. In 1996, 40 percent of the U.S. population earned $25,000 or less, 38 percent had incomes between $25,000 and $50,000, and 23 percent earned more than $50,000 annually. Household incomes are expected to increase between three and seven percent annually depending on the economic conditions of the country and specific job-related environments.

Individuals who become members of fitness centers (profit or nonprofit) have enough *discretionary*
income to afford club memberships. That is, after household expenses are paid there are enough additional funds to spend on discretionary items (i.e., personal grooming, hobbies, traveling, books, movies, etc.). Unfortunately, as household income levels decline, discretionary income also declines. Consequently, many consumers view club memberships as a luxury that they can omit if necessary.

Workout Routine Data

Once a customer has joined a health fitness center another way of obtaining important information is to become familiar with workout routines. In other words, determine the answers to such questions as the following: How long does the average member exercise each day? What type of workout do members prefer? Which pieces of cardiovascular equipment do they prefer? What time of the day do members prefer to exercise? Knowing the responses to these questions provides an understanding of member traffic patterns and personal preferences.

A segment of the Universal Gym Equipment survey (Marketing Development Consultants 1993) determined a typical member profile. The survey asked respondents to identify factors that motivated them to join a club, how often and how long they worked out, and what areas of a facility they used most.

As shown in figure 2.5, nearly 40 percent of the survey respondents work out three times a week.

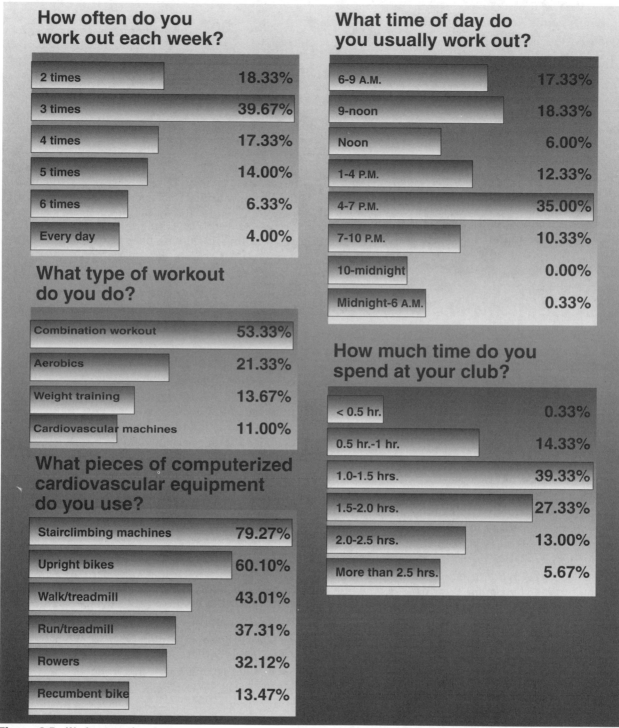

How often do you work out each week?

2 times	18.33%
3 times	39.67%
4 times	17.33%
5 times	14.00%
6 times	6.33%
Every day	4.00%

What type of workout do you do?

Combination workout	53.33%
Aerobics	21.33%
Weight training	13.67%
Cardiovascular machines	11.00%

What pieces of computerized cardiovascular equipment do you use?

Stairclimbing machines	79.27%
Upright bikes	60.10%
Walk/treadmill	43.01%
Run/treadmill	37.31%
Rowers	32.12%
Recumbent bike	13.47%

What time of day do you usually work out?

6-9 A.M.	17.33%
9-noon	18.33%
Noon	6.00%
1-4 P.M.	12.33%
4-7 P.M.	35.00%
7-10 P.M.	10.33%
10-midnight	0.00%
Midnight-6 A.M.	0.33%

How much time do you spend at your club?

< 0.5 hr.	0.33%
0.5 hr.-1 hr.	14.33%
1.0-1.5 hrs.	39.33%
1.5-2.0 hrs.	27.33%
2.0-2.5 hrs.	13.00%
More than 2.5 hrs.	5.67%

Figure 2.5 Workout routine data.

Reprinted, by permission, from Marketing Development Consultants, 1993, *Today's club members* (West Palm Beach, FL: Universal Gym Equipment, Inc.) Copyright 1993 by Universal Gym Equipment, Inc.

Ten percent of the members were hard-core exercisers who work out six to seven times per week. About one-fifth of the members exercise at their club twice a week. Fifty-eight percent of those who exercise average two to three days per week.

The most popular time of the day to work out is between 4 and 7 P.M. Thirty-five percent of members choose this time because it's the end of a workday and the location of the facility is generally between work and home. The 9 A.M. to noon period is the second busiest time (18 percent), primarily due to at-home parents and retirees. Approximately 17 percent of members get an early start and exercise between 6 A.M. and 9 A.M. The slowest time for most commercial clubs is at noon, when only 6 percent of members work out. Conversely, noon is the busiest time for the corporate sector.

As for the length of time spent at a club, it appears that members are a devoted group. Nearly 40 percent of the participants spend between 1 and 1.5 hours per club visit; about 30 percent stay from 1.5 to 2.0 hours. There is even a small group (13 percent) who stay up to 2.5 hours. However, from these periods it is difficult to distinguish how much time members actually spend working out versus socializing and grooming.

The importance of cross-training has also become apparent among exercisers. Fifty-three percent of members incorporate both cardiovascular and weight-training workouts. About 21 percent devote themselves exclusively to aerobic activities, 14 percent specifically to weight training, and 11 percent to working out with cardiovascular equipment. Nearly 35 percent of those who use cardiovascular equipment spend between 50 and 75 percent of their workout time using this equipment only.

Member Demographic Summary

To summarize the member demographic information, a fact list with comments follows:

- The number of men and women members in both the for-profit and nonprofit settings is approximately a 1:1 ratio.

    For-profit 40 percent men to 60 percent women
    Nonprofit 50 percent men to 50 percent women

- In both the for-profit and nonprofit settings, men participate more frequently than women.

    For-profit 88 days per year for men and 82 days per year for women
    Nonprofit 111 days per year for men and 89 days per year for women

- The age categories comprising the largest percent of the total membership are:

    For-profit 42 percent of the total membership for 18 to 34 year olds
    Nonprofit 33 percent of the total membership for 35 to 54 year olds

- In the for-profit settings, the senior membership (55 or more years) has the highest usage fre-

quency of any other age group (100 days per year). In the nonprofit settings, the under-18 year category has the highest usage frequency of any other age group (165 days per year for 12 to 17 year olds; 146 days per year for 6 to 11 year olds).

- With an expected growth of 37 percent in the next 10 to 15 years, the senior market should be closely watched. Estimates state that by the year 2000, 20 to 25 percent of fitness center members will be over age 50. A major emphasis should be placed on long-range forecasting and strategic planning in both the for-profit and nonprofit settings regarding the senior market. To accommodate this potential growth, consider the following areas:

1. Staffing has always been with young employees who sometimes lack people skills and do not understand the aging process. Consider hiring older employees, and spend more time training and educating personnel.

2. The need for expanded senior programming is essential. Adopt campaigns that promote overall fitness and health.

3. Be conscious of your image. Many seniors feel out of place in fitness centers because of the hard-core weightlifting mentality or the socializing aspects of young singles. Provide an atmosphere that caters to the senior market.

4. Always have employees available who can teach and explain the exercise equipment. Often the fear of getting hurt or showing their lack of athletic skills prevents seniors from using cardiovascular or strength equipment.

- Additional planning should also include the youth market (under 18 years). Focus on such issues as programming options, space availability, child care, and facility supervision.

- Always consider the average household income levels before establishing prices for membership fees, programs, and services. In the health fitness business, establishing *perceived value* always depends on what the respective target market can afford. Perceived value is the perception that a member has regarding an established service and the corresponding charge for that service. Does the service justify the price being charged?

- The average participant works out an average of three times a week (usually between 4 and 7 P.M.) with a combination of aerobic and weight-training exercises.

- Those members who weight train prefer free

weights to selectorized by a 57 percent to 40 percent margin.

• Most members (40 percent) spend 1 to 1.5 hours per day at their fitness facility.

• Men engage in weight training (24 percent) more than women (3 percent), and women are more involved in group exercise (27 percent) than men (15 percent).

• Women tend to work out in equal numbers from 9 A.M. to noon, as they do from 4 to 7 P.M.

For future planning, remember the 1:1.5 ratio of men to women members when organizing facilities, programs, and staffing. Maintain an equal balance when accommodating sexes.

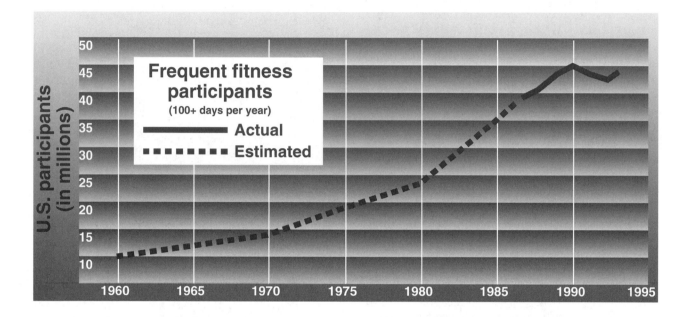

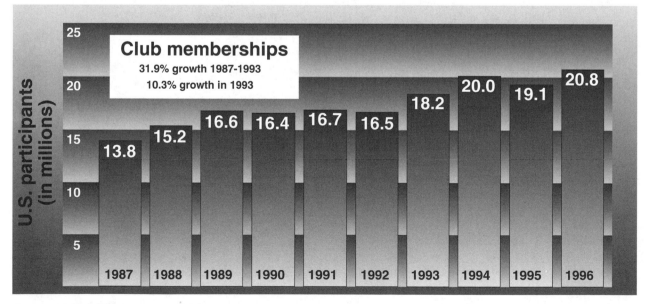

Figure 2.6 The fitness movement (1960-1996).

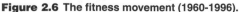

Reprinted, by permission, from American Sports Data, 1995 and 1997, *IHRSA report on the state of the health club industry* (Boston: IHRSA).

PARTICIPATION PATTERNS

The growth in fitness participation over the last three decades (1960 to 1996) has increased dramatically. According to American Sports Data, Inc., the number of Americans who participate in sport or fitness activities at least 100 days per year reached 43.9 million in 1996. As figure 2.6 illustrates, it was estimated that in 1960, 10 million Americans exercised regularly. By 1996, that figure had grown to approximately 44 million, representing a 440 percent increase in fitness participation over a 35-year period.

The largest period of growth occurred between the years 1980 and 1990. During that decade, participation grew from 25 million to 45 million exercisers. Although a temporary decline in growth occurred in 1991 and 1992, participation rebounded in 1993, grew to 20 million in 1994, and fell slightly to 19 million in 1995. Expectations for future growth appear positive according to Harvey Lauer, president of American Sports Data, Inc. (see figure 2.6). He projects that fitness enthusiasts will represent a majority of the U.S. population by the middle of the next century.

In 1996, total fitness center memberships (for-profit and nonprofit memberships combined) increased to 20.8 million members in the United States. This increase represents 9 percent growth over the previous year and reflects the highest membership level ever experienced in the fitness industry.

U.S. SPORT AND FITNESS PARTICIPATION

Monitoring sport and exercise participation is another way to learn about the customer. Obtaining data and analyzing trends on activities most preferred by Americans today is important for all fitness professionals. Information derived from this data can assist in program development, marketing plans, and fitness facility design.

In 1996, American Sports Data, Inc. conducted a national study on 15,000 households across the United States. The survey sampled three mutually exclusive populations: health club members, non-club members who frequently work out at home or outside, and sedentary individuals. The purpose of the study was to determine a ranking of sport and fitness activities preferred overall by all populations. Table 2.3 provides a summary list of the study's findings.

Table 2.3 Sports and Exercise Participation	Health club users (566)	Home/outdoors exercisers (750)	Club/home exercisers (125)
Aerobic equipment exercise	72.8%	46.6%	79.9%
Strength training	64.5	25.5	73.8
Fitness walking	49.4	64.4	58.7
Aerobics	40.8	22.2	38.2
Bicycling (fitness)	39.8	30.6	47.3
Swimming (fitness)	35.4	18.2	46.1
Running/jogging	31.0	19.1	38.9
Hiking	28.7	26.3	33.0
Basketball	23.9	19.6	27.5
Volleyball	23.4	13.1	25.9
Baseball/softball	22.0	17.7	25.2
Skiing	19.2	13.2	22.6
Tennis	15.6	9.7	17.0
Rollerblading	15.0	5.7	17.0
Racquetball	14.1	3.1	18.0
Football	13.2	8.9	10.6
Soccer	7.8	4.1	9.3

Reprinted, by permission, from IHRSA, 1995, *Why and where people exercise* (Boston: IHRSA), 15.

The top five sport and fitness activities for all groups were

1. aerobic equipment exercise,
2. strength training,
3. walking,
4. bicycling, and
5. swimming.

In terms of equipment use, the 1997 IHRSA/American Sports Data, Inc. *Health Club Trend Report* establishes that resistance machines (selectorized) lead the way as the most popular equipment in a club setting, with approximately 9.3 million participants in 1996.

Free weights and treadmill use filled the second and third positions, with 7.7 million using free weights and 7.4 million using treadmills. Stationary cycles and stairclimbers are ranked fourth and fifth in participation, with 7.4 million exercising on stationary cycles and 6.4 million on stairclimbers.

Future trend projections for exercise participants are that activities primarily being used today will continue to increase in use significantly through the year 2000. Different programs and equipment will be introduced, but few, if any, will take the place of walking, swimming, cardiovascular equipment, weight training, and cycling. These five categories will continue to dominate the interests of mainstream fitness enthusiasts.

MEMBER TRACKING

Members are considered the lifeblood of the fitness industry. The goal of every fitness professional, manager, and owner should be to maintain a membership at or near full capacity. Although attracting and obtaining new members is important and should continually be emphasized, retaining existing members is just as important or perhaps more so.

According to IHRSA's 1996 survey of the health and fitness industry, *Profiles of Success,* more than 11 million individuals are currently enrolled in commercial health fitness settings, and 34 to 38 percent drop out annually depending on the setting. To compensate for this loss, clubs routinely try to replace this number with new members. Unfortunately, little consideration is given to the actual costs involved in generating a new member. For example, if the sales and marketing expenses, salaries, commissions, and administrative costs are

totaled up for all new members, it becomes obvious that keeping existing members happy is a lot cheaper than obtaining new members.

Keeping existing member information current is one of the best methods for measuring overall customer satisfaction. Tracking membership growth and attrition allows management to gauge the organization's performance regularly. Without compiling the appropriate information first, it would be difficult to implement or even create changes within an existing program. Methods for acquiring this information should be included in the internal operations of every health fitness center.

Member tracking information should include the following:

1. Member usage
2. Member adherence and attrition
3. Average length of membership
4. Membership growth

Member Usage

Tracking daily attendance in a health fitness setting is necessary for understanding member traffic flow. Knowing the number of members who use the facility daily, the preferred time and day of the week, and activities they most often use are all factors in determining the various patterns associated with a club's membership. Analyzing this data and comparing the findings against industry standards can assist fitness professionals in implementing programs, scheduling staff, and tracking the actual number of members who use the facility regularly.

Obtaining attendance information is best accomplished through member check-in at the point of entry. Traditionally, two methods have been used to acquire this information: either a manual sign-in sheet or a computerized check-in system primarily using member ID number cards or bar code readers. With the recent advancement in technology, check-in systems will soon include on-screen photo IDs, hand scanners, and fingerprint scanners. Additional information on member tracking systems will be discussed in chapter 19, Computer Applications.

Figure 2.7 provides a weekly attendance report indicating the various subtotals and percentages of usage for the time and day of the week.

When reviewing a weekly attendance report, address the following evaluation questions:

Time of day by day of week									
Time	**Sun**	**Mon**	**Tue**	**Wed**	**Thur**	**Fri**	**Sat**	**Total**	**% of usage**
0:00	0	0	17	2	0	0	0	19	.49
0:30	0	0	12	0	0	0	0	12	.31
1:00	0	0	32	0	0	0	0	32	.83
1:30	0	5	41	0	0	0	0	46	1.19
2:00	0	3	42	0	0	0	0	45	1.16
2:30	0	9	56	0	0	0	0	65	1.68
3:00	0	8	45	28	0	0	0	81	2.09
3:30	0	6	32	24	0	0	0	62	1.60
4:00	0	18	25	48	0	0	0	91	2.35
4:30	0	14	22	30	0	0	0	66	1.70
5:00	0	27	21	73	0	0	0	121	3.13
5:30	0	49	15	47	0	0	0	111	2.87
6:00	0	20	6	39	0	0	0	65	1.68
6:30	0	22	4	22	4	0	0	52	1.34
7:00	0	6	0	41	4	0	0	51	1.32
7:30	0	21	0	23	12	0	13	69	1.78
8:00	14	49	0	19	55	0	34	171	4.42
8:30	15	52	0	12	47	0	46	172	4.44
9:00	15	54	0	5	31	0	30	135	3.49
9:30	8	51	0	4	29	1	26	119	3.07
10:00	19	67	0	0	20	13	12	131	3.38
10:30	18	56	0	0	14	19	7	114	2.94
11:00	11	32	0	0	27	38	12	120	3.10
11:30	24	45	0	9	23	16	2	119	3.07
12:00	12	44	0	14	11	7	13	101	2.61
12:30	17	26	0	9	24	12	6	94	2.43
13:00	35	15	0	10	7	3	9	79	2.04
13:30	17	6	0	9	5	3	10	50	1.29
14:00	22	7	0	9	4	16	18	76	1.96
14:30	31	0	48	3	2	15	21	120	3.10
15:00	33	0	14	0	14	2	15	78	2.01
15:30	26	0	11	0	15	14	20	86	2.22
16:00	42	6	13	0	17	5	19	102	2.63
16.30	35	10	8	0	23	15	21	112	2.89
17:00	10	25	31	0	23	6	12	107	2.76
17:30	26	16	28	25	49	20	12	176	4.55
18:00	10	35	23	19	44	20	7	158	4.08
18:30	13	7	18	7	32	43	4	124	3.20
19:00	16	0	23	0	46	22	4	111	2.87
19:30	1	0	14	0	28	22	0	65	1.68
20:00	0	0	17	0	20	29	0	66	1.70
20.30	0	0	32	0	9	9	0	50	1.29
21:00	0	0	8	0	4	0	0	12	.31
21:30	0	0	5	0	2	0	0	7	.18
22:00	0	0	10	0	0	0	0	10	.26
22:30	0	2	2	0	0	0	0	4	.10
23:00	0	6	0	0	0	0	0	6	.15
23:30	0	8	1	0	0	0	0	9	.23
Total	470	827	676	531	645	350	373	3872	
	12.14	21.36	17.46	13.71	16.66	9.04	9.63		

Figure 2.7 Weekly attendance report.

1. Is overall usage consistent with the previous week?

2. If net membership totals are similar, does weekly usage compare closely to the previous year?

3. Are the usage or traffic patterns comparable throughout the day?

4. Do the majority of members still use the facility around preestablished prime time hours?

5. Do Monday through Wednesday continue to be the highest usage days?

6. Do the usage numbers justify the hours designated for opening and closing?

7. Are staffing schedules consistent with high and low use times?

Member Adherence and Attrition

When discussing member tracking, there are two terms that we first need to define: *adherence* and *attrition*. The word adherence means to stick to something. It is often used to describe a person's continuation in an exercise program.

> *A member who is adhering to a program is someone who is devoted to what he or she is doing.*

Another word often used interchangeably with adherence is retention. Both adherence and retention apply to keeping and maintaining members. The percentage of members who retain their memberships annually is called the adherence rate.

Conversely, attrition means to wear down or tear away by friction. In a fitness setting, attrition applies to those members who have canceled their memberships. Reasons why members decide to leave a facility are varied but are usually grouped into two categories: controlled or uncontrolled. Controlled attrition includes reasons specifically related to the organization and its operations. Generally, these reasons are believed to be preventable and should rarely occur if the business is operated in a professional and proficient manner.

Examples of controllable reasons why attrition might be high include the following:

- Dirty facility, lack of maintenance
- Rude or unprofessional staff
- Poor service
- Broken equipment that is never repaired
- Club overcrowding
- Disorganized activity programs
- Management not reacting to members' needs

Uncontrolled reasons of attrition include reasons that are not in the control of operators but do affect overall attrition rates. Individual circumstances can prevent members from continuing their involve-

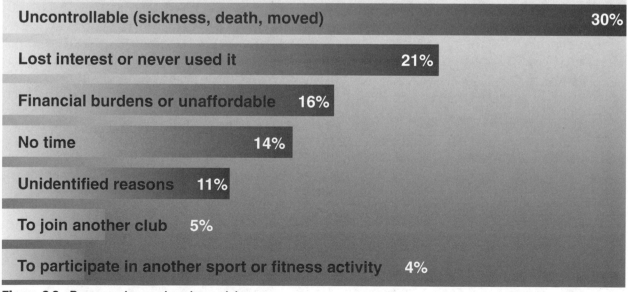

Uncontrollable (sickness, death, moved)	30%
Lost interest or never used it	21%
Financial burdens or unaffordable	16%
No time	14%
Unidentified reasons	11%
To join another club	5%
To participate in another sport or fitness activity	4%

Figure 2.8 Reasons why members leave clubs.

Reprinted, by permission, from IHRSA, 1994, *Profiles of success* (Boston: IHRSA), 42. Copyright 1994 by IHRSA.

ment with a facility. Examples of uncontrollable attrition include the following:

- Family interruptions such as moving or birth
- Injury, sickness, or death
- Change in job that causes time constraints
- Club's location inconvenient
- Financial status change

According to IHRSA's 1994 *Profiles of Success*, 30 percent of the reasons given for leaving a commercial fitness facility were considered uncontrollable; the remaining 71 percent were controllable. Figure 2.8 lists the various reasons members choose to leave commercial fitness facilities.

In 1995, the average annual attrition rate for commercial fitness clubs was 34 percent. To put this figure in perspective, consider that a club with 1,000 members at the beginning of the year would lose 340 members by the end of the year. Of those 340 members who left, 126 would have dropped for uncontrollable reasons and 214 for controllable reasons.

Member attrition rates fluctuate monthly. Rarely are two months the same when tracking attrition. Consequently, when determining member loss, the figure derived is for a given point in time only. The following formula shows how to calculate member attrition rates:

$$\text{Member attrition rate (percent)} = \frac{\text{number of members lost during period (year or month)}}{\text{number of members at start of period (year or month)}} \times 100$$

Average Length of Membership

Another indicator used by fitness operators to determine overall performance is to compute the average length of membership. Knowing the approximate length of time members maintain their membership assists in planning and projecting for the future. Using the industry's average annual member attrition rate of 34 percent, the average length of membership for 1995 was 2.94 years. The following formula shows how to calculate the average length of membership:

$$\text{Average length of membership} = \frac{1}{\text{member attrition rate}}$$

Consider a scenario in which the annual attrition rate is 25 percent instead of the industry standard 34 percent. Given the formula mentioned, the average length of a membership would be four years. If the average length of a membership was almost doubled how would profitability be affected? As mentioned earlier, the longer a business keeps a customer, the more profitable the customer is to the business. Also, as a member's lifetime value grows, the more dependent he or she becomes on a facility and the less susceptible he or she is to other club offers of a lower price.

For years, professionals in the health fitness industry have believed annual attrition rates have been too high and they should take steps to reduce the level of terminations. As a result, operators are encouraged to adopt a philosophy focused on retaining members. A strategy should be developed that involves retention in every aspect of the operation. Retaining members is a process.

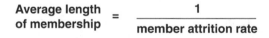

Everything from fitness programming, to hiring personnel, to facility maintenance should be based on what the member wants.

Operators need to take into account the nonexercising public's views of the fitness industry. According to Dr. Brooks' survey (1994a), member growth could accelerate significantly over the next decade if clubs successfully removed four sources of intimidation that prevent individuals from joining a club.

- Physical intimidation—nonexercisers don't have the athletic ability to belong to a club and may be injured as a result.
- Intellectual intimidation—nonexercisers find fitness equipment difficult to use.
- Psychological and social intimidation—nonexercisers believe they would be outsiders in a club full of insiders.

Little Rock Athletic Club Annual Gross Membership Attrition Report						
	Jan	Feb	Mar	Apr	May	June
Membership base at beginning of month	2,537	2,588	2,605	2,599	2,600	2,601
Memberships added	80	50	40	37	31	35
Memberships lost	29	33	46	36	30	36
Net difference	51	17	-6	1	1	-1
Membership base at end of month	2,588	2,605	2,599	2,600	2,601	2,600
% gross attrition for month	1.14%	1.28%	1.77%	1.39%	1.15%	1.38%
Estimated annual attrition (%)	13.72%	15.30%	21.19%	16.62%	13.85%	16.61%

Figure 2.9   Sample attrition report

• Ethical intimidation—nonexercisers question the honesty and integrity of club operators.

One can speculate that if nonexercisers' views could be altered or reversed immediately, memberships could increase up to 85 percent by the year 2000. To accomplish this goal, operators must familiarize themselves with the reasons given for terminating a membership, then actively follow up to prevent controllable issues from occurring.

Membership Growth

In addition to tracking member attrition and facility usage, monthly membership growth is another indicator for determining overall performance. Whether in a for-profit or nonprofit setting, a consistent membership base is needed to project and plan for the future. Unfortunately, the health fitness business is a dynamic industry, and the number of new members joining and existing members terminating varies daily, which alters the membership base. Consequently, the continuous monitoring of membership numbers is a necessary responsibility of the fitness professional.

If much fluctuation occurs in membership numbers, financial projections and long-term goals may be jeopardized.

Determining net membership growth involves adding the number of new members who join monthly and subtracting member terminations. The net difference reflects either a positive or negative growth rate. The goal for every club should be to average a positive annual growth rate. The net membership growth rate for all IHRSA clubs averages 6 percent annually. For example, a club with 1,000 members and a 6 percent growth rate would net (after subtracting terminated members) 60 new members by the end of the year.

Once all monthly membership numbers have been tabulated, a membership attrition report should be compiled to provide a summary and historical account of the monthly transactions. This report should include the total number of new members, terminated members, net member difference, membership base at the end of the month, and estimated annual attrition rate. Tracking these numbers establishes a road map for club operators to follow regarding membership growth and estimated annual attrition rates. Figure 2.9 provides an example of a membership attrition report.

Key questions to ask when analyzing a monthly membership report include the following:

1. Are actual member numbers close to membership projections from the first of the year?

2. Does the estimated annual attrition percentage coincide with national industry standards (i.e., IHRSA, YMCA, Jewish Community Centers) as in the following list?

Little Rock Athletic Club Annual Gross Membership Attrition Report *(continued)*						
July	**Aug**	**Sept**	**Oct**	**Nov**	**Dec**	**End of year**
2,600	2,602	2,615	2,605	2,607	2,606	
37	56	30	36	23	48	503
35	43	40	34	24	29	415
2	13	-10	2	-1	19	88
2,602	2,615	2,605	2,607	2,606	2,625	
1.35%	1.65%	1.53%	1.31%	0.92%	1.11%	1.33%
16.15%	19.83%	18.36%	15.66%	11.05%	13.35%	15.97%

5 to 10 percent = excellent

11 to 16 percent = very good

17 to 21 percent = good

22 to 27 percent = fair

28 percent or more = poor

3. Is there a positive net membership growth for the year?

4. Are the joining patterns of new members consistent from year to year?

5. Comparing the number of new members and terminated members, is there a positive or negative variance from the previous year?

IN CLOSING

In this chapter, we emphasized the importance of knowing and understanding the customer or member and how consumers view the fitness industry. It is important for the health fitness professional to be aware of why people choose a sedentary lifestyle and what reasons would cause them to become active. Understanding consumers' perceptions of fitness centers and what ingredients are needed to adopt the ideal club setting can also help the health fitness professional most effectively manage and operate their programs.

Health fitness professionals must recognize the importance of member demographics, including their average member's profile, participation pat-terns, and how it relates to overall U.S. sport and fitness participation. This chapter also addressed additional information on the importance of member tracking and controlling member attrition.

KEY TERMS

Adherence

Attrition

Demographics

Discretionary income

External attitudes

Internal attitudes

Perceived value

Preconditioning

Target market

RECOMMENDED READINGS

Albrecht, K., and R. Zemke. 1985. *Service America! Doing business in the new economy.* Homewood, IL: Dow Jones-Irwin.

American Sports Data, Inc. 1996. *Health club trend report.* Hartsdale, NY: American Sports Data.

Anderson, K., and R. Zemke. 1991. *Delivering knock your socks off service.* New York: Performance Research Associates.

Brehm, B. 1995. Understanding attrition: Why do clients quit? *Fitness Management* (January): 25.

Brooks, C. 1994a. *How consumers view health and sports clubs*. Ann Arbor, MI: International Health, Racquet and Sportsclub Association.

———. 1994b. Membership age wave. *Fitness Management* (March): 38-40.

Connellan, T., and R. Zemke. 1993. *Sustaining knock your socks off service*. New York: Performance Research Associates.

International Health, Racquet and Sportsclub Association. 1994. *Profiles of success*. Boston: IHRSA.

———. 1996. *Profiles of success*. Boston: IHRSA.

———. 1997. *The American health club experience*. Boston: IHRSA.

International Health, Racquet and Sportsclub Association and American Sports Data, Inc. 1996. *Why and where people exercise*. Boston: IHRSA.

———. 1997. *Health club trend reports*. Boston: IHRSA.

Marketing Development Consultants, 1993. *Today's club members*. Cedar Rapids, IA: Universal Gym Equipment.

National Sporting Goods Association. 1992. *Sports participation in 1992*. Mt. Prospect, IL: National Sporting Goods Association

Nykiel, R. 1990. *You can't lose if the customer wins*. Stamford, CT: Longmeadow Press.

Pessin, F. 1995. Calculating a member's value. *Fitness Management* (September): 40-41.

U.S. Department of Health and Human Services. 1995. *Healthy people 2000: Midcourse review and 1995 revisions*. Washington, DC: U.S. Department of Health and Human Services.

U.S. Department of Health and Human Services. 1996. *Physical activity and health: A report of the Surgeon General*. Atlanta, GA: U.S. Department of Health and Human Services, Centers for Disease Control and Prevention, National Center for Chronic Disease Prevention and Health Promotion.

Vavra, T. 1995. *Aftermarketing: How to keep customers for life through relationship marketing*. Chicago: Irwin.

Winters, C. 1994. The art of keeping members. *Club Industry* (February): 18-23.

Zemke, R. 1989. *The service edge: 101 customers that profit from customer service*. New York: New American Library.

CHAPTER 3

Organizational Development

In the first chapter we introduced you to the health fitness industry. The second chapter introduced the types of members frequenting the various settings in the industry. In this chapter we present the development and organization of the health fitness settings. Regardless of the setting, programs go through a predictable concept development process—program goals are defined, then implemented in a standardized manner. The organizational structures evolving from this concept development process are remarkably different. Because professionals in our industry frequently move across a number of settings as careers unfold, it is important to understand how the different settings are structured and organized.

The first major step in organizational development is to understand the concept development process for a health fitness organization. This is complicated and entails different procedures in various settings. Planning for a commercial program has a large financial element attached to it, whereas planning for a corporate setting often has important nonfinancial elements related to the health and fitness levels of the company employees. Planning for the clinical setting, such as a hospital-based wellness program, involves some corporate program elements concerning employee involvement in the program, but it takes on the features of a commercial program when operating as a for-profit hospital community outreach fitness center. Community programs such as YMCAs are generally nonprofit organizations concentrating on program delivery while operating under the legal constraints of nonprofit status. Each program evolves from a statement of the program's objectives and the development of its mission. The implementation of the programs is a manifestation of their stated or implied objectives. Let's explore the concept development process in each setting.

CONCEPT DEVELOPMENT

The first step in organizational development is to understand the *concept development process* for a health fitness organization. This is complicated and entails different procedures in various settings.

Commercial Setting

According to the Small Business Administration (SBA), there are distinct groupings of businesses that can be categorized by the number of employees working in their particular enterprise. Approximately 98 percent of all business firms in the United States are small—having fewer than five full-time employees. There are 19 million such businesses accounting for about half the American workforce. Regarding the health fitness industry, the rapidly expanding personal training business is an example of this size business. Budding entrepreneurs abound as contractors providing value-added expertise within larger commercial facilities or as sole proprietors of a fitness consultant business.

The next and slightly larger SBA employee grouping is the five-to-nine employee classification, accounting for almost a million businesses. The small aerobics studio or bodybuilding facility characterizes such a business grouping. These facilities fill a special niche in the marketplace by providing services to special segments of the fitness market.

The group with 10 to 19 full-time employees, the SBA's next largest category for business size, comprises approximately one-half million businesses. This is the grouping in which the average commercial health fitness business falls. Of the 12,000 commercial health fitness businesses currently in the United States, the average fitness-only club will hire approximately 10 full-time and 40 part-time employees, operate a 25,000-square-foot facility with 3,000 members, and generate over $1 million in annual revenue (IHRSA 1996; Markarian 1993).

This business grouping is changing rapidly and is in the process of maturing as an industry. One aspect of its maturity is the merging, joint venturing, and acquiring of small businesses by corporations creating large organizations, which benefit from economy of scale with centralized management. Club Corporation of America is an example of a large corporation owning or managing more than two hundred clubs throughout the United States. Although the organizational and ownership structure may change, the inherent size of the health fitness enterprise may remain within the SBA grouping of 10 to 19 full-time employees for the foreseeable future.

The number of members using the facility determines the size of a commercial health fitness business.

Although each health fitness facility and program is unique and difficult to pigeonhole, during the concept development phase of an organization, it is important to determine staff size. The following guidelines regarding staffing and facility allotments should prove helpful in planning an organizational structure:

- Each 200 members requires the addition of one full-time staff member.
- Each 50 members requires the addition of one part-time staff member.
- Each member will require approximately 10 to 20 additional square feet of facility space.

These guidelines are fitting for the average commercial, corporate, or community health fitness facility that is 3 to 5 years old with a stable membership growth rate. Early development stages for these settings and the clinical setting at any stage of development that requires more staff-intensive programming does not fit these generalizations.

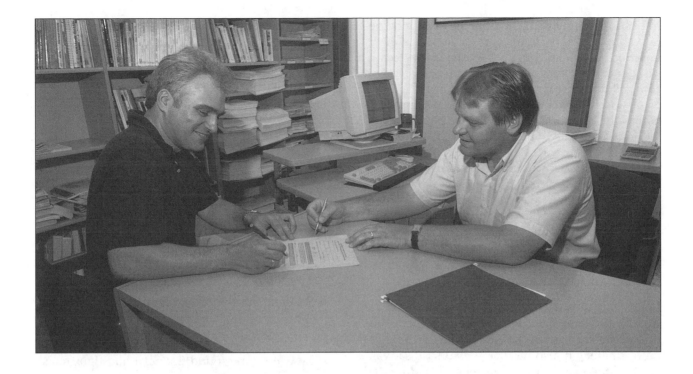

For many of us, starting a business of our own in the health and fitness industry is something frequently contemplated but rarely undertaken. Those brave individuals who bite the bullet and start their own business generally do so after accumulating several years of experience, considerable assets, and good business contacts. If you are one of these brave few determined to open your own business, the first step is to develop a *business plan*. The business plan serves many purposes, but one of the most critical is that of securing financing for the project. This is true regardless of whether you are seeking *start-up funds* through a bank loan, *venture capital*, or personal loans from family or friends.

Business planning is a complicated process and requires expertise in the areas of finance, space planning, architecture, program planning, management, and marketing, to mention a few. No one person usually has the expertise to develop every aspect of a good business plan; it usually takes a team approach and requires months of hard work. To find out more about business planning in the health fitness industry we recommend *Developing and Managing Health Fitness Facilities* (Patton et al. 1989).

In the early stages of planning a health fitness business, budding entrepreneurs are asked many questions by those experts with whom they consult. Should you buy an existing business or a franchise that has built-in marketing, management, staffing, and programming systems?

Acquiring a franchise, such as a Gold's Gym, is an appropriate approach for someone with limited experience needing proven operational systems.

Should you become a *sole proprietor* and start a health fitness business that relies entirely on your skills? The risk-reward potential is greatest in the sole proprietorship environment, but this approach should not be undertaken by anyone inexperienced or faint of heart. The freedom to call your own shots regarding business matters, reaping the rewards of your own efforts, and having the sense of accomplishment when your enterprise is flourishing can be offset by the long hours, increased liability risks, potential for bankruptcy, and not being in control of the inevitable economic cycles of the marketplace.

Should you go into a *partnership agreement* with a fellow professional or someone with the necessary capital? Your sweat equity coupled with a partner's financial equity might be a good recipe for success, especially if your partner has a good business background. Selecting the right business partner is thought to be as important a decision in your business life as selecting a spouse in your personal life. You will certainly spend as much time making significant decisions with a partner as you would with a spouse.

Should the health fitness business be incorporated into a *C- or S-corporation*? Each form of incorporation has advantages and disadvantages to consider and discuss with a competent attorney and accountant before leaping headlong into the world of business. C-corporations are legally and economically best suited for the larger players in the industry. Generally, the S-corporation, which is most commonly adopted by small health fitness businesses, has the distinct advantage of having corporate status while behaving to some extent like a partnership. Before we explore the intricacies of incorporation, let us explore the opportunities of buying an existing business within the commercial health fitness industry.

Buying an Existing Business

Purchasing an existing health fitness business, assuming it can be acquired for the right price, has some distinct advantages over starting from scratch: unfortunately, it also has some distinct disadvantages. If the health fitness business is mature and successful, it has the following advantages:

- There is a greater likelihood of continued success than a start-up from scratch.
- It has a proven location for successful operation.
- The need for thorough up-front business planning is minimized.
- The existing business has an established membership.
- The equipment and inventory are already established.
- The financing can be accomplished with a single purchase transaction.

Even if the preceding advantages stand the test of careful study on your part and scrutiny from your consultants, you should weigh them against the following disadvantages for purchasing an existing business:

- You will inherit any ill will from past members toward the previous owners.
- The existing equipment and building may not conform to current industry standards or trends.
- Staff members who are not assets are frequently inherited with the business.
- Inherited membership may not fit a changing marketplace and changing the image would be difficult.

- Policies established by the new business may not be accepted by an existing membership.

These advantages and disadvantages are helpful in considering the purchase of an existing health fitness business; however, they are not the only factors to consider and evaluate. For example, evaluate the financial status of the enterprise over the last three to five years carefully by asking the following questions:

☑ Are the financial profiles of the business consistent with industry standards?

☑ Do the balance sheet and income statement reflect a sound financial operation?

☑ Are the revenue and expenses in line with industry data?

☑ Would the investment of your resources in this business yield higher returns than a fresh start in a new business?

These are some sound financial questions to ask yourself before buying an existing business.

There are also critical marketing questions to answer before purchase.

☑ Is the market service area for the fitness center growing?

☑ What kind of competition exists or is being planned for the market service area?

☑ What is the image of the facility within the market service area?

☑ Is the reputation of the present owners tarnished?

☑ If so, will image development by your new ownership be difficult or impossible?

☑ Is the focus of programs offered consistent with industry trends?

Although not comprehensive, these questions help a prospective buyer focus on marketing issues that could impact the decision to purchase and the determination of value of an existing business.

Finally, there are operational questions to address before purchasing an existing fitness facility.

☑ Is the facility owner leasing space?

☑ If so, the details of the lease, such as the terms, renewability, pricing, liabilities, escalation, and transferability become important issues, particularly for a prime location. Secure options for renewing a lease in writing before signing a purchase agreement for the business.

If all the previous issues are overcome and you still want to buy the club, then you are well advised to seek appropriate professional advice from an attorney, accountant, architect, and other industry professionals before completing the purchase process. Obtaining professional advice is essential to avoid pitfalls and oversights commonly experienced by newcomers to the industry.

Buying a Franchise

Purchasing a franchise is becoming a popular solution to ownership in the health fitness industry. The franchise is the largest grouping of ownership types and the fastest growing business format for the health fitness industry. Accordingly, we focus much attention on this form of business structure.

A *franchise* is an arrangement between a parent company such as Gold's Gym and an entrepreneur such as yourself. The parent company has a successful history of operating health fitness businesses and has developed a formula for success, which is purchased usually by a less-experienced entrepreneur seeking an avenue into the health fitness industry. The entrepreneur receives the benefit of the experience of the parent company plus the name, logo, marketing techniques, management systems, staff training methods, and other expertise. The parent company is called the franchiser and the entrepreneur is called the franchisee. They operate under a formal franchise agreement identifying the contractual rights and obligations of both parties. The agreement is usually for an initial period with renewal provisions based on performance. There are many distinct advantages and disadvantages to both the franchiser and the franchisee.

Franchiser Advantages
- Community acceptance with local owner.
- Marketing costs shared by franchisee.
- Operating costs shared by franchisee.
- Flat fees often collected monthly.
- Selling supplies are profitable.
- Retains quality control via agreement.

Franchisee Advantages
- Sound management procedures.
- Less risk with market-tested company.
- Established marketing program.
- Membership within large industry player.
- Better credit access with franchise.
- Mass purchasing economies.

Franchiser Disadvantages
- Long distance oversight of franchisee.
- Possible credit extension to franchisee.
- Supervisory personnel expenses.
- Loss of some ownership.

Franchisee Disadvantages
- Loss of freedom in management decisions.
- Purchase obligations for supplies.
- Shared profits with franchiser.
- Franchises are expensive.

Reprinted, by permission, from D. Steinhoff and J. Burgess, 1993, *Small business management fundamentals*, 6th ed. (New York: McGraw-Hill), 79, 80. Copyright 1993 by McGraw-Hill.

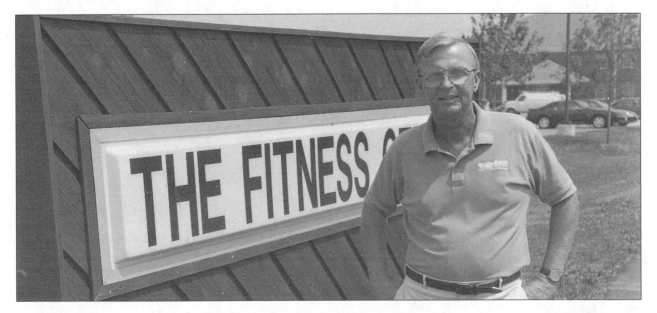

Table 3.1   Checklist for Evaluating a Franchise

The contract

1. Did your lawyer approve the franchise contract?
2. Does the franchise call upon you to take any steps that are unwise or illegal?
3. Does the franchise give you an exclusive territory for the length of the franchise?
4. Is the franchiser connected with any other franchise company?
5. If you answered yes to the last question, what is your protection from a second franchise company?
6. Under what circumstances can you terminate the franchise and at what cost?
7. If you sell your franchise, will you be compensated for your goodwill?

The franchiser

1. How many years has the firm offering you a franchise been in operation?
2. Has it a reputation for honesty among the local firms holding its franchise?
3. Has the franchiser shown you any documentable profits from an existing franchise?
4. Will the firm assist you with
   a. a management training program,
   b. an employee training program,
   c. a sales staff training program,
   d. a public relations program,
   e. capital,
   f. credit, and
   g. centralized purchasing?
5. Will the firm help you find a good location?
6. Is the franchising firm adequately financed to carry out its responsibilities?
7. Is the franchiser a large enough company to deliver on its commitments?
8. Exactly what can the franchiser do for you that you can't do for yourself?
9. Has the franchiser investigated you thoroughly to determine your potential for success?
10. Does your state have a law regulating the sale of franchises and has the franchiser complied?

You—the franchisee

1. How much equity capital will you need to purchase the franchise and operate until your income is expected to meet your expenses? Where will you get it?
2. Are you prepared to give up some independence of action to secure the franchise?
3. Do you really believe you have the ability, training, and experience to be a success?
4. Are you prepared to spend much or all of your business life with this franchise?

Your market

1. Have you made any study to determine whether the fitness services you want will be accepted in your market?
2. Will the population in your market service area increase over the next five years?
3. Will your fitness services be in greater demand in five years than at the present?
4. What competition exists for your proposed business? What is being planned?

Reprinted from U.S. Department of Commerce 1990.

Please note that each advantage and disadvantage will not necessarily exist for every franchise agreement. Historically, franchises have been successful when workable business plans have been developed during the planning process of the business. However, there are exceptions, such as the now defunct or struggling fitness business chains based on high-pressure sales with low-quality programs and staffing. Although most franchises encourage high-volume business, they now provide well-equipped facilities with improved programming and staff. It is highly likely that franchises will continue to be a viable method of getting into the health fitness business well into the 21st century. To determine if a franchise is the best for you, consult the checklist in table 3.1.

Table 3.2 lists franchising and licensing information of selected companies. As can be seen from the table, the number of franchises, costs for startup, advertising, and management support varies significantly.

Starting Your Own Business

The creation and construction of your own business is a rewarding but complicated and drawn out process. The business planning phases are similar to, but more detailed than, purchasing an existing business or buying a franchise. Because there is no history for the business, the diligence required to adequately prepare the business plan is more intensive, and acquiring the financing is more difficult. The facility construction process usually takes at least 18 to 24 months, and few have survived this experience without some serious construction delays and cost overruns.

The allocation of capital to feasibility studies, architectural, and construction costs are only part of the expenses. The wise professional sets aside enough reserve and *operating capital* to sustain the health fitness enterprise through preopening campaigns, the inevitable contingency costs associated with opening a facility, and the first six months to one year of operation costs. Inadequate construction and start-up capital is frequently a problem and usually results in dipping into *contingency capital* or reserve capital initially allocated for the start-up and early operation of the business. However, the greatest reason for failure in start-up businesses in this industry is lack of adequate reserve capital to sustain the business during the early periods when revenue is inadequate to meet expenses. Patton et al. (1989) offer suggestions for determining capital needs for starting and operating health fitness businesses, as well as setting aside capital for unforeseen contingencies.

Legal Forms of Business

The owner of a small business today must deal with myriad government rules, regulations, and laws. To ensure survival, the small business person must understand the local, state, and federal laws that impact the operation of the business. One of the first decisions is the choice of the legal structure that best suits the needs of the particular business. All forms of business have their advantages and disadvantages, and there are hundreds of laws that influence the final choice. Let's examine these different forms of business.

Sole Proprietorship

The single, or sole, proprietorship is a business owned and operated by one person. The owner and the business are synonymous in the eyes of the law. All assets in the firm are owned by the proprietor, subject only to the liabilities incurred in its establishment and operation. The proprietor is solely responsible for all personal and business debts and any losses incurred. The proprietor assumes all the risks, usually provides most of its capital, and its total management. If the owner intends to use checks, sign contracts, or obtain licenses in the name of the business, most states require a registration of a *dba* or *doing business as*. Depending on your location or locations, a sole proprietorship may need to file a dba with the city, county, or state.

The sole proprietor is the most popular form of business in America, representing approximately 75 percent of all business firms, and accounts for a sizable number of the 12,000 health fitness centers in the United States. As with any maturing industry, the sole proprietorship is being challenged by the large franchise groups and major companies. The economy of scale in marketing, purchasing, and operating larger enterprises places them at an advantage in the marketplace. The sole proprietorship manifested as single-facility owners in the health fitness industry is on the decline. However, the niche for small proprietorships remains an opportunity for the enterprising professional. This is manifested most frequently in the form of contractors providing personal training, aerobics, and other fitness services to individuals or facilities. There is no definitive data source to indicate the size of this business segment, but one might speculate that there are many contract professionals in our industry.

Table 3.2   Franchise Information for Selected Companies

Company name	Franchise (F) License (L)	Year established	Initial franchise/ license cost	Annual franchise fee/ renewal licensing fee	Annual royalties due
Gold's Gym Franchising Venice, CA 310-392-3005	F	1965	$12,000	$6,000-$50,000 (price varies depending on market area served)	None
World Gym Santa Monica, CA 310-450-0080	F	1981	$12,000	$6,500	None
Powerhouse Gyms International Farmington Hills, MI 810-476-2888	L	1975	$12,500	$5,000	None
Lady of America Ft. Lauderdale, FL 954-492-1201	F	1984	$25,000-$35,000	10 percent of then-current new franchise fee	10 percent of gross receipts; 5 percent after a certain sales level is met
LifeQuest Charleston, SC 800-264-8535	F/L	1996	$11,750	$5,750	F: 2 percent of quarterly gross L: None
Cory Everson Licensing Columbus, GA 706-321-0999	L	1995	$9,500	$5,000	None
Universal Fitness Centers Kansas City, MO 816-960-1077	L	1996	$12,500	$5,750	None
Bally Fitness Franchising, Inc. Chicago, IL 800-410-CLUB	F	1996	$40,000	Initial term is 15 years; renewed for 10 years at the cost of the then-current franchise fee	3 percent of total cash receipts; 4 percent of total membership revenues; group sales are higher

Reprinted, by permission, from data compiled by Dana Connor, 1997, *Club Industry* (March): 22. Copyright 1997 by Cardinal Business Media.

Advantages of the Sole Proprietorship

- Tax advantages.
- Simplicity of its organization.
- Owner's freedom to make all decisions.
- Owner's enjoyment of all profits.
- Lack of legal restrictions.
- Ease of its discontinuance.

Disadvantages of the Sole Proprietorship

- Owner's possible lack of ability and experience.
- Difficulty in attracting and retaining quality employees.
- Difficulty in raising capital.
- Limited life of the firm.
- Unlimited liability of the proprietor.

Because most nonfranchised and unincorporated enterprises in the health fitness industry are sole proprietorships, it would seem that the advantages outweigh the disadvantages. However, there is much to recommend other forms of business structure. Let's explore the partnership next.

Partnership

A *partnership* is defined as two or more persons acting as co-owners of a business for profit. Partnerships are based on formal and informal partnership agreements. Although it is not a legal requirement, the partnership agreement should be in writing. The agreement should define, as clearly as possible, each partner's rights, obligations, liabilities, duties, and authority, along with the limits to such authority. It should also include an agreement on how profits and losses are to be divided and what will happen if the partnership needs to be dissolved. As with anything, there are distinct advantages and disadvantages for the partnership.

Advantages of Partnerships

- Tax advantages.
- Ease of formation and dissolution.
- Ability to combine individual talents, judgment, and skills.
- Greater amounts of capital usually available to the firm.
- Definite legal status of the firm under law.

Disadvantages of Partnerships

- Unlimited and mutual liability of the partners.
- Limited life of the firm with enforced termination.
- Division of authority.
- Danger of disagreements among the partners.

Partnerships are usually either *general partnerships* or *limited partnerships*. A general partnership is one in which each partner carries unlimited liability for the firm's debts and obligations. A limited partnership is one in which some partners have their liability limited to the extent of their investment, whereas at least one general partner carries the unlimited liability obligation. For example, the general partners might manage a health fitness facility, whereas limited partners might be investors in the enterprise. Withdrawal of a limited partner does not dissolve a partnership as does withdrawal of a general partner. For limited partnership agreements, which identify the status of each partner, to have legal standing they must usually be filed with the appropriate administrative department of the partnership's home state. In Texas, for example, partnership agreements are filed with the Secretary of State. In many states the filing is with the Commerce Department.

Special types of partners may be appropriate in certain circumstances. *Secret partners* play an active role in the business but are not identified to the public as partners. *Silent partners* are not active in the operations of the business but share in its profits. *Dormant partners* are not active and are not known to the public. *Nominal partners* are not really partners at all but allow the public to think they are by their actions and words. Finally, *joint ventures* are partnerships formed by two corporations to complete a specific task (Steinhoff and Burgess 1993). The joint venture is frequently used in the health fitness industry when, for example, a hospital or corporation with fitness facilities may seek out a fitness management company to staff and operate the program.

> *Joint ventures between health care and health fitness will undoubtedly continue as managed care grows and seeks ways to curtail health care costs through preventive services.*

Corporations

Entrepreneurs who want to limit their personal liability can choose to incorporate their business. *Corporations* are recognized under state and federal law as separate legal entities. They are separate and distinct from the owners to the extent that corporations can own property, enter into contracts, and sue or be sued in their own name. Corporations are composed of shareholders who contribute capital in exchange for an opportunity to share in the profits, directors who manage the corporate board, and others who manage the day-to-day activities of the corporation. The Model Business Corporation Act, enacted in 1946 (revised subsequently) and adopted by two-thirds of the states, provides the regulations under which corporations maintain perpetual succession, can sue and be sued, have a corporate seal, acquire and sell real estate and personal property, lend money, and make and alter their bylaws. Approximately 17 percent of all businesses are corporations, accounting for 87 percent of the business volume in the country (Anderson and Dunkelberg 1993). The corporation as a form of business is growing in popularity in the health fitness industry. As the industry matures, it is inevitable that large corporate structures evolve. It is the nature of industry life cycles in this country.

Advantages of a Corporation

- Limited liability.
- Transfer of ownership.
- Stability.
- Acquisition of capital.
- Skilled managers.
- Stockholders tend to be customers.

Disadvantages of a Corporation

- Taxes.
- Rigidity.
- Shared ownership.
- Regulations.

S-Corporations

Entrepreneurs who like the limited liability of corporations but not the double taxation can choose to form an *S-corporation*. This is a hybrid corporate form that was created in the 1960s especially for small businesses. This legal form of organization allows the corporation to distribute earnings among its shareholder owners, with each shareholder paying personal income tax on his or her distribution of those earnings. At the same time, such small firms are given the advantages of limited liability, perpetual life, ease of transferring ownership, and expansion. S-corporations can have a maximum of 35 stockholders held in a domestic corporation that is separate from any holding company or affiliated group of corporations and has only one class of stock.

Advantages of an S-Corporation

- Lower income taxes—paid at personal rates rather than corporate.
- Exemption from corporate alternative minimum tax.
- Flexibility in accounting methods.

Disadvantages of an S-Corporation

- Becomes unwieldy when operating in several states.
- Capital loans are more difficult than in regular corporation.
- Rigid restrictions in some states.

Selecting the Right Business Format

Before you select a business format, you need to answer a series of questions. The answers will help you decide which format is best suited for you. Be sure to seek competent legal counsel when deliberating this issue. The following is a partial list of questions your attorney should address.

1. How big is the risk? What is the amount of the investor's liability for debts and taxes?
2. How important is the continuity of the firm? What if something happens to you or one of the other principals?
3. What legal structure insures the greatest adaptability in running the business?
4. What are the influences of applicable laws on the business?
5. What are the possibilities of additional income for the business? What about more capital?
6. What are the needs or the possibilities of attracting additional management expertise?
7. What are the costs and procedures involved in starting the proposed business?
8. What is the ultimate goal and purpose of the business, and what format is best to achieve this goal?
9. How much control of the business does each owner, partner, or investor wish to have in the long run?

The answers to these questions will provide guidance in evaluating the advantages and

Table 3.3   Summary of Business Formats

	Proprietorship	Partnership	Corporation	S-corporation
Risk	Unlimited	Share of total	Investment	Investment and loans
Continuity	Lifetime	Lifetime of one partner	Unlimited	Unlimited
Adaptability	High	Moderate	Low	Moderate
Legal requirements	Low	Moderate	High	Moderate
Capital	Owner only	Loans from partners	Sell stock or bonds	Sell stock
Staffing	Poor	Poor	Good	Fair
Cost to establish	Low	Moderate	High	Moderate
Control	High	Moderate	Depends on amount of stock	Moderate

disadvantages of the different legal formats discussed. These questions will help you focus your attention on the important aspects of running your new health fitness business. To help remind you of the advantages and disadvantages of each business format, refer to table 3.3.

Historically, the health fitness industry was dominated by sole proprietorship business formats. Approximately 80 to 90 percent of the businesses were run as single clubs with one owner. Today, the health fitness industry is becoming dominated by corporate business formats in the form of conglomerates, franchisors, or management entities. Approximately 80 to 90 percent of the health fitness businesses are now being run by a corporation either owning, franchising, or managing facilities nationwide. Yet, there are a large number of contractors providing individual services that remain important but are not counted in our industry statistics. This trend is likely to continue.

Corporate Setting

Patton et al. (1986, 1989) have developed a model for corporate health fitness program implementation.

The Association for Fitness in Business (AFB) published *Guidelines for Employee Health Promotion Programs* (1992), which serves as a definitive reference for organizing and implementing programs in the corporate setting. Regardless of the model used during conceptual development, there are some necessary steps to take.

A consultant is usually hired to facilitate concept development for corporate fitness programs and to assist the *champion* spearheading the project within the corporation. This champion is often an influential employee located within the management level who has prodded decision makers into action. This manager-champion has often been instrumental in getting the project started and gaining approval to develop or at least to explore developing a health promotion program. During the initial planning stages, it becomes critical that management support is obtained. Regardless of the nature and amount of planning that is undertaken by consultants and committees, the effort is fruitless without the support of upper management. Upper management must be involved in setting at least the broad parameters of the mission, the tangible and intangible objectives, and focus of the program (i.e., medical versus recreational).

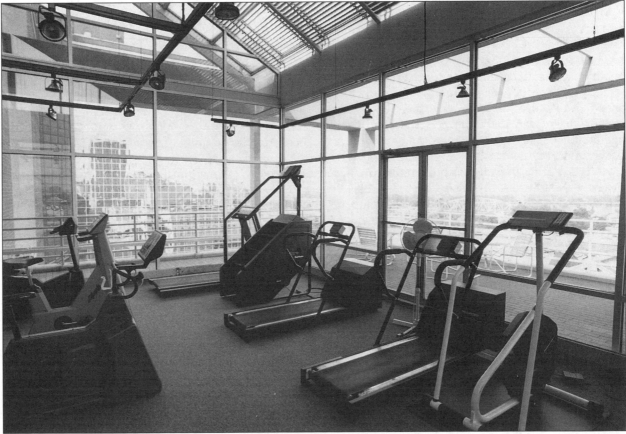

© Tom Wallace

> *Upper management must determine the objectives of the corporate health fitness program, either tangible such as reduced absenteeism and reduced health care costs or intangible such as improved employee morale.*

Once the level and nature of support from upper management is determined, it is important to identify the perceived needs of midmanagement and employees. This needs analysis can be accomplished in several ways, but usually takes the form of a questionnaire or interview. Samples of these instruments are included in chapter 8 and in the AFB's *Guidelines for Employee Health Promotion Programs.* These data collections and analyses can be performed by a committee created to chart the course of the employee health promotion program. The committee should include individuals from human resources, medical, marketing, and other departments and be supplemented by health fitness consultants. It is important to have employees and middle and upper management represented on this committee, and it is essential to have the champion for the cause on this committee. Once upper management input is received and the needs analysis is completed, you can begin the concept development for the program.

During concept development, the program takes shape and is customized to meet the needs of the organization. Early in this process, the upper management needs to develop a mission, purpose, and preliminary budget for the program. They should establish specific and measurable goals to gauge program progress. A program director is usually hired during this planning process. Program planning becomes more definitive as decisions are made regarding types of facilities, programs, staff, budgets, and other factors needed to fulfill the mission and objectives of the program. At this point, the committee is usually weaned from operationalizing the concept development and takes on an advisory role to the program director. The committee remains important because of the access to and input from all levels and types of individuals within the company. The consultant is also weaned from the program once a program director feels comfortable in administration and implementation.

An alternative solution to program development is to hire a management company or form a joint venture with some organization such as a hospital to do a turnkey implementation. Hiring the management and operations staff of your corporate health fitness program is analogous to a franchise in the commercial setting and has many of the same advantages and disadvantages.

In the final analysis, during the concept development process, a corporate health fitness program needs to achieve a minimum set of quality standards. The following is a list of quality standards provided by the Association for Worksite Health Promotion, formerly known as the AFB (1992):

1. Commitment from senior management to dedicate sufficient resources—funding, personnel time, equipment, and facilities. Ideally, management also shows support by participating in the program.

2. A clear statement of philosophy, purpose, and goals that declare the organization's commitment to motivate and assist a significant proportion of employees to practice healthier lifestyles.

3. A process of assessing organizational and individual needs, risks, and costs.

4. Leadership from well-qualified health fitness professionals in the program's design, implementation, and ongoing operations.

5. A program design that addresses the most significant health risks to our nation, specific risks within the employee population, and needs of the organization.

6. High-quality and convenient programs that motivate participants to achieve lasting behavior changes.

7. Effective marketing to achieve and maintain high participation rates.

8. Efficient systems for program operation and administration.

9. Procedures for evaluating program quality and outcomes.

10. A system for communicating the program results to employees, staff, and senior management.

Clinical Setting

Historically, the clinical health fitness centers followed the facility and program development model of commercial centers. They looked and functioned much like the commercial programs. The early concept behind a clinically-based fitness center was to serve in a community outreach capacity to increase the hospital's market share of traditional medical services. There was no urgency to make great profits, especially in nonprofit hospitals. The potential to impress the community with broad spectrum health care and access to quality health care regardless of need was most important. Some early programs extended beyond community fitness services to include outpatient cardiac rehabilitation, physical therapy, and hospital employee wellness programming. Single-purpose programs used the commercial model for concept development. However, the multipurpose programs used a complex multimodal concept development model. Each aspect of the program took on a separate dimension, often managed by different people answering to various department heads. Reporting relationships for hospital health fitness directors could conceivably include management from clinical services, marketing, outpatient services, or some executive manager such as the *CEO*. Bear in mind, these organizations are extremely varied, and the health fitness programs are equally varied, depending on the primary purpose for their existence.

Today it is different. The economics of the health care industry are rapidly changing. For the first time, hospitals have a financial incentive to keep their clientele healthy and fit. Under traditional health care, providers are paid a fee for each service performed. The more services performed, especially expensive services, the more reimbursement received. Under this system, there is no significant financial incentive for hospitals to promote health fitness programs that focus primarily on preventive care. The only exception would be programs that serve to attract more patients for traditional reimbursable services. Until the mid-1990s, this traditional fee-for-service model dominated as the form of health care delivery. Because fitness services were not a billable service to insurance companies, the hospital-based fitness services took on a commercial model in which community citizens became members in a hospital health fitness enterprise.

Health care is moving away from the traditional approach and rapidly moving toward more managed care, capitation, and risk sharing. In the mid-1990s managed care began to dominate as a form of health care delivery. In a managed care environment, hospitals may accept the financial risk of caring for a group of people for a fixed, or *capitated*, fee, creating an environment in which a hospital's fiscal fitness depends in large part on the physical fitness and health status of its patients. This new interest in patient wellness has significant financial rewards for managed care and bodes well for the health fitness industry. There are movements to create joint venture relationships between health fitness companies and health care companies in an effort to reduce costs. Managed care companies are now hiring health fitness professionals to orchestrate preventive managed care services. How this will eventually manifest in terms of organizational structure is yet to be determined. We will discuss hospital-based and health care–based issues in greater detail in the final chapter of the book.

Community Setting

There are many health fitness agencies in the community setting. The public parks and recreation agencies provide health fitness services in many community recreation centers across the country. There are many nonprofit organizations offering health fitness services, including such groups as the Boys' Clubs and Girls' Clubs. Many religious groups offer health and fitness programs. Jewish Community Centers are extremely active in this regard. However, the Y system, which includes YMCA and YWCA, is without question the largest community agency dealing with health fitness services in America. There are over 2,000 YMCA programs in the country, serving approximately 14 million members of all ages, both sexes, and without regard to religious persuasion.

The concept development process of community agencies is predetermined. The missions and program developments for YMCA programs, for example, have been extensively developed over the past 150 years in this country. There is little one need do beyond seeking help at a higher level within the Y system in order to start a new program. The same would be true to a lesser extent with many other community agencies, such as parks and recreation departments and schools.

ORGANIZATIONAL PATTERNS

Througout this chapter we have elaborated on how the programs are developed. The concept development process has been discussed for each health fitness industry setting. Regardless of the setting, as each program evolved, an organizational structure developed to reflect the hierarchy of authority and facilitate management functions. These structures are illustrated by several organizational charts (see figures 3.2 through 3.6) representing stereotypical organizational patterns in various health fitness settings. The settings are unique and inherently take on different organizational patterns; however, they are also influenced by fundamental concepts such as levels of authority, division of labor and departmentalization, span of control, and delegation of responsibility.

Levels of Authority

In the health fitness industry, three levels of authority have been customary: the *general manager* or executive director, the supervisory or middle-management level, and the health fitness instructor or direct service staff person. The lower-level health fitness instructors report to middle managers who in turn report to upper managers. However, in many larger organizations this represents an extreme oversimplification of the hierarchy of authority. In a large commercial health fitness company, for example, major influence would be wielded by a board of directors, headed by a chief executive officer. Reporting directly to the board of directors are several individuals who comprise the top management of the organization and whose primary function is to develop corporate plans and make

major policy decisions. Below the top management level are middle-management individuals who may be known as department or division heads, supervisors, or project managers. Their task is to implement the policy and plans established by top management; they do this by developing intermediate plans and maintaining control over aspects of company performance such as sales figures. Below middle management are first-level managers, such as the program managers responsible for implementing programs and maintaining facilities. These managers are responsible for developing and implementing short-range operating plans and day-to-day programming and marketing activities. Some clinical and community settings may follow similar patterns.

Division of Labor and Departmentalization

Traditional management theory stresses the need to divide work into a number of sharply defined, specialized tasks to ensure that each employee knows precisely what he or she must accomplish and to standardize work methods. Thus, with any organization, people are typically assigned to certain roles, such as front service desk receptionists, locker-room cleaning attendants, or program specialists such as aerobics coordinator.

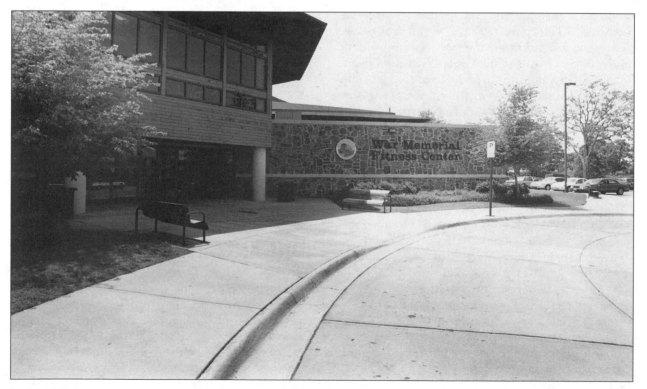

© Tom Wallace

Departmentalization consists of identifying and using the major functional areas within an organization as a basis for grouping jobs and determining the lines of managerial control and communication. In the health fitness industry, the most common manner of assignment is according to a given area of responsibility within the program. Examples of this compartmentalization would be the designation of aerobics coordinators, aquatics coordinators, special events coordinators, and sales coordinators, to mention a few. The delineation of subunits within an organizational chart is largely determined by the number of people supervised or the amount of work associated with the assigned tasks.

Span of Control

Span of control is concerned with the height and width of the organizational structures and the number of subordinate employees a supervisor or manager is expected to supervise. For example, in a wide span of control, there are few horizontal layers, and each manager supervises a large number of subordinate employees. In a narrow span of control, there are more horizontal layers of employees, and each supervisor is responsible for overseeing a smaller number of subordinates. In general, a wide span of control is appropriate for an organization in which work is clearly defined and systematized, and the work force is relatively homogeneous. A narrow span of control is more useful when the work tasks vary greatly, requiring flexibility in job performance, and when the work force is likely to be more heterogeneous. For example, if the aerobics and aquatics programs are small with only one or two instructors in each area, these program areas might be combined with other fitness services and be supervised by one fitness program manager. On the other hand, a large program with six part-time aerobics instructors might warrant designation of an aerobics coordinator dedicated to manage the aerobics program. In contrast, more regimented tasks, such as maintenance and janitorial services, may have 1 manager supervising 10 individuals.

> *Generally, in the health fitness industry it is thought that one person can supervise approximately five to seven people for a given set of related tasks.*

Delegation of Authority

Delegation of authority is concerned with the extent to which individuals are permitted to make their own decisions without having to seek approval of managers on a higher level. An organization that favors delegation of authority is generally thought of as *decentralized*; an organization that favors control over subordinates is generally thought of as *centralized*. In a decentralized organization, managers are encouraged to assume problem-solving responsibilities and develop their creativity and ingenuity. In a sense, this approach requires managers to develop broad rather than highly specialized skills, because they often are called on to deal with a wide range of problems that are not covered by program policies. In a centralized organization managers are not encouraged to assume problem-solving responsibilities. This approach does not require managers to develop broad ranges of skills, because they are not frequently called on to deal with a wide range of problems.

Generally, in the health fitness industry there is a decentralized organizational approach to management. Managers are authorized to provide a wide range of programs and activities to meet or even exceed the service expectations of their memberships. Even direct service providers, such as front desk or locker-room personnel, are given wide latitudes when it comes to providing membership services. Some environments embrace a centralized authority in which upper managers tend to *micromanage* the problems within the organization. This approach requires strict adherence to well-established policies and standards.

> *Franchise and corporate health fitness environments tend to be more centralized than sole proprietorships regarding delegation of authority.*

ORGANIZATONAL STRUCTURE

The organizational structures found in the health fitness industry are extremely variable. Although there are tendencies to have common organizational patterns within a given setting, most organizations are unique in some respects.

Many factors define the managerial style of an organizational structure. Figure 3.1 shows how organizations might fall along a continuum ranging from highly formal and structured on the left to informal and unstructured on the right. As we can see from this graphic, organizational structures will tend toward one extreme or the other along each continuum. Organizations tending toward the left are characterized as structured, bureaucratic, mechanistic, and are thought to stifle managerial creativity. Organizations tending toward the right are characterized as unstructured, nonbureaucratic, organic, and are perceived as promoting managerial creativity.

The structure of the organization determines the nature of operating units, the administrative hierarchy, reporting relationships, and formal lines of communication. An example of the health fitness program that would be highly structured and centralized would be one located on a military base in which the program director would be supervised by military personnel and operate within the guidelines advanced by military doctrine. An example of a highly unstructured and decentralized health fitness program is a university faculty fitness program in which the program director would be supervised by an academic administrator and operate within the guidelines of the university environment.

Health fitness professionals must know how the organizational structure affects them and how to derive maximum benefit from their position in the hierarchy. Where you fit in the organizational chart determines the formal communication channels and influences the power you have within the organization. In a formal system, your communication is primarily limited to your immediate supervisor. Bypassing lines of communication by going over the head of an immediate supervisor invariably creates difficulties for all concerned.

Power and Authority

Power and authority differ in that *power* is defined as influence outside the organizational unit whereas *authority* is defined as influence from within. In any case, people with power or authority have a major impact on the organization in terms of communication, job satisfaction, and the quality of interpersonal relationships. More specifically, power increases the probability that the will of an individual will be carried out despite resistance. A midmanager, for example, who is a family member of the owner of the health fitness organization will probably wield more power within the organization than most of his midmanager colleagues. Formal authority is the right to provide positive or negative input related to the behavior of others, such as promoting, demoting, hiring, firing, rewarding, and punishing (Wilson and Glaros 1994).

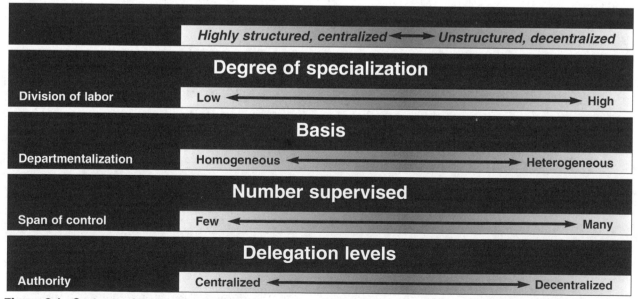

Figure 3.1 Contrasts of organizational structures.

Adapted, by permission, from R.G. Krause and J.E. Curtis, 1986, *Creative management in recreation, parks, and leisure services* (St. Louis: Times Mirror/Mosby), 69.

Line and Staff

In any organizational structure, positions can be placed in one of two categories. *Line positions* refer to functions that are directly involved with the health fitness program delivery or service provided. *Staff positions* refer to units that are service, supportive, or auxiliary in nature (Wilson and Glaros 1994). Depending on the organization, health fitness work assignments can be line or staff positions. The front office executive assistant or the night cleaning employee, for example, may be classified as a staff position. The aerobics instructor or the fitness director may be classified as a line position. Typically, the line positions are occupied by professionally educated and trained health fitness professionals. Staff employees may or may not be professionally educated or trained for their duties. Under normal circumstances, it is unimportant whether a position is line or staff. However, during the cyclical nature of business and fluctuations in the economy, if downsizing becomes inevitable, staff positions are usually the first to be eliminated. This probably is due to the less direct impact on members. When business is good and positions are eliminated it is usually a staff person. For example, when membership has reached a set cap and there is a waiting list to join the club, it is common to reduce sales staff. When business is bad the line positions tend to be eliminated. For example, when

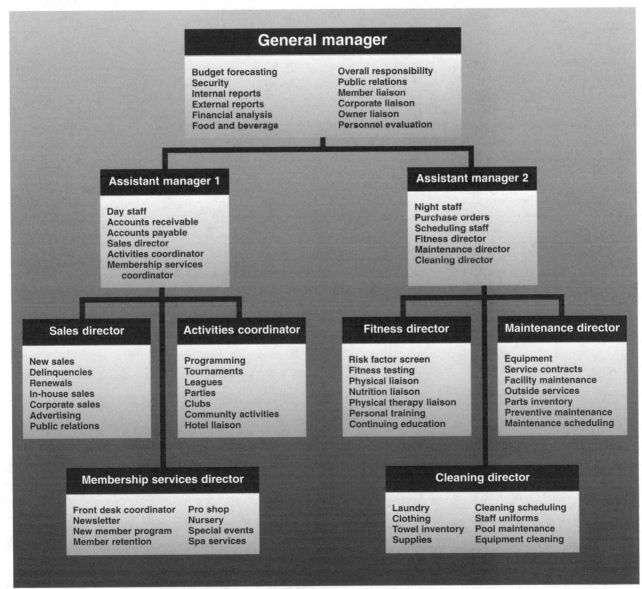

Figure 3.2   **Commercial health fitness program organizational chart.**
Adapted, with permission, from communication with Dan Lynch 1990.

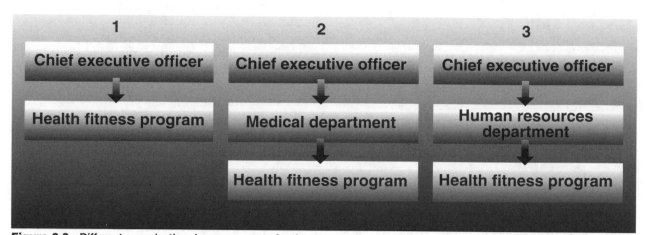

Figure 3.3 Different organizational arrangements for the corporate setting. Copyright 1997 by Cardinal Business Media.

membership is down, management can justify reducing the fitness instructor staff on the basis that fewer members are in the facility to use their services.

All people in the organization need to understand the role everyone plays in meeting its mission. It is important that they understand that an organization is likely to respond to changes in the marketplace, technology, and other influences. Evaluating your potential for promotion within the organization will always require understanding the organizational structure and the dynamics of the organization, and constantly preparing for your next career move.

ORGANIZATIONAL CHARTS

The organizational chart of an organization can illustrate the functional and communication patterns within the business. An organizational chart will only illustrate formal lines of communication and functional groupings. Informal relationships cannot be illustrated. Also, some formal reporting

relationships may not be shown on an organizational chart. For example, during an extended absence of an assistant manager, the sales director might report directly to the general manager. Despite these shortcomings, organizational charts are useful.

You can base organizational charts on different criteria. Most organizational charts in the health fitness industry are functional organizational charts. This type of chart depicts the nature of the tasks performed and the reporting channels involved. The organizational chart illustrated for the commercial setting shows both the functional tasks and reporting channels. Although you can use other criteria to develop organizational charts (geographic regions, projects undertaken, and grid associations), the functional portrayal of a health fitness business or program is most common.

Commercial Setting

To illustrate a typical organizational chart in the commercial setting we will use a full-service opera-

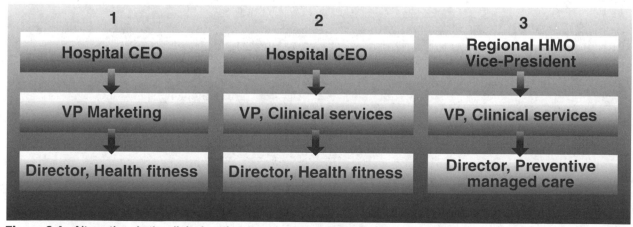

Figure 3.4 Alternatives in the clinical setting organizational chart.

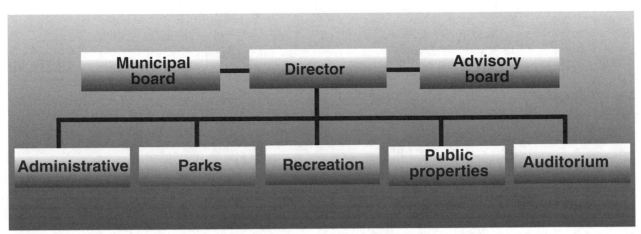

Figure 3.5   Community parks and recreation program organizational chart.

tion with 25,000 square feet, 3,000 members, 10 full-time staff and 40 part-time staff (see figure 3.2). In this case, there is a general manager with two assistant managers. One assistant manager would probably open the club; the other assistant manager would probably close at night. Their duties reflect their work hours; however, most general managers will cross train their midmanagers to have adequate supervision during contingency periods such as holidays, illnesses, and position vacancies.

Corporate Setting

In the corporate setting, the health fitness program is usually organized under the supervision of human resources or medical departments, but occasionally it is located directly below the chief executive officer. This, of course, is ideal because of the elimination of bureaucratic layers between the program and decision making (see figure 3.3).

Clinical Setting

The clinical setting is in a state of flux regarding health fitness organizational patterns. Historically, the health fitness services were organized as an entity within the marketing department or a clinical services department. In the former case, the program was viewed as a marketing arm of the hospital. In the latter, it was viewed as an extension of clinical services. As discussed earlier, the trend is toward health care services being offered in a managed care context, and the health fitness services are being viewed as preventive managed care services. Figure 3.4 illustrates these patterns.

Community Setting

There are a host of different organizations in the community setting. The local parks and recreation department is a good example of a community organization. Figure 3.5 illustrates such an orga-

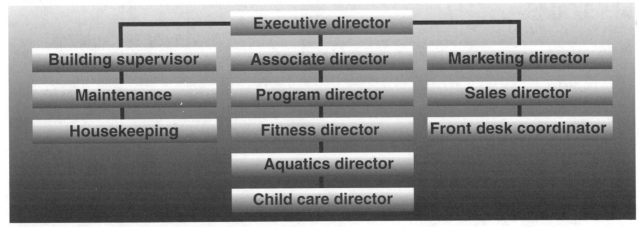

Figure 3.6   Community branch YMCA organizational chart.

nizational chart. The YMCA is also a good example of a community organization. Figure 3.6 provides an example of a Y's organizational chart.

IN CLOSING

In this chapter we introduced the process of concept development of an organization. Although the process of concept development has some generic applications, such as determining goals before building facilities or developing programs, each setting is unique. The commercial setting, for example, has profit as a fundamental goal of the business; therefore, the planning for financial aspects of the enterprise is emphasized. The corporate setting requires the support of upper management as an essential first step in the concept development. Without clear understanding of the needs and interests of upper management the corporate programs cannot proceed. The clinical and community settings also have unique features in their concept development process.

Some organizations are bureaucratic and structured, and others are less structured and organic. The organizational chart that evolves from initial planning is somewhat determined by the degree to which decision making is centralized or decentralized. It is also influenced by such factors as line of authority and span of control. The lines and staff of the organizational chart that takes shape are an effort to create optimal communication and reporting channels for individuals within the organization. Sometimes informal communications with individuals with power will yield results as much as formal communications with immediate supervisors. However, one must never undermine the formal lines of communication.

KEY TERMS

Authority
Business plan
Capitalized fee
C-corporation
Centralized
CEO
Champion
Concept development process
Contingency capital
Corporations
Decentralized

Delegation of authority
Doing business as (dba)
Dormant partners
Franchise
General manager
General partnerships
Joint ventures
Limited partnerships
Line positions
Micromanage
Nominal partners
Operating capital
Partnership
Partnership agreement
Power
S-corporation
Secret partners
Silent partners
Sole proprietor
Staff positions
Start-up funds
Venture capital

RECOMMENDED READINGS

Anderson, R.L., and J.S. Dunkelberg. 1993. *Managing small businesses*. St. Paul: West.

Association for Fitness in Business. 1992. *Guidelines for employee health promotion programs*. Champaign, IL: Human Kinetics.

Ellis, T., and R.L. Norton. 1988. *Commercial recreation*. St. Louis: Times Mirror/Mosby College.

International Health, Racquet and Sportsclub Association. 1996. *Profiles of success*. Boston: IHRSA.

Kraus, R.G., and J.E. Curtis. 1986. *Creative management*. St. Louis: Times Mirror/Mosby College.

Markarian, M. 1993. How does your club compare to the typical club? *Club Industry* (February): 23-29.

Parkhouse, B.L. 1991. *The management of sport*. St. Louis: Mosby Year Book.

Patton, R.W., J.M. Corry, L.R. Gettman, and J.S. Graf. 1986. *Implementing health/fitness programs*. Champaign, IL: Human Kinetics.

Patton, R.W., W.C. Grantham, R.F. Gerson, and L.R. Gettman. 1989. *Developing and managing health fitness facilities*. Champaign, IL: Human Kinetics.

Steinhoff, D., and J.F. Burgess. 1993. *Small business management fundamentals*. 6th ed., New York: McGraw-Hill.

Wilson, B.R.A., and T.E. Glaros. 1994. *Managing health promotion programs*. Champaign, IL: Human Kinetics.

CHAPTER 4

Management and Managers

Simply stated, management is a set of activities directed at the efficient and effective use of resources in the pursuit of an organization's goals. Frederick Taylor, known as the father of scientific management, defined management as "knowing exactly what you want [people] to do, and then seeing that they do it in the best and cheapest way." Although easy to define in the abstract, effective management is difficult to achieve because it involves a complex mix of activities that change frequently.

Health fitness operations and early management practices date back several thousand years. When Socrates and Plato ruminated on theories of management and job specialization, it is likely they did so while sitting in the spa or watching young philosophers work out in the gymnasium. Management and the field of fitness remained out of the main focus of research and publication until recent years, when health fitness operations began to evolve from small mom and pop businesses to complex facilities managed by multimillion dollar corporations.

The challenges facing modern health fitness professionals have expanded greatly. The successful health fitness manager needs experience and training in the fundamental business practice areas of management, personnel, finance, marketing, and operations. This chapter reviews issues related to managerial responsibility, knowledge, and skill. The chapter begins with a brief review of the basic management models used to define the overall scope of managerial responsibilities. Next, it presents an integrative analysis synthesizing the different managerial schools of thought. Using the *I-formation management model*, we explore the different roles health fitness managers play. The chapter presents essential skills and knowledge that every health fitness manager needs to successfully perform managerial roles. It concludes by reviewing how health fitness managers develop managerial skills and acquire managerial knowledge.

STANDING ON THE SHOULDERS OF GIANTS

Throughout this book, we discuss leading edge approaches to health fitness management. How-ever, these ideas did not develop in a vacuum. They emerged from the theory and history of management pioneers. To paraphrase Sir Isaac Newton, we have the opportunity to see farther because we stand on the shoulders of giants. By understanding historical viewpoints, modern managers not only can learn valuable lessons, but also can avoid repeating the mistakes of the past. The theories serve as a framework for understanding contemporary management and developing individual management practice skills.

We begin by establishing the historical context of management practices and identifying early management theorists of the 1800s before discussing the major management viewpoints: classical, behavioral, quantitative, and contemporary (see figure 4.1). We then review the traditional manager functions and responsibilities that are required for successful health fitness management.

Early management concepts and techniques were integral to the accomplishments of ancient civilizations. The construction of the great pyramids of Egypt, the massive military operations of Alexander the Great, and the complex road and water systems of early Greece and Rome could not have been completed without sophisticated management prac-

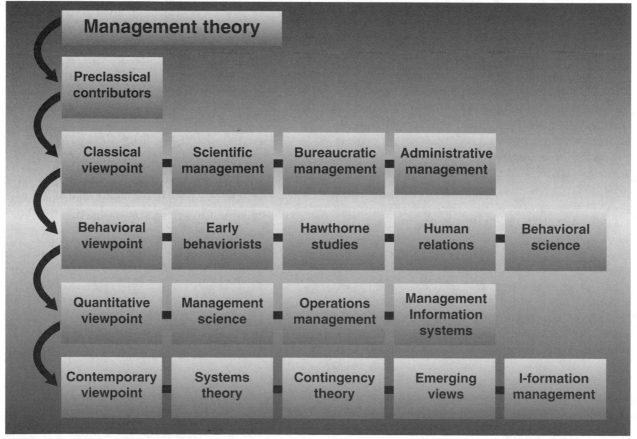

Figure 4.1 Major management viewpoints.

tices. Civil engineering projects of the ancient Babylonians, Chinese, and Venetians all applied principles of good management to solve complex problems. Socrates discussed management concepts as early as 400 B.C. and Plato outlined the theory of job specialization in 350 B.C. Yet, management as an area of formal study did not emerge until the industrial revolution during the 1800s. Before this time businesses were generally run as small family operations. Similar to many modern health fitness organizations, most operated at a subsistence level with little planning for growth or profit. The large organizations involved in commerce were either governmental or military, with vast financial, material, and human resources. These organizations had little need to concentrate on issues related to efficiency, waste, motivation, or profit.

The creation and growth of factories during the industrial revolution of the 1800s required coordination and supervision of large groups of workers performing a variety of jobs. During this period, a number of individuals—including Robert Owen, Charles Babbage, and Henry Towne—experimented with innovative approaches to factory operations. A review of their early management concepts is useful not only for historical reference but also to illustrate how many of their ideas remain applicable to modern health fitness managers.

Robert Owen (1771-1858), a British industrialist and reformer, was considered a radical for his efforts to improve the living conditions of employees, including upgrading streets, houses, sanitation, and education. He argued that improving the quality of life of workers increased productivity by 50 to 100 percent. Owen's efforts and views are considered the forerunner of modern human resources and employee welfare theories. Placed in a modern context, Robert Owen's understanding of the impact that overall quality of life had on work productivity is the same theory that supports modern employee health and wellness initiatives and work-site health promotion programs.

> *Early management theory recognized the important and influential tie between overall quality of life and worker job performance.*

Charles Babbage (1792-1871), an English mathematician, applied a practical, analytical approach to the areas of production efficiency and work specialization. His book, *On the Economy of Machinery and Manufactures* (1832), outlined and defended the concept that physical and mental work could be accomplished more efficiently if allocated to specialists. Babbage also devised a profit-sharing plan based on a combination of overall factory profits and recognition of individual suggestions that proved useful.

> *The management theory of work specialization is widely practiced in the health fitness industry where specialists are hired to teach aquatics, aerobics, personal training, and other programs requiring advanced knowledge, skills, and abilities.*

Henry Towne (1844-1924), a mechanical engineer and president of Yale and Towne Manufacturing Company, is best known for his landmark paper *The Engineer as an Economist* (1886), in which he articulated the need to consider management as a separate field of study. Towne called for the establishment of a science of management and the development of principles that could be applied across all types of management situations. In the health fitness industry it is common to see entry-level professionals trained as exercise physiologists, who apply scientific principles to testing and prescribing exercise, moving up the organizational ladder by applying problem-solving techniques in the management and operations of programs.

These three pioneers set the stage for the development of management as a separate field of study. Although many early ideas focused on solving specific problems rather than developing basic theory, it is impressive to note that many of their forward-thinking ideas continue to influence modern management theory.

CLASSICAL MANAGEMENT THEORIES

The next phase of evolution for management theory involved the development of the classical viewpoint. The perspective of the *classical viewpoint* emphasizes identifying and documenting methods to manage work and organizations more effectively. Three approaches are included in the classical viewpoint: *scientific management*, *administrative management*, and *bureaucratic management*.

Scientific Management

Scientific management emphasizes the scientific study of work methods to improve worker efficiency. The major contributors to this approach include Frederick Winslow Taylor, Frank and Lillian Gilbreth, and Henry Gantt.

Frederick Winslow Taylor (1856-1915), recognized as the father of scientific management, observed workers in his steel factories operating at less than full capacity. Taylor believed that workers gave less than full effort for three primary reasons:

- They were afraid that greater productivity would mean fewer jobs.
- They were paid in a manner that encouraged slow work.
- They were required to use work procedures that were inefficient.

> *Workers are less productive if there is a fear that increased productivity will create the need for fewer jobs, if wage and salary systems encourage or reward slow pace, and if inefficient work procedures are perpetuated over a long time.*

Taylor developed four principles of scientific management to resolve the problem.

1. Develop a science for each element of the job.
2. Scientifically select, train, and develop the worker.
3. Supervise the workers to ensure that they are using scientific methods.
4. Make management responsible for planning and the worker responsible for execution.

Taylor advocated using wage incentive plans that paid workers from 30 to 100 percent higher wages

Activity	Month 1																														Month 2												
---	1	2	3	4	5	6	7	8	9	10	11	12	13	14	15	16	17	18	19	20	21	22	23	24	25	26	27	28	29	1	2	3	4	5	6	7	8	9	10	11	12	13
Select and confirm planning committee	X	X	X	X	X																																					
Schedule weekly planning meeting					X																																					
Hold weekly planning meeting								X							X							X									X							X				X
Select preliminary date options								X																																		
Complete preliminary budget															X																											
Check with city to clear date options									X																																	
Prepare and submit permits										X	X	X	X	X	X	X	X	X																								
Prepare sponsor packets																		X	X	X	X	X	X	X																		
Distribute sponsor packets																					X	X	X	X	X	X	X	X														
Complete sponsor solicitation																									X																	
Collect all sponsor logos																																	X									
Create event logo																									X																	
Design brochure																									X																	
Design shirts																									X																	
Approve designs																											X															
Order brochures																																	X									
Order shirts																																	X									
Order race numbers																																	X									
Mail brochures																																										X

Figure 4.2   Sample Gantt chart.

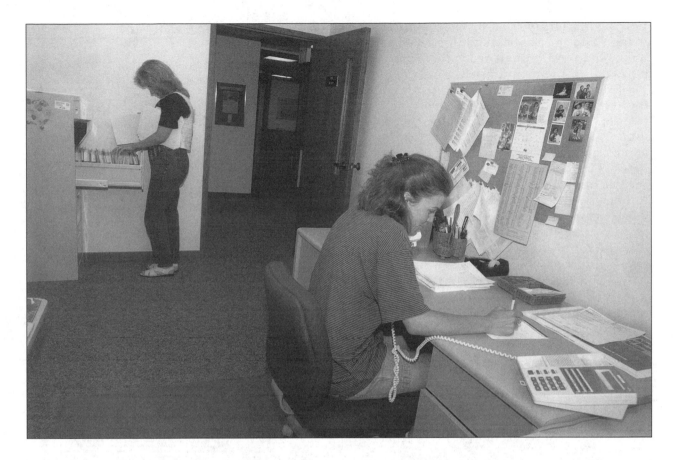

for using the scientifically developed work plans and meeting daily standards. He also implemented *time and motion studies* to break down the work task into individual elements, eliminate unnecessary motions, determine the most efficient way to do each task, and time each motion to determine the amount of production expected per day.

Although his original studies are more than 100 years old, Taylor's approach for increasing efficiency remains applicable in a modern health fitness setting to evaluate the proper location for storing equipment, supplies, and information. For example, health fitness managers should study the use and location of towels in their facility. Are the current towel storage and collection locations established to minimize the number of times a towel has to be moved by staff? Are the towel sites placed in the expected travel path of members at points where the towel is used or discarded? Will placement impact the number of towels used by members or improve security to minimize towel theft? You can answer these and similar questions by conducting basic time and motion studies that measure how long and how many steps each activity takes, then eliminate unnecessary steps. Health fitness managers can apply scientific management principles to evaluate all major activities within the health fitness setting.

Henry Gantt (1861-1919), a contemporary and close associate of Taylor, is best remembered for developing the *Gantt chart*, a graphic aid to planning, scheduling, and control. Modern organizations still use Gantt charts to schedule work flow over time and to identify the sequencing of work tasks. Consider in figure 4.2 the first page of a Gantt chart tracking the activities related to organizing a fun run.

Although he is best known for his scheduling systems, Gantt also devised a unique system that paid workers based on reaching defined standards in allotted time and paid bonuses to supervisors of successful workers. Gantt's system was one of the first to encourage supervisors to coach and train workers to improve performance. Gantt's planning and employee pay concepts continue to be excellent tools for health fitness managers.

Frank (1868-1924) and Lillian (1878-1972) Gilbreth, a husband and wife team of industrial engineers, were also noted contributors to the field of scientific management. Using bricklaying as his research environment, Frank Gilbreth proved that job efficiency could be improved by almost two hundred percent by implementing changes determined by time and motion studies.

Lillian Gilbreth focused on the welfare of the worker and the application of scientific methods to help individuals reach their maximum potential. Lillian's published doctoral thesis, *The Psychology of Management* (1914), is one of the first applications of psychology to the workplace. Lillian Gilbreth contributed to the definition of scientific management by focusing on and refining the concepts of analysis and synthesis. First, analysis breaks down a task into the essential parts. Second, through synthesis, the task is reconstituted to include only the most essential elements. Applying state-of-the-art technology to study efficiency, the Gilbreths pioneered the use of motion pictures to study job tasks.

How can health fitness managers apply the scientific management approach to managing a modern health fitness organization? Using the scientific management approach, managers should break down each major operational aspect of the organization into detailed lists of specific tasks. Then assign each task to specific individuals throughout the organization with checklists and timetables to track completion.

Bureaucratic Management

The bureaucratic management approach emphasizes operating in a rational manner with a system of rules and guidelines based on technical competence. Max Weber (1864-1920), consultant, professor, and author, was the first to describe the concept of bureaucracy as it applies to management. Weber formulated the characteristics of an ideal organization, operated on a purely rational basis, without regard to individual personality or personal considerations. In his model, the ideal bureaucracy has

- the division of labor clearly defined;
- one consistent set of rules for all workers;
- a clear chain of command and communication;
- a businesslike, impersonal manner;
- advancement based solely on experience and performance; and
- careful record keeping for organizational learning.

Weber coined the term bureaucracy from the German word *büro*, meaning "office." The health fitness

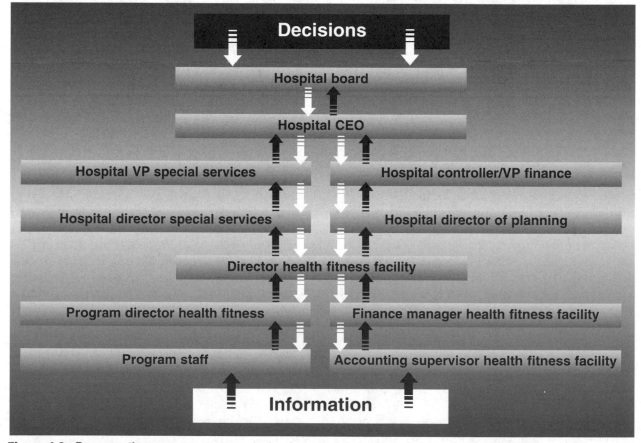

Figure 4.3   Bureaucratic management approach showing a decision path for large budget expenditures.

setting most likely to encompass a bureaucratic management approach is a large hospital-based facility with many layers of departments and supervisors (see figure 4.3). Although bureaucratic management systems have fallen out of favor because of their impersonal and inflexible reputation, modern health fitness managers should still consider the important efficiency gains that a well-designed bureaucracy achieves.

Administrative Management

Administrative management theory is based on a set of principles that coordinate the internal activities of organizations. Two major contributors to administrative management theory are Henri Fayol and Chester Barnard.

Henri Fayol (1841-1925), a French industrialist, believed that universal theories of management should be developed that could be taught to all individuals with administrative responsibilities. By isolating the main types of activities involved in industry, Fayol developed a functional definition of management that remains in widespread use today.

Fayol's definition of managerial activities is divided into five primary functions: planning, organizing, commanding, coordinating, and controlling.

Fayol also developed 14 general management guidelines that he believed to be universally valid, and if followed, would always enhance managerial effectiveness.

Fayol's General Principles of Management

1. *Division of work.* Work specialization can result in efficiencies and is applicable to both management and technical functions.

2. *Authority.* Authority is the right to give orders and the power to exact obedience. It derives from the formal authority of the office and from personal authority based on factors such as intelligence and experience. With authority comes responsibility.

3. *Discipline.* Discipline is absolutely necessary for the smooth running of an organization, but the state of discipline depends essentially on the worthiness of the leaders.

4. *Unity of command.* An employee should receive orders from one superior only.

5. *Unity of direction.* Activities aimed at the same objective should be organized so that there is one plan and one person in charge.

6. *Subordination of individual interest to general interest.* The interests of one employee or group should not prevail over the interests and goals of the organization.

7. *Remuneration.* Compensation should be fair to both the employee and the employer.

8. *Centralization.* The proper amount of centralization or decentralization depends on the situation. The objective is the optimum use of personnel capabilities.

9. *Scalar chain.* A scalar (hierarchical) chain of authority extends from the top to the bottom of an organization and defines the communication path. Horizontal communication is also encouraged as long as the managers in the chain of authority are kept informed.

10. *Order.* Materials should be kept in well-chosen places that facilitate activities. Similarly, due to proper organization and selection, the right person should be in the right place.

11. *Equity.* Employees should be treated with kindness and justice.

12. *Stability of personnel tenure.* High turnover should be prevented because employees require time and expense to become effective in new jobs.

13. *Initiative.* Managers should encourage and develop subordinate initiative to the fullest.

14. *Esprit de corps.* Because union produces strength, harmony and teamwork are essential.

Chester Barnard (1886-1961), president of New Jersey Bell Telephone Company, published one of the classic administrative management books, *The Functions of the Executive* (1938), in which he presented his theory that authority does not depend on who gives orders, but on the willingness of those who receive the orders to comply. In Barnard's theory, it is the employees who decide whether directions will be followed, not the managers or supervisors. Employees are willing to accept directions from a manager under the following conditions:

1. They understand the communication.
2. They see the communication is consistent with the purposes of the organization.
3. They feel that actions indicated are in line with their needs and those of other employees.
4. They view themselves as mentally and physically able to comply.

> *Employees are willing to accept directions from a manager if they understand the communication, see that the communication is consistent with the purposes of the organization, feel that the directions meet their needs and those of other employees, and view themselves as mentally and physically able to comply.*

Fayol's 14 points and Barnard's theory of authority provide the health fitness manager with valuable insight into management approaches that work.

BEHAVIORAL MANAGEMENT THEORIES

The classical management approach provided the theoretical structure that allowed the study of management to be recognized as a valid scientific discipline. It also provided innovative insights into organizational structure and operational efficiency that are as helpful today as they were more than 100 years ago. The limitation of the classical approach is the reluctance to consider psychological influences on human behavior as relevant to performance efficiency. In contrast, the *behavioral viewpoint* focuses on the human element in the workplace. Psychologist Hugo Munsterberg and political scientist Mary Parker Follett were two early pioneers in developing the behavioral management perspective.

Hugo Munsterberg (1863-1916) set up a psychological lab at Harvard in 1892 and began working on practical applications of psychology. In 1913 he published *Psychology and Industrial Efficiency* in which he outlined the three major ways psychologists could help industry: (1) they could study jobs and find ways of identifying individuals best suited to particular jobs; (2) they could identify the psychological conditions under which individuals are most likely to do their best work; and (3) they could develop strategies that would influence employees to behave in ways compatible with management interests.

Mary Parker Follett (1868-1933) was an early behaviorist who became interested in employment and workplace issues while working as a social worker. Her focus on group dynamics led her to believe that groups have the capacity to effectively exercise control over themselves and their activities. The fact that self-directed work teams and quality circles are considered contemporary management theories is a reflection of how forward-thinking she was in the early 1900s. Follett's approach reinforces the importance of effective staff meetings and ongoing internal training programs for the health fitness employee group.

Following the lead of behavioral managers, health fitness managers have responsibility to set up specific, active mechanisms for receiving feedback from employees at all levels of the organization. Internal suggestion boxes, idea memos to the top, periodic staff focus groups or brainstorming sessions, and a specific time scheduled on the agenda during regular staff meetings to discuss new ideas are all ways for the health fitness manager to reinforce the importance of group participation in solving problems and creating new opportunities. Some health fitness organizations provide cash incentives and staff awards for new ideas that are implemented. Others provide the manager with the authority to hand out impromptu certificates for nominal gifts, such as movie theater passes or food coupons, when they get a good idea from an employee about solving a problem, resolving a conflict, or suggesting a new program.

Hawthorne Studies

A series of research studies conducted at the Hawthorne plant of Western Electric Company between 1924 and 1932 provided the catalyst for the behavioral viewpoint and ultimately the development of the human relations model of management. Known as the *Hawthorne studies*, the three separate sets of experiments investigated (1) the relationship between lighting and productivity; (2) the impact of workday length, rest periods, pay, free lunches, and supervisory arrangements on productivity; and (3) the impact of pay system on group standards and performance. The most lasting impact of the studies was the recognition that a variety of social factors, including level of personal attention, group acceptance, and other positively perceived changes, significantly impact work productivity.

> *A variety of social factors at the workplace, including level of personal attention, group acceptance, and other positively perceived changes, significantly impact work productivity.*

Human Relations

The Hawthorne research created an intense interest in the social dimension of human behavior in organizations. Developing a viewpoint that considers human relations gives an alternative to the classical viewpoint of the worker in a rational, systematic, economic context. The human relations model recognizes the unique needs and motives each individual brings to the workplace. Two noted academicians, Abraham Maslow and Douglas McGregor, developed innovative models to help managers understand the complex nature of workers and motivation.

Abraham Maslow (1908-1970), chairman of the psychology department of Brandeis University, developed a theory of human motivation incorporating workers' having a range of needs beyond the basic desire to earn a wage for food and housing. *Maslow's need hierarchy* (see figure 4.4) is based on three assumptions: (1) human beings have needs that are never completely satisfied; (2) human action is directed toward fulfilling unsatisfied needs at a given point in time; and (3) needs fit into a predictable hierarchy.

The hierarchy outlined by Maslow has five levels of needs: physiological, security, social, esteem, and self-actualization. The lowest tier of needs are physiological and include basic survival requirements such as food, air, and adequate warmth. In the health fitness workplace, these basic needs are satisfied with adequate wages to meet the employee's need for food,

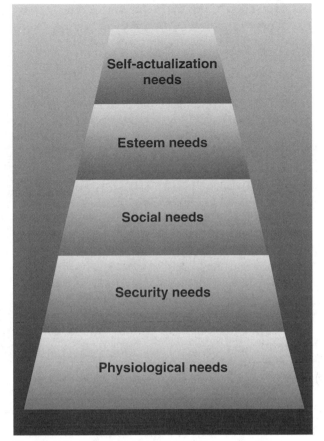

Figure 4.4 Maslow's need hierarchy.

clothing, and housing. The next level of needs are security requirements for a safe physical and emotional environment. Providing employees with job stability; a safe work environment; fair grievance procedures; and employee health, welfare, and retirement plans are elements of meeting work-based security needs. Social needs include the need for belonging, love, affection, and peer acceptance. The health fitness organization's ability to promote teamwork and to support employee group activities are elements of fulfilling the social needs. Esteem needs combine the need for respect and recognition from others and the need for self-respect and a positive self-image. Job titles, office size and location, company awards and recognition, and opportunities for advancement provide support of the external esteem needs at work. Accomplishment of personal goals plays an important role in meeting internal esteem needs. Finally, the highest level of needs are self-actualizing needs. These include the need to continue personal development, expand individual skills, and achieve important personal and business milestones. Maslow's theory is a dramatic departure from the one-dimensional scientific management viewpoint that pay is the primary motivation for work. In fact, many elements of modern corporate wellness programs are directed at fulfilling the employee needs identified by Maslow's research.

Douglas McGregor (1906-1964), a professor of industrial management at the Massachusetts Institute of Technology, developed the dichotomy of Theory X versus Theory Y managers. Theory X typifies pessimistic managerial thinking and assumes that workers are basically lazy, need to be coerced, have little ambition, and are motivated primarily by security needs. In contrast, Theory Y represents an optimistic managerial viewpoint in which workers have the potential for integrating personal and organizational goals and respond positively to creativity, innovation, and the opportunity for personal achievement. McGregor believed that managers treat workers in a manner consistent with their Theory X or Theory Y assumptions (see table 4.1). In response, workers are likely to react in a manner that reinforces the manager's assumptions.

The health fitness manager can learn from the human resources viewpoint that each individual brings unique needs and motives to the job. The health fitness manager becomes a more effective manager by learning to use this information to improve communications within the organization, match individuals to appropriate jobs, and create a more humanistic and personal approach to management.

Behavioral Science

The behavioral science approach to management uses scientific research to establish practical guidelines for managers. Behavioral science research includes the disciplines of management, sociology, psychology, anthropology, and economics. Concepts developed from research are tested in laboratory settings and in actual business organizations before they are considered valid management tools. The objective of the behavioral science approach is to develop theories that provide managers with specific guidelines, alternatives, and contingencies rather than simple, universal principles. Many health fitness organizations use techniques such as management by objectives, total quality management, employee stock ownership, employee assistance programs, and other employer-sponsored programs that have been developed on the basis of behavioral science research.

QUANTITATIVE MANAGEMENT THEORIES

The quantitative management viewpoint focuses on quantitative techniques such as mathematics, statistics, and information aids to support managerial functions, decision making, and organiza-

---

Table 4.1 Theory X and Theory Y Assumptions

Theory X

1. The average person dislikes work and will try to avoid it.

2. Most people need to be coerced, controlled, directed, and threatened with punishment to get them to work toward organizational goals.

3. The average person wants to be directed, shuns responsibility, has little ambition, and seeks security above all.

Theory Y

1. Most people do not inherently dislike work; the physical and mental effort involved is as natural as play or rest.

2. People will exercise self-direction and self-control to reach goals to which they are committed; external control and threat of punishment are not the only means for ensuring effort toward goals.

3. Commitment to goals is a function of the rewards available, particularly rewards that satisfy esteem and self-actualization needs.

4. When conditions are favorable, the average person will seek and accept responsibility.

5. Many people have the capacity to exercise a high degree of creativity and innovation in solving organizational problems.

6. The intellectual potential of most individuals is only partially used in most organizations.

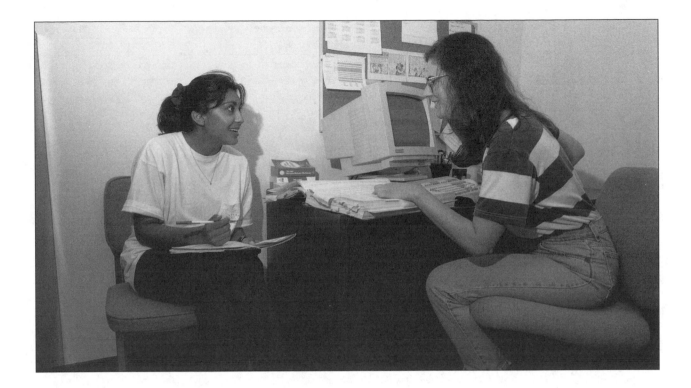

tional effectiveness. The principle value of the quantitative management viewpoint is the wide range of tools it provides for management. These tools can significantly enhance managerial decision making, planning, and control.

Management Science

Management science is the development of mathematical models and statistical methods to increase management decision-making effectiveness. The availability of personal computers and user-friendly software has dramatically increased the opportunity to use these tools in organizations. Management science models in a health fitness setting are used to design facilities, set pricing, maintain inventory, schedule personnel, order supplies, replace and maintain equipment, evaluate acquisitions, and improve many other important health fitness management functions.

Operations Management

Operations management uses mathematical and statistical tools to improve the processes and systems that produce and deliver a health fitness organization's products and services. Examples of operations management in a health fitness setting

include inventory management, work scheduling, facility development and design, and quality assurance. Figure 4.5 illustrates how you can organize an operations management approach to planning an new facility using a planning and scheduling model.

Management Information Systems

Management information systems (MIS) focus on developing, installing, and maintaining computer-based information systems. Information consists of data organized in a meaningful way. Data are merely facts and figures identified without specific organization or application. From a management standpoint, data are useless until they are organized, processed, and reported meaningfully. Every information system has five basic components: (1) a method to get data into the system; (2) a central processing unit to organize, analyze, and summarize data; (3) storage capability for data and information; (4) a method to make information available to users; and (5) an overall control system.

The development of an effective management information system for a health fitness organization requires matching information needs with various computer system options. Data within a health fitness organization includes membership information, health screening records, employment data,

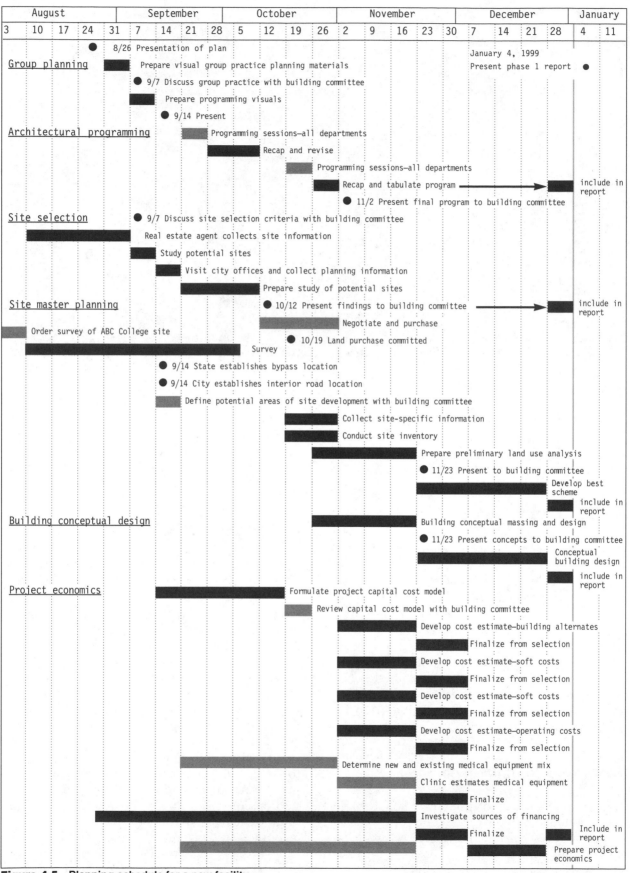

Figure 4.5   Planning schedule for a new facility.

financial data, marketing data, vendor and supplier information, programming information, and many other data sources. The matching process involves the health fitness manager's leading the organization through a series of questions designed to identify organizational information goals; management requirements; cost-benefit analysis; hardware and software evaluation and selction; and system design, installation, and testing. Figure 4.6 illustrates the process of evaluating and selecting data-based systems. Management science systems affect the performance of an organization, the organization's structure and design, and the people within the organization. For example, service desk access to membership data that works in conjunction with an electronic screening and access system at the control desk requires a more complex computer network than a manual membership card system in a small club that limits computer uses to back office financial support. The only constant for health fitness organizations of all sizes is that the rapid expansion of management science information resources will continue to challenge management's ability to keep current in technology, equipment, and personnel skills.

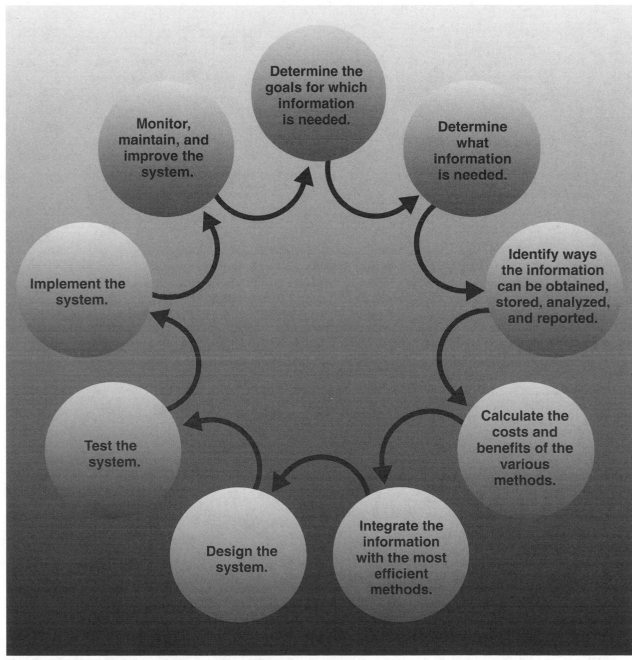

Figure 4.6   Matching information needs to an information system.

CONTEMPORARY MANAGEMENT THEORIES

Innovations in management theory continue to evolve from earlier viewpoints and from new and unique ideas. Although many new ideas do not yet have the stature of representing a school of thought, the emerging views may provide managers with useful tools for addressing contemporary challenges.

Systems Theory

Systems theory is based on the premise that we can visualize organizations as systems. A system is a series of interrelated parts that operate as a whole in pursuit of common goals. An organizational system has four major components, as we see in figure 4.7.

Inputs are the various human, material, financial, equipment, and informational resources required to produce goods and services. Transformational processes are the organization's managerial and technological abilities that convert inputs into out-

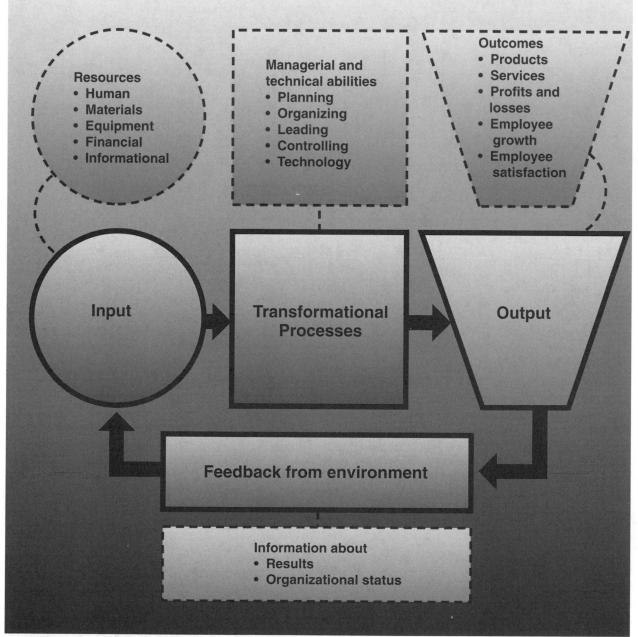

Figure 4.7 Systems view of organizations.

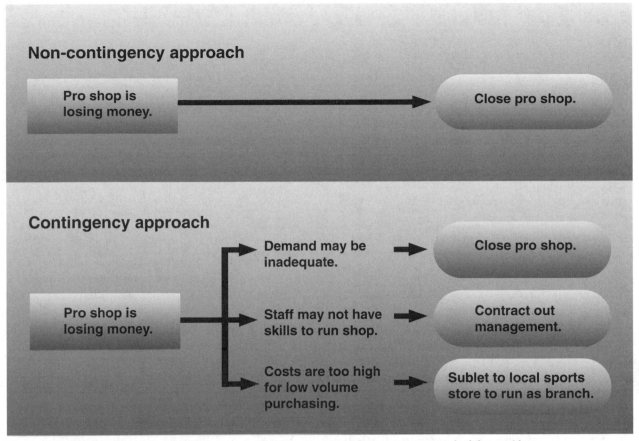

Figure 4.8 Non-contingency approach versus contingency approach to management decision making.

puts. Outputs are the products, services, and other outcomes produced by the organization. Feedback is information about results and the organization's status related to the external environment. There are four major advantages to systems theory. First, it allows a manager to evaluate systems at different levels. Second, it provides a framework for assessing the extent to which various parts of an organization are working together to achieve a common purpose. Third, it highlights that changes in one part of a system may affect other parts. Fourth, the systems approach considers how well an organization interacts with the external environment.

Systems can be open or closed to external influence. An open system is one that operates with continuous interaction with the external environment. The interaction provides new input and feedback in response to system output. For example, the evolution of managed care has created opportunities for some health fitness organizations to create partnerships with primary care providers, employers, and third-party administrators. By serving as the preventive care component in the larger community health and wellness environment, the organization becomes part of the mainstream market, rather than an isolated specialty provider.

In contrast, a closed system operates independently and by doing so takes the risk of suffering damaging or fatal results from external factors of which it is unaware. A specific example is an employer-based health fitness facility that fails to monitor corporate profits, employment needs, and market competition. These external factors are likely to have more impact on the facility's budgeting and future than any specific programming results.

A closed system is at risk from entropy, the tendency for systems to decay over time. Without new energy in the form of input and feedback from the environment, closed systems falter and die. From a systems management viewpoint, health fitness organizations operating in an open system model have a significantly greater chance of success and growth.

Table 4.2   Evolution of TQM in an Organization

Phase 1	Phase 2	Phase 3
- Organization begins to learn about quality.	- Workers focus on increased efficiencies.	- Self-directed work teams take over operations.
- Emphasis is placed on training.	- Organization identifies world-class companies and tries to emulate them.	- Team members develop and implement training.
- Organization tries to emulate major competitors.	- Suppliers are selected primarily on the basis of quality and secondarily on the basis of price.	- Emulating the world's best companies becomes the °standard method of operation.
- Suppliers are selected on the basis of price and reliability.		
- Service orientation becomes the primary focus of the organization.	- Quality enhancement becomes a fundamental part of the organization's culture.	- Continuous improvement becomes a routine and ongoing part of the organization's business.

Contingency Theory

Contingency theory is based on the assumption that appropriate managerial actions are contingent or depend on elements of each specific situation. The theory recommends that when health fitness managers face a problem or situation, they examine important contingencies to determine which of several potential solutions may be most appropriate. The contingency theory does not suggest that every situation requires a unique response. Even though situations may vary, a manager may solve different problems by a similar solution or action. An example in a health fitness setting of contingency theory in practice is illustrated in figure 4.8.

Total Quality Management

Total quality management (TQM) is a comprehensive, organization-wide strategy to improve product or service quality continuously. TQM is based on a strategic commitment to quality and, as illustrated in table 4.2, relies on employee involvement, materials, methods, and technology to achieve the designated levels of improved quality. W. Edwards Deming (1900-1993) reintroduced his theory of TQM to American management in 1980, more than 45 years after he first presented the concepts to an uninterested business community. In the intervening years, Deming's philosophy became one of the pivotal theories in Japanese management. Deming's TQM philosophy centers on 14 points:

1. Plan for the future.
2. Realize the need for change.
3. Build quality into products and services.
4. Build preferred vendor relationships.
5. Improve every process.
6. Institute on-the-job training.
7. Institute leadership.
8. Drive out fear.

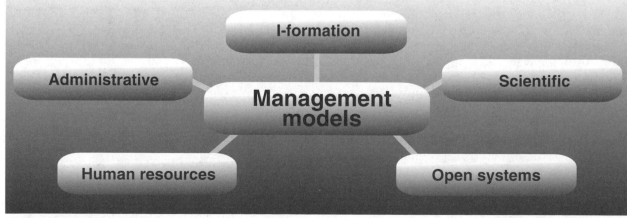

Figure 4.9   Management models.

9. Break down barriers.

10. Eliminate "work harder" posters or slogans.

11. Eliminate arbitrary numerical targets.

12. Push pride on the job.

13. Encourage education.

14. Define top management's commitment to quality.

High Involvement Management

High involvement management is a category of management approaches that includes a variety of participative management techniques. High involvement management relies on the principles of self-control and self-management at all levels of the organization. Specific techniques include quality circles, self-directed work teams, quality-of-life programs, gain sharing, job sharing, and new design plans. High involvement management theories and techniques continue to be in a rapid state of development and implementation.

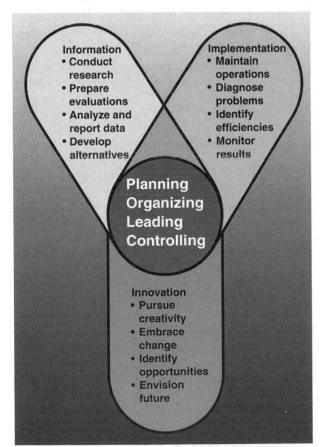

Figure 4.10 I-formation management model.

DEFINING MANAGEMENT RESPONSIBILITY USING MODELS

Perhaps it is easier to understand the value of each theory if we think of them as *management models*. Models provide a representation of a more complex reality. For example, a toy car may serve as a physical model of a new concept vehicle. Having a model to twist and turn and view from different perspectives makes it easier to understand the function, limitations, and potential of the original idea. In a similar manner, the managerial schools of thought, as management models illustrated in figure 4.9, represent a set of assumptions and a way of viewing concepts related to management responsibility. The overall area of study becomes complicated because each management model explains only one part or one perspective of the management process.

I-Formation Management Model

The management process involves four basic functions: planning and decision making, organizing, leading, and controlling. Because these are the central functions around which the *I-formation management model* is developed, we introduce them here. However, we include a more complete discussion later in the chapter. For an understanding of the I-formation management model, the abbreviated definitions are as follows: *planning* is identifying an organization's goals and deciding how to achieve them; *organizing* is the grouping of activities and resources in a logical manner; *leading* is the process of getting people to work together to achieve the organization's goals; and *controlling* is the monitoring of the organization's progress toward the goals.

Health fitness managers must develop the tools and skills to perform the basic management functions and be prepared to face the challenges of a rapidly changing industry. The I-formation management model defines the functions of management as a dynamic relationship involving three dimensions: information, implementation, and innovation. We can use the I-formation model to define and evaluate the overall organization, subgroups within the organization, and individual managers. The model is represented graphically in figure 4.10 by three overlapping spheres, indicating the interrelationship of the three dimensions.

The I-formation model illustrates that effective organizations must consistently focus on three separate but related dimensions of management responsibility to effectively perform the four primary managerial functions. The dynamic characteristic of the model comes from the aspect that each of the three dimensions requires continuous input from the other two in order to be effective. The following three I-formation questions should challenge every level of the management process:

1. **Information**—Is appropriate information available and being used in support of the decision, action, and goal?

2. **Implementation**—Is the most efficient and effective approach to implementation in place or planned?

3. **Innovation**—Have the existing assumptions been confronted by and survived the challenge of innovative ideas?

Let's use the example of tracking the development of a new program in a health fitness setting. Observing that more members are bringing children to the facility could trigger an innovative idea to develop a separate children's program. The concept makes sense but requires considerable planning and research to determine if it is a viable idea from facility use and financial aspects. By gathering *information* you may begin to see if other facilities have tried the concept. You may evaluate whether members might pay an additional fee for special children's programming. You may then research what resources are necessary to deliver the programming. If the idea continues to appear viable, the health fitness manager may choose to test the idea by *implementing* a prototype or pilot program. By collecting information as the pilot program is implemented, you may obtain valuable insight about the current effort and possible innovations that could make a larger program more successful. This approach is effective when you apply it to new programs and when you evaluate existing programs.

We use the I-formation model throughout this book to define standards related to the traditional managerial responsibilities of marketing, administration, finance, operations, and human resources. You can also apply the I-formation model to each employee's role in the organization. Do employees understand their responsibilities in contributing to enhancing innovation, information gathering and analysis, and effective implementation throughout the organization? It is the role of the health fitness manager to create the framework within which all employees understand the I-formation elements of their jobs and the I-formation objectives of the organization. To emphasize these elements, we use I-formation icons throughout the book to call out management and operational points related to information, implementation, and innovation.

Scientific Model

The scientific management model focuses on making the best product in the most efficient way. In some ways, it was a forerunner to the current quality movement. The central idea of this model is to identify the best way to do a task, then to make sure the task is done that way. One reason for delivering a service as efficiently as possible is to keep the cost low. By doing so, the service is more attractive to customers.

> *The health fitness manager's primary responsibility in the scientific management model is to satisfy the customer (an external focus) by delivering a service the best way possible at the lowest cost.*

The health fitness manager using the scientific model should continually look for ways to cut costs and increase efficiency without lowering the quality below members' expectations. The health fitness manager should study issues, such as contracting out facility maintenance, laundry services, food services, and pro shop operations, to determine whether the opportunity exists to lower cost and improve service by bringing in vendors who specialize in their respective service areas.

Administrative Model

The administrative management model focuses on the internal operation of the organization. It attempts to make administrative procedures more efficient by finding better ways to coordinate and monitor the work of the organization. If successful, the organization becomes more stable and predictable. Whereas the scientific management model has an external focus on pleasing the customer, the

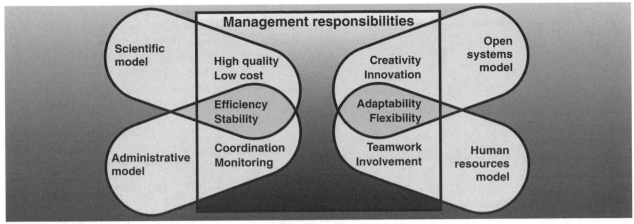

Figure 4.11   Comparison of management models' definitions of responsibilities.

administrative management model has an internal focus on improving systems and operations.

> By making the work of the organization as predictable as possible, health fitness managers can easily evaluate the productivity and success of the various activities occurring throughout the organization. If results are predictable, it is clear when health fitness managers must take action to correct deficiencies.

Examples of effective administrative managing by health fitness managers include computerizing membership records; installing point of purchase terminals that capture and provide centralized reports on food, beverage, and product sales; standardizing cleaning and maintenance programs; and implementing mandatory member orientation programs. The primary objective of all administrative management efforts is to increase efficiency and standardize quality.

Human Resources Model

The *human resources model* emphasizes flexibility by focusing on the people inside the organization. A health fitness manager's responsibility in a human resources model is to build team orientation and employee involvement through-

out the organization. Under the model, if employees are committed to the health fitness organization and willing to adapt to organizational changes, the organization becomes more cohesive and reacts positively to internal and external challenges. The human resources model emphasizes satisfaction of the people within the organization. A satisfied employee provides excellent service and feels encouraged to help the organization improve.

> Using the human resources model, the health fitness manager establishes and maintains an open dialog with employees at all levels of the organization.

Staff meetings, departmental meetings, multi-departmental planning teams, employee incentive programs, award and recognition programs, and personal and professional training programs are all important elements of this model.

Open Systems Model

The *open systems model* focuses on developing adaptability to external changes. The objective is to create a health fitness organization capable of reacting quickly and creatively to forces outside the organization. Outside forces include new technology, changing market demographics, new competitors, and social and lifestyle changes.

> *The open system model challenges the health fitness manager to develop entrepreneurial capabilities and a supportive environment for new ideas throughout the organization.*

Health fitness management activities that promote an open system management model include conducting regular membership and client surveys, performing competitor shopping, attending industry and trade shows, circulating news and information from trade journals and other sources throughout the organization, and establishing regular opportunities for staff and members to contribute new ideas for improving the organization.

APPLYING MANAGEMENT MODELS

After considering each management model, it becomes clear that several models overlap in their definitions of management responsibilities (see figure 4.11). For example, the administrative management and the scientific models both emphasize the manager's responsibility to establish and maintain efficiency and stability. The human resources and open system models share an emphasis on flexibility and adaptation. The human resources and administrative management models focus on internal processes in the organization. The open systems and scientific management models both focus on external forces and their effect on the organization.

Several models have opposing points of view. The human resources model, with its emphasis on team orientation and employee involvement, clashes with the scientific management model, which emphasizes worker efficiency and task simplification. Likewise, the models of administrative management standardization and open systems flexibility are opposed. The administrative management model encourages health fitness managers to develop stable and efficient organizations, whereas the open systems model argues for an adaptive and fluid organization. These differences among managerial models reflect the challenges

health fitness managers face every day. The question is how can health fitness managers resolve the obvious differences in the models to select appropriate actions that will make them successful? The answer is that they all contribute to the managers' understanding of how to make their organizations succeed, yet no one model can solve every managerial problem.

> *Remember that no single model is absolutely right or wrong. Because management is a fluid and dynamic process, successful health fitness managers continuously evaluate the various functions of their jobs and select different managerial models to address changing needs within the organization.*

UNDERSTANDING TRADITIONAL MANAGER FUNCTIONS

Fayol's definition of four primary management functions—planning, organizing, leading, and controlling—has evolved into the traditional measure of manager responsibility. The introduction of the I-formation management model expands Fayol's definition by requiring managers to focus on information, implementation, and innovation to effectively perform the four primary managerial functions. In both cases, the process of management is an ongoing activity, entails reaching important goals, and involves knowing how to perform these four functions. Let's look at these functions and consider how they relate to the roles, skills, and operational responsibilities of a health fitness manager.

Planning

Management planning involves setting goals and deciding how best to achieve them. It implies that effective health fitness managers think through goals and actions in advance and move forward with a method or logic rather than at random.

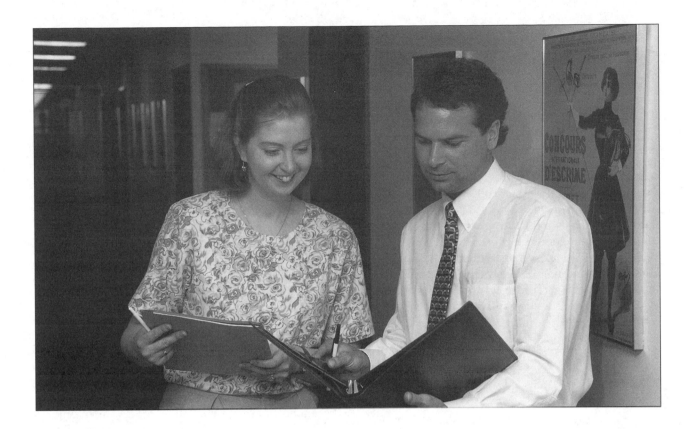

Managers spend a significant part of the planning process gathering and evaluating information. Information they use in planning is likely to span historical, current, and future time and include past implementation results as well as future innovation opportunities. The information dimension of the I-formation management model plays a primary role in the planning function.

Organizing

The function of organizing refers to the allocation and arrangement of human and nonhuman resources to successfully carry out planned goals and objectives. The process of organizing includes defining the tasks, timetables, resources, and responsibilities that make up the structure of an organization; implementing planned actions; and recording and reporting information related to this implementation.

Leading

The leading function includes directing, influencing, and motivating individuals and groups to engage in essential behavior necessary to reach organizational goals. By using a variety of communication methods to define vision, provide direction, and motivate performance, leadership requires disseminating information effectively, motivating actions that facilitate implementation, and creating an environment that encourages innovation and creative problem solving. All three dimensions of the I-formation management model are important in successfully leading an organization.

Controlling

Controlling means regulating activities to ensure that actual performance conforms to expected organizational standards and goals. To do the necessary regulating, managers must monitor ongoing activities, compare results with expected standards, and take corrective action as needed. Quality control and total quality management (TQM) are examples of implementing the controlling function. Operational standards and measurements, financial reporting, performance evaluations, employee surveys, and member surveys are also part of the overall controlling function. The information and implementation dimensions of the I-formation management model support the controlling function.

IMPLEMENTING THE MANAGEMENT PROCESS

The four management functions explain and define the most basic elements of the managerial process. However, a more detailed look at the day-to-day activities of managers illustrates how difficult it can be to clearly define management in these simple terms. Management scholar Henry Mintzberg, on the basis of several classic studies presented in *The Nature of Managerial Work* (1973), observed that managers were not reflective, systematic planners who base management decisions on thoughtful review of formal management and financial reports. He observed managers functioning at an unrelenting pace, dealing rapidly with a wide variety of issues, using fragmented information, and relying on a network of people to accomplish their individual and organizational objectives.

Managers' Roles

To make sense of the reams of data he collected, rather than define management by the four traditional functions, Mintzberg attempted to categorize the managers' various activities into roles. He defined a role as an organized set of behaviors associated with a particular position and identified three roles played by managers: interpersonal, informational, and decisional. Within these role types, Mintzberg outlined 10 more specific roles that managers play (see table 4.3). Mintzberg's categorization of managerial activities into roles provides valuable insight into the daily activities of a typical manager. More importantly, the roles provide information about the kinds of skills required to effectively perform the functions of a health fitness manager. Note how each role fits within the traditional management functions of planning, controlling, organizing, and leading (included in parentheses).

Interpersonal

Interpersonal roles grow directly out of the authority of a health fitness manager's position and involve developing and maintaining positive relationships with people. There are three interpersonal roles in the health fitness manager's job:

1. *Figurehead*. A health fitness manager serves as a figurehead when an appearance without serious communication or decision making meets the needs of the situation. For example, the general manager of a facility may periodically greet members at the front desk, attend special events organized and coordinated by other managers, or serve in a volunteer capacity for other organizations. By making a personal appearance, the general manager is symbolizing the importance of maintaining personal contacts with members and potential members, even if her primary responsibility as a manager is limited to administrative and operational functions. This role can help emphasize the value of an activity by the manager's mere presence. It can be effective in internal and external settings (leading).

2. *Leader*. As a leader, the health fitness manager hires, coordinates, and motivates employees. The health fitness manager is enacting the leadership role when working with employees to teach the importance of high quality performance and to help define and clarify the roles of each worker (leading).

3. *Liaison*. Managers regularly deal with people outside the organization. Health fitness managers must be able to work well with outside agencies that can help them achieve their organizational goals. Managers perform the liaison role by developing a network of contacts throughout the health fitness industry and within the community (organizing).

Informational

Informational roles pertain to receiving and transmitting information that allows the health fitness manager to serve as the nerve center of an organization. The three informational roles in the health fitness manager's job are as follows:

1. *Monitor*. As a monitor, the health fitness manager seeks information from outside sources—trade journals, newspapers, television, or discussions with vendors, competitors, or other professionals—that may be useful to the organization. Successful health fitness managers maintain a high level of awareness of information from a variety of sources (organizing and planning).

2. *Disseminator*. A health fitness manager actively collecting information as a monitor also has the responsibility to disseminate the information to appropriate people in the organization. The health fitness manager serves as an informational switchboard, routing useful information from one source to another throughout the organization (controlling and organizing).

3. *Spokesperson*. The spokesperson role is similar to the figurehead, but different in that the spokes-

person is expected to provide meaningful information about, or on behalf of, the organization. As a spokesperson, the health fitness manager has the authority to speak as the organization's formal representative (leading).

Decisional

Decisional roles involve making significant decisions that affect the organization. Collectively these roles represent some of the most important and challenging aspects of successful management.

1. *Entrepreneur.* As an entrepreneur, the health fitness manager is constantly looking for opportunities to try new ideas and use creative solutions. In organizations encouraging the open system model of management, the health fitness manager is responsible for striking the careful balance between encouraging and pursuing entrepreneurial ideas and wasting time and resources by attempting too many high risk or ill-advised endeavors (planning and leading).

2. *Disturbance handler.* This role serves to resolve disputes within the organization and between the organization and outsiders. To be effective, a health fitness manager must be able to collect information regarding a dispute, evaluate the consequences, and communicate the decision and reasoning to all involved parties. As a disturbance handler, the health fitness manager must be willing and able to step in between staff and members to resolve disputes, disagreements, and miscommunications (leading and controlling).

3. *Resource allocator.* The resource allocator role requires a health fitness manager to make decisions about dividing limited resources among many possible users. Money, personnel, supplies, information, facility space, and time are all part of the pool of limited resources that a health fitness manager must use efficiently (controlling).

4. *Negotiator.* In this role, the health fitness manager attempts to work out agreements and contracts that protect the best interests of the organization. Agreements requiring negotiation fall into a wide range of circumstances; employment agreements, purchasing contracts, facility and equipment leases, sales contracts, warranty agreements and claims, member and guest claims, and vendor relationships all require certain levels of negotiation talent. (Chapter 17 reviews in more detail how to select and work with attorneys in circumstances that involve a high level of potential liability or serious financial risk.) The

negotiator's role occurs both inside and outside the organization. For example, a general manager may negotiate a contract with a consulting firm, or an operations manager may negotiate for janitorial services for the organization. Inside the organization, a health fitness manager will frequently negotiate staff scheduling, vacations, and overtime requests. Each activity requires the health fitness manager to serve in the negotiator role (leading and controlling).

Mintzberg's role descriptions provide a more complex definition of managerial roles and responsibilities than the traditional division into four basic management functions. In fact, Mintzberg's findings appear incompatible with the view that planning, organizing, leading, and controlling are the most effective ways to define and understand the management process. However, it is important to note that Mintzberg's study did not attempt to explain *why* managers engage in different roles. For example, a health fitness manager may periodically perform the role of negotiator as defined by Mintzberg when dealing with outside vendors. With no additional information, it would be expected that negotiating skills should therefore be included in the qualifications for becoming a health fitness manager. However, the relative importance of a health fitness manager's negotiation skills is not apparent unless the tasks related to the job are measured and defined as part of the organizing function of management. It is only after specific job tasks are reviewed, and responsibilities assigned, that we can determine the importance of each potential management role. In this example, if the primary vendor negotiations are actually assigned to an assistant manager, hiring health fitness managers on the basis of their negotiating skills may be a mistake. It is the process of defining jobs by task and frequency (organizing) that identifies the relative priority that you should place on specific manager roles.

Roles and functions may help define the overall management process. However, health fitness managers still require a method for focusing their individual efforts to achieve their goals and objectives. One effective method is using well-planned manager work agendas to allocate limited time to the most important management responsibilities.

Manager Work Agenda

A work agenda is a loosely connected set of tentative tasks that a manager is attempting to

Table 4.3   Mintzberg's 10 Managerial Roles

Roles/categories	Description	Activities
Interpersonal		
Figurehead	Symbolic head, performs routine legal or social duties	Ceremony, status requests, solicitations
Leader	Responsible for motivating subordinates; responsible for staffing, training, and associated duties	Virtually all managerial activities involving subordinates
Liaison	Maintains self-developed network that provides favors and information	Acknowledgments of mail, external board work, other activities involving outsiders
Informational		
Monitor	Seeks and receives wide variety of special information (much of it current) to develop thorough understanding of organization and environment, emerges as nerve center of internal and external information of the organization	Handling all mail and contact concerned primarily with receiving information (e.g., periodical news, observational tours)
Disseminator	Transmits information received from outsiders or from other subordinates to members of the organization; some information factual, some involving interpretation and integration of diverse value positions of organizational influencers	Forwarding mail into organization for informational purposes, verbal contacts involving information flow to subordinates (e.g., review sessions, instant communication flows)
Spokesperson	Transmits information to outsiders on organization's plans, policies, actions, results, and serves as expert on organization's industry	Board meetings, handling mail and contact involving transmission of information to outsiders
Decisional		
Entrepreneur	Searches organization and its environment for opportunities and initiates improvement projects to bring about change, supervises design of certain projects	Strategy and review sessions involving initiation or design of improvement projects
Disturbance handler	Responsible for corrective action when organization faces important, unexpected disturbances	Strategy and review sessions involving disturbances and crises
Resource allocator	Responsible for allocating organizational resources of all kinds	Scheduling, requests for authorization, any activity involving budgeting and the programming of subordinates' work
Negotiator	Responsible for representing the organization at major negotiations	Negotiation

accomplish. It is less formal than an annual plan and is continually reassessed in the face of changing circumstances and emerging opportunities. By using work agendas and networking strategies, health fitness managers are able to engage in short, seemingly disjointed activities throughout the day and still accomplish their larger management goals and objectives. Rosemary Stewart, a British expert on managerial work, suggests that there are three main factors that impact a manager's work agenda:

• *Job demands*—the activities a health fitness manager must do. For example, health fitness managers usually have responsibilities related to the major goals and plans of the organization (such as achieving a 10 percent increase in membership sales). Ignoring these responsibilities creates a high risk of failing to perform the job adequately.

• *Job constraints*—the factors, both inside and outside the organization, that limit what a health fitness manager can do. Constraints include such variables as budget limits, legal restrictions, facility limitations, market factors, staff training, equipment quality, external schedules, and the presence or lack of realistic planning.

• *Job choices*—work activities that the health fitness manager can do but does not have to do. For example, a health fitness manager might initiate a program to revise the computerized membership tracking system, even though the current system is adequate but limited for future uses.

It becomes clear that defining the responsibilities of health fitness managers by looking at their management roles and work agendas is not in conflict with the traditional definition of management function as planning, controlling, leading, and organizing. In fact, we can see it as a way to better understand the day-to-day methods that managers use to perform their functions.

MANAGERIAL KNOWLEDGE BASE AND SKILLS

Throughout their careers, health fitness managers are likely to change companies and possibly move between different specialty areas within the health fitness industry. Effectiveness in successive management positions requires an extensive knowledge base relevant to each managerial job. A knowledge base can include information about a specific specialty, new technology, changing market factors, competitor policies and practices, geographic and demographic characteristics, the new company's goals and plans, company culture, the personalities of key organization members, and important suppliers and customers.

In addition to having a knowledge base, successful health fitness managers need certain skills, as illustrated in figure 4.12, to carry out the various functions of management. For health fitness managers, three types of skills are necessary: technical, human, and conceptual.

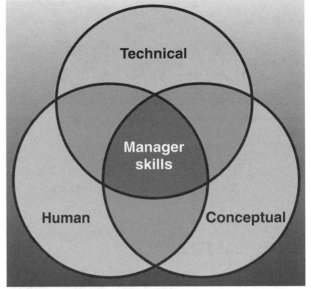

Figure 4.12   Managerial skills.

A skill is the ability to engage in a set of behaviors that are functionally related to one another and that lead to a desired performance.

Technical Skills

Technical skills help managers perform specialized tasks. For example, depending on the setting in which the health fitness manager works, the various technical skills required to perform all the functions of top management may include cardiac rehabilitation; exercise physiology; physical therapy; nutrition; stress management; weight management; psychology; and business-related skills such as accounting, finance, marketing, employee relations, and computer science. Throughout a health fitness manager's career, it is likely that additional education and training will be needed to remain current in the wide range of skill areas required to be successful.

Human Skills

Human skills refer to a manager's ability to work well with others, both as a member of a group and as a leader who gets things done through others.

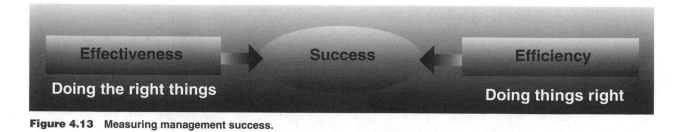

Figure 4.13 Measuring management success.

Health fitness managers with effective human relation skills are typically adept at communicating with others and motivating them to perform well in pursuit of organizational goals.

Conceptual Skills

Conceptual skills are related to the ability to visualize the organization as a whole; discern interrelationships among organizational parts; and understand how the organization fits into the wider context of the health fitness industry, community, and world.

> *Conceptual skills, coupled with technical skills, human skills, and a knowledge base, are the important ingredients that health fitness managers must have to consistently achieve high levels of organizational performance.*

MEASURING MANAGEMENT SUCCESS

How do you measure management success? On an individual level, successful managers develop specific job goals and objectives, put them in writing, then measure their results in completing each element quarterly and annually. On an organizational level, successful management is measured by the organization's ability to balance overall efficiency and effectiveness (see figure 4.13). Effectiveness is the ability to choose appropriate goals and achieve them. Efficiency is the ability to make the best use of available resources in the process of achieving goals. In essence, organizations need to exhibit both effectiveness (doing the right things) and efficiency (doing things right) to be good performers.

> *The right combination of efficiency and effectiveness is generally considered the highest level of organizational and management achievement.*

An effective organization reflects an environment of dynamic change: doing the right things at the right time in the right way. Effectiveness is measured in a longer time frame than efficiency. Maintaining a constant view to the future and changes in the marketplace is an important element of an effective organization.

> *Effective managers frequently question not only whether something was done right, but whether the right thing was done.*

An efficient health fitness manager will use available personnel, financial, informational, and facility resources to minimize waste, limit downtime, and eliminate unnecessary repetition. In an efficient organization, facility staffing will be based on an analysis of peak-time needs. Training will be implemented to minimize mistakes and provide management and administrative tools that match job responsibilities. Equipment and supplies will be purchased at quantities and prices that maximize financial resources. Information about members, guests, programming, staffing, and pricing will be distributed in a timely manner to all individuals needing access to the information. An efficient organization is one sign of successful management.

LEVELS OF MANAGERIAL RESPONSIBILITY

Historically, most health fitness organizations have been small, privately owned companies. In these companies, top management either serves as, or answers directly to, the business owners. There are a growing number of public companies and hospital corporations involved in the health fitness industry. In these companies, multiple levels of management exist that are generally defined as top, middle, and first-line management as shown in figure 4.14.

Although the same managerial process applies to all three levels of management, there are differences in levels of responsibility. Each health fitness managerial level has planning, organizing, leading, and controlling functions. However, as illustrated in figure 4.14, the scope of the responsibilities and skills increases as a health fitness manager moves upward through the organization.

Management Functions by Level

Planning tends to be more important for senior managers than for middle-level or first-line managers. This is primarily because top managers are responsible for determining the overall direction of the health fitness organization, an effort that requires extensive planning. Organizing is somewhat more important for top and middle managers than for first-line managers. This stems from the fact that top and middle levels of management are responsible for allocating and arranging resources, even though organizing is performed by first-line supervisors to a limited extent.

Much to the surprise of many management students, leading is substantially more important for first-line supervisors than for health fitness managers at higher levels. First-line managers and supervisors are charged with the direct responsibility of motivating employees to perform the tasks required by their jobs. Many first-line managers must engage in substantial amounts of communicating, motivating, directing, and supporting—all areas associated with leading.

Lastly, controlling is emphasized at all three health fitness management levels. This similarity reflects the degree to which all management levels play a role in monitoring activities, maintaining standards, and taking corrective action as needed.

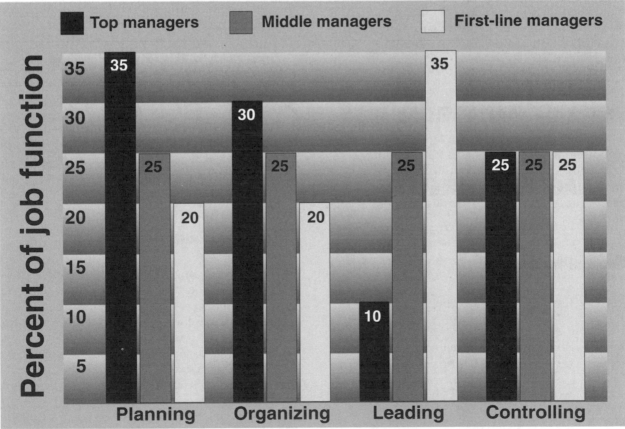

Figure 4.14 Managerial functions by level. Bar graphs show percentage of function by level.

Management Skills by Level

The three levels of management are also differentiated by the importance attached to the skills discussed earlier: technical, human, and conceptual. Conceptual skills are most important at the top levels of health fitness management. Senior managers have the greatest need to see the health fitness organization as a whole, as well as understand how its various parts relate to one another and to the world outside. In contrast, first-line managers have the greatest need for technical skills. First-line health fitness managers directly supervise most of the technical and professional employees. In addition, they frequently need sufficient technical skills to communicate with subordinates, recognize major problems, and act as liaisons between technical staff, members, guests, vendors, and other nontechnical employees. Not surprisingly, all three levels of management require strong human skills. Each management level, by definition, is working with people. Ironically, in many organizations, management promotions are based on academic or technical competence, with little consideration of human skills abilities. Sometimes this oversight can be addressed through training, but without improvement, health fitness managers lacking in sufficient human skills usually run into serious difficulties both inside and outside the organization.

TYPES OF MANAGERIAL JOBS

Another way to define health fitness managers is to identify and group jobs by the scope of management responsibility. Three broad groups define health fitness manager job types—general, functional, and project.

General Managers

General managers are responsible for an entire organization or a separate facility that includes most of the specialized management areas. The general manager presides over several functional areas. A health fitness facility will usually have only one general manager. However, a multisite health fitness organization may have general managers at each location in addition to centralized corporate senior managers.

Functional Managers

Functional managers are responsible for a specific, specialized area (often called a functional area) of the organization and supervise individuals with expertise and training in that area. Administrative functional areas include finance, operations, marketing, human resources management, accounting, quality assurance, and engineering. Special health fitness functional areas include aquatics, aerobics, racquet sports, food and beverage, senior and children programs, pro shop, and front desk.

Project Managers

Project managers are responsible for coordinating efforts and resources to accomplish a particular project. Because individuals assigned to work on special projects often remain responsible for primary job duties, project managers must have extremely strong interpersonal skills to keep things moving smoothly. Project managers are frequently selected to develop and implement a new program or to stay on top of market development for specific programming areas. Examples might include developing a special senior fitness program or integrating health fitness services into a managed care program.

LEARNING TO BE AN EFFECTIVE MANAGER

How can one learn to be an effective health fitness manager? Most observers agree that becoming an effective health fitness manager takes a combination of education and experience.

Managerial Education

For most health fitness managers, education does not end with college or graduate school degrees. Instead, managers usually take additional management-related courses as part of special programs offered through colleges and universities and by a wide range of professional associations. Health fitness managers also have the opportunity to achieve recognition for their professional expertise by becoming certified by the American College of Sports Medicine (ACSM) as a Certified Health Fitness Director.

As the demands of the health fitness management role become more complex, many managers consider management education as a process that continues throughout their careers.

Premanagement Experience

Not surprisingly, experience is a major factor in learning to be an effective health fitness manager. In a survey of CEOs for 800 large U.S. companies, work experience for the eventual CEOs started in high school (79 percent worked during high school) and largely continued in college (56 percent worked during college). Another early source of management experience was holding office in college organizations. Approximately 70 percent of the CEOs held at least one office in a club, fraternity, or other campus organization while in college. A number of the CEOs (38 percent) reported that participating in intercollegiate sport helped them learn teamwork and interpersonal skills that served them well in managerial positions. In a similar manner, individuals aspiring to health fitness management positions should seek out leadership roles in college and in professional organizations and look for opportunities to acquire progressively more demanding management positions as they build their professional resume.

Understanding Business Trends

A solid understanding of business trends is important to those preparing for a career in health fitness management. Although it is always difficult to make predictions, three trends are likely to impact health fitness managerial work in the future: the focus on quality, public concern for ethics, and the diversity of the workforce.

Increasing Importance of Quality

Health fitness organizations are becoming more concerned with quality in line with a general trend in business and industry. Known under the category of total quality management, discussed earlier in the chapter, the focus on quality performance and service involves a commitment to improve quality in every aspect of the organization's opera-

tions. With the relative ease of transferring membership between facilities, health fitness organizations are particularly vulnerable to demands from members to increase or modify services and products. Health fitness organizations known for their responsiveness to members' needs are frequently the most successful from the standpoint of profit, turnover, and referral activity from current members.

Public Concern With Managerial Ethics

Ethical concerns have arisen from the increase in white collar crimes and the perceived lack of professional ethics in modern business operations. Health fitness organizations are responding by placing greater emphasis on social responsibility and internal training and procedures to ensure compliance with corporate standards. Many health fitness organizations are developing organizational mission statements that include commitments to professional integrity and community leadership.

Diversity of the Workforce

The impact of demographic diversity on organizations and their managers continues to create new challenges. According to estimates by the U.S. Bureau of Labor Statistics in the publication *Occupational Outlook Handbook* (1990-1991), women will constitute about 47 percent of the workforce and minorities and immigrants about 26 percent by the year 2000. Health fitness managers in the 21st century will be faced with the challenge of addressing cultural and social issues with modifications in hiring and selection criteria, training programs, and employee benefits.

Issues related to two-income families and single-parent families are going to continue to impact work-related policies for family leave, insurance, child care, absenteeism, job sharing, flextime, and other benefits. The aging of the American workforce will also create challenges for retirement funding and changing job criteria as many workers choose to remain working past the current age standards for retirement.

IN CLOSING

Health fitness operations have evolved from small mom and pop businesses to complex facilities managed by multimillion dollar corporations. The challenges facing modern health fitness professionals have also expanded greatly. The successful health fitness manager needs experience and training in fundamental business practice areas of management, personnel, finance, marketing, and operations. This chapter has provided health fitness managers with a foundation for understanding contemporary management by reviewing the evolution of management theory. Health fitness managers should use the theories as a framework for developing individual management practice skills. By understanding historical viewpoints, modern managers can not only learn valuable lessons, but also avoid repeating the mistakes of the past. This chapter has introduced current and future health fitness managers to I-formation management theory as a theoretical model that defines and evaluates the health fitness management responsibilities.

Management is the process of achieving organizational goals by engaging in the functions of planning, organizing, leading, and controlling. Although these functions form the basis of the managerial process, several other elements contribute to an understanding of how health fitness managers operate. The I-formation management model suggests that skills related to information, implementation, and innovation are key elements of management success. In addition, health fitness managerial roles, as well as work agendas, prior managerial experience, and individual skills all are important elements in the complex and varied responsibilities of management. The combination of these factors impact the health fitness organization's ability to achieve effective and efficient performance. A solid understanding of business trends is important to those preparing for a career in management. Although it is always difficult to make predictions, three trends are likely to impact health fitness managerial work in the future: the increasing importance of quality, the expanding public concern with managerial ethics, and the diversity of the workforce.

KEY TERMS

Administrative management

Behavioral viewpoint

Bureaucratic management

Classical viewpoint

Controlling

Disseminator

Figurehead

Gantt chart

Hawthorne studies

High involvement management

Human resources model

I-formation management model

Leader

Leading

Liaison

Management information systems (MIS)

Management models

Maslow's need hierarchy

Monitor

Open systems model

Organizing

Planning

Scientific management

Spokesperson

Time and motion studies

Total quality management (TQM)

RECOMMENDED READINGS

Babbage, C. 1832. *On the economy of machinery and manufactures.* London: Charles Knight.

Barnard, C. 1938. *The functions of the executive.* Cambridge: Harvard University Press.

Bartol, K., and D. Martin. 1994. *Management.* 2nd ed. New York: McGraw-Hill.

Boone, L., and D.L. Kurtz. 1994. *Contemporary business communication.* Englewood Cliffs, NJ: Prentice Hall.

Deming, W.E. 1986. *Out of the crisis.* Cambridge: MIT Press.

Gilbreth, L. 1914. *The psychology of management.* New York: Sturgis and Walton.

Griffin, R.W. 1996. *Management.* Boston: Houghton Mifflin.

McGregor, D. 1960. *The human side of enterprise.* New York: McGraw-Hill.

Mayo, E. 1933. *The human problems of an industrial civilization.* New York: Macmillan.

Mintzberg, H. 1973. *The nature of managerial work.* New York: Harper & Row.

Munsterberg, H. 1913. *Psychology and industrial efficiency.* Boston: Houghton Mifflin.

Scholtes, P. 1988. *The team handbook.* Madison, WI: Joiner.

Stoner, J., A.E. Freeman, and D.A. Gilbert. 1995. *Management.* 6th ed. Englewood Cliffs, NJ: Prentice Hall.

Towne, H.R. 1886. The engineer as an economist. *Transactions of the American Society of Mechanical Engineers* 7: 428-432.

Van Fleet, D., and T. Peterson. 1994. *Contemporary management.* 3rd ed. Boston: Houghton Mifflin.

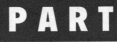

FRONT-OF-THE-HOUSE MANAGEMENT

Marketing and Sales

The purpose of this chapter is to present an overview of the marketing and sales process and to outline the marketing and sales responsibilities of health fitness managers. The chapters related to products and profit centers (chapter 10) and programming (chapters 8 and 9) include specific examples of marketing and sales initiatives.

Marketing, advertising, and selling are not the same. Distinguishing between these three overlapping activities is an important beginning to understanding the marketing process. Although commonly interchanged, we will use these terms in the following way:

- *Marketing* is the process of identifying what the public needs and determining whether you can provide it at a price that will produce a profit.

- *Advertising* is alerting the public that you have something to sell.

- *Selling* is the exchange of money for an existing product, service, or program.

A health fitness manager does not need a degree in marketing to create, implement, and manage an effective marketing and sales program. However, understanding fundamental marketing principles is necessary to be a successful manager.

MARKETING, ADVERTISING, AND SALES RESPONSIBILITIES

The health fitness manager has the primary responsibility to create, implement, and manage a process that achieves the following:

Marketing—identifying the specific needs of potential members and developing products and services to meet those needs.

Advertising—communicating information about the organization that addresses the identified needs.

Sales—selling programs, products, and services that fulfill the identified needs at a price that reflects the value to the member and results in a profit for the organization.

Figure 5.1 illustrates the proper sequence for a successful health fitness marketing and sales program. If the result of the marketing process is a steady stream of new members, the process is operating effectively. If a significant percentage of potential members fail to join the facility after engaging in the marketing process, it is a clear indication that some aspect of the process is inadequate. This chapter follows the sequence in looking at the three major elements of the marketing and sales process: marketing, advertising, and sales.

MARKETING AND SALES PROCESS

The marketing and sales process begins by defining a health fitness organization's philosophy as it relates to the marketplace. An organization achieves this first step by defining its *mission statement*. Every health fitness organization has a relationship with the marketplace that is defined by elements such as location, facility amenities, staffing, profit motive, and management or ownership priorities. For example, compare a hospital-based nonprofit health fitness center with a local for-profit commercial fitness center. Although physical facilities, staffing, and programming may appear similar, it is likely that one marketing priority, or mission, of the hospital-based facility is to attract members that are also potential clients for future primary medical care. In comparison, the for-profit fitness center has a more singular mission of providing fitness services that meet the needs of local members regardless of their potential medical needs. You would expect the mission statements of these two organizations to reflect their distinctly different relationship to the marketplace.

The second critical element of the marketing process is understanding the needs of the marketplace. From the standpoint of a health fitness organization, the needs of the marketplace translate into the needs of potential members. The principle objective of the marketing and sales process is not to manipulate members into accepting facilities, products, services, and programs that meet the sales needs of the health fitness organization, but to find effective and efficient means of allowing the organization to meet the needs of members.

The third element of the marketing and sales process is developing methods for effectively communicating to potential members the organization's ability to meet their needs. Advertising, membership referral programs, and sales promotions are several examples of methods for communicating with potential members.

The fourth element of the marketing and sales process is sales, receiving money for providing facilities, services, programs, and products that meet the needs and desires of members. Without an effective sales program, no health fitness organization will survive unless the organization is solely a charitable program without revenue expectations.

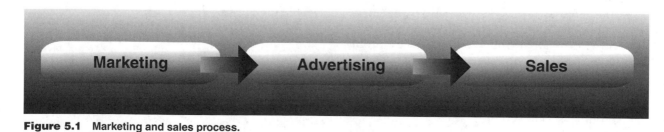

Figure 5.1   Marketing and sales process.

MARKETING

The marketing process focuses the attention of the health fitness manager and staff on understanding and serving member needs, rather than selling products, services, or programs.

> ▼ *The process of marketing involves (1) defining the health fitness organization's relationship with the marketplace, (2) determining what members and potential members want and need, and (3) identifying how those wants and needs can be most effectively fulfilled by the organization.*

These three elements of the marketing process are defined in terms of the health fitness organization's mission statement, *goals, objectives,* and *strategies.* The entire process is documented and monitored by detailing each element in a written marketing plan.

Mission Statement

Simply stated, a health fitness organization's *mission statement* defines the operational, philosophical, and financial direction of the organization. To be effective, the mission statement should be straightforward and easily understood. Although the identification of a clear-cut mission statement seems like a simple step in the marketing process, it is often misunderstood, forgotten, or overlooked.

The mission statement should define the long-term vision of the organization and identify unique qualities that differentiate the organization from others in the marketplace. The stated mission should provide direction and significance to all employees in the organization, regardless of their level of responsibility.

The basic questions that an organization must answer when it decides to examine and restate its mission are, "What is our business?" "Who are we serving?" "What should our product be?" and "Who should our customers be?" Although such questions may appear simple, they are in fact such difficult and critical questions that the major responsibility for answering them falls on senior management. In developing a statement of mission, management must

first consider the more global issues that define the organization, including history, distinctive competencies, and overall environment.

• *The organization's history.* Every health fitness organization, large or small, profit or nonprofit, has a history of objectives, accomplishments, mistakes, and policies. In formulating a mission statement, consider the critical characteristics and events of the past. For example, a local one-site fitness center may be considering a mission statement that focuses on expanding to multiple locations to serve a countywide area. However, a review of club history indicates frequent turnover of managers and difficulty in finding and keeping competent staff. In this example, a growth-focused mission is not realistic until the organization can demonstrate an ability to attract and maintain the managers and staff that will be necessary to open and operate multiple locations.

• *The organization's distinctive competencies.* Although there are many things an organization may be able to do, it should seek to do what it can do best. Distinctive competencies are things that an organization does well—so well in fact that they give it an advantage over similar organizations.

• *The organization's environment.* The organization's environment dictates the opportunities, constraints, and threats that must be identified before a mission statement is developed. For example, an organization's demographic environment may create opportunities to focus on special populations; the geographic location may require programs and schedules that cater to working members; and the area's *economic environment* may impact pricing and membership turnover.

> ▼ *When completed, an effective mission statement focuses on market and member needs rather than products. It is achievable, motivating, and specific. The mission statement should have an external rather than an internal focus.*

You can measure a successful mission statement by asking the following five questions:

1. Does the mission statement focus on the identified needs of the members?

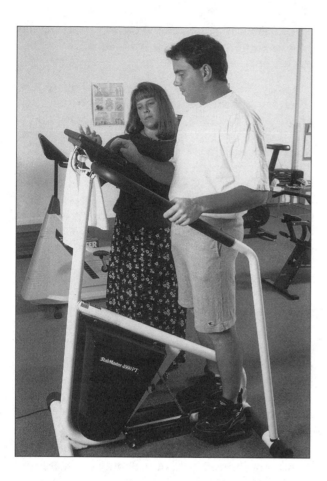

2. Is the mission clearly stated in a manner that is easily understood by everyone in the organization and by potential members?

3. Does the mission statement provide direction for developing new products, services, and programs?

4. Are performance objectives and other measurements of success in the organization based on the key elements of the mission statement?

5. Has the mission statement been reviewed lately, and does it still reflect the principle focus of the organization and the external market?

Mission Statement Viewpoints

Mission statements frequently reflect a specific orientation of the health fitness organization's ownership or management. Three common categories for mission statement approaches are product orientation, sales orientation, and marketing orientation.

Product Orientation

Health fitness organizations that are *product oriented* define their mission in terms of delivering products and services. Within these organizations, every deliverable aspect of the organization is viewed as a separate product. Aerobics classes, tennis lessons, snack bar services, locker room services, child care, service desk activities, weight room, racquet courts, wet areas, spa services, and so on are evaluated in terms of delivering the best product to members. Managers in a product-based organization frequently believe that future success is determined by increasing the quality and quantity of products available for members. For example, an aerobics studio with a product orientation will evaluate its success based on the number and range of classes offered. Each class is a different product that is reviewed independently for attendance, popularity, and effectiveness.

An example of a product-oriented mission statement is the following:

> *In partnership with our members, we will provide programming, products, and services to enhance the richly textured experience of a healthy lifestyle.*

Sales Orientation

Sales-oriented health fitness organizations define their missions in terms of increasing or maintaining a forecast rate of new membership sales. In these types of organizations, sales and service are frequently considered unrelated activities. As many health fitness organizations have discovered, long-term success is rarely achieved by a singular focus on sales that is not closely tied to the organization's service (product) orientation. Aggressive sales efforts for a poorly run organization may generate an infusion of short-term revenue. However, unless members are satisfied by the resulting level of service and programming, turnover and poor reputation will ultimately diminish the effectiveness of even the most aggressive sales efforts.

An example of a sales-oriented mission statement (for a publicly traded company) is as follows:

> *ACME Health Fitness Corporation is dedicated to maintaining its position as a growing, profitable organization and a leader in the health fitness industry. In this way we provide our shareholders a solid return on their investment, our employees with the benefits of gainful employment, and our members with the resources of a world-class organization.*

Marketing Orientation

Health fitness organizations that define their mission from a marketing orientation focus all their efforts on satisfying member's needs. In these organizations, the twin goals of member satisfaction and profit are reflected in every aspect of the organization. All activities—membership sales, program implementation, finance, membership services, and operations—are devoted to identifying the needs of current and potential members, then creating an organization that supports the delivery of the programs, facilities, products, and services to satisfy those needs. The underlying principle of a marketing-based mission statement is that if the needs and wants of its members are satisfied, a profit will result. By focusing on the needs of their members, a marketing-oriented organization will also reflect the changes in the marketplace. As member needs change, such as the trend toward family programs from the previous single adult focus, the organization also changes focus by modifying its mission.

An example of a marketing-oriented mission statement is the following:

We are in the business to please our members by providing a healthy lifestyle environment that meets or exceeds their expectations. Our primary measures of success are member satisfaction, low turnover, and a high number of referrals from existing members.

Goals and Objectives

A successful marketing process achieves an equilibrium between the short and the long term by balancing historical information with preparation for the inevitable changes in markets, technology, and competition. The output of the marketing process is developing a written marketing plan. Completing the marketing plan requires several steps: setting goals, establishing objectives, and determining action strategies.

Setting Goals

Goals are three-to-five-year milestones that are measurable or observable. Primary and secondary research (as described later in this chapter) provides the underlying support for selecting goals. The shorter-term focus of the goals distinguishes them from the long-term focus of the mission statement. If formulated properly, they can accomplish the following:

1. They can be converted into specific objectives.
2. They will provide clear-cut direction.
3. They can establish long-run (three-to-five-year) priorities.
4. They can facilitate management control by setting organizational standards.

Examples of health fitness organization goals include the following:

To provide members with programs and services that meet or exceed expectations as measured by our annual membership survey.

To provide a safe environment for our employees and members that is reflected by no injuries within the facility or on the property.

To provide a rewarding working environment for employees that promotes low turnover and high levels of personal challenge and satisfaction.

Establishing Objectives

Objectives are more specific than goals and should be achievable within one year. The organization's objectives should be quantifiable or measurable. As with the statement of mission and goals, organizational objectives must be more than good intentions or vague references to a management wish list. Management must translate the organizational mission into clear-cut goals, specific objectives, and ultimately, practical action strategies to support the realization of the mission.

The following list presents examples of organizational objectives. Note that they are specific statements of a continuing nature. They specify the end points of an organization's mission and the results that it seeks, both externally and internally. Most important, the following objectives are measurable commitments on the part of the organization.

Table 5.1   Organizational Strategy Matrix

	Present program	New programs
Present members	Market penetration	Program development
New members	Market expansion	Program diversification

Sample Objectives

Market standing—to make our organization number one in the market by achieving a 20 percent market share

Innovations—to be a leader in introducing new services by investing a minimum of 10 percent of annual revenue into developing new programs and services

Productivity—to service more members per employee and per square foot while raising membership annual satisfaction ratings

Physical resources—to lower replacement costs 15 percent by increasing maintenance budget by 10 percent

Profitability—to achieve an annual rate of return on investment of at least 15 percent

Manager performance—to reduce manager turnover and increase specific management skills in the areas of financial analysis and employee motivation

Employee performance—to reduce employee turnover and maintain levels of employee satisfaction

Social responsibility—to receive recognition as a corporate leader in the community by sponsoring healthy lifestyle community events and supporting volunteerism in civic organizations by managers, employees, and members

Developing Strategies

The challenge for health fitness organizations throughout the remainder of the 1990s and into the 21st century will be to develop strategies that reflect an accurate measurement of the needs and desires of the marketplace. There are four types of growth strategies a health and fitness facility can consider: market penetration, market expansion, new program development, and program diversification. As we discuss in the following examples, organizations may use a variety of approaches to achieve strategic growth.

Table 5.1 illustrates a program and market matrix showing the strategic alternatives available to a health fitness organization for achieving its objectives. An organization can grow in a variety of ways, by concentrating on present or new programs, by acquiring more of the same type of members, or by attracting different types of new members.

Market Penetration

The first growth strategy deals with attracting more participants to your established programs. This is termed *market penetration* and consists of two plans of action:

1. Attracting participants who are in other programs or who are working out at home

2. Encouraging existing participants to expand their current participation into new areas

Using a market penetration strategy, the health fitness manager is saying, "Let's keep doing what we have done in the past, just more of it." The manager takes a low risk by selling current services to similar buyers. Examples of market penetration strategy include increasing direct mail efforts, changing advertising medium, and making minor changes to programs and personnel.

A market penetration strategy is effective as long as membership is growing at an increasing rate.

Market Expansion

At some point, every market achieves a certain level of saturation. The majority of potential new members has been reached and turnover has been minimized. Health fitness organizations that find themselves in this market condition may need to identify and consider new products, services, or programs. By initiating a *market expansion* strategy, the health fitness manager is saying, "Let's take the programs we have and go after new target markets." The health fitness manager is recommending a moderate marketing risk by attempting to sell current products and services to new target markets.

> *If membership growth of an organization is less than 5 percent per year, a market expansion effort is a prudent strategy.*

As part of the strategy, the organization should consider adjustments to methods of promotion, modest changes in programs, and possible alternatives, such as offering programs in other locations as outreach programs. Perhaps changing or adding personnel will also help in expanding into new markets. For example, without building any new facilities, a health fitness club could consider adding children's programming, summer camps, and special sport clinics to expand into a new market for individuals with young adolescent children—same club, new target markets.

> *A market expansion strategy is effective as long as growth in the new markets continues at an increasing rate each year. Once the number of new members from the expanded market begins to dwindle, the organization needs to consider either new market targets or new program development.*

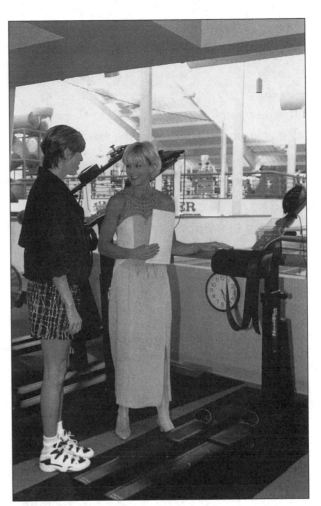

© Tom Wallace

New Program Development

There are predictable cycles in the life of every health fitness program, during which participants become bored with the same old routine. To secure a foothold in an existing market, a successful health fitness organization needs to develop new variations of existing programs. The transition from high- and low-impact aerobics, to step aerobics, to funk, to slide, and the many other variations are examples of new ways to vary existing group exercise class workout programs. Using a strategy of new program development, the health fitness manager is saying, "Let's do whatever it takes to update our programs to meet the needs of our current members." Programs, services, people, and pricing will be modified to reflect their current interest. Examples of this approach may include modifying facilities to add programming such as rock climbing, challenge courses, or completely replacing old resistance training equipment with interactive computerized equipment.

Market expansion frequently requires in-depth research to identify and estimate the demand for potential new markets and to determine the most effective manner of promoting the new products or services.

Most health fitness managers continually vary all aspects of their programs to maintain an overall growth policy. "Let's face it, eventually everyone gets bored with exercise. Fitness buffs are always looking for something different," one health fitness manager recently commented. "If we can constantly provide our clients with innovative programs, they are not likely to look elsewhere. If a client tells us of a new trend or a new service another club is offering, we realize we have to offer something comparable or they may be tempted to switch clubs."

In mature markets, without constant program innovation, health fitness organizations cannot respond to the changing needs of consumers or to the threats from competitors.

Diversification

To remain competitive in the future, health fitness organizations will need to search for methods of diversifying products and services. One method of achieving diversity is to create a network of services by combining the resources of a primary facility with other area programs. Examples of this type of networking *diversification* include combining access to swim clubs, golf clubs, dance facilities, and preventive health services through a single membership. The combined resources may be far more valuable to a potential member than the individual facility. Cross-selling services provides diversification without adding costly capital expenditures.

Another diversification strategy can be to take the extreme risk of creating untested, new

Evaluating Risk

Is there a method of selecting market strategies that will reduce risk? The most cost-effective route is to concentrate on market penetration first. When the growth rate of new members or revenue slows below 5 percent per year, modify the strategic plan to focus on market development. As growth of new markets diminishes, either try another form of market development or move to new program development. The most risky strategy, diversification, should be based on extensive market research and analysis. Moreover, it is important that all decisions related to strategies be based on the answers to the basic four questions:

1. What is the target market?

2. How big is it?

3. How does it behave?

4. Who are the existing competitors?

What other characteristics should you consider in developing specific strategies? Management should select strategies that are consistent with their mission and that capitalize on unique characteristics to create a competitive advantage. Unique programming, a high value-to-cost ratio, reputation for member service, convenient location, well-directed financial resources, continued program innovation, and effective marketing efforts are examples of distinctive competencies that can lead to a sustainable competitive advantage. Below are 10 principles for developing market strategies.

Ten Principles for Developing Marketing Strategies

1. Create member satisfaction.

2. Know your member characteristics.

3. Divide the market into specific segments.

4. Strive for a high market share.

5. Develop deep and wide products, programs, and services.

6. Use pricing to position products and services.

7. Use service to distinguish from competitors.

8. Promote and support member referrals.

9. Reward staff performance and encourage innovation.

10. Use information to improve decisions.

Table 5.2   A Comparison of Product-, Sales-, and Marketing-Oriented Strategies

	Product orientation	Sales orientation	Marketing orientation
Basic philosophy	Focus on development; sell what you can develop.	Focus on sales; more is better.	Focus on members; develop what they want to buy.
Product	Emphasize new product features.	Emphasize getting more sales for existing products.	Emphasize developing products based on members' needs and wants.
View of members	Get more products for them.	Get them to buy more.	Identify products and services to meet members' needs and wants.
Market research	Get member reaction to product.	Identify how to increase sales.	Identify members' needs and wants.
Profit	Emphasize profit potential of new products.	Increase sales leads to increase volume.	Provide products and services that have premium value to members.
Sales force	Roll out new products; use add-on pricing.	Sell more products; use special promotions.	Facilitate member purchase if product meets their needs; coordinate sales/service.
Promotion	Emphasize value of the product.	Emphasize product features and improvement over competition.	Emphasize benefits of product to meet members' needs and wants.
Internal organization	Focus on product development and the facilities for making the product available.	Focus on advertising, direct sales, and promotion.	Focus on integrating/coordinating all business activities.

products and services and attempting to sell them to new markets. For example, a decision to remodel an indoor tennis court into a boxing ring and martial arts training facility would constitute diversification and require a significant revision of promotion, programs, personnel, and pricing. To minimize the risk of total disaster, diversification requires in-depth research to identify and estimate the potential demand for new products, services, and facilities and to determine the most effective methods of promotion and pricing.

Table 5.2 compares product-, sales-, and marketing-oriented growth strategies. As the table illustrates, perhaps the most distinctive difference among the three approaches is in primary focus. Product growth focuses on developing new products, services, and programs. Sales growth focuses on selling more of the existing products, services, and programs. Finally, marketing growth focuses on developing the prod-

ucts, programs, and services that members want to buy.

Written Marketing Plan

The marketing process can be an impossible management challenge unless it is organized and monitored using a written plan. There are two important aspects of having a written plan versus a verbal plan that is never formally documented. First, the written plan document provides a resource to use as a checklist for evaluating its success or failure over time. Second, the written plan is the communication vehicle for notifying all personnel about the specific mission, goals, and objectives of the organization. As new employees join the organization, the plan document is the most accurate summary information about the organization.

The major elements of a marketing plan include

Task name	Start	End	Duration	Note	1997		1998				
					Nov	Dec	Jan	Feb	Mar	Apr	May
Marketing plan	22/Nov/97	21/Dec/97	21.00 d								
Market analysis	22/Nov/97	29/Nov/97	40.00 h								
Target market	22/Nov/97	24/Nov/97	24.00 h								
Competitive analysis	22/Nov/97	29/Nov/97	40.00 h								
Establish objectives	30/Nov/97	01/Dec/97	16.00 h								
Develop tactics	02/Dec/97	08/Dec/97	5.00 d								
Sales forecasts	09/Dec/97	13/Dec/97	24.00 h								
Staffing requirements	14/Dec/97	14/Dec/97	8.00 h								
Draft complete	14/Dec/97	14/Dec/97	0.00 h								
Review plan	15/Dec/97	21/Dec/97	5.00 d								
Advertising plan	21/Dec/97	08/Feb/98	30.00 d								
Meet with ad agency	21/Dec/97	21/Dec/97	0.00 h								
Sample ads from agency	22/Dec/97	06/Jan/98	10.00 d								
Review	07/Jan/98	13/Jan/98	5.00 d								
Approval	13/Jan/98	13/Jan/98	0.00 h								
Final layout	14/Jan/98	25/Jan/98	5.00 d								
Develop media schedule	26/Jan/98	08/Feb/98	10.00 d								
Send to periodicals	08/Feb/98	08/Feb/98	0.00 h								
Press release sent	06/Jan/98	06/Jan/98	0.00 h								
Present sales promotion	08/Feb/98	08/Feb/98	0.00 h								
Public relations	22/Dec/97	25/Jan/98	20.00 d								
Press tour	22/Dec/97	25/Jan/98	20.00 d								
Secure speakers	22/Dec/97	06/Jan/98	10.00 d								
Travel arrangements	07/Jan/98	13/Jan/98	5.00.d								
Prepare presentation	14/Jan/98	25/Jan/98	5.00 d								
Press release	22/Dec/97	06/Jan/98	10.00 d								
Write copy	22/Dec/97	29/Dec/97	5.00 d								
Review	30/Dec/97	06/Jan/98	5.00 d								
Approval	06/Jan/98	06/Jan/98	0.00 h								
Product brochure	22/Dec/97	09/Mar/98	50.00 d								
Read product spec	22/Dec/97	29/Dec/97	5.00 d								
Develop first draft of copy	30/Dec/97	13/Jan/98	10.00 d								
Technical review	14/Jan/98	25/Jan/98	5.00 d								
Final draft of copy	26/Jan/98	01/Feb/98	5.00 d								
Create graphics	02/Feb/98	15/Feb/98	10.00 d								
Page layout	16/Feb/98	23/Feb/98	5.00 d								
Printing	24/Feb/98	09/Mar/98	10.00 d								
Product brochure complete	09/Mar/98	09/Mar/98	0.00 h								
Customer mailing	22/Dec/97	15/Feb/98	35.00 d								
Develop copy	22/Dec/97	29/Dec/97	5.00 d								
Samples from ad agency	30/Dec/97	13/Jan/98	10.00 d								
Final format decisions	14/Jan/98	25/Jan/98	5.00 d								
Printing	26/Jan/98	08/Feb/98	10.00 d								
Materials to mail house	09/Feb/98	15/Feb/98	5.00 d								
Customer mailing sent	15/Feb/98	15/Feb/98	0.00 h								
Sales Promotion	22/Dec/97	11/Apr/98	14.40 w								
Develop promotional piece	22/Dec/97	01/Feb/98	25.00 d								
Copy	22/Dec/97	29/Dec/97	5.00 d								
Samples from agency	30/Dec/97	13/Jan/98	10.00 d								
Printing	14/Jan/98	01/Feb/98	10.00 d								
Distribution	02/Feb/98	08/Feb/98	5.00 d								
Ad campaign begins	11/Apr/98	11/Apr/98	0.00 w								
Video project	22/Dec/97	23/Feb/98	40.00 d								
Script	22/Dec/97	29/Dec/97	5.00 d								
Production	30/Dec/97	25/Jan/98	15.00 d								
Editing	26/Jan/98	08/Feb/98	10.00 d								
Duplicate masters	09/Feb/98	23/Feb/98	10.00 d								
Send video to sales	23/Feb/98	23/Feb/98	0.00 h								

Figure 5.2 Time line and deadlines for media marketing plan.

the following:

I. Organizational mission statement
II. Three-to-five-year goals
III. One-year objectives
IV. Specific action strategies
   A. Deadlines
   B. Responsibilities
   C. Budget requirements
   D. Measurable results
V. Barriers to success
   A. Staffing
   B. Market factors
   C. Financial resources
   D. Organizational issues

VI. Unique strengths of the organization
   A. Staffing
   B. Market factors
   C. Financial resources
   D. Organizational issues
VII. Other considerations

Within the marketing plan, create project time lines and develop deadlines for specific marketing action items that have many steps and need to be monitored over a period of months. As an example, figure 5.2 illustrates a detailed planning diagram for a multiple media marketing program.

Figure 5.3 shows an example of the section of a marketing plan outlining the specific marketing model used for a saturation direct mail campaign.

Marketing model for saturation use of flyers in primary zip code areas

1. Repeat flyers to target homes: one per week for 4-6 weeks.
2. Suggest flyers versus direct mail based on cost. Can get twice the coverage using flyers.
3. Select primary zip codes (14 areas) based on 90-day sales history.
4. Consider expanding to secondary zip codes (28 total) during grand opening weeks.
5. Support flyer program with newspaper ads. Consider repeat daily ads during a grand opening week versus spreading limited ads across all 4 weeks.

Club	Target homes	Tls / week	Jan Tls @ 1.5%	Appts. @ 95%/Tls	Closes @ 75%/apt.	Close % Tls/target	Jan $s @ $750
Arlington	10,000	38	150	135	100	66/1	75,000
Carrolton	20,000	75	300	285	200	66/1	150,000
DeSoto	10,000	38	150	135	100	66/1	75,000
Hulen	10,000	38	150	135	100	66/1	75,000
Mesquite	14,000	50	200	190	125	66/1	95,000
N.R. Hills	10,000	38	150	135	100	66/1	75,000
Oakridge	10,000	38	150	135	100	66/1	75,000
Plano	10,000	38	150	135	100	66/1	75,000
Preston	6,000	25	100	95	75	66/1	57,000
Total	**100,000**	**375**	**1,500**	**1,425**	**1,000**	**66%/1%**	**$752,000**

Expenses

100,000 flyers per week for 4 weeks = 400,000 flyers
400,000 flyers @ $400 per 5,000 = $32,000 distribution

Distribution	$32,000	
Printing	5,000	(?)
Newspaper ads	13,000	(?)
Total	$50,000	

Assumptions (These are for discussion and should be modified by actual club results.)
% of TI responses over one month	1.5%
% of TI scheduled appointments who show up for tour	95.0%
% of closes following tour	75.0%
% of closes from target homes	1.0%
Average value of memberships sold during January	$750

Figure 5.3 Marketing model for direct mail saturation campaign.

Marketing Research

Market research identifies potential clients, competitors, geographic and demographic data, industry data, management and marketing methodologies, pricing, historical trends, and future opportunities. Throughout the marketing process, current, reliable, and valid information is needed to make effective marketing decisions. The health fitness manager must develop access to useful information related to both internal and external positions of the organization. In some cases, managers and staff can conduct market research to avoid the cost of consultants.

Census reports and demographic information available through the local chamber of commerce and business bureau can yield a wealth of information. As part of your monthly activity, collect and maintain client-based information from a wide range of sources, including published reports, client surveys, personal contacts, and personal experience.

Success in a competitive market requires a systematic, professional approach to gathering information.

Understanding the External Market

You can evaluate the external factors that impact an organization by looking at six areas of concern: (1) the cooperative environment, (2) the competitive environment, (3) the economic environment, (4) the social environment, (5) the political environment, and (6) the legal environment. In analyzing each environment, the health fitness manager must search for opportunities and constraints or threats that impact the organization's objectives. Opportunities for profitable marketing often arise from changes in these environments that bring about new needs to satisfy. Constraints on marketing activities, such as unemployment in the local economy or the opening of a nearby competitor, also arise from these environments.

Cooperative Environment

The *cooperative environment* includes all firms and individuals who have a vested interest in the organization accomplishing its objectives: suppliers, vendors, contract service providers, and network partners within the community. Marketing opportunities in this environment are primarily related to methods of increasing efficiency. For example, a health fitness organization might decide to contract out or develop a cooperative arrangement with local food service or pro shop organizations. By taking advantage of these cooperative relationships, the club can focus its marketing efforts on its primary areas of business while continuing to have a broad range of services and products available to members. Considering the resources available in the cooperative environment as part of the marketing strategy may allow the health fitness organization to significantly reduce risks and costs for inventory overhead, supplies, and personnel in areas that are not part of the primary business.

Competitive Environment

The *competitive environment* includes other facilities, activities, and organizations in the market area that rival the health fitness organization for both resources and members. Opportunities in this environment include such things as (1) acquiring competing firms, (2) offering better value to members and attracting them away from competitors, (3) driving competitors out of the market, and (4) establishing cooperative programs with potential competitors. It is important to realize that competition for health fitness organizations comes from a wide range of demands on leisure-time activity and disposable income. In many market areas, after-school and weekend children's sport, religious, and social organizations, and free or nominally priced community or college facilities provide competition for the time and money of potential members. As part of the overall marketing strategy, the health fitness organization should understand the impact of each primary competitive market factor and develop positive, specific strategies that respond to them. Pricing, scheduling, products, and services are all influenced by the competitive environment.

Economic Environment

The state of the economy also creates marketing opportunities and constraints. For example, factors such as high inflation and unemployment can limit the available disposable income in a market area. Lower amounts of disposable income correlate to lower membership sales for health fitness services. At the same time, these factors may offer a profitable opportunity to expand into the corporate fitness market and look for other buyers of group services. In addition, changes in technology can provide significant threats and opportunities. For example, each time new, unique fitness-related equipment

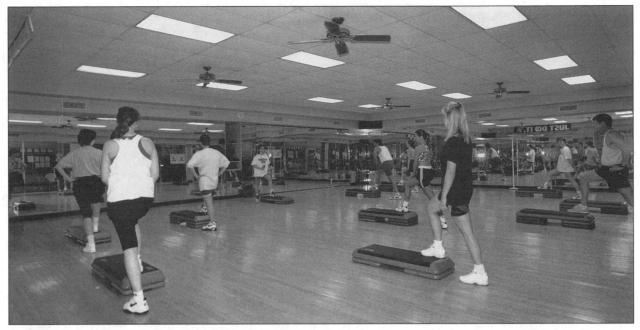

© Tom Wallace

becomes available, an opportunity is created to capture member interest in a new area of fitness. However, it may require more capital than an organization can afford and create a threat when competitors upgrade first.

Social Environment

The social environment includes cultural and social traditions, norms, and attitudes. Although these values change slowly, such changes often bring about the need for new programs and services. For example, healthier eating habits increase the desirability of healthy snack bars in clubs. Baby boomer members demand greater alternatives for children's programming and child care. The aging population has created new demands for senior programs. Health fitness organizations must maintain a forward-looking view to identify these trends. Although they may create profit opportunities, the organization must be in a position to plan for possible facility remodeling expenses to deliver new services.

Political Environment

The *political environment* includes the attitudes and reactions of the general public, social and business critics, and other professional organizations, such as the American College of Sports Medicine (ACSM), the American Heart Association, and the U.S. Surgeon General's Report (1996). Changes in the political environment frequently are the impetus for external guidelines, regulations, and operational standards. For example, a new no-smoking ordinance in a city or county

could create opportunities to aggressively market smoking cessation programs. A governmental report on the fitness level of children in public schools might create the opportunity to provide contract programs to train teachers or coaches in the local school district.

Legal Environment

The *legal environment* includes federal, state, and local laws; administrative rules; permits; licensing; and other government inspections. Legal regulatory issues for health fitness operations include health and safety regulations, food and beverage permits, specialty licensing requirements, child care regulations, fire and building code issues, tax permits and reports, disability accessibility regulations, and many other governmental standards. Legal liability issues for health fitness organizations include standards of care for negligence, contract law, uniform commercial code (sales) warranties, the Fair Credit Reporting Act (credit card sales), and a wide range of employment-related claims. Review chapter 17 for a more detailed discussion of legal issues for health fitness organizations.

Using Demographic Data

You can use *demographic data* to define the primary market area for a health fitness facility. Based on industry standards, analyzing demographic and economic data within a 5-mile radius is a conservative measure of the primary market for a health club. The accepted standard for evaluating the

Table 5.3   External Market Questions

The environment

1. What is the state of the economy, and are there any trends that could affect the industry, organization, or previous marketing strategy?

2. What are current trends in cultural and social values, and how do these affect the industry, organization, or marketing strategy?

3. What are current political values and trends, and how do they affect the industry, organization, or marketing strategy?

4. Is there any current or pending federal, state, or local legislation that could change the industry, organization, or marketing strategy?

5. Overall, are there any threats or opportunities in the environment that could influence the industry, organization, or marketing strategy?

The marketplace

1. What is the geographic definition of the market area?

2. Who are the major competitors in the market area, and what are their annual sales, market share, and growth profile?

3. What strategies have competitors in the market area been using, and what has been their success with them?

4. What are the relative strengths and weaknesses of competitors in the industry?

5. How much threat is there of new competitors coming into the market area, and what are the major entry barriers?

primary market for a residential area or suburban facility is a 15-minute drive time radius. The following are examples of demographic data that define a primary market:

Primary market area—total population, 18 years or older, within a 5-mile radius

Primary market size—total number of households within the primary market area

Age distribution by gender—distribution by age groups, 18 to 24, 25 to 39, 40 to 49, 50 or older

Household family types—percent of households with single adult or couples, with or without children

Female family work status—evaluation of working versus nonworking women, with or without children

Household income—percent of households with $35,000 income or greater and average household income

Single versus multifamily—distribution of housing by type occupied

Owner versus renter—percent distribution of housing by owner versus renter

Table 5.3 is a checklist of questions that you should use to direct an analysis of the external market.

Understanding the Internal Market

Consumer demand is considered the driving force behind the majority of industrial innovation. In addition, one of the most frequent reasons members give for leaving a facility is management's unwillingness to listen and respond to their needs. These combined factors point out that in the health fitness industry, as in any other industry, the most valuable feedback comes from the consumer.

Keep in mind that what may be new and innovative programming today will eventually become commonplace. In your client interviews and surveys, be sure to ask which programs your members feel are the most valuable, and take action in your organization based on this feedback. Underused programs should be either replaced or updated. For example, by conducting a simple membership survey, one club discovered that the declining participation in their exercise classes was because of the club's failure to update the music selection available for the instructors. The members were burned out on the old music and began seeking other programs. With a small investment, the club was able to invigorate the exercise program and show a direct response to member preferences.

Member Surveys

Successful clubs make it a priority to maintain an open dialogue with members and guests by using suggestion boxes, distributing *membership surveys*, publishing monthly newsletters, and conducting focus groups. Client surveys can be an effective tool for tapping into new markets. One club reported that a membership survey conducted several years ago indicated a large group of members with special medical and orthopedic needs. In response, the staff developed guidelines for trainers to follow when dealing with problems such as continuing knee and shoulder rehabilitation, hypertension, diabetes, and exercise for pre- and postnatal women. The club has gained a reputation in the community for specialized care, which has become their specialty niche. In recent years the club has been developing asthma, adolescent, and sport-specific protocols.

Membership Databases

There is an old marketing adage that states, "Your next member will most likely look like your last new member." This is the principle for developing and maintaining a functional *membership database*. A good system should provide a variety of demographic information about an organization's member base and produce regular reports to indicate important trends. For example, a health fitness manager should be concerned if membership analysis indicates unusual departures or turnover within a specific age group or from a particular geographic area. Frequently these trends indicate an area that should receive immediate attention or at least become the focus of investigation.

Membership management software programs effectively record and report information in these categories. However, consider integrating membership accounting and demographic information. Not all systems automatically provide a comprehensive or interactive relationship between these areas. A common error in managing membership information is establishing separate systems for storing data, for example, keeping one set of membership names and addresses on an accounting system for billing purposes and a separate set for mailing list and marketing programs. The result is that modifying name or address information on one record does not update the other. In a surprisingly short time it is impossible to generate accurate membership information from either system.

Developing membership data systems should be a process that involves all departments of the organization to ensure compatibility and appropriate access.

Other Sources of Information

A wide variety of information sources are available to the creative health fitness manager. Secondary research (already published) sources are usually free or nominally priced, provided by government agencies, industry groups, trade magazines, bar associations, chambers of commerce, economic development organizations, community organizations, university publications, national and regional magazines, and on-line research databases.

In some cases, primary research (collection of original data using techniques such as questionnaires, surveys, interviews, and focus groups) is the most effective source of information. Reviewing the results of another club's published client survey results is helpful for broad issues, but does not specifically identify what *your* clients or prospective clients want. Employee feedback at staff meetings is a common source of suggestions for improvements in member services, cost savings, and profitability. Primary research can be formal or informal, based on your budget, timing, or the critical impact the results will have on decisions and planning. Formal primary research includes developing a structured questionnaire, identifying a representative sample group, and obtaining responses to the questionnaire in person, on the telephone, or through the mail. It is common to use outside consultants to help with a formal primary research effort. However, formal primary research does not need to be complicated or time consuming. It can be as simple as implementing the following *Rule of 10*. The Rule of 10 is a process of developing 10 specific questions to be answered by 10 individuals on a selected topic. To implement the Rule of 10, use the following directions.

1. Develop 10 questions on a specific topic that individuals can answer by rating the response on a scale of 1 to 10, with 10 being "most important" or "strongly agree."

2. Prepare a simple survey form that has each question and a place to record the 1-to-10 rating for each question. Include a header with spaces for the date, name of the person interviewed, and information such as company, title, address, telephone number, and fax number.

3. Leave blank space at the bottom of the page to record additional comments.

4. Identify 10 individuals who can provide useful input on the topic you have selected.

5. Schedule an appointment to spend 10 minutes with each individual. Tell them the topic ahead of time, and briefly describe why you are gathering the information.

6. Meet with each individual, briefly review the topic and why you are gathering the information, then go through the questions. Try to keep the entire process to 10 minutes, as promised.

7. However, once you have completed the questionnaire, thank the respondent for his help, sit back, then ask a final open-ended question such as, "Is there anything else I should consider about [this topic]?" or "Do you have any other suggestions for me related to [this topic]?" This is the point at which some of the best feedback, ideas, and recommendations are given.

8. Record the information in the blank space at the bottom of the survey form. You may want to wait until after the interview to summarize the comments if taking notes will distract from the conversation.

9. When you have completed all 10 interviews, tally the results, determine the average score for each question, and rank the questions in order of importance.

10. In addition to the numerical ranking, combine and list all other comments in appropriate topic groups.

Applying the Rule of 10 requires a total expenditure of less than two days' effort. Using this direct, but effective, approach will generate valuable, client-based, marketing information on almost any topic.

Obtaining Informal Opinions

Lack of resources or time to complete a formal primary research effort are not sufficient reasons to abandon all efforts to obtain external input. Informal primary research can be quick, effective, and provide a valuable snapshot of a specific issue. Informal primary research includes brainstorming sessions, organized focus groups, and discussions with knowledgeable or experienced individuals. To be effective, organized discussion sessions need to have an identified leader, focus on a specific topic, and summarize information obtained during the session. Individual discussions should also focus on a specific issue with comments and opinions summarized in writing.

Information-Gathering Summary

A combination of formal and informal information-gathering techniques should be part of an ongoing marketing process to identify potential clients, individual client needs and priorities, specialty practice niches, competition, and trends in the marketplace. This information provides the basis to define services from the standpoint of the client and the marketplace. As a summary of the market research process, table 5.4 provides a checklist that leads you through the four major steps to follow.

Table 5.4   Checklist for Market Research Process

Define external market	Use demographic research.
	Conduct market studies.
	Identify niche markets and opportunities.
	Look for market trends.
Define internal market	Conduct personal interviews.
	Develop and distribute client surveys.
	Use suggestion boxes.
	Involve staff.
	Track member demographics.
Consider options	Get feedback from all involved parties.
	Research other similar programs.
	Weigh advantages versus disadvantages.
	Communicate and explain decisions.
Implement plan	Involve staff.
	Be flexible.
	Look for early successes.
	Follow up.
	Collect regular feedback.
	Monitor results.
	Make adjustments.

Table 5.5 Relative Cost and Impact of Advertising			
Method	**Type**	**Cost**	**Impact**
Advertising	Television	$$$$$	!!!!
	Radio	$$$$	!!!
	Direct mail	$$	!!!
	Newspapers	$$	!!
	Billboards	$$	!
Personal contact	Referrals		
	Friends/relatives	$	!!!!!
	Other members	$	!!!!!
	Selective calling		
	Special lists	$$	!!
	Cold calling	$$	!
Special events	Receptions/parties	$$$	!
	Sponsored events	$$$$$	!

$$$$$ = most expensive

Developing a Marketing Budget

There are no fixed rules for allocating money or time for marketing activities. Unfortunately, little objective data is available. The primary reason is that many health fitness organizations are privately held organizations and, as such, have no reason to share any significant financial information. IHRSA data and limited reports from Club Industry Magazine are the most reliable sources.

Start with a budget that you estimate will provide adequate resources to achieve your goals and objectives. Modify the budget based on annual results. Remember, most marketing activities take six months to a year to show results. Do not abandon your plan too early. Complete at least six months to a year before making major changes. As a rule, monitor marketing plans and budgets quarterly and thoroughly review and revise annually.

ADVERTISING

The second major element of the marketing and sales process is developing communication strategies that involve advertising and promotions. Although the number of media and media combinations available for advertising is overwhelming at first glance, four interrelated factors limit the number of practical alternatives. First, the nature of the specific health fitness organization may limit the number of practical and efficient alternatives. Second, the nature and size of the target market also limits appropriate advertising media. Third, the organization's advertising budget may restrict the use of expensive media, such as television. Although these factors reduce media alternatives to a more manageable number, specific media must still be selected. A primary consideration at this point is media effectiveness or efficiency.

Measuring Advertising Productivity

In the advertising industry, a common measure of efficiency or productivity is *cost per thousand* or CPMs. This figure refers to the dollar cost of reaching 1,000 prospects, and its chief advantage lies in its simplicity and allowance for a common base of comparison among differing media types. The major disadvantage of using CPMs also relates to its simplicity. CPMs do not reflect the demographic differences of the audience.

Measuring Advertising Impact

Table 5.5 compares the relative costs of various advertising alternatives. The chart also includes an estimate of the relative impact each advertising alternative has on potential members. The ratings are based on observations and do not represent a formal study. However, the comparisons provide a base from which to begin your evaluation of appropriate types of advertising activities.

Table 5.6 Advantages and Disadvantages of Selected Media

Media	Advantages	Disadvantages
Newspapers	Flexible and timely. Intense coverage of local markets. Broad acceptance and use. High believability of printed word.	Short life. Read quickly. Small pass-along audience.
Radio	Large, broad audience. Audience selectivity via station format. Low cost (per unit of time). Geographic flexibility.	Audio presentation only. Less attention than TV. Wide range of rates. Short life.
Outdoor signage	Flexible. Relative absence of competing advertisements. Repeat exposure. Relatively inexpensive.	Creative limitations. Many distractions for viewer. Limited selectivity of audience.
Television	Multimedia impact. Appeals to senses. Mass audience coverage.	Nonselectivity of audience. Fleeting impressions. Short life. Very expensive.
Magazines	High geographic and demographic selectivity. Quality of reproduction. Pass-along readership.	Long closing periods (6 to 8 weeks before publication). Some waste circulation. No guarantee of position (unless premium is paid).
Direct mail	Audience selectivity. Flexible. Low cost.	Consumers often pay little attention and throw it away.

Advantages and Disadvantages of Selected Media

Selecting specific advertising methods will require careful analysis of your organization's market, programs, and services. Although each market will be different, there are certain characteristics that allow a health fitness manager to evaluate the strengths and weaknesses of specific types of advertising. In most cases, mounting a successful advertising campaign requires the assistance of an advertising or public relations firm. Although their fees may appear prohibitive initially, there is little value in spending media placement dollars to send out an ineffective message. Table 5.6 compares the advantages and disadvantages of different types of media advertising.

Member Promotions

Member promotions can fulfill several distinct objectives. Some more commonly sought-after objectives include (1) inducing the member to try a new program, (2) encouraging and rewarding referrals, and (3) developing opportunities for members to trade up to higher value memberships. Examples of member promotions include the following:

1. **Credits**—providing a credit or cash bonus for bringing in a referral
2. **Sweepstakes and contests**—offering cash or prizes during a membership drive
3. **Premiums**—giving rewards or gifts
4. **Coupons**—providing discounts for future programs or services

Example of Existing Member Promotion

The elements of a membership promotion for a new one-on-one fitness training program for women members only are given on the next page.. Current members would be charged a sign-up fee in addition to dues to join the special program.

Membership promotions are also effective for new members. Some forms of new member promotion activities include the following:

1. *Sampling*—offering trial memberships either free or at a nominal price
2. *Pricing specials*—providing discounts from the regular price

---

Name of the promotion: LadyWorks Premier!

Pricing: Multisession package fee

Premiums for participating

LadyWorks Premier warm-up and oversized T-shirt

LadyWorks Premier tote bag

LadyWorks Premier diary

Specially designated lockers and baskets for participants while in the program

Reserved parking at front door for LadyWorks Premier

Special punch cards to keep track of LadyWorks Premier workouts

Postprogram shopping spree with promotional discounts

Promotions and advertising

Badges for all fitness staff, "Ask me about LadyWorks Premier!"

Posters to place at check-in area and locker rooms

Flyers for lockers and baskets

Information for service desk and all program personnel

Mannequin for front door with sample outfit

---

3. *Bonus deals*—adding extra months or years to initial membership terms at no additional charge

Example of a New Member Promotion

Figure 5.4 shows an example of a New Year's promotion for a local women-only health fitness facility. The promotion used local mailing lists to create a personalized letter to women in the primary market area. It is an excellent example of using a calendar event as the focus of a membership promotional strategy.

SALES

The third element of the health fitness marketing and sales process is the actual sale of memberships, services, programs, and products. One primary responsibility of the health fitness man-

ager is to oversee the sales process. The goal of the sales process is threefold: (1) to create an environment in which sales and service are the primary responsibilities of every employee, (2) to develop and schedule training programs in which every employee participates, and (3) to establish and communicate sales-specific objectives that are understood throughout the organization.

Sales Training

Each organization needs to develop a sales training program that meets the specific needs of the organization. Although each program will be unique, there are common characteristics observed in many successful sales training programs, including the following:

- 100 percent training for all staff
- System of retraining for those who fall below sales goals
- Consistent delivery from every sales person throughout the organization
- Limited- or no-variation step-by-step sales protocol
- Training-practice-evaluation-correction-feedback-retraining process
- Opportunities to advance to sales management
- Systems to ensure minimization of record-keeping errors
- Maximum follow-up for noncloses
- Heavy focus on referrals from existing members

Table 5.7 provides a checklist of elements for a sales training program.

Developing Successful Sales Strategies

Develop specific sales strategies as part of your marketing and planning process. Some common categories of sales strategies include special pricing for group and corporate sales, use-based pricing for access during restricted times or for selective parts of the facility, and add-on pricing that increases the basic membership fee revenue from special programs or products.

Timing throughout the year is also an important element for sales strategies. In the northern United States, special membership promotions generally precede the cold winter months. In the southern parts of the country, summer heat increases demand

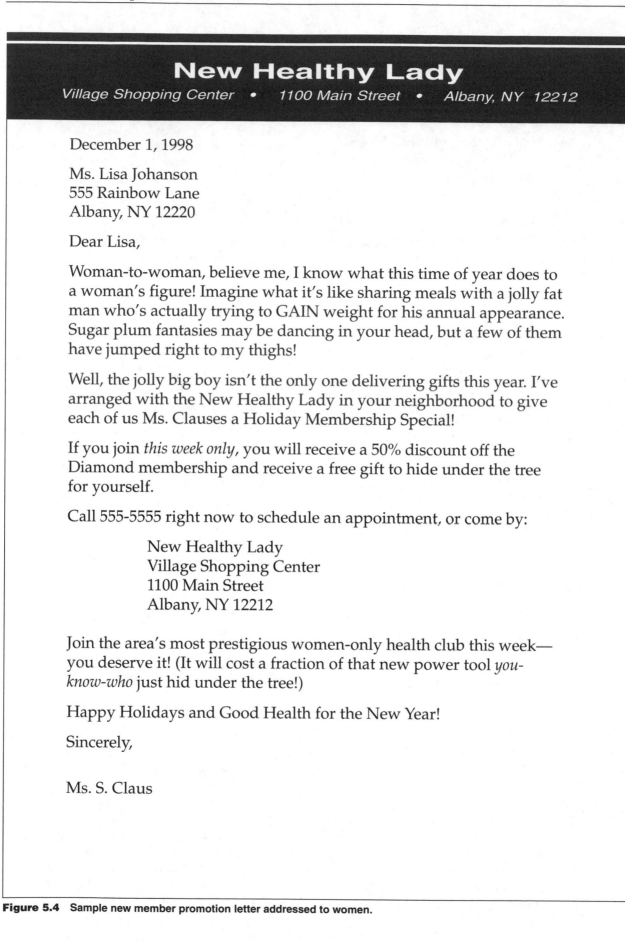

New Healthy Lady

Village Shopping Center   •   1100 Main Street   •   Albany, NY 12212

December 1, 1998

Ms. Lisa Johanson
555 Rainbow Lane
Albany, NY 12220

Dear Lisa,

Woman-to-woman, believe me, I know what this time of year does to a woman's figure! Imagine what it's like sharing meals with a jolly fat man who's actually trying to GAIN weight for his annual appearance. Sugar plum fantasies may be dancing in your head, but a few of them have jumped right to my thighs!

Well, the jolly big boy isn't the only one delivering gifts this year. I've arranged with the New Healthy Lady in your neighborhood to give each of us Ms. Clauses a Holiday Membership Special!

If you join *this week only*, you will receive a 50% discount off the Diamond membership and receive a free gift to hide under the tree for yourself.

Call 555-5555 right now to schedule an appointment, or come by:

> New Healthy Lady
> Village Shopping Center
> 1100 Main Street
> Albany, NY 12212

Join the area's most prestigious women-only health club this week— you deserve it! (It will cost a fraction of that new power tool *you-know-who* just hid under the tree!)

Happy Holidays and Good Health for the New Year!

Sincerely,

Ms. S. Claus

Figure 5.4   Sample new member promotion letter addressed to women.

Table 5.7   Checklist for Sales Training Program

A. Information and facts regarding the club
____ All rules, regulations, and policies
____ Guest policies
____ Membership types
____ Club schedule
____ Facilities
____ Size
____ Daily usage procedures
____ Reservation policies
____ In-house mail and communications procedures
____ Program schedules and availabilities
____ Fee collection procedures
____ Teamwork approach
____ Fitness staff and qualifications

B. Club sales presentation
____ Club story
____ Handling objections
____ Price presentation
____ Closing procedures
____ Finding selling points
____ Giving the tour
____ Using audiovisual aids
____ Sales presentation scripts

C. Sales process
____ Overall selling plan
____ Using the phones
____ Prospecting
____ Handling guests
____ Using the mail
____ How to use scripts
____ Time management and utilization
____ Professional standards
____ Self-attitude
____ Motivating
____ Questioning techniques
____ Listening techniques
____ Prospect motivation
____ How to work at full capacity
____ Problem solving
____ Industry knowledge
____ Communication skills
____ Sales language
____ Using a prospect card (to be developed)

D. Membership administration
____ Handling applications
____ Collecting money
____ Paperwork procedures
____ Reporting forms and systems

for swimming programs and inside sport and exercise alternatives. Throughout the country, New Year's resolutions are common incentives for new members and should be the focus of at least one major membership drive. Each health fitness manager will need to evaluate the seasonal impact on various programs and services and continually look for ways to use the seasons to positively impact membership sales and program participation.

Results From a Successful Sales Program

Evaluate the sales process from the standpoint of specific, observable, measurable, and predictable results. The following are examples of results that you can achieve with an effective sales process:

1. Higher percentage of closes for trained sales personnel
2. Improved sales staff morale across the board
3. Lower turnover of sales staff
4. Higher quality new sales staff
5. Reduction in crisis management

6. Improved planning due to data (sales and demographic) accuracy
7. Increased training allowing for upward mobility for successful personnel

Establishing a Standardized Sales Process

Regardless whether the primary source of new member sales is from the telephone, walk-ins, appointments, or referrals, the sales process must be standardized to maintain long-term effectiveness. The following sales training program outline includes examples of standardized procedures.

Sales Training Program Outline

Session I

A. Club orientation.
   1. Pass out rules and regulations and discuss them.
   2. Review guest policies.
   3. Present membership prices and types.

4. Take tour of facilities.

5. Discuss club teamwork.

B. Sales process.

1. Handling guests.

2. Other prospecting.

3. Overall club sales process.

4. Professionalism.

C. Club sales presentation.

1. Stage a mock membership sale between two people who know what's going on.

2. Introduce sales presentation; review all sections. Briefly relate to mock membership sale.

3. Pass out sales presentation scripts; instruct individuals to read and memorize them.

Session II

A. Review club orientations from last session and start new material.

1. Reservation procedures.

2. Daily usage procedures.

3. Review club programs.

B. Sales process.

1. Demonstrate the proper way to tour.

2. Discuss questioning and listening techniques.

C. Sales presentation.

1. Practice sections of sales presentation, the club story, benefit search, and club tour.

Session III

A. Club orientation written test—membership coordinator should be responsible for all materials presented.

1. Correct test out loud; give the right answers.

B. Building success.

1. Time management.

2. Setting goals.

3. Money management.

4. Striving to do more.

C. Sales presentation.

1. Practice handling objections.

2. Review last session's work.

Session IV

A. Problem solving.

1. Create situational problems for membership coordinators to solve.

2. Discuss dealing with tough guest situations.

B. Administration.

1. Introduce tracking system.

2. Discuss new member setup and administration.

3. Discuss prospecting.

C. Sales work.

1. Practice membership closes.

2. Practice handling objections.

3. Review the rest of the presentation.

Session V

A. Practice making presentations.

1. Theater environment.

2. Using mirror.

3. Group evaluations.

B. Show inspirational film or play tape.

1. Start on motivational work.

2. Demonstrate what success can do.

Tools and Systems to Use in the Training Process

We remember 20 percent of what we hear, 40 percent of what we see, and 60 percent of what we hear and see.

Visual aids

1. Movies and films

2. Video cassettes

3. Slide shows

4. Flip charts

5. Flash cards

Audio aids

1. Cassette tapes

2. Live telephone conversations

Written aids

1. Magazine articles

2. Books

3. Workbooks

Live presentations

1. Lectures

2. Question and answer periods

3. Role playing sessions

4. Simulated sales situations

5. Miniconferences and round table meetings

6. Scripted play acting

7. Group evaluations

8. Mirror selling

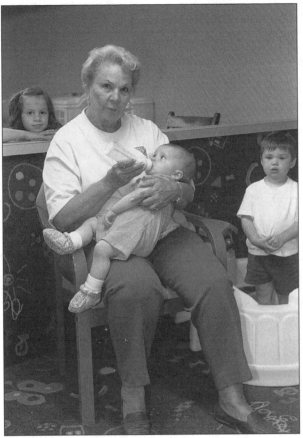

© Tom Wallace

There are several methods for establishing sales goals and keeping track of sales results. Most programs center on detailed record keeping of the sales goals, activities, and results on a daily, weekly, and monthly basis. Figures 5.5, 5.6, and 5.7 illustrate examples of simple sales tracking forms.

The first level of record keeping is the daily sales record. Figure 5.5 is an example of a daily production sheet that records the goals and production for prospect phone calls, member phone calls, appointments made, presentations made, mailings completed, and total sales made for the day. In a single sheet, goals, results, and the specific names of appointments and prospects are recorded.

At the end of the week, each sales person should complete a weekly report. Figure 5.6 provides an example of a weekly sales production sheet. The weekly report summarizes the goals for every day of the upcoming week.

To manage the club's overall sales progress, maintain a monthly sales production record on a week-by-week basis. Figure 5.7 provides an example of a sales production record that provides a running month-to-date record of each salesperson's results from the previous week, the current week, and the

total to date. This report is repeated every week during the month to allow the manager to track overall performance.

For most organizations, using results-oriented measures will be more effective than using the traditional effort-oriented measurements.

Compensation for Sales Personnel

Compensation is an important aspect of recruiting and retaining an effective sales force. Devising a compensation plan for a sales department is a technical matter, but there are some general guidelines in formulating such a plan. First, the compensation system should make sense to both management and the sales force. Second, the system should be fair and equitable and reward performance in proportion to results. Third, the system should allow the salesperson to earn a competitive salary to comparable sales positions in other businesses. Fourth, the system should attempt to minimize attrition by providing a long-term opportunity to grow within the organization. Finally, and perhaps most important, the system must support the overall marketing and sales plan for the organization.

The two types of sales compensation are salary and commission. Salary usually refers to a specific amount of monetary compensation at an agreed rate for definite time periods. Commission is usually monetary compensation based on number or volume of sales. It is common to mix a base salary with a commission program to create sales incentives.

PUBLIC RELATIONS

It is easy to confuse advertising and public relations activities because both share the objective of placing information into the public media. The simple distinction is that advertising is paid placement of information, whereas *public relations* information, if newsworthy, is placed at no charge. The benefit of good public relations coverage is that the health fitness organization may get thousands of dollars worth of coverage free. The limitation is that the information must be deemed newsworthy by the media before it will be printed or broadcast. The activities that might generate public relations coverage include speeches, sponsorships of nonprofit fundraising events, grand openings of new facilities, special contests, awards, and other meaningful human interest stories.

My Daily Individual Production Sheet
(to be filled in daily)

Employee name: _____

Club: _____

My goals today	Goal	Actual
Phone calls to prospects		
Phone calls to members		
Appointments to set		
Presentations to make		
Mailings to go out		
Other sales phone calls		
Total number of sales		

Today's Work Summary

Appointments		Calls to make		Other work notes
Name	**Time**			
1.		1.	11.	
2.		2.	12.	
3.		3.	13.	
4.		4.	14.	
5.		5.	15.	
6.		6.	16.	
7.		7.	17.	
8.		8.	18.	
9.		9.	19.	
10.		10.	20.	
11.				
12.				

Figure 5.5   Daily sales production sheet.

My Weekly Individual Goal Sheet
(to be filled in at the end of each week in preparation for next week)

Employee name: _____

Club: _____

My weekly goals	Mon	Tue	Wed	Thurs	Fri	Sat	Totals
Prospect phone calls to make							
Prospect phone calls to members							
Appointments to set							
Presentations to be made							
Mailings to go out							
Total number of sales							

To help me reach my goals this week I need to:

1.	7.
2.	8.
3.	9.
4.	10.
5.	11.
6.	12.

Figure 5.6 Weekly sales production sheet.

Public relations information is disseminated to the media using press releases and press packets. Included in a press release packet is usually a brief (1/2 to 2 pages) written story of the subject, photos, audio- or videotapes (depending on whether the target is print, radio, or television media), background information, and lists of contacts for additional information. Present all information in a format and tone that generates interest in the subject and creates the image that the public would either be interested in the story or would benefit by knowing the information. Some health fitness organizations retain the services of a public relations firm to assist in developing the press information and to actively promote media placement.

IN CLOSING

This chapter provided an overview of the marketing and sales process and responsibilities of health fitness managers. A health fitness manager does not need a degree in marketing to create, implement, and manage an effective marketing and sales program. However, understanding fundamental marketing concepts and principles is necessary to be a successful manager.

KEY TERMS

Advertising
Competitive environment
Cooperative environment
Cost per thousand

Weekly Sales Chart

Club: _____   Club quota: _____   Week ending: _____

Name	Sales last week	Goal last week	Mon	Tue	Wed	Thur	Fri	Sat	This week's total	Sales this month	Goal this month

Figure 5.7 Monthly sales production record.

Demographic data
Diversification
Economic environment
Goals
Legal environment
Market expansion
Marketing
Market penetration
Market research
Membership database
Membership surveys
Mission statement
Objectives
Political environment
Product oriented
Public relations
Rule of 10
Sales oriented
Selling
Social environment
Strategies

RECOMMENDED READINGS

Anderson, R.L., and J.S. Dunkelberg. 1993. *Managing small businesses*. St. Paul: West.

Corman, J., and R.N. Lussier. 1996. *Small business management*. Chicago: Irwin.

Drucker, P.F. 1985. *Innovation and entrepreneurship, practice and principles*. New York: Harper & Row.

King, J.B. 1996. *Business plans to game plans*. Santa Monica, CA: Merritt.

Peter, J.P., and J.H. Donnelly, Jr. 1994. *A preface to marketing management*. 6th ed. Chicago: Irwin.

Timmons, J.A. 1994. *New venture creation*. Chicago: Irwin.

U.S. Department of Health and Human Services. 1996. *Physical activity and health: A report of the Surgeon General*. Atlanta, Georgia: U.S. Department of Health and Human Services, Centers for Disease Control and Prevention, National Center for Chronic Disease Prevention and Health Promotion.

Member Management

Control and maintenance of the *membership database* is an important task in the daily operation of a health fitness facility. The membership database contains vital information for many of the club's operational departments. Membership sales teams need accurate information to continue their marketing efforts; accounting requires up-to-date records to continue the billing cycle without interruption; and the programming departments require accurate demographic information to invite members to participate. Is the membership database current and accurate in your facility? Is the information contained in the database mined for meaningful marketing information? Is the database information secured from unauthorized access? Find out how to get the most out of your membership database from the following information.

The membership database in each facility holds a wealth of information for the enterprising health fitness manager.

Proper database management includes the responsibility of not only maintaining secure, accurate, and complete demographic and billing information, but also gathering and using the wealth of information to optimize retention.

Vital to the profitability of the organization is a secure, accurate, and comprehensive membership database.

In this chapter we examine the many aspects of a complete membership database and the ways in which the resourceful health fitness manager can use this information to attract solid prospects, offer popular programming, optimize payroll spending through efficient scheduling, and retain a solid dues-paying membership (see figure 6.1). We discuss specifics regarding database maintenance, access, and security. Finally, we consider some reporting techniques that will assist the health fitness manager in the ongoing challenge of anticipating membership demands and desires in this day of dynamic industry change.

IMPORTANCE OF MEMBER MANAGEMENT

Database management is an important function of club operations. Information should be readily available to assist management in the day-to-day decision making that governs both short- and long-term strategic planning.

Database management is a full-time effort. Information in the database must be constantly and meticulously maintained. The accuracy of the information is imperative to the success of the operation. Demographic information changes must be tracked carefully to ensure accurate billing and accounting. Programming and member usage information should be continually monitored to examine trends in participation. Health history information must be available to assist in the event of an emergency. Focused attention must be given to this area of club management to ensure operational efficiency.

Manual Record Keeping

Although most facilities use computers to assist in the overwhelming task of membership database maintenance, some facilities employ manual systems. These systems, typically handwritten records maintained in a member file, function well in many small health fitness operations. These manual systems, often refined over time, offer management specific information needed on a member at any given time. Manual systems do not, however, allow management to examine trends, large amounts of data, or produce reports detailing any of hundreds of points of interest. Investigation of and investment in a computerized database maintenance system is warranted for any health fitness organization desiring to remain competitive.

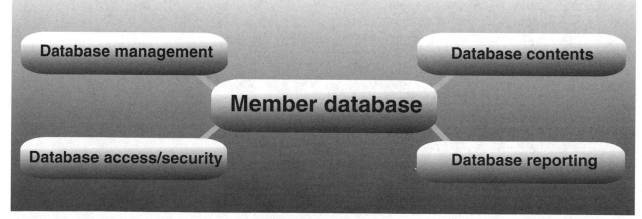

Figure 6.1 The many aspects of a complete member database.

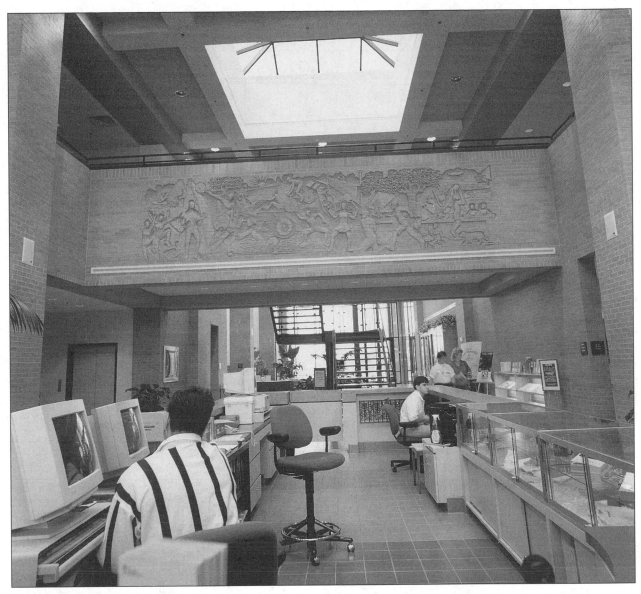

Courtesy of the Dallas Texins Association

Computer Record Keeping

Establishing a membership database on computer is easily one of the most cost-effective investments conceivable for any health fitness organization. Using the computer to do tedious number-crunching efforts, search and retrieve a desired group of members (i.e., smokers) from thousands of health history questionnaires, or prepare mailing labels for a special promotion saves many hours of staff time. The long-term labor expense savings attained following computerization will pay for its cost many times over.

The true value of *computerized records* is not in the day-to-day inquiries of a single member, but in the ability to access large amounts of data stored for purposeful intent, such as determining the average demographics of the existing membership. You can then use this information to direct future marketing efforts. You can examine programming and usage trends at the tap of a key. A sales force targeting a prospective population can easily establish demographic profiles of the current membership population. Staff can accurately maintain billing and address information, allowing monthly billing to take place with minimal effort and ensuring a constant revenue stream. (See chapter 19 for additional information regarding advantages of computerization and programs available to the health fitness industry.)

Membership Application

Name: _____   Spouse's name: _____

Primary member's SSN: _____   Date of birth: _____

Spouse's SSN: _____   Date of birth: _____

Home address: _____

_____

Home telephone number: _____   E-mail: _____

Business address: _____

_____

Work telephone number: _____   E-mail: _____

Type of membership you are applying for:

        Individual   Family   Corporate   Off-peak   Senior

Initiation fee: $_____   Monthly dues: $_____

Bank affiliation: _____

    I agree to abide by the membership bylaws and club policies and procedures. I understand that my membership may be terminated at any time should I not adhere to said bylaws, policies, and procedures. I also understand that these policies and procedures may be amended at the discretion of the club management.

    I understand that in order to terminate my membership, I must provide the ABC Club membership department with thirty (30) days written notification. I also understand that I am responsible for any charges incurred up to the termination date of my membership.

Signature: _____   Date: _____

Sales manager: _____   Date: _____

Membership director: _____   Date: _____

Figure 6.2   Basic membership application form.

Many companies offer computer software to assist with establishing a membership database. Review these companies and their products based on information provided in this chapter and chapter 19 if your organization is establishing a new computerized record system or optimizing your existing system.

Membership Application

Name: _____   Spouse's name: _____

Primary member's SSN: _____   Date of birth: _____

Spouse's SSN: _____   Date of birth: _____

Names and birth dates of children:

Name: _____   Birth date: _____

Name: _____   Birth date: _____

Name: _____   Birth date: _____

Name: _____   Birth date: _____

Anniversary date: _____

Home address: _____

_____

Home telephone number: _____   E-mail: _____

Business address: _____

_____

Work telephone number: _____   E-mail: _____

Do you prefer club mail to be sent to your home or work? _____

Company name: _____   Title: _____

Assistant's name: _____   Phone number: _____

Type of membership you are applying for:

          Individual   Family   Corporate   Off-peak   Senior

Initiation fee: $_____   Monthly dues: $_____

Bank affiliation: _____   Account number(s): _____

_____

Other club affiliations and length of membership:

Club: _____   Date joined: _____

Club: _____   Date joined: _____

(continued)

Figure 6.3 **Expanded membership application form.**

Personal health information: (Please complete supplemental forms for each member of the family.)

Name: _____   Age: _____

1.   Check if you have ever had any of the following conditions:

_____ heart disease   _____ high blood pressure   _____ heart attack

_____ heart surgery   _____ stroke   _____ emphysema

_____ chronic bronchitis   _____ arthritis   _____ diabetes

_____ ulcer   _____ epilepsy   _____ anemia

_____ kidney disease   _____ liver disease   _____ cancer

_____ asthma   _____ sports-related injury: _____

Other: _____

2.   Is there a history of heart disease in your immediate family?   _____ Yes   _____ No

3.   Are you presently on any medications?   _____ Yes   _____ No

     If yes, please specify and for what purpose: _____

4.   Current weight: _____   Ideal weight: _____

5.   Are you following a special diet?   _____ Yes   _____ No

     If yes, what type? _____

6.   Do you smoke? _____ Yes   _____ No   If yes, how much? _____

7.   How would you rank your level of stress?

                    (Low)   1   2   3   4   5   (High)

     I agree to abide by the membership bylaws and club policies and procedures. I understand that my membership may be terminated at any time should I not adhere to said bylaws, policies, and procedures. I also understand that these policies and procedures may be amended at the discretion of the club management.

     I understand that in order to terminate my membership, I must provide the ABC Club membership department with thirty (30) days written notification. I also understand that I am responsible for any charges incurred up to the termination date of my membership.

Signature: _____   Date: _____

Sales manager: _____   Date: _____

Membership director: _____   Date: _____

ESTABLISHING A COMPLETE DATABASE

A key to successfully using the membership database is in its establishment. Predetermining the information to be captured should not be taken lightly. This specific information, when collected on each member, sets the foundation for the long-term management of the database. Key personnel should spend time detailing a wish list of reports and information they would like to monitor to ensure that the necessary data points are distinguished as fields in the database. Programming managers should think of long-term efforts when creating their list in order to capture members who possess a specific trait or medical condition on which the programming efforts may target. Sales and marketing personnel should consider demographic information that will assist them in defining the current membership. Once this group is demographically defined, you can focus marketing and sales efforts to find similar prospects. When you have created this wish list or data field listing, provide it to several computer software vendors to assess their products' ability to meet your needs.

Membership Data

The sales force charged to maintain certain membership sales figures and retention percentages is interested in specific pieces of data to achieve their goals. Detailed here are some of the commonly used tools in membership sales departments to continually gather information vital to the sales process.

Membership Application

The membership application is a legally binding document detailing a great deal of information. Membership applications differ from facility to facility due to differing informational needs. At a minimum, this application should state the terms of membership; parties subscribing to the membership agreement; applicable legal demographic information such as full names, birth dates, addresses, telephone numbers, and so on; personal financial data such as bank affiliations and account numbers; the binding length of the membership agreement; and required termination policies and procedures. (See chapter 17 for more information on membership contracts.) Most facilities supplement this base level data with information that allows them to better meet the needs of each client. Information

such as professional field of work, title, work demographic information, spousal or partner information, children's names and ages, other club affiliations, referral source or member, physician name and telephone number, rules and regulations, and much more can be useful information to add to a membership application. You can collect these data as fields in the membership contract or on additional forms completed as a part of the joining process. Samples of basic and expanded membership applications are provided in figures 6.2 and 6.3. Keep in mind that you should determine the contents of your facility's membership application with the organization's legal counsel.

Financial Records

Often collecting financial information is required to complete the membership application process. As mentioned previously, financial data such as bank affiliation, account numbers, and credit references are necessary to ensure a solid credit rating. This rating can provide the controller, credit manager, or general manager a certain degree of comfort in extending charging privileges at the club or immediately inform the operator of a potential credit risk. Local, state, and federal regulations exist regarding the collection of financial data on persons making application for membership. It is prudent to review these regulations and all plans regarding financial information with financial and legal counsel.

New Member Interviews

New member interviews are a valuable way to quickly facilitate a new member's assimilation into the activities of the club. Typically the membership sales associate completing the sales transaction will initiate the new member interview and complete appropriate interest survey documentation. See figure 6.4 for a sample interest survey form. Operating department managers can use this documentation to place telephone calls or write notes to new members introducing them to specific programs, activities, or events either occurring in the club currently or planned in the near future.

The departmental manager should extend a special invitation to new members to attend activities or programs of interest and inform the sales associate of their intent to attend. Both the departmental manager and sales associate should greet new members upon arrival and introduce them to others who share similar interests so the new members feel welcome and quickly feel a part of the club. Keep the new member interview information in the member

New Member Interest Survey

Please indicate the activities that may be of interest to you, your spouse, or children. A member of the staff will be contacting you to assist in your introduction to the programs indicated below. We look forward to serving you.

Activity	Male	Female	Child 1	Child 2	Child 3	Child 4
Name:	_____	_____	_____	_____	_____	_____
Fitness assessment:	_____	_____	_____	_____	_____	_____
Personal training:	_____	_____	_____	_____	_____	_____
Child care:	_____	_____	_____	_____	_____	_____
Group exercise classes:	_____	_____	_____	_____	_____	_____
Tennis leagues:	_____	_____	_____	_____	_____	_____
Racquetball lessons:	_____	_____	_____	_____	_____	_____
Swimming team (kids):	_____	_____	_____	_____	_____	_____
Masters swimming:	_____	_____	_____	_____	_____	_____
Swimming lessons:	_____	_____	_____	_____	_____	_____
Junior tennis camp:	_____	_____	_____	_____	_____	_____
Junior fitness camp:	_____	_____	_____	_____	_____	_____
Birthday parties:	_____	_____	_____	_____	_____	_____
Workout partner:	_____	_____	_____	_____	_____	_____
Cooking classes:	_____	_____	_____	_____	_____	_____
Other: _____	_____	_____	_____	_____	_____	_____
Other: _____	_____	_____	_____	_____	_____	_____
Other: _____	_____	_____	_____	_____	_____	_____
Other: _____	_____	_____	_____	_____	_____	_____
Other: _____	_____	_____	_____	_____	_____	_____

Member name: _____   Telephone number: _____

When is the best time to contact you? _____

Figure 6.4 New member interest survey.

file and so the sales associate can use it in scheduled follow-up calls to ensure the new member is comfortable and active in the club. Periodic review of this information by department managers with appropriate follow-up calls and invitations shows continued interest in the new member, decreasing the risk of a membership cancellation.

Many facilities track new member interview information and interest surveys by computer through fields in the membership database. Tracking in this manner optimizes the ability to continue periodic follow-up and invitations to events or programs of interest. For example, if a new member is interested in racquetball, the fitness director or programming manager can pull a list of all individuals with these interests and extend telephone or written invitations to events such as an upcoming club league, tournament, clinic, professional tournament, or exhibition.

Leads and Referrals

Sales associates spend a great deal of time procuring and qualifying leads for new member prospects. Enlisting the current membership to assist in producing quality leads is a sure way to enhance membership. Members who are pleased with the quality of the club, its services, and programs are the best source for qualified leads and referrals. Many health fitness programs in all settings employ periodic promotions to entice existing members to assist the membership sales force in acquiring leads and referrals. Discount offers, dues credits, and special prizes are examples of rewards offered to existing members who provide a referral who joins the membership. Close tracking of membership referral efforts in the membership database ensures proper rewards and recognition. This positive reinforcement of members' assistance can encourage them to continue assisting the membership sales force in acquiring leads and referrals.

Guest Tracking

Equally beneficial to the membership sales effort is the member who brings a guest on property to experience the club. Many members in programs are first introduced to the facility as a guest. Diligently follow up with guests to assess interest in membership and to ensure club security and membership integrity. Tracking guests through written and signed guest registration forms (see figure 13.6) allows for timely follow-up. Later, entering guests'

information and tracking their visits by computer allows the membership sales team to examine all guest visits during a specified period, the number of visits a particular guest has been to the club, and the names of sponsoring members.

Mailing List

Maintaining an accurate and complete mailing list is an essential function of the membership database. Computerization eases this task by allowing all members of the staff access to make necessary changes. Whether the member notifies the club of an address change by noting it on a payment remittance, stopping at the service desk to verbally communicate the change, or sending it via e-mail, updating the database ensures all functional areas of the club are notified and necessary modifications to the mailing list are automatically completed. The membership database should contain both home and work street addresses and e-mail addresses for those members who wish to receive information via the Internet.

Exit Interviews

When members choose to relinquish their memberships, important data should be obtained.

Careful tracking and analysis of exit interview information assists the departmental and program managers in continuing to improve facilities and programs.

A sample exit interview form can be found in figure 6.5. Carefully monitor reasons the member is leaving the club, and statistically calculate and track both controllable and uncontrollable reasons. The membership sales force and general manager should watch for controllable deletion trends such as cleanliness concerns, poor equipment maintenance, or lack of staff training so that such concerns can be rectified immediately.

The membership sales force should occasionally review exit interview information for possible return members following correction of their primary reason for deletion. Any club renovation or new service should be a cue for the membership sales force to revisit exit interviews for persons who may now be interested in rejoining.

The staff at ABC Club would appreciate it if you would take a moment to complete this resignation inquiry. Read each question carefully and circle the most appropriate answer. Any comments you could provide will assist us in providing a better club for our members and would be greatly appreciated. Please return this form to ABC Club in the enclosed self-addressed, stamped envelope. Thank you for your input and for allowing us to serve you at ABC Club.

1. How long were you a member of ABC Club? _____

2. What is your overall rating of the ABC Club as a health/fitness facility?

    1 (worst)   2   3   4   5 (best)

3. Why did you resign from ABC Club?

    Relocation   Travel   New job   Lack of use

    Personal illness   Family illness   Financial   Lack of time

    Other: _____

4. Please list the most enjoyable aspects of ABC Club.

    1. _____

    2. _____

    3. _____

5. Please list the aspects of ABC Club that could be improved.

    1. _____

    2. _____

    3. _____

6. Did you leave ABC Club because you were dissatisfied with some aspect of the club?

                Yes   No

    If yes, please specify: _____

    _____

7. Are there any conditions under which you would rejoin ABC Club? _____

    _____

Optional information:

Name: _____   Member number: _____

Thank you for your time!

Figure 6.5   Exit interview form.

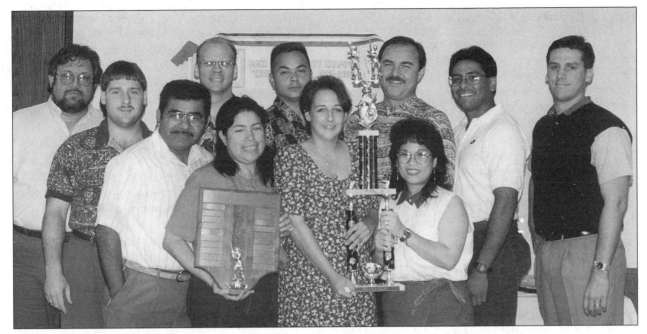

Courtesy of NCH Corporation, Dallas, Texas

Member Adherence Data

Health fitness literature often cites that the cost of acquiring a new member is five to six times higher than the cost of retaining a current member (Winters 1994). Staggering figures such as these force prudent health fitness managers to place high priority on membership retention efforts. Information

gathering begins during the membership application process and should never cease.

As previously covered, we can classify reasons for deletions as controllable and uncontrollable. Samples of controllable and uncontrollable reasons are provided in table 6.1. Tracking this information will assist departmental and program managers in preventing controllable membership deletions.

Table 6.1 Controllable and Uncontrollable Deletion Reasons

Controllable reasons	Uncontrollable reasons
Lost interest	Moving away from area
Lack of use	Financial burden or affordability
No time	Extended illness
Poor facility or equipment maintenance	No longer with sponsoring company
Poor cleanliness	Death of member or family member
Lack of trained staff to assist with questions and concerns	Accounting deletion (nonpayment)
Lack of child care or children's programming	Asked to leave club membership for rules infraction or poor conduct
Lack of expected results	
Poor motivation	
Lack of creative and motivating programs	
Overcrowding	
Feel uncomfortable in club atmosphere	

Health History Review

Discussed at length in chapter 13, the health history review serves as an important retention tool. Health fitness managers and staff should review the health history questionnaire not only for conditions that may limit or restrict certain activities, but also for personal goals and objectives related to an exercise and wellness program. For example, review of a health history questionnaire may indicate a member's recent knee injury requiring surgery. Although the health fitness manager must be aware of the potential for reinjury and program modifications necessitated by the injury, she must also be aware if rehabilitation of the knee injury is in order. This rehabilitation may allow the member to return to a loved activity or sport, which may be the individual's primary objective in joining the club. The possibility for member retention is enhanced when goals, objectives, and results are met and achieved at the health fitness facility. Review of the health history questionnaire will provide valuable insight into these goals and objectives to assist and motivate the member.

Interest Survey

Although the new member interview is the perfect time to begin the process of welcoming and as-similating a new member into the club's membership, an interest survey taken of new and existing members provides feedback useful in retaining these members. Tailor the interest survey form in figure 6.4 to fit the activities, programs, and events available in the facility. Program managers should be accountable for regular telephone calls and invitations to new and existing members. Many clubs now have programs in which they provide the new member interest survey to the department manager of the areas of greatest interest. The department manager, following a welcome telephone call to the new member, assigns a staff member to the new member. The staff member is responsible for overseeing the scheduling of any new member consultations or assessments, providing an orientation of the facility and equipment, and assisting new members in any way possible. This personal service touch for the first six months to one year of membership enhances retention efforts.

Annual Member Surveys

Member surveys provide health fitness organizations with a vast amount of data regarding all aspects of program operations. Annual surveys offer members the opportunity to provide their opinions regarding what they most enjoy about the

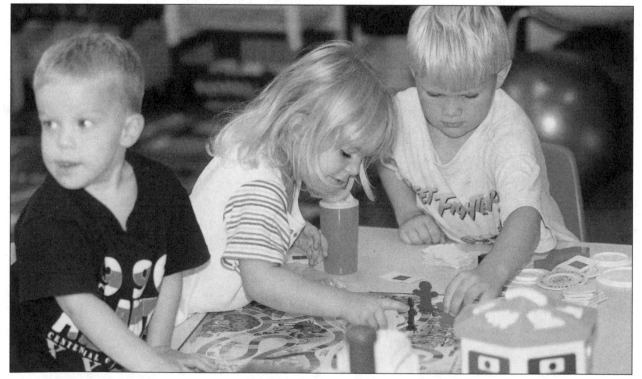

Courtesy of Dallas Texins Association

program and issues or concerns they feel should be addressed. This information, when used proactively, can demonstrate to the members the program commitment to service and quality. Discuss results of member surveys openly and honestly among staff and membership. Address issues identified in a straightforward manner. Monitor intervention programs closely to ensure desired change is taking place. Finally, publish all efforts to the membership through bulletin boards, newsletters, and any other viable means of communication. Don't waste the time, energy, and cost of producing a quality member survey through inadequate or half-hearted attempts to rectify issues identified. A member survey provides management and membership with a win-win situation when you offer honest efforts.

Birthdays and Anniversaries

Special occasions such as birthdays and anniversaries are easily tracked through a membership database. Special occasions provide an excellent opportunity for the organization to recognize a member on a special day through a card or telephone greeting. Often, gifts are extended to members, such as a complimentary dessert with dinner in the restaurant anytime throughout their birthday or anniversary month.

Computers allow easy tracking of these special occasions. A list of members with a birthday or anniversary in a given month can be printed along with mailing labels. A short note from an appropriate staff member adds a personal touch to a greeting from the entire staff.

Special Accomplishments

Special accomplishments achieved by members should never go unnoticed. Whether the accomplishment is the completion of a 10K race, the loss of a desired amount of weight, or an award or recognition earned in school or business, the health fitness manager must recognize and note these efforts. Establishing a goals or notes field in the member database with a goal date of achievement can flag the alert fitness manager to check the progress of the member. A monthly Thumbs Up column in the member newsletter is an excellent way to recognize members for their special achievements. Noting these accomplishments in the member database allows the conscientious staff the opportunity for timely acknowledgment of such achievements.

DATABASE ACCESS

Security is a major concern of individuals as the computer becomes ingrained in our personal and professional lives. Important personal data is maintained in databases of all kinds. Day in and day out we read articles in the popular press detailing the illegal access of a computer hacker into some of the most highly secured databases in the world. How then can health fitness managers ensure the wary member that data collected, such as addresses, telephone numbers, bank affiliation and account numbers, or highly personalized data, such as drivers license or social security numbers, will be kept secure? Personal data should be secured from all unauthorized queries. Careful procedures must be in place and enforced to ensure membership database integrity.

Database security should be a high priority, from selecting the vendor, product, and installation to training all new staff.

Management

Senior management and department heads need to be trained regarding the importance of membership database security. They should in turn impart this importance to their staff. Management should be issued or should select a *personal password* that allows them access to vital database information as needed. Take special care to ensure that passwords remain private and are changed frequently. Management should never share password information or sensitive member information with any staff member.

Service Desk

Service desk staff members often need access to nonsecured information, such as family member's names and ages, address, and telephone number (if published), but should not have access to sensitive and secured information. The ability to access this nonsecured information to make changes at the member's request is often necessary. Service desk

ABC Club Membership Demographic Profile Report					
Date: 1/1/97	**Percentage**		**Age breakdown**	**Males**	**Females**
Total population = 2,104	100%		0-5 years	81	92
Adult population (n = 1,562; 15 years)	74.2%		6-10 years	25	48
Child population (n = 542; < 15 years of age)	25.7%		11-15 years	120	176
			16-20 years	90	45
Gender			21-30 years	125	168
Adult males	852	54.5%	31-40 years	458	410
Adult females	710	45.5%	41-50 years	156	67
Child males	226	41.6%	51-60 years	15	11
Child females	316	58.3%	60+	8	9

Figure 6.6   Demographic membership profile.

staff may also obtain access to club-related information such as join date, usage data, or membership type. Through integration of the membership database with other software components, such as accounting software, the service desk staff can see if membership dues for a particular account are in arrears without access to sensitive accounting information. This integration ensures important information is provided to the service desk responsible for facility control without allowing access to sensitive information.

Most software programs available today assist the health fitness manager with controlling access to this sensitive information. The administrator of the software program should be able to establish authorizations for each staff member delineating specifically which areas of information that particular staff member can access. This allows the service desk personnel the ability to access the areas they need, yet maintains the security of other information.

Fitness Professionals

The professional fitness staff should also have access to the nonsecured information available to the service staff. In addition, designated fitness staff members should be able to gain access to personal health history information through assigned or selected passwords. Management can guarantee care-

ful control of sensitive health history information by setting and enforcing strict guidelines.

Membership

The membership should *never* have access to the membership database. Under no circumstance should a member be allowed access to or be provided with information on another member. Even seemingly harmless inquiries such as addresses or telephone numbers should be denied. Staff can offer a membership directory if such a directory exists. As a secondary offer, staff could contact the member to obtain permission to provide another with the requested information or could dial the number and connect them.

REPORTING

The standard reports available in most commercial software programs offer management a great deal of valuable information. The addition of a report generator to software programs allows health fitness managers the opportunity to generate any report for which data has been captured. Managers can then use these data to monitor club sales and retention activity in order to continually improve the offerings and operations of the facility.

> *The reporting capabilities of a computerized membership database is the most valuable, yet underused, tool in the long-term strategic planning effort of any health fitness organization.*

Listed here are some reports that will help you optimize the reporting capabilities of a membership database.

1. Retention report—monthly or annually
2. Attrition report—monthly or annually
3. Membership sales report—weekly, monthly, or annually
4. Leads report
5. Referral report
6. Exit reasons report
7. Dependent report
8. Corporate affiliation report
9. Sales statistics flash report
10. Member count by membership type
11. Lead generation source report

Membership Profile

The continual goal of the membership sales team is to identify the target market, invite qualified prospects to visit the facility, and add their names to the membership roster. A computerized database can clarify the current membership demographics to provide a clear picture of others who may fit the facility's target market. The manager can monitor information such as age, gender, marital status, number of persons in household, annual income, years of membership, distance of residence from club, distance of workplace from club, and more to provide insight to the membership sales team. You can review an example of a demographic member profile in figure 6.6. If the data is collected during the membership sales process, statistical reporting of that data should be available. Maintaining a clear picture of the constantly changing membership is important for long-term growth of the club.

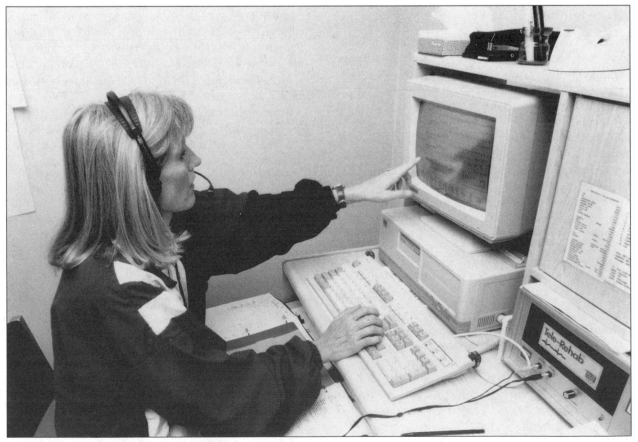

Courtesy of Medical City Dallas, Cardiac Rehabilitation

Attrition

Carefully monitored attrition information can assist the membership sales process. You can make changes in scheduling, marketing, and programming following analysis of an attrition report. An attrition report can detail membership statistics month by month to monitor trends. You can review a sample membership attrition report in figure 2.9. Managers can identify trends negatively affecting membership growth in early stages so they can implement intervention techniques and strategies. Capitalize on positive membership growth trends to continue the positive cycle. Additionally, close analysis of the previous year's data can help accurately predict monthly and annual sales and retention forecasts.

> *Membership reporting should assist the alert sales manager to identify a target market, qualify prospective members, and stay ahead of the current membership trends.*

New Member Profiles

Managers can generate new member profiles, similar to a full membership profile, so they can compare the demographics of new members joining the facility in the previous month or quarter to the general membership profile. This comparison can provide additional information to the sales team regarding sales trends, changing demographics in the area, new companies entering the region, or the impact of a new program offering, such as child care, to the sales effort. Changing demographics will dictate changing needs. Maintaining a clear picture of membership changes is vital to continued success.

Programming Profile

You can also use information captured in the membership database to further the efforts of the programming department. Information on usage patterns, cursory medical history, and family demographics can provide the innovative program manager with a wealth of information from which to draw creative programming ideas. The health fitness programming staff can use the membership database in the following ways.

Usage Patterns

Many membership databases are configured with accompanying software programs such as front desk check-in or exercise logging. These software programs are detailed in chapter 19. For the club that incorporates a membership database, exercise logging, and front desk check-in programs into the operation of their facility, a great deal of data revealing the exercise patterns of the membership is available. Good questions to ask about your club's usage patterns include the following:

- What time is the club in greatest use?
- On average, how many people participate weekly in group exercise?
- When are most mothers of young children on property?
- Who is not using the facility regularly and why?
- How do usage patterns on holidays and weekends differ from weekday usage?
- Which group exercise classes and teachers draw the largest participation?

You can use this information to enhance participation in programs during the peak usage periods and offer other high interest programs in nonpeak times to encourage greater club usage at this time. Program managers can incorporate programming for the new mother and young children concurrently to heighten member satisfaction. You can promote leagues and tournaments through telephone invitations to a predetermined list of racquetball enthusiasts. The membership database contains a great deal of information for the programming manager willing to pay attention.

Intervention Programs

You can also determine the need for certain intervention or wellness programs through reporting on certain data in the health history of each member. For example, the membership database may contain information regarding the smoking habits of individuals in the membership. A simple report can tell the programming manager the number of members who currently smoke, their names, and telephone numbers. Although not all members who smoke will be interested in a smoking cessation program, simply determining the potential target group for such a program provides the programming manager with a statement of potential need. The same can be said for programs that positively affect hypertension. You can determine the need for classes such as exercising and hypertension, low fat and low cholesterol cooking, or home blood pressure monitoring.

A common complaint among programming managers continues to be that quality programs are offered and no one attends. Ascertaining the need and target market through membership database reporting, followed by a personal invitation and aggressive promotion to participate, will enhance participation and silence this common complaint.

IN CLOSING

This chapter has examined the membership database and the many ways that you can use the data it contains to further the successful management and operation of the club. We discussed the contents of a useful database and how to select a computerized database that will most appropriately fit the needs of your facility. We examined membership database access and security, because this issue continues to rise as a member concern. We discussed reporting capabilities of membership database software in an effort to enhance membership retention and programming. Chapter 8, Program Management, provides additional programming information in hopes that the program manager can plan and implement the foundation for selective program development and design laid out in this chapter through techniques offered in the following chapters.

KEY TERMS

Computerized records

Membership database

Personal password

RECOMMENDED READINGS

Pessin, F. 1995. Put a lid on attrition with your computer. *Fitness Management* (November): 24-27.

Winters, C. 1994. The art of keeping members. *Club Industry* (February): 18-23.

Service Desk Management

The front-of-the-house discussions continue appropriately with a look at the service desk. Is the service desk in your facility inviting for members and guests? Is the staff friendly and welcoming? Are responsibilities of the service desk staff clearly defined? Is there an ongoing training program to refine the interpersonal skills of the service desk receptionists? Discover some effective suggestions for managing your service desk in this chapter.

The service desk, or front desk, has a vital role to play in the success or failure of a program (see figure 7.1). Service to members will continue to be a critical element as the customer-driven evolution of the industry continues. However, member satisfaction and retention will be less of a challenge if managers spend the time and energy required to assemble and train a professional, service-directed desk staff. A service desk that consistently surpasses the needs and expectations of members and guests cannot be measured by conventional tools. The successful service desk must provide consistent, quality service with efficiency and friendliness.

> *Outstanding member service must begin at the service desk.*

As the old saying goes, you never get a second chance to make a first impression. First impressions have immeasurable value to prospective and long-term members. Going to a club for the first time is much like going to a party by yourself. The awkward and often intimidating first moment in a facility is minimized or eliminated by the welcome provided by friendly and attentive service desk personnel. Long-time members greeted by name will feel welcome and appreciated. This initial contact is the first step in building essential camaraderie between staff and members. The warm welcome and pleasant atmosphere are important responsibilities of the service desk, an area of the club often overlooked and underappreciated.

WHAT IS THE SERVICE DESK'S FUNCTION?

The primary control point is located immediately inside the front door of the facility, thereby obtaining the common name, front desk. Successful facilities enhance the responsibilities assigned to the front desk to create a more properly named *service desk*. Although the service desk has a long list of specific tasks and responsibilities, a warm welcome and fond farewell for each member and guest is one of the most important. All too often, nonpeople-related tasks at the service desk are given priority

over membership service. Creating a culture of outstanding member service begins by redirecting the attention and energy of service desk personnel to anticipating and serving member needs. Specifically assigning all nonpeople-related responsibilities a lower priority demonstrates the importance of service to members and staff. Remember, it is a service desk, not simply a front desk.

SERVICE DESK STRATEGIES

The service desk is responsible for creating the culture of member service for the entire program. A service-directed staff does this by using many strategies. However, the methods used to achieve superior customer appreciation are not as important as consistent delivery. A *service culture* is created by setting high standards that fit the unique environment of the facility. The following are examples of customer service methods that have proven successful in creating this service culture.

Staffing

The characteristics of individuals hired to staff the service desk can make or break the service culture. A facility with the best equipment and most lavish amenities will not appeal to the consumer if the first interaction that individual has with personnel is with an indifferent, unmotivated staff person. The challenge facing health fitness managers is to hire bright, enthusiastic, service-minded individuals, often for little compensation. Service desk personnel are often the lowest paid front-of-the-house staff members. If the goal of the program is to create an outstanding service culture, rethinking the value of

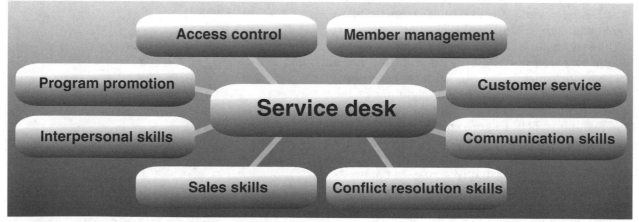

Figure 7.1   The skills and roles of a health fitness service desk.

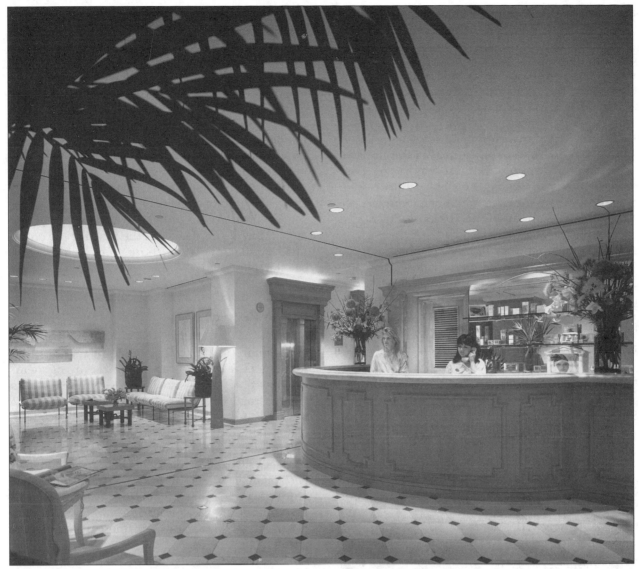

Courtesy of The Spa at the Crescent, Dallas, Texas

Desirable Characteristics of Service Desk Personnel

Professional

Energetic

Good role model

Healthy appearance

Quick smile

Dependable

Outgoing and upbeat

Intelligent

Friendly

Strong communication skills

Positive attitude

Organized

Strong computer skills

Decision maker

Confident

Detail oriented

Not afraid of conflict

Strong telephone skills

Capable of handling multiple tasks at once

Strong name recognition skills

A variety of ages to reflect club's member demographics

the service desk staff may be in order. Creation of profit sharing or incentive programs based on retail sales, member retention, name recognition, or a number of other alternatives are creative ways that you can enhance the compensation package for service desk personnel. Managers should encourage these individuals, as much as any other club employee, to become long-term employees. Programs that allow promising service desk personnel to cross train in other areas of the club can offer long-term options for these employees. Constant turnover in this high-visibility area is often frustrating to members. Remember, members see the club as a second home and become attached to the people they see each day.

The characteristics of the service desk staff are similar to those in any service business. The personnel must be qualified, energetic, service-oriented individuals who are quick with a smile. In IRSA's (now called IHRSA) 1994 study, *How Consumers View Health and Sports Clubs*, prospective members often cited their impression of the staff as "indifferent" to those who were not fit or in shape. A successful operation often depends on the intangible qualities of staff members who can make everyone feel welcome. Communication and human relations skills, friendliness, willingness to help, and professionalism, are important factors in creating and maintaining a service culture. Some specific desirable characteristics of service desk personnel are listed on the previous page. The image these individuals create will reflect the image of the entire club.

The IRSA report also noted that the most important factor for members who discontinued their membership affiliation with a club was an inability to adjust to the club's atmosphere; these members stated they simply did not feel welcome or comfortable in the facility. This information reflects the importance of a friendly, welcoming service desk. An organized and professional image at the service desk sets the tone for the entire facility and strongly affects member retention and satisfaction.

Name Recognition

Encouraging staff to call members by name consistently ranks as a top strategy for improving member retention. An effective service culture conveys the message to all members that the staff looks forward to their visit each day. What better welcome than to address all members by name, not only as they walk in the door, but as they come in contact with a staff member. Being interested in each member as an individual can make him or her feel more welcome and at home. It is the manager's responsibility to encourage the staff to make each member feel like a guest in the staff member's home.

> *Name recognition is one of the most powerful tools available to create a service culture.*

Clubs have a variety of methods available to teach staff the names of participants using the facility. The only limiting factor is creativity. One of the most effective methods gaining popularity and visibility in the industry is a computerized front desk check-in system with video capability. These systems display a video image of the member on the screen, making identification and name recognition easy. A second, more conventional method is to make a copy of the new member identification card photo available to staff mem-

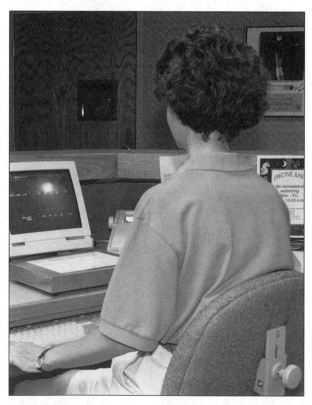

© Tom Wallace

Name Recognition Contest Example

The goal is to create a contest that will positively reinforce the efforts of every employee to learn *and use* the names of members. Remember, these are only suggestions; modify them to best fit your facility and keep it fun.

1. Create or purchase tickets to hand out to staff heard using a member's name.

2. Give the tickets to supervisory and management staff and direct them to immediately reward a staff member using a member's name by signing and dating a ticket and presenting it to the employee with a positive message like "great job." The signature and date eliminates any possibilities of duplication of tickets. Create different types of tickets or *money* for each departmental supervisor. For example, *muscle money* for the fitness staff, *game, set, and match* money for the tennis staff, *membership money* for the membership department, and so on.

3. Give *mystery money* to any other individuals you think would support your efforts. This way the staff members will try to use names all the time and not simply in the presence of a manager or supervisor.

4. Create a tote board or contest chart listing the names of every staff member who has daily contact with club members. Hang the contest chart in a prominent staff area so that all staff can monitor their progress.

5. The staff member presents the money they have accumulated to their manager, who then places a star by the name of the staff member on the contest chart for each ticket earned. This provides the manager with an excellent opportunity to offer personal words of positive reinforcement for the effort.

6. The grand prize winner is the individual who collects the greatest amount of money based on the number of hours worked during the contest period.

7. Hold a meeting with the staff to unveil the contest. Explain the rules, duration for the contest, and the prizes. Offer a grand prize winner as well as department winners so each employee has an opportunity for success.

8. Hold an entire club staff meeting to award the prizes. Display the names of the winners prominently in the club or publish the names in your club newsletter. The greater the positive reinforcement the better.

9. Have fun.

bers during daily or weekly training meetings. Placing a bulletin board in a staff area with pictures and names of both new and existing members is a powerful training tool. Devise games and contests to motivate the staff and make learning names fun. Shown here is an example of such a contest.

Maintaining a photo of each member in their membership record file can clarify disputes over the identity of a member and provide a wealth of training opportunities for name recognition. Knowing members by name will not only make a member's visit to the facility more enjoyable, it will increase job satisfaction for employees by giving them an opportunity to know the members they see and assist each day. Another method that staff can use daily is simple, direct, and effective. Encourage staff to introduce themselves to each person they speak with if they do not know his or her name. This exchange of names provides the opportunity to continuously learn and retain more names. Set a standard to learn three names daily. Name recognition is not easy with hundreds or perhaps thousands of members, but it is worth the effort.

Every new staff member must understand that member name recognition is a primary job responsibility.

Scheduling Information

Another way to create a powerful service culture at the service desk is to ensure that staff is well informed about scheduled programs and events. Because the service desk is where members go when they have a question—whether by phone call or in person—members expect the service desk to be current on all events in the club. Depending on the size and activity level of the program, maintaining this service can be a major undertaking. Where is the stress-management class meeting tonight? Who is teaching the 6:00 A.M. group exercise class on Wednesday? What are the holiday hours for the club? How do I sign up for a fitness evaluation? What is the charge for a personal training session with Tom? Who is the best swimming teacher for a small child? The service desk is expected to have all the answers.

> *Solid communication between operational departments and the service desk is crucial to creating a service culture.*

Creating general information and special events notebooks is one way to provide answers to the most common questions efficiently and accurately. Following is a listing of information to include in the general information book for a multipurpose facility. Boldly label these standard three-ring binders and make them easily accessible for the service desk personnel. Department managers should review and update these books daily. The service desk supervisor should also meet periodically with each departmental manager to review the information for accuracy and completeness.

The special events book will change daily and must be reviewed and updated regularly. This book should include the details of each event and provide a sign-up or reservation sheet for the function, if needed. Figure 7.2 provides an example of an *event order*. Organize these event orders by department and, within each department, by date. It is important to place the event

---

Special Event Order

Special event: _____

Department: _____ Date of event: _____ Time: _____

Description of event: _____

_____

_____

Contact person: _____ Phone number: _____

Member contact (if applicable): _____ Phone number: _____

Details of event:

    Date: _____

    Time: _____

    Location: _____

        Contingency location: _____

    Cost: _____

Members only?	Yes	No
Additional cost for non-members?	Yes	No
Charge to membership account or credit card?	Yes	No
Age requirement?	Yes	No

        If yes, age required: _____

    How to register: _____

Registration/reservation required?	Yes	No
Registration/reservation for attached?	Yes	No

        If no, location of reservation form: _____

Cancellation policy in effect?	Yes	No
Food and beverage/catering order necessary?	Yes	No

        Name of catering staff assisting: _____

Additional information/notes: _____

_____

_____

Style of dress for event: _____

Figure 7.2   Special event order form.

General Information Book Topics

Facility hours

Facility address

Facility phone numbers

Facility fax numbers

Phone numbers for direct lines to departments

E-mail address (if applicable)

Emergency phone numbers

Emergency plan

List of commonly called phone numbers

Names of key personnel with phone numbers

Names and phone numbers of personnel employed by department

Certifications of employees

Hours and availability of staff members

Calendar of events

Hours of departments (if they vary from facility hours)

Blank originals of forms or checklists

Menus from the restaurant

Menus of services, their hours, and price lists of facility outlets, such as salon, laundry service, airport shuttle, spa services

Listing of membership types and pricing

Pool temperature

Procedures for shipping packages or overnight mail

Listings of reciprocal clubs

Ongoing services, such as personal training or private swim lessons, and their fees

Weekly group exercise schedules with instructors

Descriptions of the types of classes offered

Membership listing

Computer instructions and service telephone numbers

orders in the special events book well before the event. Planning ahead is critical in creating and maintaining a service culture. This allows service desk personnel to access information on every event in the club without asking the members to wait or to check back later. The accurately in-

formed service desk personnel who can respond quickly assists the department manager in the difficult task of promotion while presenting a professional image. Again, make it the responsibility of the service desk supervisor and each departmental manager to ensure the special events book is accurate and complete.

Service Desk Organization

Finally, the service desk itself can positively affect the creation of a service culture. The structure, organization, appearance, and efficiency of the service desk can offer a professional, warm, hassle-free welcome or it can be cold and disorganized. The design of the service desk should offer easy entrance to the club while controlling access. Using natural and direct lighting will provide a bright and energetic entrance.

The most qualified staff cannot make up for an inefficient service desk.

The desk should be organized to minimize delays for members entering or leaving the club. Front desk terminals, access control systems, and staffing levels during peak times should not cause delays. Designate separate areas for member access, guest registration, pro shop purchases, and staff interacting with members. Give much care and effort to the design and functionality of the service desk area. Efficiency and control are key elements of a service culture.

The basis of a service culture is an attitude that service to members is the top priority.

It is an attitude that management leads and supports. Each interaction with a member, whether it is issuing a daily locker key and towel or correcting a billing error, must be positive, friendly, and professional. The service desk has the responsibility of creating a positive first and last impression for every member, every day.

Every contact with a member is an opportunity to create a positive or negative impression.

TRAINING BASICS

How does a manager begin developing individuals for the difficult position of service desk receptionist? An important first step is knowing that training is an ongoing process. It does not end after the new hire orientation; ongoing training should be a top priority in the scheme of daily operations. Management must acknowledge the importance and value of consistent, quality training.

Orientation is one of the first steps in hiring and training a new employee. Orientation typically takes place as soon as possible after hiring and covers issues such as company philosophy, organizational structure, policies and procedures, safety guidelines, and job responsibilities. The initial training process optimally takes a few weeks to complete as the new hire assimilates into the position. As orientation is completed, the next challenge is the ongoing refinement of task performance, while trying to learn the names and faces of hundreds of people. Unfortunately, in many facilities, training ends with orientation, leaving the employee and the organization short of reaching potential. Although orientation is vital to the initial success of the new employee, it must be consistently reinforced through daily and weekly training.

Continual training and reinforcement of that training are key to a successful organization, regardless of the experience or educational background of the staff. Training sets the standard for performance of each individual task an employee tackles. An organization must integrate training, supervision, and growth into a total developmental package to ensure consistent staff development efforts. Failure to support a staff member with ongoing training is shortsighted and eventually costly.

Effective training, coaching, and counseling builds an organization of highly skilled individuals who convey self-confidence, teamwork, and professionalism.

Establishing training as a top priority in the daily operations of the club is a difficult task. Training becomes more difficult when things get busy. In the short run, it is much easier to do it yourself than to train a new employee. However, even though the initial effort to create and conduct training may seem overwhelming, once the systems and priorities are in place, the process becomes a natural part of daily operations.

Constructing an Effective Training Session

Developing standards for job performance, a consistent method for delivering each training session, and strategies for daily reinforcement will reduce the overwhelming burden of ongoing training. A technique long recognized by many service industries is developing standards for each task an employee performs daily. This provides guidelines for performing the task that are both specific and measurable. Breaking down a job into smaller, specific tasks provides a clear picture of the level of performance you expect. (See tables 7.5 and 7.6 for examples of task breakdowns and resulting standards.) Additionally, these standards establish performance expectations that raise the level of service in the facility. For example, if every employee working at the service desk specifically understands the procedure for answering the telephone, a uniform, high level of service becomes the standard. Dividing each job into small, achievable tasks provides the employee a clear opportunity for success.

Developing a training delivery system allows club management staff to efficiently prepare and conduct ongoing training sessions. The employee also benefits from this delivery system through an enhanced learning curve. Whether training is in a one-on-one or group setting, whether formal or informal, a consistant delivery system will enhance training for both the employee and the organization. In developing a training delivery system that will best fit the needs of your facility and staff, consider the following elements.

- Each training session should last no more than 10 to 15 minutes.

- The task must have specific and measurable standards of performance.

- The employee must have an opportunity to practice the new skill.

- The employee must have the opportunity to ask questions.

- Positive reinforcement throughout the session is crucial.
- The employee must experience success.

The training delivery system must be clear, concise, and consistent. A format developed by the Freeman Group and used by Rosewood Hotels and Resorts, operators of five-star hotel properties such as The Mansion on Turtle Creek, is displayed at right. The delivery system will differ for each organization and must be developed to fit the service culture the facility strives to attain.

A 15-minute training session on a particular task will not necessarily ensure the employee has mastered the skill. It is important in putting systems in place to continually remind the staff of the training session and the standard of performance expected. Management must continually evaluate the staff on the new task and provide ongoing coaching and counseling with positive reinforcement. This ongoing training is typically informal, but it conveys the message that management is serious about each employee successfully achieving the standard level of performance. Powerful methods of sustaining training include placing reminders on bulletin boards in staff areas as well as quizzing the employees during daily rounds of the club.

Focusing on Specific Service Skills

An effective service desk staff member must be trained in a variety of service-specific skills. Member service will be enhanced when the following service skills are included in the orientation training program and modeled by health fitness managers.

People skills are vital ingredients to the formula of a successful service desk. Training can enhance effective communication, successful negotiation, conflict resolution, and sales skills. Include an element of interpersonal skills training during all task training sessions.

Communication

Open lines of communication between management and staff, management and members, and staff and members are important to the success of the operation. Health fitness managers typically spend a great deal of time and effort preparing, planning, and executing programs to enhance the member experience. However, the best laid plans and most creative programs will not be effectively communicated to the member if the tone is not professional.

Training Delivery System Used by Rosewood Hotels and Resorts

The Rosewood training program consists of three areas: the introduction, the development or body of the training session, and the consolidation. Using the key word, *Intro*, Rosewood continually reminds its management staff of the simple yet effective structure for introducing each training session.

Interest—Capture the trainees' interest by showing a finished product of the task to be learned, asking an open-ended question, or telling a story.

Need—Why is it important for the trainee to know this particular task? Reasons could be a change in job description, change in policy, or a legal or safety concern.

Title—The precise name of the task to be learned.

Range—How the trainee will be involved in the training session. He or she will be involved through asking and answering several questions and performing the task step by step.

Objective—What will the trainee be able to do after completing the training session?

Developing the training session consists of the trainer breaking the task down into logical and learnable steps. This part of the training will include

1. the trainer asking questions of the trainee,
2. the trainee asking questions of the trainer,
3. a step-by-step demonstration of the task by the trainer,
4. participation by the trainee in the step-by-step-process, and
5. praise of the trainee for his/her successful efforts.

The consolidation of the training session is important in that it confirms that the trainee has learned the task and understands the information taught. Consolidation is accomplished by

1. answering any additional questions the trainee might have,
2. having the trainee perform the task alone,
3. praising and coaching, if needed, and
4. making a link forward to the next training session.

Table 7.1 Professional Wording Alternatives	
Words to avoid	**Use instead**
You have it all wrong.	There has been a miscommunication.
It's not my job.	Let me see what I can do to help.
Someone else messed up again.	I'm sorry for your inconvenience.
It's the computer again.	It appears an error has been made.
I don't know.	Let me find out for you.
You'll have to . . .	May I suggest . . .
	Would you mind . . .
I've never heard of that happening before.	Thank you for telling me . . .
Have a nice day.	Thank you for . . .
	Come back again . . .
Phrases to use	
• I can see how . . .	
• I understand what an inconvenience . . .	
• I can appreciate what you're saying . . .	
• Perhaps I misunderstood . . .	
• Let's see what we can work out together . . .	
• We realize this is an inconvenience . . .	
• Please allow me to give you more information . . .	

Adapted, by permission, from JJ Lauderbaugh 1995.

It is not so much what is said, as how it is said.

The tone of voice, selection of words, and delivery of the message can either motivate and encourage members to participate or offend them in a way that they may consider not only skipping the event, but also canceling their memberships. Training the staff with the necessary skill to promote effective communication at the service desk gives a level of confidence in both pleasant and unpleasant circumstances.

The importance of using professional and helpful language when communicating with members cannot be overestimated.

Professional communication positively impacts the customer service image of the program. As illustrated in table 7.1, word choices and service-directed phrases can be implemented to improve the customer service impact in day-to-day communications.

Positive, professional communication can be ensured if the following simple strategies are used.

• *Use professional language.* Replacing slang terminology with professional language presents a polished image. For example, replace "yep" or "you bet" with "certainly" or "right away."

• *Use a pleasant, reassuring, and confident tone of voice.* Never be sarcastic or derogatory in conversations with members.

• *Listen attentively.* Lean forward and actively listen to the member. Offer periodic comments such as "I see" or nod occasionally to let the speaker know you understand and are interested in what he/she is saying.

• *Maintain eye contact.* Do not let outside distractions interfere with the conversation. Maintain eye contact and actively listen.

- *Use open body language.* Lean toward the speaker with a smile letting the speaker know you are involved in the conversation. Avoid defensive body language such as leaning back or crossing your arms.

Conflict Resolution

Like it or not, service desk personnel often hear from disgruntled members. Although the support of management in these situations is welcome and warranted, understanding basic conflict resolution skills is an asset for every service desk staff member. Using the communication and interpersonal skills we have discussed, a simple formula for conflict resolution will be effective in most circumstances. This formula is a common sense approach to conflict resolution. Follow the steps and make adjustments to fit the situation.

- *Defuse the discontent.* Talk to the member and explain to him that you are interested in what he is saying. Agree with him that this situation has inconvenienced or angered him, and assure him that the situation will be researched.

- *Agree on the problem.* Once the member is rational and can discuss the issue calmly, restate the problem as you understand it. Agree on the issue and let the member know that a representative of the club, if it is not yourself, will be in touch to follow up on the matter.

- *Gather facts.* Research the issue. Find all the details relating to what happened, how it happened, why it happened, who was involved, and what possibly could be done to prevent it from reoccurring.

- *Establish a solution.* Whether a system is created or a new policy or procedure is put in place, establish a solution to the situation. This solution may not be the long-term answer, but may be a first step that you can refine. Ensuring the situation does not occur again is critical to member and staff confidence.

- *Train on the solution.* Meet with staff members to inform them of the new system or policy. Explain to them the reasons for the action and ask them to offer suggestions. Go over the solution in detail so every staff member understands the policy and why it is now in effect.

- *Follow up with the member.* This is the most important and unfortunately the most neglected step. A great deal of effort has been expended to research the problem, find a solution, and train on the solution. Be sure to let the member know you have heard the complaint and have taken action. A personal phone call or note from the management team will go a long way in establishing member confidence.

Sales

The service desk staff is not often thought of in terms of sales. However, every member of the staff should be taught basic sales skills. Whether the product is a tangible item such as a retail product, or as intangible as an upcoming event, basic sales training is essential for the organization to succeed. How detailed the training program is depends on the job description of the staff involved. The personnel selling memberships need more in-depth sales training than the person supervising the exercise floor. Some sales training for the fitness floor supervisor will assist in selling a program to the member, enhancing member involvement and enjoyment. Basic selling skills will teach each staff member to identify the member's need and fill the need with a product or service available at the club.

Member questions and requests are two opportune times to sell the member on available programs or events or on the quality and comprehensiveness of the facility and programming. Keep in mind the following issues when responding to a member question or request.

- *Need.* A great deal of the sales process is correctly identifying the needs of the member or prospective member. If a prospective member enters the club and the first person he comes in contact with at the service desk is not trained or interested in why he came to visit the club, consider the sale lost. Train the service desk staff to ask leading questions and listen carefully to identify the need. This information can then be passed to the membership sales team.

- *Listen for objections.* Every person who enters the club is interested in joining or he would not have spent the time to visit. Often, the sale comes down to confirming for the prospective member this is a good idea. Listen carefully for objections or excuses the prospective member may offer and work to overcome those objections with positive attributes of your facility or program.

- *Presentation.* Present the facility and programming in a way that responds to the individual's needs while positively overcoming objections defined in earlier discussions.

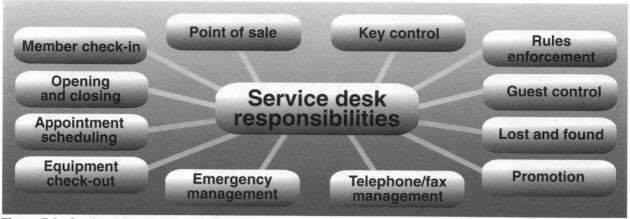

Figure 7.3   Service desk personnel roles.

• *Ask for the sale; close the sale.* Whether it is a membership or a personal training client, ask for the sale by saying something like, "Can I schedule your first appointment?"

• *Service.* Now that the person has committed and made the purchase, give her more than she would normally expect. Make a call to her home or business to welcome her and check on her progress in the club. Offer her a complimentary T-shirt as a token of appreciation. Offer an orientation personal training session or fitness assessment to immediately provide value for the dollar spent.

All these skills will contribute to the customer experience. Using these skills will build a relationship with the members that will last. To deliver consistent, quality service, the management and staff must make a commitment to offering the best services and products available. Anticipating needs, listening attentively and actively, finding workable solutions, and communicating those solutions to both membership and staff are skills indicating an organization committed to quality member service.

SERVICE DESK RESPONSIBILITIES

The list of daily responsibilities of the service desk staff never ends (see figure 7.3). This position carries a great deal of responsibility. A brief review of some common tasks and ideas to improve their efficiency follows. By no means is this list finite; responsibilities differ in every facility. Successful and efficient completion of these tasks will enhance the professionalism of the service desk and the organization.

Opening Procedures

The responsibility for opening the club in the early morning hours often falls squarely on the shoulders of the service desk staff. The staff member who holds this responsibility must be highly dependable. The club must be opened and ready to operate at the scheduled opening time without fail. Typically, the performance of opening checklist duties (see, for example, table 7.2) takes between 15 and 30 minutes. This list must be complete, the club ready, and the front door unlocked on time. Hold staff responsible for the opening checklist by requiring them to initial each task, instead of simply checking it off. This will provide a degree of accountability.

Closing Procedures

As important as the opening responsibilities are the closing responsibilities. As with the opening procedures, the service desk staff often perform most of these duties. Closing and securing the club is an important task. Again an initialed checklist, with all evening shift responsibilities along with tasks specific to closing the club, will provide accountability and consistency to the closing procedures. Table 7.3 offers a typical closing checklist.

Service Desk Check-In

The primary responsibility of every service desk is to ensure the exclusivity of the club. Controlling access to only qualified members and their guests is a difficult job. Many systems, both manual and computerized, are available to assist the service desk staff in this task. However, these systems simply assist the staff, they do not replace them.

Table 7.2   Opening Checklist

Instructions: Please *initial* each task when complete and give this to the general manager at the end of your shift.

_____ 1. Ensure alarm is turned off as you enter the building.

_____ 2. Turn on all lights in the facility.

_____ 3. Walk through the entire facility to ensure its cleanliness and order. Report any cleanliness issues on the bottom of this form.

_____ 4. Turn on or initialize the computer system.

_____ 5. Retrieve all computer reports printed overnight and place them in the bookkeeper's box.

_____ 6. Turn on the music systems.

_____ 7. Turn on the television systems.

_____ 8. Retrieve your cash bank from the safety deposit box and ensure it has exactly $150.00 in small bills and change. Obtain change if necessary.

_____ 9. Activate the point of sale system.

_____ 10. Unlock all equipment cabinets, retail cabinets, and locker key drawers.

_____ 11. Ensure all staff members are in place and prepared for opening.

_____ 12. Check facility appointment books for potential errors or problems.

_____ 13. Arrange sign-in sheet and computer magnetic strip reader. Ensure the proper day and date are recorded on the top of the page and screen.

_____ 14. Ensure all paper products such as note pads, stationery, tickets, cash register tape, credit card vouchers, and so on are stocked.

_____ 15. Go to locker rooms and ensure wet areas are in working order.

_____ 16. Ensure locker room amenities are well stocked.

_____ 17. Take the telephones off Do Not Disturb or deactivate the answering system.

_____ 18. Unlock the doors *on time*.

Notes, maintenance needs, issues for management follow-up

Manual systems for controlling access to the facility are considered less effective than computerized check-in systems. In some facilities, however, manual systems have proven effective. A manual system may involve tendering a picture identification card to gain access. In others simply signing in on a registration pad will gain access. Whatever the method of manual member check-in, the integrity of control for the facility rests heavily on the service desk staff. With the many responsibilities the service desk staff must complete, a nonregistered guest may enter the facility while the staff is distracted. Properly staffing the service desk to prevent such distractions will improve control over the facility.

With the rapid advancement of computer technology and the resultant decrease in costs for computer hardware and software, many clubs are now using computerized front desk check-in systems. These systems increase control of the facility while minimizing inconveniences and delays for members entering and leaving the club.

Basic programs simply log the member in by reading a bar code or magnetic strip off the member identification card. If the member is in good standing with the facility, access is granted. If the person is no longer a member or his/her account is in arrears, access is denied. As mentioned earlier, some of the more deluxe systems display video images of

Table 7.3   Closing Checklist

Instructions: Please *initial* each task when complete and give this to the general manager at the end of your shift.

_____ 1. Secure all doors after all members have departed.

_____ 2. Place telephones on Do Not Disturb and activate answering service.

_____ 3. Complete roll-out and bank deposit procedures.

_____ 4. Start the overnight computer reporting process.

_____ 5. Check each area of the club before staff departs.

_____ 6. Fitness floor   _____ All small equipment arranged neatly.
                                       _____ All equipment aligned and arranged neatly.
                                       _____ Trash containers emptied.
                                       _____ Soiled towels to laundry and clean towels stocked.
                                       _____ Water cups stocked.
                                       _____ All plates returned to racks.
                                       _____ All newspapers recycled and magazines straightened.

_____ 7. Tennis courts   _____ Cup dispenser stocked.
                                       _____ Chairs and tables neatly arranged.
                                       _____ Tennis equipment put away.
                                       _____ Trash containers emptied.
                                       _____ Soiled towels to laundry and clean towels restocked.

_____ 8. Pool   _____ All furniture neatly arranged.
                                       _____ Soiled towels to laundry and clean towels stocked.
                                       _____ All pool equipment stored neatly.
                                       _____ Chemical balance charts reviewed.

_____ 9. Locker rooms   _____ All areas neat and tidy.
                                       _____ All amenities restocked.
                                       _____ Pick up temperature charts for the wet areas.
                                       _____ All lockers secured or empty.
                                       _____ Lost and found items returned to service desk.
                                       _____ Soiled towels to laundry and clean towels stocked.

_____ 10. Turn off point of sale system.

_____ 11. Turn off music systems.

_____ 12. Turn off television systems.

_____ 13. Turn off computer systems.

_____ 14. Lock all equipment closets and display cabinets.

_____ 15. Perform audit of daily locker keys and secure key drawer.

_____ 16. Collect all daily tickets and place in bookkeeper's box.

_____ 17. Review appointment books for potential problems.

_____ 18. Ensure all lost and found items have been logged and secured.

_____ 19. Walk through the entire club for maintenance issues. Write notes on back of this form.

_____ 20. Turn off lights.

_____ 21. Set alarm system and lock all doors.

the member on the screen as his/her ID card is scanned, making identification and verification an easy task. Whether basic or deluxe, these computerized programs can provide a wealth of decision-making information to the management of the club. (See chapter 19 for a more detailed discussion regarding the capability of front desk and other software systems.) Although these systems are only as effective as the staff operating them, computerized check-in has the potential to enhance service delivery by freeing the staff to focus attention on member service.

Point of Sale

The service desk staff is often the primary point of sale for the club. Responsibilities may include cash transactions such as sale of pro shop items, collecting fees for services, or simply making change. Maintaining a balanced cash bank takes a great deal of effort and concentration. To ensure accountability, each staff member must keep his or her personal bank in a locked cash drawer. The only person who should have access to that bank is the person responsible for its accuracy. By maintaining tight controls over cash banks and assigning cashier numbers to each staff member, management with the help of point of sale systems can track every sale.

Standardize and strictly enforce procedures for accepting any form of payment from a member or nonmember for products or services rendered. Common payment methods include signing to their membership account, cash, credit cards, check, or rendering a gift certificate. Specific procedures for accepting payment will differ at each facility. Consult with a CPA to establish strict guidelines for handling cash, credit card, or check payments; bank integrity; as well as close out and bank deposit procedures at the end of each shift.

Key Control and Locker Rental

The control of daily locker keys and the permanent locker rental program often fall on the service desk. Control of daily locker keys is an important task that could prove costly if you don't maintain tight control. Strict procedures must be in place if a daily locker key is lost or removed from the club. The possibility that a duplicate key to any locker exists eliminates the integrity of the locker system and places the club in a liability position should items in the locker be stolen. Periodic reviews of the lock and

key mechanism by a qualified locksmith will ensure the pins located in the core are in good working order.

New lock and key systems designed specifically for the health fitness industry are available from many manufacturers to remove this responsibility from the service desk. The club is freed of this liability by replacing traditional locks and keys with special release mechanisms that prevent the loss of the locker key. Review one of the many industry source guides to find potential vendors.

Permanent locker rentals offer the opportunity for significant revenue. Assessing a monthly locker rental charge to members who wish to keep personal items at the club can prove beneficial to the bottom line while offering a convenience to the member. Permanent locker rental programs can be as basic as offering the key to the member and charging the member account a nominal fee per month, or as elaborate as mounting the member's name on the locker and providing that member with laundry service for a higher monthly fee. Whatever the extent of the locker rental program, developing a low-maintenance control system, in close cooperation with the accounting department, is essential for its success. The service desk can maintain a running list of locker changes, additions, deletions, and moves and can provide it at month end to the accounting department for appropriate billing. The system need not be complicated to be effective. A brief review of possible locker rental procedures can be found on the following page.

Enforcing House Rules and Regulations

The service desk is the front line defense for enforcing house rules and regulations, whether the issue is dress code, guest registration, or conduct unbecoming a member. Strong training in conflict resolution skills will assist the service desk staff by giving them the confidence to confront members who are not in compliance with the rules. Staff can successfully enforce the rules with the following tips:

• *Never embarrass or harass the member.* Take the member aside to discuss the issue instead of announcing the rule violation in front of other members. It is important to turn this potentially negative situation into a positive one by maintaining the integrity of the member.

• *Management should never overturn a judgment call made by service staff.* Nothing will kill the motivation

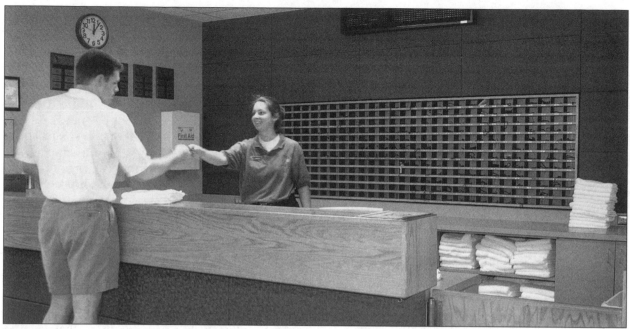

© Tom Wallace

of the service staff to enforce the rules quicker than having a manager or supervisor who is not comfortable with conflict let the rule violation pass, even if it is "just this time."

• *Create a win-win situation.* If the member's T-shirt violates the club dress code, instead of turning the member away from the club angry, offer to provide him with another T-shirt. Anticipate the problem and have win-win solutions prepared.

• *Be consistent with rules enforcement.* Nothing more, nothing less—consistency is the key to member respect.

Guest Control and Check-In

The professional handling of guests and prospective members in any facility has a tremendous impact on new member sales, and the membership sales department should assist with its development. When a member brings a guest to the facility, she expects her guest to be treated courteously and professionally. Programs to efficiently register the guest or prospect with the club, offer him a tour of the facility, and familiarize him with the exercise equipment will pay dividends when this guest considers a new club affiliation. The importance of complete registration with the facility cannot be overly stressed. It is important not only to gather the necessary information, such as name and phone number, so the membership de-

Permanent Locker Rental Procedures

1. Maintain a single accurate listing of all available lockers for permanent rental.

2. List the name of the person renting the locker beside the specific locker they are renting.

3. Provide this current list of locker rentals to accounting for billing.

4. Audit the monthly billing to ensure all permanent locker holders have been billed.

5. Standardize the procedure for permanent locker changes at the service desk (i.e., maintain a singular location and procedure for all locker inquiries and modifications).

6. Prepare a summary listing at the front of the locker listing for all modifications during the present month. This listing includes lockers issued, deleted, moved, and so on.

7. Compare the modifications listing, which has been verified during the previous month's audit (see step 4), with the master listing kept by the service desk manager.

8. Prepare a complete listing of all locker changes and update accounting as needed.

Note: It is helpful if all locker rental procedures are handled by one or, at most, two individuals.

Table 7.4   The PAR-Q (Physical Activity Readiness Questionnaire)

PAR-Q & YOU
(a questionnaire for people aged 15 to 69)

Yes	No	
☐	☐	1. Has your doctor ever said that you have a heart condition and that you should only do physical activity recommended by a doctor?
☐	☐	2. Do you feel pain in your chest when you do physical activity?
☐	☐	3. In the past month, have you had chest pain when you were not doing physical activity?
☐	☐	4. Do you lose your balance because of dizziness or do you ever lose consciousness?
☐	☐	5. Do you have a bone or joint problem that could be made worse by a change in your physical activity?
☐	☐	6. Is your doctor currently prescribing drugs (for example, water pills) for your blood pressure or heart condition?
☐	☐	7. Do you know of *any other reason* why you should not do physical activity?

If you answered **YES** to one or more questions

Talk with your doctor by phone or in person BEFORE you start becoming much more physically active or BEFORE you have a fitness appraisal. Tell your doctor about the PAR-Q and which questions you answered YES to.

- You may be able to do any activity you want—as long as you start slowly and build up gradually. Or, you may need to restrict your activities to those that are safe for you. Talk with your doctor about the kinds of activities you wish to participate in and follow his/her advice.

- Find out which community programs are safe and helpful for you.

If you answered **NO** to all questions

If you answered NO honestly to *all* PAR-Q questions, you can be reasonably sure that you can:

- start becoming much more physically active—begin slowly and build up gradually. This is the safest and easiest way to go.

- take part in a fitness appraisal—this is an excellent way to determine your basic fitness so that you can plan the best way for you to live actively.

DELAY BECOMING MUCH MORE ACTIVE:

- if you are not feeling well because of a temporary illness such as a cold or a fever—wait until you feel better; or

- if you are or may be pregnant—talk to your doctor before you start becoming more active.

Please note: If your health changes so that you then answer YES to any of the above questions, tell your fitness or health professional. Ask whether you should change your physical activity plan.

Reprinted, by permission, from the 1994 revised version of the Physical Activity Readiness Questionnaire (PAR-Q and You). The Par-Q and You is a copyrighted, pre-exercise screen owned by the Canadian Society for Exercise Physiology.

partment can make a follow-up call, but also to have the guest complete a waiver or release of liability for the facility. The most commonly used instrument is the PAR-Q (see table 7.4). These instruments will not release the facility in cases of gross negligence, but they will ensure the guest understands and accepts his limitations and the potential risks involved.

Telephone Etiquette, Message Handling, and Fax Management

Professional telephone skills should be stressed in every customer-service facility. Developing standardized methods for answering the telephone; transferring a call, message, or fax handling; and paging of members should be a priority. Variances in techniques and terminology in answering the telephone gives the caller the impression the facility is unorganized and unprofessional. Table 7.5 details possible standards for this important area of customer service.

Emergency Procedures

The staff of the service desk must be well trained and well practiced in handling emergency situations. It should be the service desk staff that communicates with the emergency management service for the community during times of medical or other crisis. Although specific responsibilities will differ from facility to facility, the service staff should be prepared to handle the following issues during an emergency situation. Refer to chapter 13 for

additional discussions regarding emergency response management.

• *Know all emergency exits.* The service staff should assist in evacuating all members and guests who are close to the service desk.

• *Evacuate with daily sign-in records.* Should the need arise to evacuate the building, the service staff should quickly gather all the records available that indicate who had visited the club that day. This information is important when emergency officials are attempting to account for all individuals in the facility.

• *Gather any specific records as directed by the general manager.* There will be valuable information located behind the service desk. With prior discussions and practice, it will become reactionary for the service desk staff to locate and remove any necessary information during the evacuation process.

Table 7.5   Telephone Etiquette Standard of Service

Procedure	Standard
1. Answer the phone promptly.	• Answer phones with a smile in your voice.
2. State time of day, department, and name.	• Answer all phones in three rings with "Good morning, afternoon, or evening, (club name), (your name) speaking. How may I help you?"
3. Speak in a clear voice.	
4. Use professional language.	
5. Use a comfortable speed; never rush.	
6. Use caller's name when known.	
7. Listen carefully and do not interrupt.	
8. Never chew gum while speaking on the phone.	
9. When placing a call on hold do the following:	
Ask for caller's permission to place on hold. If yes, say "Thank you."	• Give callers an opportunity to respond before placing them on hold.
If caller refuses, handle immediately and reassure waiting members that you will be with them momentarily.	
Return to calls on hold within 45 seconds.	• Callers are not on hold longer than 60 seconds.
Thank callers for holding when returning to assist them.	
10. Take messages legibly and completely, including the following:	
• Caller's complete name.	• Offer to take messages before caller asks.
• Caller's phone number.	• Write message legibly and completely.
• Day and time of call.	
• Message.	
• Your initials.	
11. Allow caller to disconnect line before you hang up.	• Place telephone gently in cradle.

- *Work comfortably and calmly with emergency services.* During an emergency, the staff must be well prepared and calm. Critical information must be related to emergency personnel efficiently and precisely. Include the service staff in the monthly practice of the medical emergency plan to prevent costly chaos and delays.

- *Know vital information.* The service desk will be looked upon to provide information to emergency services. Information such as the club address and telephone number as well as statistics, such as age, allergies to medications, and the person to contact in case of such an emergency, on any individual needing medical attention. This information must be available or easily attainable for the staff.

Special Events Promotion

As discussed earlier in this chapter, the service desk could also be called the information desk. The service desk is a key player in recruiting members for programs and events occurring in the club. Service desk staff should promote upcoming events enthusiastically to encourage attendance.

Equipment Checkout

Equipment checkout procedures are required in every facility to ensure the return of property owned by the club. Items such as locker keys, towels, workout uniforms, basketballs, racquets, weight-training belts, pool buoys, and so on may be the responsibility of the service desk staff. Procedures as simple as rendering an ID card or driver's license will ensure the items are returned or the individual responsible for their loss will be identified and charged. Well-defined procedures that are strictly enforced will ensure expensive equipment remains in the club.

Lost and Found

Procedures to log and secure lost and found items will ensure any items misplaced by members are quickly returned presents a professional and organized image of the club. The service desk staff should log all items found in the club or turned in to a staff member and quickly secure them behind lock and key. When a member inquires whether an item has been found, a quick review of the log book will allow the service staff to respond efficiently to the inquiry. Likewise, staff can log items that members have misplaced but have not yet been turned in to ensure a quick return if they are found later.

Appointment Scheduling

Appointment scheduling can be a simple or complex task, depending on the number of services available. Services such as massage, manicures, tanning, personal training, fitness assessments, and more may all be available to members through the service desk. Whether staff uses conventional appointment books or computer systems, appointment scheduling has the potential to positively affect the bottom line of the club. Systems to carefully book the appointment and confirm the time, date, service, and service provider with the client before terminating the telephone call or conversation show professionalism and organization. A reminder telephone call one day before the event will prove profitable. Professional and efficient handling of the appointment process will result in return clients, referrals, and greater profitability.

ADMINISTRATIVE CONCERNS

The presence of a concerned health fitness manager who oversees the operation of the service desk can greatly enhance the quality of the work environment for the staff and the service for the member. Careful preparation of staff schedules and standards for conduct should be on the top of the list of areas for administrative assistance.

Staff Scheduling

Staffing the service desk is an important management task. Efficiency of service to members who are hustling to fit in a workout during their busy days is mandatory. With the numerous tasks the service desk is responsible for, staffing becomes crucial. Evaluating the daily traffic patterns to ensure adequate staffing during the busy hours is an ongoing task. Cross-training several members of the staff to assist during times of heavy usage is a wise management strategy. Popular staffing strategies include overlapping staff during prime time hours to ensure proper coverage. As any manager is aware, personnel costs must be tightly controlled; however, inadequate staffing at the service desk may prove much more costly in terms of membership dissatisfaction and attrition.

Table 7.6 Grooming Standard	
Procedure	**Standard**
• Maintain good personal hygiene at all times	• Appearance makes a positive impression on the members.
1. Shower or bathe daily.	• Take pride and great care in your personal appearance.
2. Use deodorant daily.	• Strict adherence to grooming and uniform standards is expected.
3. Brush teeth regularly.	
4. Keep breath fresh.	
5. Use perfume or cologne sparingly.	• Use fragrances only to complement overall appearance, never offensive.
6. Keep hands and nails clean at all times.	• Be sure nail length does not interfere with work.
7. Maintain regular haircuts and daily cleaning and conditioning of hair.	• Keep hairstyles attractive, neatly styled, and professional in appearance.
	• Employees returning from smoking are to ensure that no smoke smell is present on clothing, hands, or breath.
• Guidelines for women	
1. Use makeup conservatively.	
2. Keep hair out of face.	
• Guidelines for men	
1. Keep hair neatly trimmed.	
2. Keep mustaches neatly trimmed above upper lip.	

Dress Code and Grooming

Setting standards for the grooming and professional dress of the staff of the service desk is important. The presentation of these individuals speaks volumes about the professionalism of the entire organization. Decisions regarding hair length and style, jewelry, clothing, and hygiene should be predetermined and strictly enforced. Individuals not dressed or groomed properly have no business behind the service desk for any reason. Image and service are important and cannot afford to be compromised. A sample grooming standard can be seen in table 7.6.

IN CLOSING

In this chapter, we presented an operational overview of the service desk. Creating a service culture through such practices as name recognition, task efficiency, and well-informed, outgoing, and professional staff makes an important first impression on anyone who walks in the door. Effective new employee training programs and ongoing training for club employees are an important part of consistently delivering superior service. Although specific tasks related to service desk operations and administration vary from club to club, one consistent fact remains: the optimal service desk of every club should be operated and managed with professionalism and friendliness.

KEY TERMS

Event order

Service culture

Service desk

RECOMMENDED READINGS

Boccafogli, P. 1995. *Rosewood Hotels and Resorts training program*. Dallas: Rosewood Hotels and Resorts.

IRSA (now IHRSA). 1994. How consumers view health and sports clubs. An IRSA Vanguard study conducted by the University of Michigan Center for Research on Active Lifestyle Behavior.

Lauderbaugh, JJ. 1995. *Winning with teamwork*. Seminar presented at the International Health, Racquet and Sportsclub Association conference and trade show, March, San Francisco.

Morris, B. 1994. Front and center. *Club Industry* (October): 33-34, 37-43.

Nash, M. 1985. *Making people productive*. San Francisco: Jossey-Bass.

Pacetta, F., and R. Gittines. 1994. *Don't fire them, fire them up*. New York: Simon & Schuster.

Patton, R.W., W.C. Grantham, R.F. Gerson, and L.R. Gettman. 1989. *Developing and managing health/fitness facilities*. Champaign, IL: Human Kinetics.

Sattker, T., and J. Mullen. 1995. Winning the sales war, peacefully. *Fitness Management* (February): 48-50.

Program Management

A focal point of every club is the ongoing activities and events that create member excitement. All too often in the health fitness industry, program planning is secondary to crisis management. Clubs with health fitness managers who carefully plan, implement, and evaluate their activities and special events will develop a successful member following. Do you prioritize appropriate program planning time in your schedule? Do you carefully implement programs with a thorough marketing and public relations effort? Following the event, do you hold a staff debriefing to evaluate the success of the program so constant improvement of programs is the norm? If the answer to any of these questions is not overwhelmingly positive, consider the following information as you plan your programming calendar for the next month, quarter, or year.

The term *program* has been used interchangeably to define the total health fitness wellness concept initiated within the commercial, corporate, clinical, or community setting and the individual contests, leagues, special events, and so on that are planned within the health fitness setting. For background purposes, the distinguishing features, specific purposes, and target markets of each setting were discussed in chapter 1. This chapter, however, and chapter 9 deal specifically with planning, implementing, and evaluating the programs or *programming* that occurs within the different health fitness settings (see figure 8.1).

> *Developing quality programming within a health fitness setting is often cited as a major factor in the successful retention of members and thus the profitability of a club (Coffman 1994; IHRSA 1994b; Lynch 1990; Patton et al. 1989).*

Programming that is professionally planned and implemented will keep the membership active in a facility long after the initial wave of good intentions has passed. Quality programming that offers opportunities for fun and social interaction, while enhancing the probability of meeting personal fitness and wellness goals, will keep the member in the club and on the dues-paying membership roster. Innovative programming that is professionally delivered is a powerful weapon in the ongoing battle for membership retention.

As stated in chapter 1, each unique health fitness setting caters to a specific target population to achieve the goals and objectives of the organization. To meet these predetermined objectives, the program must have participants. Quality programming is the key to attracting and keeping members active in the facility. In the commercial setting, the primary goal is to generate a profit. If members are active in the facility and make the club a part of their weekly routine because of quality programming, they retain their memberships, thus providing the club operator with membership dues and other incidental revenues. In the corporate environment, the primary goal is to improve the quality of life of the workforce and, therefore, positively affect the organization's bottom line by decreasing health care costs, increasing productivity, and improving morale. If programming offered in the corporate environment educates and motivates the workforce to make positive lifestyle changes, and thus decreases the likelihood of disease, the corporate objective is met. Within the community setting, service programs are designed to reach as many people as possible with the message of health, wellness, or recreation. Sources of the service message may come from many voluntary health agencies, such as the American Heart Association, YMCA, YWCA, or JCC. The clinical setting, with its varied objectives and goals, can reach many people through high-quality, medically-based programming. The planning and implementation of motivating, entertaining, and educational programming that is in compliance with the organization's mission is the key to reaching and retaining members while meeting the organizational objectives. Table 8.1 compares programming goals and outcomes.

Whatever the setting, the primary focus of the health fitness manager should be developing and implementing innovative programming that meets the changing needs of the member population. Industry reports and journals often discuss current trends in programming. According to a recent IHRSA report (IHRSA 1995), "programming in the 1990s will be kinder and gentler to meet the needs of an older health club member, and more diverse to meet

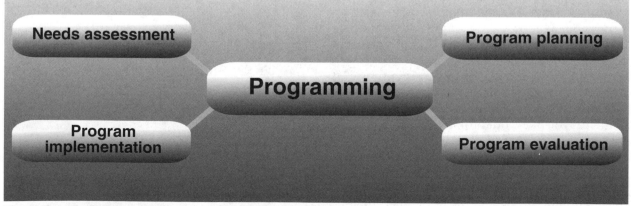

Figure 8.1 Basic components of successful programming.

Table 8.1	Contrasting the Goals, Programs, and Outcomes of Health Fitness Settings		
Setting	**Primary goals**	**Quality programs**	**Outcomes**
Commercial	Profit.	Personal training. Private instruction.	Increased dues. Retain members. Increased service revenue.
Corporate	Improve employee health and quality of life to decrease health care spending.	Smoking cessation. Back safety. Stress management.	Better employee health. Positive attitudes. Reduced stress.
Clinical	Market to apparently healthy population. High quality programs.	Cardiac rehabilitation. Physical therapy. Older adult care.	Reach market for later health care services.
Community	Reach public with wellness message.	Child care. Children's programs. Family programs.	Educate public. Family events.

the changing needs of a population that is more interested in a holistic approach to health which encompasses, but is not limited to, physical activity." This projection forces the health fitness manager to learn about several new areas to meet the growing needs of the active older adult. We must educate ourselves about complementary care techniques for stress management and optimal health, such as yoga, relaxation, meditation, and deep breathing. We must become knowledgeable about current research regarding the changing physiological demands of exercise as we age. As health fitness professionals, we must also evaluate what psychological barriers to exercise and health now present themselves as the population ages. This trend presents a challenge to the traditionally trained health fitness manager, who must develop or acquire the knowledge and management skills necessary to meet the needs of a rapidly changing industry.

The I-formation management model presented in chapter 4 provides managers with a foundation for acquiring the skills necessary to retrain and reeducate ourselves to meet the needs of the aging population. We must gather information to understand the trends in this dynamic industry. Innovative thinking is mandatory in developing programs and services demanded by the educated consumer. Professional implementation of these innovative ideas will meet the needs of the consumer and continue the cycle of growth and change in the industry. Managers must continually gather and evaluate information throughout the process so we can refine and implement a continual pool of innovative ideas in a manner best suited to meet the objectives of the program. In an enterprising facility staffed with energetic managers, the cycle of refinement, growth, and change never ends.

CONTRASTING PROGRAMMING IN HEALTH FITNESS SETTINGS

Chapter 1 discussed in detail the objectives and target population of programs in the different health fitness settings. In this discussion we learned that each setting has compelling reasons for developing a health promotion program within the boundaries of its global mission and that no two programs, although some similarities do exist, are exactly alike. We can also say this for the programming each setting offers. The organization must design the

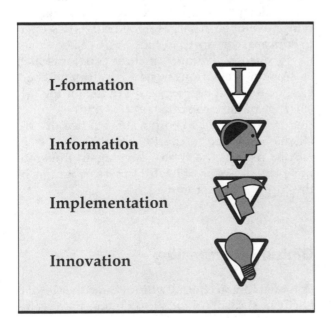

I-formation

Information

Implementation

Innovation

leagues, contests, classes, and special events to meet the global mission of the setting as well as the needs and objectives of the target population within that setting. In the following sections, we will examine the different programming these distinct environments typically offer.

Commercial Programming

The programming this setting offers must either independently generate a profit or contribute to the professionalism and profitability of the club through intangible means, such as member satisfaction and retention. Programs, such as classes in martial arts and yoga, or services, such as massage therapy, have the ability to independently produce a profit while offering a service to the membership.

Top 20 Club Programs (programs most commonly offered by clubs)

Program*	Percent
1. **Fitness evaluation**	**87**
2. Step and bench aerobics	84
3. **Personal training**	**81**
4. Strength training	78
5. **Child care**	**66**
6. Cross-training	62
7. **Weight control**	**61**
8. **Nutritional counseling**	**61**
9. **Massage**	**60**
10. **Corporate programming**	**56**
11. Exercise prescriptions	51
12. Seniors' programming	46
13. Aquatic exercise	45
14. **Special programs, diabetes**	**43**
15. Juniors' programming	40
16. Competitive sports	40
17. **Martial arts**	**38**
18. **Yoga**	**38**
19. Health-education programs	34
20. Children's programming	31

* Potentially profit-generating programs are in bold.

Reprinted, by permission, from IHRSA, 1994, *Profiles of success* (Boston: IHRSA).

In fact, of the top 20 club programs listed in the 1994 IHRSA *Profiles of Success* report, several could easily produce a profit for the club (see list to the left). The remainder of the programs on the list would certainly enhance member satisfaction and retention by meeting the needs of an aging population interested in prevention programs. The challenge of the health fitness manager is to select, market, and professionally implement the programs that fit the needs and desires of their specific member population and objectives of the organization.

> *The primary goal of every commercial fitness center is profit.*

Corporate Programming

Programming in the corporate sector is designed to offer health promotion opportunities for the workforce with the intent to control health care spending. One method of achieving these health promotion goals is put forth by Opatz in *A Primer of Health Promotion* (1985): "the systematic efforts of an organization to enhance the wellness of its members through education, behavioral change, and cultural support." Through education, behavior change, and peer support, corporations that develop health fitness programs will fight the rising costs of health care with awareness and prevention of disease. Therefore, most programming developed in corporate settings is designed to educate workers to induce positive health behavior change. Examples include programs such as smoking cessation, weight control and exercise, or recreation programs. We list on the following page programs and services most frequently offered to corporate and health care clients according to the 1994 IHRSA *Profiles in Success* report. These programs again illustrate this primary focus of health fitness programs in the corporate environment.

Clinical Programming

Programming in clinical settings can either be distinctly medical or can mimic programs in the com-

Programs and Services Most Frequently Offered to Corporate and Health Care Clients (percent of clubs offering)

Program or service	Percent
1. Initial fitness assessments	70
2. Body-composition analysis	61
3. Follow-up fitness assessments	58
4. Wellness education	53
5. Employee participation tracking	53
6. Health fairs	52
7. Back programs	36
8. Companywide health history evaluations	35
9. Physical therapy and rehabilitation	29
10. Blood pressure screening and treatment	29
11. Pre- and postnatal programs	27
12. Stress management	25
13. Nutritional disorders	23
14. Arthritis	23

Reprinted from IHRSA 1994.

mercial, corporate, or community settings. Medically-based programs, such as physical therapy, cardiac rehabilitation, or diabetes education, although no longer the exclusive domain of clinical settings, are primarily offered through hospitals or outpatient clinics. As the clinical setting grows and adapts to the changes in the health care system, programming similar to that found in other settings is common. For example, the clinical setting can take on the properties of a commercial setting when it sells memberships to the fitness facility. When this occurs, programming appropriate for an apparently healthy population, such as group exercise classes and personal training, must be offered.

When the clinical setting offers wellness and health promotion programs for its employee base, it must consider education and behavior modification programs that will offset rising health care costs. Similarly, if the clinical setting offers educational support programs to the community to increase visibility and improve the image of the hospital or clinic in the eyes of the consumer, programming will be similar to that found in community settings. Thus, it should not surprise the consumer to find a variety of programs available through a local hospital-based fitness center.

Community Programming

Programs in the community sector are as varied as those in the clinical setting. However, these programs share a common goal of reaching and serving the public. Community-based programming, such as after-school child care programs offered through the local YMCA or YWCA, CPR classes taught by the American Heart Association or American Red Cross, or multisport recreational leagues organized by local parks and recreation departments, demonstrates that these organizations reach out to educate and serve the community. Community organizations are reaching the family more effectively than any other setting. Organizations such as the YMCA and YWCA are actively designing and marketing programs to meet the growing needs of families with little discretionary time. Program offerings in this setting often reflect this trend.

Examples of some typical annual programming calendars for the commercial, corporate, community, and clinical environments can be found in tables 8.2 through 8.5.

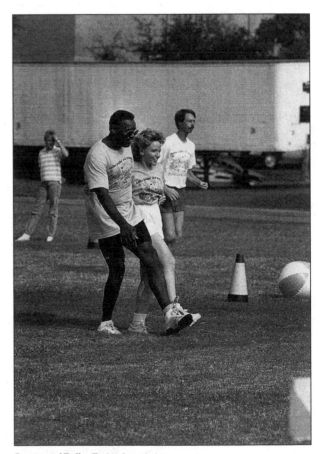

Courtesy of Dallas Texins Association

Table 8.2   Annual Programming Calendar for a Commercial Setting

January	Resolution month fitness contest Health fair Basketball leagues—children and adults Superbowl party
February	Healthy heart cooking class Body fat screening Heart attack master aerobics class American Heart Association charity fund-raising silent auction Children's Valentine's Day cookie decorating contest
March	Swimsuit season weight-management seminar series Spring training softball conditioning program Spring tennis league championships Spring break kids' camp
April	Golf club tournament of champions Night out at the symphony Aerobic marathon (two-hour master class) Stress-management dine and de-stress dinner Annual family picnic at Gateway Park
May	Rock climbing weekend getaway Memorial Day tennis tournament Swimming for fitness clinic Cycling club meeting Children's tennis lessons begin Children's swimming lessons—session I begins
June	Hike and bike family outing at Hideaway Lake Water exercise classes begin—outdoor pool Kids' camp—session I Hope community service project Splashfest—family swimming party
July	Fourth of July annual picnic and fireworks display Bingo night party Family night at the Texas Ranger game Kids' camp—session II Children's swimming lessons—session II begins
August	Wallyball league begins Fantasy football league begins Casino night party Weight-training seminar Club scuba trip to the Bahamas
September	Jazz on the terrace happy hour Murder mystery dinner Community CPR certification Fall fitness fest—group exercise and fun walk Skin care and makeup seminar
October	Flu shots Couples massage seminar Video golf swing analysis with the golf pros Volleyball league begins Chili cook-off and picnic Children's Halloween party
November	Wine tasting social and dinner Surviving the holidays—shopping strategies and gift-giving seminar Home for the holidays canned food drive for charity Healthy holiday cooking classes Annual turkey shoot basketball classic
December	Club gift wrapping service with proceeds for charity Children's holiday party Holiday party New Year's Eve party

Table 8.3   Annual Programming Calendar for a Corporate Setting

January	Fresh start New Year's resolution program Body fat testing and counseling Weight-loss program begins Introduction to group exercise classes Superbowl party
February	Heart test—risk factor screening Healthy treats cooking seminar Strength-training clinic Heart healthy lunch and learn—heart healthy eating
March	Spring into fitness Nutrition trivia contest Outdoor walking program begins Gardening seminar Volleyball league begins
April	Outdoor sport challenge Power walking seminar Quarterly blood pressure screening Body fat reevaluation
May	Stress-management seminar Company picnic—bring the family Health and safety in the workplace fair Softball league begins
June	Cycling trip to Austin Flexibility clinic Back care clinic Family play day
July	Fourth of July party Firecracker stress-reduction class Biofeedback seminar Swimsuit season master class
August	Self-defense classes begin Kick boxing aerobics master class Quarterly blood pressure screening Ergonomics at work seminar—back care
September	Outdoor walk/hike club registration Fall fitness wear fashion show Nutrition seminar—label reading SMAC 28—screening
October	Fall fitness fest Cancer awareness month Mammogram screening for women PSA screening for men Halloween party and master class
November	Great American Smokeout—smoking cessation class Quarterly blood pressure screening Maintain, no-gain holiday weight-control program begins
December	Healthy holiday cooking class Ski conditioning clinic Holiday family party New Year's resolution goal-setting counseling

Table 8.4   Annual Programming Calendar for a Clinical Setting

January	New Year cardiac risk profile Monthly luncheon—exercise and the cardiac-pulmonary patient Tour of Texas walkathon for points—restaurant tour
February	Healthy heart month Blood pressure/resting heart rate screening Monthly luncheon—heart healthy nutrition choices
March	Patient and family health fair Monthly luncheon—stress management Quarterly cardiac-pulmonary support group meeting
April	CPR certification classes Monthly luncheon—20 ways to simplify your life Checkers or chess social
May	Great American Heart Walk (employees) Monthly luncheon—heart healthy summer cooking class Cardiac-pulmonary support group picnic
June	Quarterly cardiac-pulmonary support group meeting Monthly luncheon—exercising in the heat Nutrition trivia contest
July	Fourth of July firecracker stress-management seminar Monthly luncheon—personal safety skills Power walking seminar
August	Cholesterol screening program SMAC 28 blood profiles Monthly luncheon—interpreting your blood test results
September	Bingo night Quarterly cardiac-pulmonary support group meeting Monthly luncheon—fad diets and other nutritional myths
October	Healthy back seminar Monthly luncheon—healthy bones and preventing osteoporosis Halloween party
November	Great American Smokeout—smoking cessation program Monthly luncheon—surviving the holidays Thanksgiving social
December	Monthly luncheon—creative holiday gifts you can make Quarterly cardiac-pulmonary support group meeting Cardiac-pulmonary support group secret Santa

INTRODUCTION TO QUALITY PROGRAM DEVELOPMENT

With an understanding of the typical programming in the different health fitness settings, let us discuss the planning and implementation process. Strategic planning is vital as it helps the health fitness manager identify and meet the market's changing demands for health promotion programs. Managers in corporate, community, clinical, or commercial settings must be innovative to meet the current and future demands of their customers, whether they are employees, citizens, patients, or members. Unfortunately, many managers do not follow the necessary steps in planning and implementation to produce consistent, quality programs. Sandy Coffman (1994) has provided an example of the typical faulty program planning and implementation process found in many clubs: "For many [managers], the programming scenario has sounded something like this: (1) get an idea, (2) put out a sign-up sheet, (3) announce the program in the club newsletter, (4) 'talk it up,' and (5) sit back and hope it flies." This haphazard approach to programming will not produce consistent, high-quality programs.

> *A systematic approach to the planning, implementation, and evaluation of program development is necessary.*

Patton et al. (1986) produced a generic model that delineates the steps of a strategic management plan necessary to consistently produce quality programming. This four-stage management plan involves the following steps:

1. Assessing needs and interests

2. Planning the programs

3. Implementing the programs

4. Evaluating the programs to ensure that the organization's health and fitness mission is well organized and purposeful

To produce consistent high quality programming, constantly cycle these steps. As you implement and evaluate programs in the third and fourth stages, gather information relating to how you can better offer future programs. Use information obtained on one program to design a follow-up program.

Table 8.5   Annual Programming Calendar for a Community Setting

January	Basketball leagues begin—boy's, girl's, men's, women's, and coed Indian guide/Indian princess meeting Country western dance lessons First aid classes taught by American Red Cross
February	National heart attack risk study screening CPR classes taught by American Heart Association Tae kwon do classes begin—session I Fitness committee meeting
March	Roller hockey league begins Senior citizen's tai chi classes begin Women on weights classes begin Spring family picnic and volleyball tournament
April	Soccer leagues begin—children and adults Healthy cooking on a budget seminar Little tots track meet Gymnastics classes begin
May	Weight-control program begins Children's swimming lessons—session I Little League baseball begins Family health and safety fair sponsored by city fire department Fitness committee meeting
June	Tae kwon do classes begin—session II Summer kids camp
July	Fourth of July family picnic First aid classes Indian guide/Indian princess camping trip
August	After–school care programs begin Healthy cooking classes—quick and easy healthy meals Fitness committee meeting CPR classes
September	Tennis lessons—children and adults Annual find-raising dinner and silent auction Flag football season begins
October	Golf lessons—children and adults Flu shots provided at low cost Family Halloween party Basic training—weight-training seminar
November	Give a turkey food drive Fitness committee meeting Holiday stress-management seminar
December	Secret Santa program to benefit the Boys' and Girls' Clubs Children's holiday party Wrap a gift holiday fund raiser for charity

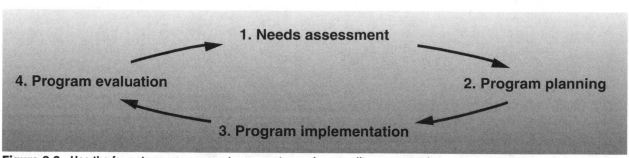

Figure 8.2   Use the four-stage management process to produce quality programming.

Adapted, by permission, from R.W. Patton, W.C. Grantham, R.F. Gerson, and L.R. Gettman, 1989, *Developing and managing health/fitness facilities* (Champaign, IL: Human Kinetics), 202.

Then cycle through the four stages during the follow-up process and so on. The four-stage management process is illustrated in figure 8.2.

A sound strategic plan has built-in flexibility to change if needed. The following are some questions to ask and issues to explore in planning and developing health fitness programs:

- What is the market demand?
- What are the needs and interests of the participants?
- How will the market change?
- How is the competition positioning itself?
- What are the organization's capabilities?
- How will the programs be evaluated?

Let's examine these questions using the four-stage management process.

Needs Assessment

The first stage in planning and developing health fitness programs is to decide what programs will fulfill the needs and interests of the clients. After all, the clients support the program and there will be no

program without them. Regardless of the setting, conduct a *needs assessment* to discover what programs will interest the clients. The types of needs assessments that you could conduct in the various settings are illustrated in table 8.6.

Commercial

In a start-up commercial setting, conduct a market analysis to determine which specific health fitness services the clients will purchase. An outline of the essential items used in a market analysis follows. A market analysis can cost between five thousand and hundreds of thousands of dollars, depending on the scope of the project and how well you have defined the objectives before hiring the marketing consultant. The more information you provide to the consultant, the less the cost will be.

Outline of Essential Items for a Market Analysis

A. Demographic analysis
   1. Service area
   2. Population data—age, gender, income, family dwellings
   3. Employment—major employers, growth, major occupations

Table 8.6   Program Needs Assessments

Commercial setting	Community/clinical setting	Corporate setting
1. Conduct a market survey.	1. Conduct a market survey.	1. Management's perception of needs.
2. Owner(s)' perception of needs.	2. Input from AHA, ACS, ALA, Red Cross, and so forth.	2. Employees' interests/health habits.
3. Investor(s)' perception of needs.	3. Physician(s)' perception of needs.	3. Input from advisory committee.
4. Board of directors' perception of needs.	4. Feedback from existing programs (parks and recreation)	4. Results from health screening, medical evaluation, fitness test.
5. Survey current members.	5. Survey current participants.	

Adapted, by permission, from R.W. Patton, W.C. Grantham, R.F. Gerson, and L.R. Gettman, *Developing and managing health/fitness facilities* (Champaign, IL: Human Kinetics) 1989, 203.

4. Travel time—to work, to health fitness center

B. Competitor analysis

1. Types of competitors—multipurpose clubs, fitness centers, sport clubs, personal training centers, hospital wellness centers, clinics, community programs, and the like

2. Size of competitors—number of participants

3. Location

4. Membership characteristics

5. Competitive success factors

6. Staffing qualifications and facility requirements

C. Primary market analysis—consumer survey

1. Current participation

a. Type, frequency, duration of exercise

b. Time of day

c. Place of exercise

d. Reasons for exercise (health, fitness, fun, etc.)

e. Number of current club memberships

f. Amount an individual will pay for membership fees and dues

g. Appealing features of a health fitness program

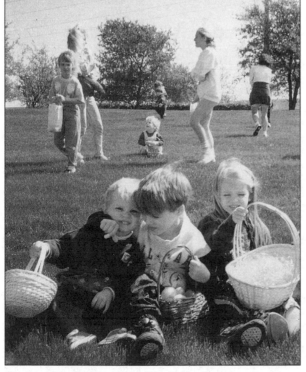

Courtesy of North Dallas Athletic Club, Dallas, Texas

2. Screening

a. Testing

b. Counseling

c. Health promotion programs (weight control, nutrition counseling, smoking cessation, stress management, etc.)

d. Leadership qualifications

e. Full-service facility—equipment, child care, food and beverage, and so on

f. Structured group programs

g. Individual programs

h. Family programs

i. Location

j. Cost

k. Other

3. Demographics of individuals surveyed

a. Age, gender

b. Education, occupation, income

c. Marital status, children

d. Zip code

D. Secondary market analysis—referral sources

1. Physicians

2. Hospitals

3. Physical therapy and rehabilitation

4. Other

E. Demand projections

1. Consumer membership

2. Referrals—source and mechanism

3. Turnover

F. Financial considerations

1. Product design

a. Programs and services (fees, dues, testing, rehabilitation, classes, food and beverage, guest fees, personal training, pro shop, other)

b. Operating expenses (salaries, benefits, taxes, rent, utilities, equipment, advertising, administrative, and general)

c. Nonoperating revenues and expenses (interest income and expense, depreciation, amortization)

2. Market strategy

a. To consumers

b. To referrals

c. Pricing and discount programs

3. Preliminary financial analysis—pro forma

G. Recommendations—plan of action

Table 8.7   Sample Interest Survey for Current Program Participants

ATTENTION MEMBERS!

Karen Bankle joins The Sporting Club as member services manager/event planner. She will be responsible for coordinating member services and organizing a number of special events throughout the year. To help Karen effectively meet member needs and plan future activities, we need your feedback. Please complete the following questionnaire and return it to the service desk by May 20th, or mail it to Karen at The Sporting Club, 220-224 South Broad St., Philadelphia, PA 19102.

Name _____   Phone _____

Please circle the number that best indicates your rating of the club in the following areas:

	Poor				Excellent
Service (athletics, fitness)	1	2	3	4	5
Friendliness of staff	1	2	3	4	5
Cleanliness/maintenance	1	2	3	4	5

Please put a check next to the activities in which you usually participate and those you are interested in learning more about:

	Usually participate	Learn more about
Basketball	_____	_____
Squash	_____	_____
Racquetball	_____	_____
Aquatics	_____	_____
Volleyball	_____	_____
Running	_____	_____
Aerobics	_____	_____
Cross-training	_____	_____
Weight training	_____	_____
Personal training	_____	_____
Sports nutrition	_____	_____
Massage	_____	_____

Please put a check next to the social events you are most interested in attending:

Theme parties (i.e., Caribbean)	_____
Sports tournaments	_____
Cultural (music, art)	_____
Guest speakers (food, fashion, business)	_____
Outside trips (biking, hiking, rafting)	_____

Please put a check next to the special-interest clubs you would like to join:

Running	_____	Dinner	_____	Chess	_____
Biking	_____	Travel	_____	Music/theater	_____
Hiking	_____	Ski	_____	Hunting/shooting	_____
Triathlon	_____	Sailing	_____	Rafting	_____
Swimming	_____	Softball	_____		

Are you familiar with our member referral bonus program?   Yes _____   No _____

Please add any comments or suggestions:

_____

_____

Reprinted, by permission, from S. Nottingham, 1992, "Diversification," *Fitness Management* 8(9): 34. Copyright 1992 by Fitness Management, Los Angeles, Ca.

In addition to market analysis, the organization's owner(s), investor(s), and board of directors generate programming ideas in the needs assessment of commercial programs. For existing commercial programs, survey current members (see table 8.7) to establish the needs and interest levels for future programming.

Corporate

In the corporate setting, needs are identified by a combination of management's perception of those needs, results from employee surveys, and input from a company advisory committee. This advisory committee should consist of a top management member who will support the program (the champion of the program), interested employees (both management and line staff from a variety of departments with all shifts represented), as well as an expert in health fitness. Results from health screening programs may also assist management in defining the needs, and not simply the desires, of the

employee population. Still, the areas of interest override the areas of need because the interest selections reflect what programs the participants might attend. This type of health screening and interest survey is also appropriate for use in the commercial, clinical, and community settings in identifying participants for various programs.

Additionally, corporate environments have a distinct benefit of access to personnel records. Although the corporation must be extremely careful to conceal the identity of the employee population, trends regarding absenteeism, turnover, and insurance costs can be beneficial in the needs assessment stage of program planning. A listing of some potential sources for valuable data to consider in the needs assessment stage is listed in table 8.8.

Community and Clinical

In community and clinical settings, the needs and interests of the potential clients are also discovered through market surveys and analyses. You could

Table 8.8 Sources of Data for Needs Analysis by Impact Area

Impact area	Source of data
1. Employees' needs/interests	
a. Health risks	Health risk profile
b. Health habits	Needs/interest survey
c. Program interests	Needs/interest survey
d. Work partners	Needs/interest survey
e. Facility usage patterns	Needs/interest survey
2. Health benefit	
a. Medical care costs	Personnel records
b. Type of medical claims	Employee health services
c. Worker's compensation claims	Personnel records and employee health services
d. Health crises	Employee health services and anecdotes from managers
e. Life insurance costs	Personnel records
f. Other insurance costs	Personnel records
3. Productivity	
a. Morale	Employee opinion survey
b. Turnover	Personnel turnover reports
	Interviews with employment representatives
c. Recruiting success	Interviews with employment representatives
d. Absenteeism	Personnel records
e. Physical and emotional disabilities	Personnel records
	Employee health services records
f. Desire to work	Employee opinion survey

Reprinted, by permission, from M. O'Donnell, 1986, "Design of workplace health promotion programs," *American Journal of Health Promotion* 1: 10-11, 18-22, 27, and Association for Fitness in Business 1992.

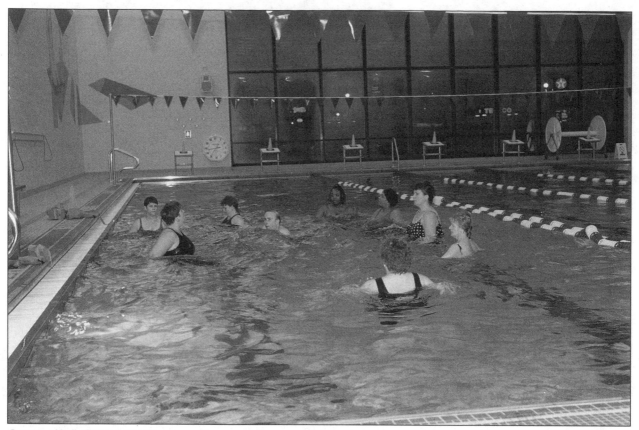

Courtesy of Dallas Texins Association

use the same essential items shown in the market analysis here. In addition, needs of the community are identified by the local health agencies such as the public health department, American Heart Association, American Cancer Society, and American Red Cross, as well as the physicians practicing in that community. Community programs offered through parks and recreation departments and special events, such as health fairs, also provide channels of feedback in identifying community needs and interests in health and wellness. Another source of needs and interest information is participants in existing health fitness programs.

Program Planning

Program planning involves using the information from the needs and interest assessments to define specific program goals and objectives from which you can establish programs. Involve all health fitness staff members in program planning, primarily because they are responsible for carrying out these programs. Their input as to whether a program will work is valuable. The manager should hold several staff meetings to review survey results and other information from the needs assessment process. Questions to answer in the planning process include the following:

- Who is interested in the program?
- What long-term and short-term goals should we achieve?
- What are the internal and external resources?
- What are the staffing needs?
- What are the program options?
- Who will develop the programs?
- How will we market and promote the programs?
- How will we deliver the programs?
- Who will supervise the programs?
- How and when will we enroll participants and will there be a cost to the participant?
- What medical screening procedures will we use, if any?
- How will we give feedback to the participants?
- What follow-up procedures will we use?
- What motivational techniques will we use?

- What special events will we conduct?
- What are the anticipated obstacles to program implementation?
- What is the estimated budget?
- What is the timing of program implementation?
- What are the adherence motives and incentives?
- How will we evaluate the programs?

These questions will give rise to others as you initiate the detailed planning of programs. Any health fitness manager proposing a program for the first time or assuming responsibility for a repeat program should be well organized and careful to consider all possible program variances, such as the timing of the program, the number of members expected to participate, or subtle changes in the program operation, to improve the outcome. A well-constructed programming proposal, such as the one used at the Cooper Fitness Center, will help the health fitness manager consider the vital aspects of the program. A sample programming proposal, adapted from the Cooper Fitness Center proposal, can be found in table 8.9.

Program Organization

For programming to be successful, it must be well organized. Structure and outline in detail the planning process for every program, whether it is a one-hour blood pressure screening or a citywide fun run that consumed months in planning. Constructing critical paths or time lines ensures that you handle important issues in a timely manner, eliminating the last minute scrambling to pull together staff, supplies, or participants.

Constructing a critical path time line assists the health fitness manager in organizing the event and delegating duties vital to the event's success. The steps necessary to create a working critical path include the following:

- *Hold a brainstorming meeting.* Create a comprehensive list of tasks that personnel must complete for the event to be successful. Using previous events as guides and involving all key personnel will typically produce a complete task listing.

- *Prioritize tasks.* Place issues and tasks in order of necessary completion date, with the items needing to be addressed first listed first. For example, a permit from the city to hold a fun run must be obtained before printing the race brochure.

- *Assign completion date goals.* First place the date of the event as the final listing of the prioritized tasks. Then work backward from that point assigning dates for completion. Allow a buffer of at least one week to accommodate any unforeseen delays or additional tasks not initially listed.

- *Assign staff responsibility.* Once again, hold a meeting of all key personnel. Distribute the prioritized task listing, complete with goal dates. Assign a staff person to each task. Some tasks will naturally lend themselves to a particular individual or department, whereas others you must divide among personnel. Be careful not to assign multiple tasks with similar completion dates to one individual. Attempt to provide each team member with only one to three tasks per week.

- *Set meeting dates.* Before adjourning the staff meeting, agree on weekly meeting times and dates to commence immediately. These meetings are vital to ensure planning is going as scheduled, to address any complications that have arisen, and to keep all team members informed on the progress of the event. As the event nears, it may be necessary to schedule meetings more frequently.

Several computer programs are available through retail computer software stores that assist with critical path development and tracking. Note an example of a complete critical path in table 8.10.

Program Timing

Organizing the programming calendar to take advantage of peak and off-peak times in daily traffic as well as high and low seasonal traffic will enhance the success of the programs. Schedule impulse events, such as flu shots or blood pressure screenings, which do not take a great deal of the members' time or energy, before or after work during high-traffic periods. Use special events, such as a lecture series or special children's programs, to bring people to the club when traffic typically would be minimal, such as midmorning or late evening. Create programming diversity to appeal to all participants throughout the year. Research done in Scotland on 7,202 men and 9,284 women demonstrates clearly that seasonal changes make a difference in exercise participation (Brehm 1993). This study showed that exercise volume peaked in July and dropped dramatically during the winter. Researchers cited the summer heat and humidity, the challenges of exercising outdoors in the winter, and daylight savings time ending as major contributors to the cessation of regular exercise. Create programs that will help

Table 8.9   Sample Programming Proposal

Purpose of event _____

Name of program _____

Program director _____

Dates of program _____ Rain date _____

Program description _____

_____

Participant profile

The participants in this program include the following (check all that apply):

Projected		Actual	
_____ Members	_____ 18 and under	_____ Members	_____ 18 and under
_____ Nonmembers	_____ 19-29 years	_____ Nonmembers	_____ 19-29 years
_____ Families	_____ 30-49 years	_____ Families	_____ 30-49 years
_____ Individual	_____ 50 plus	_____ Individual	_____ 50 plus
_____ Children only		_____ Children only	

Budget

Income	Projected	Actual
Sponsors	_____	_____
Entry fees	_____	_____
Rental fees	_____	_____
Spectator fees	_____	_____
F&B	_____	_____
T-shirts	_____	_____
_____	_____	_____
_____	_____	_____
_____	_____	_____
Total income	_____	_____

Expenditures	Projected	Actual
Office supplies	_____	_____
Prizes/trophies	_____	_____
T-shirts	_____	_____
Printing	_____	_____
Staff costs	_____	_____
Equipment	_____	_____
F&B	_____	_____
Postage	_____	_____
Advertising	_____	_____
Decorations	_____	_____
Total expenditures	_____	_____

Reprinted, by permission, from Cooper Fitness Center, Dallas, Texas.

members overcome these obstacles, such as an indoor triathlon during the heat of the summer, holiday weight-control programs or healthy cooking classes in the winter, and group exercise classes to overcome the difficulties of early darkness in the evenings. Creative programming will keep the members active and in the club year round.

Marketing and Promotions

Developing the strategic plan for marketing and promoting programs is an important step. In the past, health fitness specialists have been trained to know program content and delivery. They have not been trained in marketing and promoting programs. An increasing number of health fitness professionals are becoming proficient at marketing and promotion. ·

The best programs will not succeed if nobody knows they exist.

Use the same careful planning methods in program implementation as you used for marketing programs. Generally, the marketing plan should include the following:

• Objectives
• Strategies for program promotion
• Staff assignments in the promotional efforts
• Target dates and a timetable of tasks
• Resources to use in promoting programs

Table 8.10   Sample Critical Path Time Line

Fall fitfest critical path

Date	Activity	Key team member
June	Set event date	AS
	Block space for event	AS
July	Determine logo	AS
	Prepare information packet	RT
	Prepare printed materials	RT
August		
8-10	Design invitation	RT
8-10	Schedule guest speaker	BL
8-25	Confirm room	AS
8-25	Schedule entertainment	AS
8-25	Prepare newsletter article	RT
September		
9-1	Order invitations and printed material	RT
9-1	Purchase decorations	BL
9-1	Order trophies and plaques	BL
9-8	Schedule photographer	BL
9-8	Order F&B through catering	AS
9-8	Order radios	AS
9-8	Arrange AV for music	RT
9-15	Place promotional material	ALL
9-15	Mail invitations	JD
9-15	Staff meeting	JD
9-15	Begin registration	RT
9-15	Present training for the fall fitfest seminar	SH
9-15	Place newsletter article	RT
9-22	Order T-shirts	AS
9-22	Pick up awards	AS
9-22	Confirm equipment inventory	SH
9-22	Schedule staff	SH
9-29	Memo to all staff/security	AS
9-29	Solicit volunteers	AS

Fall fitfest critical path

Date	Activity	Key team member
October		
10-1	Confirm staffing/schedules	SH
10-1	Reconfirm speaker and entertainment	AS
10-1	Reconfirm photographer	AS
10-1	Invitations at service desk	AS
10-8	Pick up all supplies	AS
10-8	Measure and mark course	SH
10-8	Confirm room and F&B with catering	AS
10-10	Hold packet pickup	ALL
10-10	Volunteer training	AS
10-12	Clean grounds/maintenance	SH
10-12	Gather all equipment	JD
10-12	Test all equipment	JD
10-12	Reminder calls to members	JD
10-14	Decorate—balloons, streamers	ALL
10-14	Set up equipment room	AS
10-14	Assign radios	AS
10-14	Mark course	SH
10-15	Set up room—F&B	Catering
10-15	Set up course	SH
10-15	Welcome speaker	AS
10-15	Welcome entertainment	AS
10-15	Welcome members	ALL
10-15	Fall fitfest	ALL
Postevent		
10-15	Secure all equipment	ALL
10-15	Assist with clean-up	ALL
10-15	Complete postevent evaluation	ALL

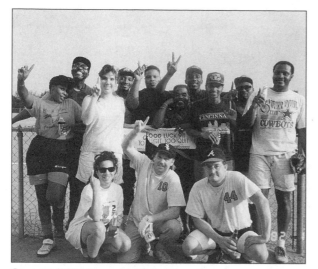

Courtesy of NCH Corporation, Dallas, Texas

Basically, the task of marketing is to show clients what you have. Therefore, design promotional efforts to reveal the main features of your services and products. Make the theme of your organization evident in your marketing materials. Illustrate the quality of your staff, programs, facilities, and equipment in your promotional information. Marketing involves projecting the image of how you want the clients to perceive your program or organization. As discussed in chapter 5, there are several promotional techniques used in marketing: brochures, print advertisements, direct mail, and so on. Use the same type of marketing effort within the club to promote upcoming events. Use marketing vehicles such as newsletters, fliers, bulletin boards, and personal invitations to boost participation in your events.

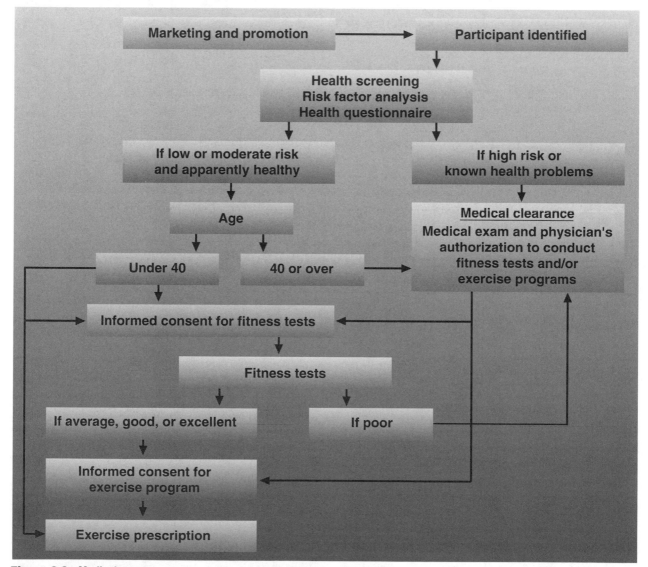

Figure 8.3   **Medical management model for handling program participants.**

Reprinted, by permission, from R.W. Patton, W.C. Grantham, R.F. Gerson, and L.R. Gettman, 1989, *Developing and managing health/fitness facilities* (Champaign, IL: Human Kinetics), 209.

When promoting a new program, the health fitness manager should consider doing an in-house pilot project to provide the staff with an opportunity to become familiar with the new program before promoting and delivering it to consumers.

Participant Screening

In any health fitness program, pay careful attention to the procedures for prescreening participants and handling individuals identified as potentially high risk. Safety of the members is of the utmost importance! Because health fitness programs usually involve exercise, there should be a medical management model for handling high-risk participants identified during the membership joining process.

Guidelines for exercise testing and prescription have been published by the American College of Sports Medicine (1995). A joint task force of the American College of Cardiology and the American Heart Association has also published guidelines for exercise testing (Schlant et al. 1986). Patton et al. (1989) combined recommendations from these two sources and presented a medical management model for handling clients, as shown in figure 8.3.

In this medical management model, the membership sales, marketing, and promotional efforts identify participants, who are then screened by a health questionnaire and risk factor analysis. The Health Screen Form the YMCA of the USA uses is a good example of a health screening questionnaire (see table 8.11). It addresses the major factors involved in potential cardiovascular problems. Another widely used screening tool is the Physical Activity Readiness Questionnaire (PAR-Q) presented in chapter 7.

In the medical management model, results of the health screening are examined to see if the participant is apparently healthy or if the participant is high risk. Any participant deemed high risk through screening procedures should seek medical clearance before undertaking an exercise program or participating in special events, leagues, tournaments, and so on. The form in table 8.12 is one that the YMCA of the USA uses for medical clearance. This is one example of how you can provide medical clearance in a program. Your medical director and attorneys should establish the exact medical clearance policy your program uses (see chapter 17).

In the planning phase of the management process, determine how to evaluate the programs you choose to implement. Later in this chapter we explain some evaluation procedures that you could use.

Program Implementation

The implementation of health fitness programs in the corporate, community, clinical, and commercial settings involve the following:

- Reviewing the planned objectives for the program
- Scheduling the program tasks to meet those objectives
- Marketing and promoting the programs
- Carrying out the assigned tasks
- Examining staff leadership, marketing and promotions, internal and external resources, and follow-up plans

Leadership

Obviously, the program tasks do not occur by themselves; professional health fitness staff members need to lead and carry out tasks properly.

If all aspects of a health fitness center in any setting were ranked in order of importance, leadership by the professional staff would be the key to a successful program.

The consumer, whether in a corporate, community, clinical, or commercial setting, responds positively to professional leaders who show a caring attitude and an expertise in assisting and offering motivation. For this reason, health fitness professionals should be skilled at motivating and guiding members. The participant doesn't always know what to do or how to get started. Herein lies the challenge for the health fitness professional—to motivate that member to action.

Well-qualified professional leaders generally know what programs are best for the various settings. However, the staff should work hard at carefully implementing the program plans to ensure success. Under these circumstances, the member often considers less-developed facilities and equipment acceptable, provided the staff is well organized in implementing programs. Too often, organizations developing health fitness centers decide on the gadgets, bells, and whistles to build or purchase for a facility without considering program needs. Then,

Table 8.11   Health Screen Form Used by YMCA of the USA

Name _____   Date _____

Male _____   Female _____   Age _____   Height _____   Weight _____

This form is intended to obtain relevant information about your health that will assist the staff in helping you with your program. Please answer all questions to the best of your knowledge.

1. Weight

  According to the attached recommended weight chart, which describes your current body weight?

  _____ Underweight (more than 5 lb. under ideal)

  _____ Normal (± 5 lb. of ideal)

  _____ 5 to 10 lb. overweight

  _____ More than 20 lb. overweight

2. Blood pressure

  Do you have high blood pressure?   Yes   No

  Have you had high blood pressure in the past?   Yes   No

  Are you on medication for high blood pressure?   Yes   No

3. Smoking

  Do you smoke?   Yes   No

  Are you a former smoker?   Yes   No

  If yes, please give the date you quit. _____

4. Diabetes

  Do you have diabetes?   Yes   No

5. Heart problems

  Have you ever had a heart attack?   Yes   No

  Heart surgery?   Yes   No

  Angina?   Yes   No

6. Family history

  Have any of your blood relatives had heart disease, heart surgery, or angina?   Yes   No

7. Orthopedic problems

  Do you have any serious orthopedic problems that would prevent you
  from exercising?   Yes   No

  If yes, please explain.

  _____

  _____

8. Other problems

  Do you have any reason to believe you should not exercise?   Yes   No

  If yes, please explain.

  _____

  _____

9. Emergency

  Please list a relative we may contact in case of an emergency.

  Name_____   Telephone _____

  Relation _____

  _____

Reprinted from *Health enhancement for America's work force: Program guide* with permission of the YMCA of the USA, 101 N. Wacker Drive, Chicago, IL 60606.

Table 8.12 Medical Clearance Form

Dear Doctor:

_____ has applied for enrollment in the fitness testing or exercise programs at the YMCA. The fitness testing program involves a submaximal test for cardiorespiratory fitness, body composition analysis, flexibility test, and muscular strength and endurance tests. The exercise programs are designed to start easy and become progressively more difficult over time. Qualified personnel trained in conducting exercise tests and exercise programs will administer all fitness tests and exercise programs.

By completing the following form, however, you are not assuming any responsibility for our administration of the fitness testing or exercise programs. If you know of any medical or other reasons why participation in the fitness testing or exercise programs by the applicant would be unwise, please indicate so on this form.

If you have any questions about the YMCA fitness testing or exercise programs, please call.

Report of physician

_____ I know of no reason why the applicant cannot participate.

_____ I believe the applicant can participate, but I urge caution because of the following:

_____

_____

_____ The applicant should not engage in the following activities:

_____

_____

_____ I recommend that the applicant *not* participate.

Physician signature _____ Date _____

Address _____ Telephone _____

City and state _____ Zip _____

Reprinted from *Health enhancement for America's work force: Program guide* with permission of the YMCA of the USA, 101 N. Wacker Drive, Chicago, IL 60606.

after the facility and fancy equipment priorities are achieved, the staff is hired to oversee the programs. These priorities are backward. Selection of professional staff must be considered first.

The staff should then conduct the needs assessments and carefully plan the proper programs to achieve the mission of the health fitness center. With this knowledge in hand, the professional staff can help design facilities and equipment to carry out those programs. Health promotion is competitive—programs must have the right kind of people with the right kind of expertise to keep pace with the demands of the marketplace.

Marketing and Promotions

In implementing programs, the timing of the marketing and promotional efforts is critical. Mar-ket and promote programs in advance to allow participants to plan their schedules accordingly. However, the time between the intensive marketing and promotional efforts and the start of the program should not be too long or too short. Scheduling the exact amount of time between the two is an art. Although it depends on the nature and the setting of the program, some common sense principles prevail. For example, in some commercial settings, a new racquetball league should be advertised and promoted three to four weeks in advance. However, a special event involving a racquetball tournament may have to be announced and promoted months ahead of the scheduled date. The program planning for any special event should begin a minimum of four to six weeks before the event to allow sufficient time for organization and promotion.

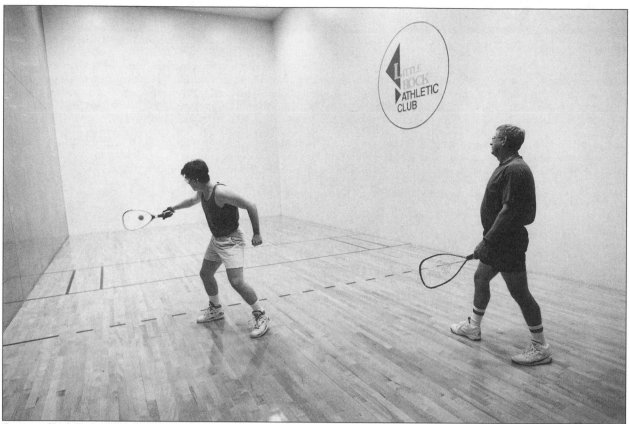

Courtesy of Little Rock Athletic Club

Internal and External Resources

Implementing a health fitness program in the corporate setting raises the question of whether to develop in-house expertise or purchase outside provider services. In most cases both internal and external resources are combined to implement a cost-effective program. For example, a program coordinator within a company may be selected to coordinate all the available resources to implement the program. Some internal experts may be hired to supervise exercise programs (e.g., exercise instructors), whereas other health promotion specialists like psychologists may be contracted to deliver stress-management programs. Developing internal expertise to conduct all aspects of a health fitness program is expensive and for small- to medium-sized companies is cost prohibitive. For the most part, this is feasible only in large corporations.

Consider that specific medical or health fitness professional certifications or licenses are required to conduct health screening, medical evaluations, fitness tests, and exercise programs. In addition, various health promotion specialists, such as degreed or licensed psychologists, dietitians, nurses,

and physical therapists, are required to conduct professional weight-control, nutrition, back care, stress-management, and smoking cessation programs. It is easy to see the extensive personnel costs involved in developing internal resources to conduct these programs. It is more cost-effective to use many of these resources as fee-for-service programs. They already exist as providers in the community, and thus you may not need to reinvent the wheel in these or other program areas. To be cost efficient, many providers in the community, clinical, and commercial settings are joining forces to reduce overhead and offer reasonably priced services.

As an example, many hospitals are joint-venturing with health clubs. The hospital provides the evaluation, prescription, and behavior modification aspects of the health fitness program. The health club provides the fitness facilities for carrying out the exercise programs. Some hospital wellness centers are built to be comprehensive providers of health fitness programs by including the exercise facilities as well as all the other aspects of the program. These centers can be costly however, due to the comprehensiveness of the program offerings.

Selecting an outside resource and purchasing the provider service to implement a health fitness program, or parts thereof, requires careful planning. The American Heart Association (1984) separates outside resources into low-, medium-, and high-cost categories. According to these guidelines, it is apparent that exercise programs can be implemented at virtually no cost by using existing facilities in the community. For example, walking, jogging, and cycling paths in parks and around lakes are now available at no charge in many communities. Par course systems are also included with many jogging trails for strength, flexibility, and endurance development. Some public schools open their facilities, such as outdoor tracks, to the public at no charge.

Many colleges and universities now offer health fitness programs through their continuing education or health, physical education, and recreation departments. Because the schools provide the programs as part of their commitment to community service, the fees are usually reasonable and would fit into the low- to medium-cost categories.

Contract exercise instructors, hospital wellness centers, and YMCA health fitness centers are ex-amples of outside resources that fit into the medium-cost category. Contract exercise instructors are now available to implement fitness programs for organizations. Check the instructor's credentials carefully to ensure the person is professionally qualified to provide a safe program.

Hospital wellness centers usually have professionally qualified personnel to conduct comprehensive health fitness programs. Many offer their preventive medicine services in the medium-cost range to promote good public relations in the community and encourage use of the hospital when treatment of illness is required.

Private fitness centers and health clubs also serve as outside resources for implementing health fitness programs for other organizations. Their primary emphasis is usually on high-tech equipment or classes for exercise and whirlpools, saunas, steam rooms, and massage for relaxation.

The American Heart Association (1984) provides an excellent summary that health fitness operators can use to evaluate outside resources before purchasing their services. When seeking help from an outside provider to implement a health fitness program, ask the following questions to evaluate the provider:

Provider Evaluation Questions

Staff

- Are staff members professionally trained in physical education, exercise science, health promotion, or medicine?

- Are staff members certified by a national organization such as the ACSM?

- Do staff members have consulting expertise?

- Do staff members have experience administering exercise programs?

Programs

- What program components are offered?

- Will the program components meet the goals and objectives set for the buyer of the services?

Facilities

- What facilities does the outside provider offer?

- Will the facilities meet program requirements?

References

- What previous and present clients has the outside resource serviced?

- Will a list be provided for a reference check?

Ownership

- Who owns the organization providing the service?

- How long has the current ownership been in place?

- What is the turnover rate in ownership and staff at the outside resource?

In addition to answering these questions, the buyer of a service should consult legal counsel before signing any agreements. The providers of health fitness programs in the community, clinical, and commercial settings would be wise to meet the following qualifications listed and be able to answer the previous questions positively.

Guidelines for Evaluating Outside Providers of Health Fitness Programs

Staff Qualifications

- Physical education or exercise science degree
- ACSM or other medical certification
- Health promotion or medical specialty
- Recreation specialty
- Program administration expertise

Program Components

- Evaluation—health screening, medical clearance, fitness testing
- Exercise prescription—cardiorespiratory, flexibility, strength, individual programs, group programs
- Back care
- Weight control
- Nutrition
- Stress management
- Smoking cessation
- Follow-up
- Documentation

Facilities

- Locker and shower rooms
- Exercise areas
- Gymnasium
- Weight-training room
- Outdoor and indoor tracks
- Courts
- Swimming pool
- Classroom(s)
- Child care center
- Medical clinic

Follow-Up

Health fitness programs should provide feedback and scheduled follow-up sessions for motivating the members. Follow-up sessions may include repeating a fitness profile, reviewing progress in an exercise program, or counseling in a behavior modification program.

> *Follow-up is an important part of program implementation that is often overlooked, especially in commercial settings.*

In the process of follow-up fitness testing, the evidence of change in fitness level can serve as important reinforcement to the participant. Reviewing progress in an exercise program can be an excellent opportunity to recognize individual achievements. Incentives, rewards, and special events serve as excellent motivators in the follow-up system. You can use shirts, equipment bags, warm-up suits, plaques, trophies, tournaments, leagues, fitness months, fitness days, and recognition banquets to motivate participants to higher levels of activity.

The follow-up component of program implementation is the bridge to evaluating the program. In fact, some managers believe that follow-up is part of the evaluation process. Either way, it is an important part of the overall program and should be carefully planned.

Program Evaluation

The fourth stage in the iterative process of managing a program involves evaluation. You can use both types of program evaluation—process evaluation and outcome evaluation—in any corporate, community, clinical, or commercial setting. These two types of evaluation involve analyzing implementation tasks that were assigned to the staff to see (a) if the tasks were accomplished (process evaluation), and (b) if the objectives of the program were met (outcome evaluation). A summary of the process and outcome evaluation techniques is presented in table 8.13.

Health fitness staff members should meet and discuss the program evaluation periodically throughout and immediately after completing the

Table 8.13   Summary of the Process and Outcome Evaluation Techniques

Monitor program implementation	
Process evaluation	**Outcome evaluation**
1. Were the program operations efficient?	1. Were the programs fun?
2. Were the time schedules reasonable?	2. Were program objectives met?
3. Were the staff members prepared properly to conduct the programs?	3. How many people participated in each program?
4. Were staff members dependable?	4. Were the programs cost effective? (corporate setting)
5. Were the resources adequate to conduct the program?	5. Were the time and money worth the effort? (community setting)
6. Was the budget adequate?	6. Were the profits worth the effort? (clinical and commercial setting)
7. Were the programs accessible to the participants?	7. Did the programs have a positive effect on the organization?
8. Did the programs have both personal and group options?	
9. Did the programs have a positive effect on the organization?	

Adapted, by permission, from R.W. Patton, W.C. Grantham, R.F. Gerson, and L.R. Gettman, 1989, *Developing and managing health/fitness facilities* (Champaign, IL; Human Kinetics), 221.

program. Keep careful records during each program to evaluate it accurately. Personal computers and software are now available to facilitate documenting and evaluating programs. We strongly recommend that you computerize all participant records and registrations, screening, and testing forms for ease of data analysis. Assign staff members specific tasks in the evaluation process. Those assignments might include keeping various records and evaluating the resultant data.

The outcome evaluation usually depends on the process. If a program is conducted well, the outcome will reveal this fact. Sometimes, however, the outcome (e.g., how many individuals participated in each program) doesn't seem to be impressive, although the process of offering and conducting the program was deemed quite successful. In this case, the process evaluation is viewed separately from the outcome evaluation. Occasionally, a popular program may be well attended (good outcome evaluation) in spite of a poorly conducted program (process). The manager does gain valuable information from the process evaluation and can then plan to conduct the program differently next time to solve the problems.

In other cases, both the process and the outcome evaluations are viewed together to see if a particular program was successful. If the program was well conducted and there were an acceptable number of participants, the program is considered successful. Examining the results from the evaluations then determines which procedures to use next for

assessing needs, planning, and implementing a new or different program in the iterative management process.

IN CLOSING

This chapter outlined the processes used in planning and implementing health fitness programs in the corporate, community, commercial, and clinical settings. The program development in each setting depends on the mission of the organization, the objectives of the program, and the target market for which the program is intended. The ultimate success of the center often depends on the quality of the personnel planning and on effectively implementing the programming for the facility.

The major function of management is administrative planning and implementation of programs to meet the organization's objectives. Effective management involves a four-stage iterative process that includes needs assessment, planning, implementation, and evaluation.

KEY TERMS

Needs assessment

Program

Programming

RECOMMENDED READINGS

American College of Sports Medicine. 1995. *ACSM's guidelines for exercise testing and prescription*. 5th ed. Baltimore: Williams & Wilkins.

American Heart Association. 1984. *Heart at work: Exercise program*. Dallas, TX: American Heart Association.

Association for Fitness in Business, 1992, *Guidelines for employee health promotion programs*. Champaign, IL: Human Kinetics.

Brehm, B.A. 1993. Exercise diversity: The fitness center advantage. *Fitness Management* (October): 27-29.

Coffman, S. 1994. Programs. *Club Business International* 15(3): 91-96.

International Health, Racquet and Sportsclub Association. 1994a. *1994 profiles of success report*. Boston: IHRSA.

———. 1994b. *The IHRSA report on the state of the health club industry*. Boston: IHRSA.

———. 1995. *The 1995 IHRSA report on the state of the health club industry*. Boston: IHRSA

Lynch, D.J. 1990. Programming success. *Fitness Management* (August): 12-13.

Opatz, J.P. 1985. *A primer of health promotion*. Washington, DC: Oryn.

Patton, R.W., J.M. Corry, L.R. Gettman, and J.S. Graf. 1986. *Implementing health/fitness programs*. Champaign, IL: Human Kinetics.

Patton, R.W., W.C. Grantham, R.F. Gerson, and L.R. Gettman. 1989. *Developing and managing health/fitness facilities*. Champaign, IL: Human Kinetics.

Schlant, R.C., et al. 1986. Guidelines for exercise testing: A report of the American College of Cardiology / American Heart Association Task Force on Assessment of Cardiovascular Procedures (Subcommittee on Exercise Testing). *Journal of the American College of Cardiology* 8: 725-738.

Specialized Programs

In the previous chapter we discussed the process involved when developing, implementing, and evaluating programming. In this chapter we examine some popular programs offered in clubs. Is your club meeting the programming needs of both the active older adult and the growing child? Is the fitness programming based on sound recommendations from an authoritative organization? Are the group exercise classes maturing to meet the needs of an aging baby boomer population? Are the aquatic programs offering a new exercise environment for those who have never ventured near the water? Find out how to implement specialty programming in this chapter.

This chapter discusses the specific types of programming popular in the different health fitness settings and the trends impacting programming decisions (see figure 9.1). The type and quality of programs and services offered positively or negatively influences the member's feelings of satisfaction and perceived value of membership. Offering a variety of cutting edge and time-tested programs

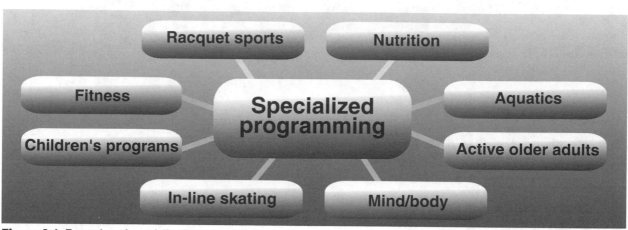

Figure 9.1 Examples of specialized programming.

gives the operator the lift needed for success. This chapter also discusses the current trends, the influential industry data, and the implementation procedures necessary to create a dynamic programming calendar.

Today's health fitness programming reflects a member-driven maturation of activities and events offered by creative health fitness managers. Annual surveys conducted by national organizations illustrate this trend in programming. The surveys conducted by American Sports Data and the Fitness Products Council, as well as the National Sporting Goods Association, provide valuable data for the club operator or program manager. The surveys analyze consumer behavior from different viewpoints. The study conducted by American Sports Data and the Fitness Products Council and cited in *Club Industry* (Loyle 1995a) examines the individual motivating factors behind regular exercise. The 1994 survey found that people were more motivated by how exercise made them feel than by developing a perfect physique. Respondents suggested that exercise is necessary to improve energy, decrease stress,

provide time for self, and improve self-esteem. Although responses are somewhat similar for men and women, the priority of the responses differ. Women, for example, are motivated by weight-control goals, a positive feeling following exercise, and increased energy. Men work out to increase muscle tone, increase energy, and improve their cardiovascular systems. This trend shows a sharp change in the reasons people exercise from years past. As baby boomers age, the reasons people exercise will continue to mature as evidenced in this study. A complete listing of the 10 most popular responses to this survey can be reviewed in table 9.1.

The survey conducted by the National Sporting Goods Association, also cited in *Club Industry* (Connor 1995), evaluated sport participation from an activity standpoint. In this survey, physical activities are ranked in order of the greatest number of participants. It also notes a comparison with the previous year. This survey found activities such as using resistance machines, free weights, treadmills, and rowing machines and participating in gym exercise, fitness swimming, and tennis showed in-

Table 9.1 Why Men and Women Exercise	
Women	**Men**
1. Weight control	1. Increase muscle tone
2. Feeling good afterward	2. Increase energy
3. Increase energy	3. Cardiovascular benefits
4. Increase muscle tone	4. Weight control
5. Cardiovascular benefits	5. Feeling good afterward
6. Keep flexibility	6. Reduce stress
7. Reduce stress	7. Build strength
8. Time for self	8. Enjoy exercise
9. Enjoy exercise	9. Keep flexibility
10. Improve self-esteem	10. Time for self

Reprinted, by permission, from D. Loyle, 1995, "Feeling well prompts exercise as much as looking good," *Club Industry* 11(10): 9. Copyright 1995 by Club Industry.

Table 9.2 Fast-Growing Club Sports			
Sport /activities	1994 participation levels*	1995 participation levels*	% change
Resistance machines	18.5	22.9	+23.6
Home gym exercise	10.2	12.2	+20.6
Treadmill exercise	26.5	29.6	+11.6
Free weights	35.9	39.7	+10.5
Fitness swimming	22.9	24.7	+7.8
Rowing machines	10.1	10.4	+3.4
Tennis	17.9	18.5	+3.1
*Data in millions			

Reprinted, by permission, from D. Connor, 1995, "Walking, swimming top list of favorite fitness activities," *Club Industry* (June): 9.

creases in participation from 1994 to 1995. Table 9.2 summarizes the growth of these activities.

These and other surveys assist the club operator and program manager in directing future programming efforts. With this data the fitness manager should develop programs that reinforce the initial motivation to exercise with activities that prove popular with the members. Programming trends such as mind-body alternative exercise and in-line skating classes reflect wisely used industry data.

Developing programming ideas that meet the needs of the consumer is the first step to assuring a popular and successful program. Surveys assist the fitness manager in the needs assessment aspect of program planning.

According to *The 1995 IHRSA Report on the State of the Health Club Industry*

Club programming is no longer limited to physical fitness activities. Wellness education, nutrition counseling, and weight-management programs are becoming as prevalent in the health club setting as cardiovascular equipment and weight machines. The swimming pool, once the domain of the lone lap swimmer, has become the setting for water walking and low-impact aerobic classes. Special programs are being developed for seniors as well as children, whose health-conscious parents are seeking to instill in them the practice of regular exercise. Overall programming is increasingly emphasizing the connection between the mind and the body, most notable with the return of yoga, which was popular during the 1970s.

These changes and others will position the health club as an important partner in the health and well-being of the active older adult as programming matures to meet member needs in the 21st century.

In the 1990s and beyond, programming will be kinder and gentler to meet the needs of an older health club member and more diverse to meet the changing needs of a population that is interested in a holistic approach to health, encompassing but not limited to physical activity. (IHRSA 1995)

FITNESS PROGRAMMING

Traditional programming in health clubs is often the foundation on which creative programming is built. Although new and exciting programs are constantly being developed, the standard fitness programming in many cases is what brings members through the health club door. Activities such as personal training, fitness testing, and general exercise prescriptions demonstrate fitness programming that may not be exciting or new, yet is fundamental to many members' goals. A cursory review of some traditional fitness programming offerings follow.

Fitness Assessments

Long considered a standard in fitness centers, the importance and value of mandatory exercise testing has fluctuated in recent years. Throughout the 1980s and early 1990s, submaximal exercise testing on all participants initiating an exercise program, with periodic reevaluations to measure improvement, was considered the norm. Data from these evaluations were considered vital for screening participants and motivating the participant through measured improvement. Particularly in the corporate environment, evaluation data were used to justify the health fitness program by demonstrating the tangible profitability of a well workforce. However, in the early 1990s, fitness professionals realized that most of the American population who were not regularly active were not motivated by exercise testing, but intimidated by it. This sedentary population, who invariably score lower on conventional health assessment batteries, is not interested in exercise if it means being embarrassed and humiliated during an exercise testing session before being allowed to participate. This population knows they are out of shape and overweight and do not need that fact proven through quantitative means.

Led by the Association for Worksite Health Promotion (formerly known as the Association for Fitness in Business), a trend introducing a softer and less intimidating invitation to exercise and wellness became prevalent and is now widely accepted. Exercise testing, although not discontinued totally, is no longer a mandatory step to exercise participation in many fitness centers. Instructors who formerly wore skintight spandex clothing to serve as role models for the perfect physique are now wearing loose-fitting exercise wear so members won't feel intimidated and inadequate. Members are encouraged initially to simply be more active instead of receiving the regimented exercise guidelines of the 1980s, which consisted of a specific target heart rate goal and minimum time requirements that were often difficult to understand and measure.

These trends and others, such as the reemergence of yoga and other *mind-body programs* that do not concentrate so heavily on vigorous exercise, are changing the way the fitness industry markets to the majority of the population who do

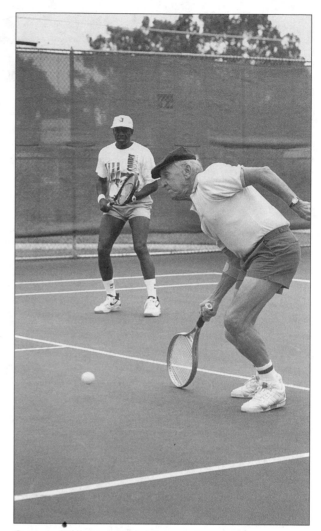

Courtesy of Dallas Texins Association

not currently exercise. Fitness assessments and health risk appraisals are still valuable program offerings in fitness centers. However, the marketing and positioning of submaximal fitness assessments continues to evolve. Fitness centers must continue to offer testing to those members who recognize its value and voluntarily undergo an assessment, while also introducing the beginning exerciser to the benefit and value of fitness testing.

Health Risk Appraisals

Health risk appraisals are paper and pencil evaluations that quantify an individual's risk of death compared to normative data for persons of the same gender, race, and age. Health risk appraisals evaluate responses to questions regarding family history of disease; personal health and wellness habits such as exercise, smoking, or alcohol consumption; as

Developing a Fitness Assessment Program

For those members who remain motivated by quantitative goals and fitness levels measured via a scientific fitness assessment, a high-quality, professional fitness testing program is essential if it is to accomplish the primary purpose and member benefits inherent to it.

The fitness assessment should present a professional image of the organization, provide the member with valuable health screening and fitness normative data, and give the fitness professional and member the opportunity to establish a friendly relationship in a caring atmosphere, enhancing retention.

Developing a quality fitness assessment program begins with hiring a qualified fitness professional who is highly trained, educated, certified, and exhibits solid interpersonal skills. He or she should have experience administering a variety of submaximal fitness assessment protocols on people who are apparently healthy. Ideally these professionals should also be certified through the American College of Sports Medicine or other governing body. The test technician should also have experience or be trained in the art of providing the member feedback from the assessment. This counseling session can either build the confidence of the member in himself and the organization or it can negatively impact the member and the club. Presenting personal information and fitness assessment data must be done cautiously and with care for the member to have a positive experience.

The professional must use the data from the assessment and information the member provides regarding his/her fitness interests and wellness goals to construct a personalized exercise prescription that will enhance participation and satisfaction with the club.

The components of a fitness assessment and the protocols used to measure fitness variables differ from facility to facility. According to the *ACSM's Guidelines for Exercise Testing and Prescription* (1995), a complete assessment of health-related physical fitness includes the following:

- *Pretest evaluation.* Depending on the preliminary assessment of cardiovascular risk factors present (see table 9.3 for a list of potential risk factors), this pretest evaluation may require a complete medical evaluation for those with elevated risk. This complete medical evaluation includes medical history review; physical examination; evaluation of blood pressure, serum cholesterol, lipoproteins, and additional blood variables; and pulmonary function. For those who are not at high risk, the pretest evaluation may consist of medical history review, measurement of resting blood pressure and heart rate, and exercise history review. Table 9.4 outlines the components of the medical history. (For a detailed discussion regarding pretest evaluation and risk factor stratification beyond the scope of this text, refer to ACSM [1995].)

- *Informed consent.* An informed consent is a valuable tool in preparing the client for the assessment. This tool ensures the client is fully aware of the procedures about to take place and his or her ability to discontinue the assessment at any time. Discussion with your legal advisor regarding an informed consent is warranted.

- *Client instructions.* Give specific instructions to members to prepare them for the fitness assessment. Following these instructions is necessary for the accuracy and validity of test results. Instruct members well in advance of the assessment so they are prepared. Specific instructions include the following:

  1. Avoid food, alcohol, caffeine, or tobacco for three hours before testing.

  2. Avoid exercise or strenuous physical activity the day of the assessment.

  3. Wear comfortable, loose-fitting clothing.

  4. Drink plenty of fluids over the 24-hour period before the test.

(continued)

5. Get enough sleep (six to eight hours) the night before the test.

- *Cardiorespiratory endurance.* Cardiorespiratory endurance is the ability to perform large muscle, dynamic, moderate-to-high intensity exercise for prolonged periods, evaluated via a treadmill, cycle, or field test protocol.

- *Body composition and body weight.* Body composition refers to the relative percentages of body weight comprised of fat and fat-free body tissue. This assessment is typically done with the use of calibrated skinfold calipers in the health club setting.

- *Muscular strength.* Muscular strength refers to the maximal force that a specific muscle or muscle group can generate. A variety of strength assessment protocols exist to measure muscular strength. Carefully select the protocol based on the member to be tested.

- *Muscular endurance.* Muscular endurance is the ability of a muscle group to execute repeated contractions over a period sufficient to cause muscular fatigue or to statically maintain a specific percentage of maximum voluntary contraction (MVC) for a prolonged time. As with muscular strength, a variety of protocols exist to measure muscular endurance.

Select the most appropriate protocol considering the age, fitness level, experience, and motivation of the member.

- *Flexibility.* Flexibility is the maximum ability to move a joint through a range of motion. A sit-and-reach protocol is most commonly used to measure this component of fitness.

You can enter quantitative data from these assessment components into one of many available fitness assessment and exercise prescription software programs (see chapter 19), providing a detailed and educational record of the fitness assessment results. You can use this data, along with the personal wellness goals of the member, to develop a detailed exercise prescription. This consultation session should educate and motivate the member by informing her of her current fitness level and what steps are necessary to reach and maintain her goals. Follow this consultation with a hands-on orientation to the exercise equipment so the member knows how to safely operate all equipment.

For more information regarding fitness assessments and certification contact the American College of Sports Medicine (ACSM) Certification Resource Center at 800-486-5643 or http://www.acsm.org/sportsmed/.

well as many other lifestyle factors. These data are then evaluated and compared with data maintained by the Centers for Disease Control and Prevention to provide the individual with his risk factor score for each of the leading 10 or 12 causes of death for individuals of the same gender, age, and race. You can use these scores to educate members regarding the effect controllable risk factors, such as smoking, obesity, or a sedentary lifestyle, have on their health status.

Most computerized health risk appraisals (see chapter 19) provide the member with valuable health information. Typically these assessments compare the individual's chronological age with *risk* age and an *achievable* age. For example, the assessment for a white male, 45 years of age may show a risk age of 56 years due to poor health and lifestyle habits. However, if controllable risk factors are modified, this member can bring his risk age to an achievable age of 42 years. With this information in hand and the guidance of a fitness professional, motivated individuals can take positive steps to improve their risk age.

Health risk appraisals provide an excellent opportunity to counsel the member on positive wellness and lifestyle change.

Group Exercise Classes

Group exercise or aerobics classes have long been a popular program in fitness centers. These programs attract members, typically women, who enjoy the social and motivating atmosphere of group exercise. The quality of these programs is often a factor in membership sales figures as well as member retention and attrition rates.

Simply offering a group exercise program is not enough. The program must continually grow to meet the changing needs of the membership. To offer a high-quality group exercise program, you need a group exercise director motivated to oversee

Table 9.3   Coronary Artery Disease Risk Factors

Positive risk factors	Defining criteria
1. Age	Men > 45 years; women > 55 or premature menopause without estrogen therapy.
2. Family history	Myocardial infarction or sudden death before 55 years of age in father or other male first-degree relative, or before 65 years of age in mother or other female first-degree relative.
3. Current cigarette smoking	
4. Hypertension	Blood pressure ≥ 140/90 mmHg confirmed by measurements on at least 2 separate occasions, or on antihypertensive medication.
5. Hypercholesterolemia	Total serum cholesterol > 200 mg/dL or HDL < 35 mg/dL.
6. Diabetes mellitus	Persons with insulin dependent diabetes mellitus who are < 30 years of age, or have had IDDM for > 15 years, and persons with noninsulin dependent diabetes who are > 35 years of age should be classified as patients with disease.
7. Sedentary lifestyle	Persons comprising the least active 25 percent of the physical inactivity population, as defined by the combination of sedentary jobs involving sitting for a large part of the day and no regular exercise or active recreational pursuits.

Reprinted, by permission, from ACSM, 1995, *ACSM's guidelines for exercise testing and prescription*, 5th ed. (Baltimore: Williams & Wilkins), 18. Copyright 1995 by Williams & Wilkins.

the continual improvement of the instructors and classes. Without a group exercise program director charged with offering an innovative and quality program, the group exercise program often languishes in mediocrity. This ongoing program, more than any other in the fitness area, requires constant attention to detail. This is the primary responsibility of the program director. The director must oversee the continued improvement of classes, research new offerings and trends in group exercise, continue the education and development of instructors and classes, and meet regularly with members to determine if the program is meeting their needs. The director must also handle the administrative aspect of group exercise, including scheduling, hiring and evaluating instructors, and interfacing with other club management personnel.

Table 9.4   Components of the Medical History

1. Medical diagnosis
   Cardiovascular disease including myocardial infarction, angioplasty, cardiac surgery, coronary artery disease, angina, and hypertension; pulmonary disease including asthma, emphysema, and bronchitis; cerebrovascular disease including stroke; diabetes; peripheral vascular disease; anemia; phlebitis or emboli; cancer; pregnancy; osteoporosis; emotional disorders; eating disorders

2. Previous physical examination findings
   Murmurs, clicks, other abnormal heart sounds, other unusual cardiac findings, abnormal blood lipids and lipoproteins, high blood pressure, or edema

3. History of symptoms
   Discomfort (pressure, tingling, pain, heaviness, burning, numbness in the chest, jaw, neck, or arms); lightheadedness, dizziness, or fainting; shortness of breath; rapid heart beats or palpitations, especially if associated with physical activity, eating a large meal, emotional upset, or exposure to cold

4. Recent illness, hospitalization, or surgical procedures

5. Orthopedic problems
   Arthritis, joint swelling, any condition that would make ambulation or use of certain test modalities difficult

6. Medication use, drug allergies

7. Other habits
   Caffeine, alcohol, tobacco, or recreational drug use

8. Exercise history
   Information on habitual level of activity; type of exercise, frequency, duration, and intensity

9. Work history
   Current or expected physical demands, noting upper and lower extremity requirements

10. Family history
    Cardiac, pulmonary, or metabolic disease, stroke, sudden death

Reprinted, by permission, from ACSM, 1995, *ACSM's guidelines for exercise testing and prescription*, 5th ed. (Baltimore: Williams & Wilkins), 30. Copyright 1995 by Williams & Wilkins.

Clubs that do not have the staff expertise, resources, or desire to oversee a group exercise program should consider outsourcing or contracting with a company specializing in group exercise. Although there are inherent advantages and disadvantages to using outside vendors, the value of offering a quality program must be the primary consideration. These outside entities perform responsibilities typically handled by the group exercise program director, including scheduling, providing quality instructors, overseeing ongoing education and certification courses, and administrative responsibilities, including payroll. The club operator must carefully weigh the value of the program and the quality with which it is run against the loss of control and accountability. The club operator must be confident the outside vendor will operate with the clubs' best interest in mind.

Whether the club hires a staff group exercise director or contracts with an outside vendor, there are challenges opposing consistent, quality program development. Daniel Kosich, PhD, the Senior Director of Professional Development for International Association of Fitness Professionals (IDEA), cited in the May 1994 issue of *Fitness Management* (Broderick 1994) the following challenges facing the program director:

1. Design of classes that enable people of various fitness levels to come to the same class and all get an appropriate workout

2. Taking enough time to consider program safety when new formats or choreographies come into vogue

3. Keeping up with new information as it emerges and addressing any new issues before introducing a new class

Meeting these challenges and others provides the club operator with a quality program.

Developing a Quality Group Exercise Program

Most professionals in the fitness industry agree that a quality group exercise program begins with the instructors. Instructors often develop close relationships with members who frequent their classes and have a powerful position in presenting a positive image of the facility. Unfortunately, group exercise instructors are often underappreciated and poorly compensated. Facilities and program directors who recognize the value of these individuals and the potential impact they have on membership retention will be rewarded with a quality program, a great reputation, memberships, and profitability.

Developing a quality group exercise program begins with the acquisition, training, and continued education of qualified group exercise leaders.

When developing a group exercise program, consider the following issues:

• *Hire dynamic instructors.* Quality instructors are hard to find but are worth the search. Instructors must possess a variety of qualities to be successful; they must be professional, qualified, innovative, motivating, enthusiastic, friendly, possess leadership qualities, understand the value of customer service and name recognition, possess solid communication skills, be well prepared, dependable, confident, and approachable.

• *Certification of group exercise instructors.* Certification is a standard expectation of quality instructors. Certifications are available through American Council on Exercise (ACE), Aerobics and Fitness Association of America (AFAA), ACSM, and other governing bodies.

• *Current cardiopulmonary resuscitation (CPR) certification.* Although required by all governing bodies before awarding any certification, the club operator or program director should ensure instructors maintain current CPR certification.

• *Ongoing training.* A program to ensure ongoing training of instructors is a must. Several seminars are offered throughout the year in many areas of the country to enhance the teaching skills and choreography in a variety of class types. Consider requiring instructors to attend periodic workshops, paying for workshop attendance, and compensating the instructor for increased knowledge.

• *Evaluating instructors.* Setting up a system of periodic evaluation provides the instructors with the constructive criticism and recognition they need to continually improve their skills. Consider bringing in recognized instructors from throughout the city or state to evaluate the class and instructor. Providing the instructor with any member feedback regarding their class is also helpful.

- *Variety of class types.* Often traditional classes are removed from the class schedule to add classes featuring the new trends in group exercise. Although continually updating the class schedule is a wise idea, carefully consider the impact of removing a class to which members have been loyal. Offering a variety of classes, such as step aerobics, circuit, low-impact aerobics, stretch and flex, boot camp, box aerobics, body toning, and so on will meet the needs of both the traditional member and the member always looking for something new.

- *Class times.* It is impossible to make everyone happy, but varying the class schedule to offer the right classes at the right time of the day is crucial to success. Consider offering abbreviated classes or circuit type classes during the lunch hour when members typically have time limitations. Consider offering the most popular class during off-peak hours to encourage members to come to the club when it typically would not be busy, reducing the crunch during peak times.

- *Variety of music.* It is without question that the music used during the class is second only to the instructor in terms of importance. Encourage instructors to use a variety of music, appropriately paced throughout their exercise class. Music must be carefully selected to fit the atmosphere of the class and should be changed often.

- *Cross train instructors.* The risk of injury and burnout is high for the group exercise instructor. Cross train the instructor, not only to teach a wide variety of class types, but also to work in other areas of the facility, so you can increase the value of that individual to the organization and keep the instructor motivated and injury free.

- *Compensate instructors as professionals.* The value of these individuals has been established; compensate these professionals accordingly. Conduct a compensation survey in the local area to ensure you are competitive. Recognize the value of these individuals to the bottom line and compensate them in a way that will encourage them to become long-term staff members. Consider compensating the instructors based on class attendance or on their continued education and expertise versus years of experience.

- *Involve instructors in program development.* Instructors often provide valuable information and creative ideas to keep the group exercise program innovative. Encourage their participation in decision making and program development.

For information regarding group exercise leadership and certification contact the following:

The International Association of Fitness Professionals (IDEA) 619-535-8979

Aerobics and Fitness Association of America (AFAA) 800-445-5950

American Council on Exercise (ACE) 800-529-8227 or http://www.acefitness.org/

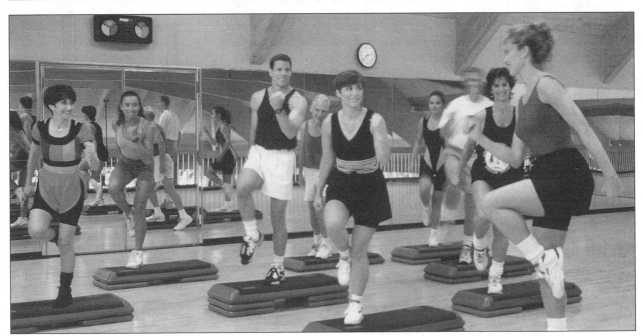

Courtesy of Cooper Fitness Center, Dallas, Texas

Personal Training

The abundance of research showing the value and health benefits of strength training has resulted in consistent growth in the number of individuals who regularly exercise with weight equipment. According to the National Sporting Goods Association, (NSGA 1995) using resistance equipment, home gyms, and free weights showed dramatic increases in participation in 1995. The study revealed the number of females who exercised with weights in 1995 rose 77 percent between 1987 and 1995, from 6.5 million to 11.5 million. The number of males using weight machines increased 30 percent in the same period, from 8.8 million to 11.4 million. Studies have shown that regular resistance training produces many positive health benefits including the following:

- Slowing of muscle loss associated with aging
- Prevention of yearly loss in metabolic rate
- Reduction in body fat
- Reduction in the risk of osteoporosis by building bone density
- Reduction of risk of heart disease
- Reduction of risk for low-back pain

These facts are good news for the club operator who offers resistance training as a primary program in the club. The consistent growth in the number of adults who exercise with weights has given rise to the popularity of personal training. Members use personal trainers for a variety of reasons. Some have set high fitness goals and want a personal coach to assist them in achieving these goals, whereas others are new to exercise and do not feel confident on their own. Some use a personal trainer to push themselves; others know they may not make exercise a priority without an appointment to keep. Busy members want the most out of a short time, and others may have physical conditions requiring intensive supervision. Personal trainers are also popular for the social aspect or status associated with having an exercise coach giving him/her undivided attention. Whatever the reason, personal training services have grown dramatically in fitness centers across the country, providing a new and valuable service for members and a constant revenue stream for both the trainer and the club operator.

Table 9.5   Advantages and Disadvantages of Contract Versus Staff Personal Trainers

Advantages of using contract personal trainers
1. Reduction in payroll taxes.
2. Not required to provide any employee benefits.
3. Little program administration time required.
4. Not required to provide ongoing training and current certification.
5. Production of revenues with little overhead expense.

Disadvantages of using contract personal trainers
1. Loss of control and accountability.
2. Trainers have little commitment to the organization.
3. Difficulty tracking sessions and accounting for all revenues owed.
4. No control over continuing education of trainer.
5. Possible legal liability for negligence by trainer.
6. High turnover of trainers likely.

Advantages of using staff personal trainers
1. Total control and accountability of trainer and training program.
2. Complete commitment of staff to program and organization.
3. Ensured of commitment to continuing education and current certification.
4. Positive member interaction reflects positively on organization.
5. Commitment to trainer encourages long-term employees.
6. Revenues easily tracked through payroll procedures.
7. Trainers may be covered by professional liability insurance held by the club.

Disadvantages of using staff personal trainers
1. Organization responsible for payroll taxes.
2. Organization may be required to provide benefit package.
3. Program administration may be time consuming.

Developing a Personal Training Program

Trainers must be knowledgeable, professional, certified, personable, motivating, and committed to the achievement of their clients' wellness goals and to the continued success of the facility.

Much like group exercise instructors, the quality of the personal trainer is the most important consideration in developing a personal training program. In addition to staff, consider the following issues when developing a quality personal training program:

- *Trainers must be good coaches and teachers.* In addition to being educated and certified, trainers must possess solid coaching skills. They must create a comfortable environment so the client is never intimidated. The trainer must help the client set realistic wellness goals and foster successful experiences. He must teach logical, safe movement patterns that the client can easily learn and build upon. The trainer must demonstrate movements, offer encouragement and feedback, be empathetic to client concerns, and provide heavy doses of positive feedback. Above all, the trainer must be knowledgeable about exercise and other wellness topics.

- *Hire trainer as a staff member or contractor?* The club operator must determine whether to hire the personal training staff as employees or independent contractors. Consider and discuss the inherent advantages and disadvantages of both with outside resources, such as consultants, accountants, and legal representation. Some possible advantages and disadvantages for the club operator are listed in table 9.5.

- *Qualifications of trainers.* Whether independent contractors or staff, determine strict criteria regarding qualifications. Make and strictly enforce decisions regarding required educational level, training certifications, CPR certification, continuing education, in-house training programs, and professional insurance liability coverage.

- *Employment rules and regulations.* Predetermine employment rules, such as dress codes, timeliness, call-in procedures, safety guidelines, phone etiquette, and more. Provide them in writing to the trainer and enforce them with a graded disciplinary process.

- *Accounting procedures.* Determine procedures for recording the revenues and paying agreed upon compensation. Will trainers present a charge ticket for each session conducted? How are cancellation and no-shows handled? Consider also time lines for payment for services rendered.

- *Compensation guidelines.* Will the trainer be paid an hourly rate, an hourly rate plus commission, an incentive based on performance, or a percentage of total revenues collected? Several payment methods are possible; consult with the organization's CPA and legal representative to determine payment methods.

- *Marketing and packaging personal training sessions.* How will personal training services be marketed and packaged? These issues are primary factors in the financial success of the program. Are trainers responsible for building their own clientele or are referrals to trainers made following an interest survey or fitness assessment? Will packages of services be offered to lower the price per session or will each session be sold separately? Will a complimentary session or two be offered to new members or prospects? Make the pricing and marketing decisions in concert with the overall strategy of the program and the operation. The club operator, head trainer, and sales personnel should assist in developing a marketing strategy that is consistent with the mission of the organization.

For information regarding personal training programs and certifications contact the following:

The Cooper Institute for Aerobics Research 800-635-7050 or http://www.cooperinst.org/

The National Strength and Conditioning Association (NSCA) 719-632-6722 or http://www.nsca-cc.org/

American Council on Exercise (ACE) 800-529-8227 or http://www.acefitness.org/

Exercise Lite

In early 1995 the Centers for Disease Control and Prevention and the American College of Sports Medicine put forth new guidelines regarding the quantity and quality of exercise needed to produce desirable health outcomes. The recommendation states, "accumulate 30 minutes or more of moderate-intensity physical activity on most preferably, all days of the week." This recommendation should be studied and implemented by professionals attempting to reach the large percentage of American adults who are currently sedentary.

Recent data from the U.S. Department of Health and Human Services indicate that only 22 percent of American adults engage regularly in enough physical activity to produce health benefits (Herbert and Ribisi 1995). With increasing health care costs, the burden of the sedentary population continues to grow. These new guidelines encourage sedentary people who may have been intimidated by previous stringent guidelines for exercise to become more active. The goal of these recommendations is to gradually move the most sedentary population to become moderately active and the moderately active to become more vigorously active.

Implement programming using the new Exercise Lite guidelines. Members who may have felt intimidated and guilty by their inability to achieve the previous guidelines for exercise frequency and intensity will be more comfortable in a club that recognizes their needs and sponsors programs for them. Gradually increasing the involvement of these members in different programs and improving their fitness levels and self-confidence will build long-term relationships and render positive results to the operation's bottom line.

Nutrition Counseling and Weight-Control Programs

Healthy People 2000, a program implemented by the U.S. Department of Health and Human Services, set an objective to reduce the prevalence of overweight adults in the United States from its current 30 percent to 20 percent by the year 2000 through sponsoring educational programs on the value of regular exercise and a healthy, balanced diet. Although it is unlikely this objective will be met, as advertising dollars promoting less than healthy food choices are far greater than the promotional dollars for the Healthy People 2000 program, it certainly isn't because the American population is not trying. Statistics show that during any period, 25 percent of male and 50 percent of female adults in the United States are trying to lose weight. Unfortunately, these efforts are not proving successful. New guidelines released in 1996 by the U.S. Department of Agriculture and the Department of Health and Human Services no longer permit an increase in weight with age, as with previous guidelines. Currently 34 percent of U.S. men and women are considered overweight. These new guidelines, however, are expected to push a majority of Americans into this category. With statistics such as these, it is no surprise that nutrition counseling and weight-management services are in high demand. Many fitness and wellness centers that offer these services to meet this member demand work closely with managed care operators to provide an additional revenue stream for the club.

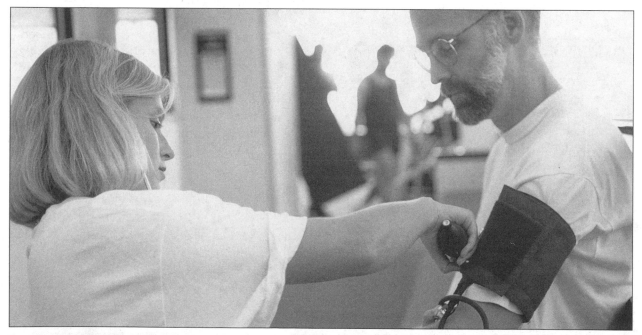

Courtesy of Dallas Texins Association

Developing Nutrition Counseling and Weight-Management Programs

Whether you offer the nutrition counseling and weight-management programs exclusively to existing members or market them throughout the community to attract new members, you must use qualified professionals to implement a quality program.

Many facilities that lack the resources and professional staff to implement an in-house nutrition service contract with outside vendors to offer this high-demand program. As with any service or program managed by an independent contractor, advantages and disadvantages exist. The club operator must determine what direction is most beneficial for the organization and the membership. The operator must address the following concerns and issues to develop a quality nutrition program.

- *In-house or independent contractor.* The number of independent companies offering nutrition-based programming to fitness centers continues to grow. These vendors offer marketing and promotional assistance, collateral materials, a predetermined weight-management system, and professional assistance in return for a percentage of revenues or profits. As fitness centers enter the weight-control business, they should give careful consideration to the blueprint for program design. Will the vendor represent the professionalism of the facility? Is it worth giving up control and accountability to offer a proven product to your membership with little or no administrative hassle? Does the club have access to nutrition professionals who would allow the creation of an in-house program? What are the time and cost limitations, if any? Consider partnering with local health practitioners or hospitals.

- *Program goal.* Determine the primary and secondary goals behind implementing nutrition services. Will the program be offered to members only to increase member satisfaction and retention? Will the program be offered year round? Will local health care professionals offer referrals to the program? Can individuals in the community join only the weight-control program initially and later decide on club membership? Is the primary goal of the program to drive revenues through membership sales, supplement sales, and program

membership fees? The answer to these questions may assist you in deciding whether to develop an in-house program or hire an independent contractor.

- *Space allocation.* Ideally the club sets aside dedicated space for private nutrition consultations and educational sessions.

- *Qualified staff.* Hiring qualified staff must be a priority for the club operator. Directors of nutrition and weight-management centers should be registered or licensed by the American Dietetic Association. These individuals should have knowledge of nutrition and understand the interaction between exercise and nutrition. Consider appointing a nutrition expert, fitness expert, and perhaps a behavioral counselor to the staff of the weight-management program.

- *Address nutrition, fitness, and behavioral factors.* For weight-management programs to be successful, you must address all dimensions of the weight-control problem. In addition to offering seminars regarding food selection, label reading, and one-on-one exercise sessions, consider support groups and counseling to address personal issues that lead to overeating.

- *Program format and pricing.* Determine the format of the program. Will the program last 6, 8, or 12 weeks? How many individual nutrition counseling sessions with the dietitian will occur during the program and at what frequency? How will you price the program? Will you offer a pricing discount to dues-paying members? Determining specifics of the program will assist in setting pricing. Consider pricing on auxiliary services or products, such as books, tapes, personal training, and so on. Also determine sales at the conclusion of the weight-control program. Can the member purchase periodic reevaluations? Is there an ongoing program for maintenance? Be sure the program format is well organized before determining marketing strategies.

- *Financial pro forma.* Once you decide on the specifics of the program, prepare detailed financial projections determining break-even point and cost-benefit analysis. The pro forma should include all potential sources of revenue conservatively projected; all overhead expenses, including utilities, marketing, legal and accounting advice; and staffing and associated labor costs.

- *Marketing strategy.* When you have set and confirmed all program specifics and pricing structures by the financial pro forma, develop and implement an aggressive marketing strategy. Determine your use of terms such as *weight control* versus *lifestyle management.* Be sure marketing strategies do not guarantee specific results in a specific period. Members who do not achieve expected results will not adhere to the program or retain their club membership.

For information regarding nutrition counseling and weight control contact the following:

The American Dietetic Association (ADA) 800-366-1655 or http://www.eatright.org/

Sports, Cardiovascular, and Wellness Nutritionist (SCAN) 303-779-1950

AQUATIC PROGRAMMING

The pool has always been considered an excellent selling tool. Only recently have club operators begun viewing the pool as an aquatic fitness center capable of expanding the service and program offerings of the club. The number of water exercise classes in the United States rose 20 percent in 1995, according to a recent study by the U.S. Water Fitness Association (Gerson 1995). With trends such as these, club operators and program managers are well advised to explore the wealth of programming opportunities available in aquatics.

With fitness trends moving toward a kinder and gentler type of exercise catering to the aging baby boomers, the aquatic fitness arena takes on a higher level of importance in the scheme of club operations.

The aquatic environment naturally caters to many different populations for several reasons. Factors such as increased buoyancy, that eliminates stress on the joints thus reducing the injury potential, are appealing to the overweight and underconditioned market, those rehabilitating from injury, arthritis sufferers, and baby boomers concerned about joint stress. The heat dissipation aspect of aquatics also appeals to the pregnant woman concerned about raising her core body temperature and the older adult or child who is susceptible to heat-related stress. The increased difficulty of movement against water resistance is attractive to the serious athlete who is looking for a low-impact cross-training method. In fact, aquatic exercise with its many program opportunities can benefit every age group and fitness level.

The number of possible programs using the pool is limited only by creativity. Aquatic programming opportunities include, but are not limited to, the following:

- Swimming lessons for adults and children
- Water exercise classes
- Masters swimming programs
- Water walking and running programs
- Deep water exercise
- Scuba diving lessons
- Water volleyball leagues
- Birthday parties
- Physical therapy and rehabilitation programs
- Family activities
- Older adult exercise programs
- Specialty programs for arthritic, overweight, physically challenged, or injured members
- Prenatal and postpartum classes
- High-intensity, low-impact, cross-training classes
- Children's programs
- Water-based personal training workouts
- Lap swimming
- Children's swim teams

The possibilities are limitless. Use creativity and offer more than one program at a time. Offer programming throughout the day for best space use. With the demand for this type of programming growing, the wise club operator will take the steps necessary to develop and maintain a quality aquatic program.

Developing Aquatics Programs

As with any other type of program, the aquatics offerings in the club should be well planned and implemented. Conduct member surveys to determine the scope and breadth of desired program offerings. Start small and build a quality program with the backing of active members. The following are issues you should consider when developing an aquatic program.

- *Hire qualified professionals.* For a program to be successful, you must hire an experienced aquatic director. This individual oversees all programming and ensures other personnel hired are qualified and well trained. Club operators should employ only certified water safety instructors, lifeguards, and water exercise instructors for all aquatic programs. Certifications can be obtained from the American Red Cross, YMCA, U.S. Water Fitness Association, and Aquatic Exercise Association.

- *Develop safety guidelines.* Strictly enforce rules and regulations protecting the safety of those participating in aquatic programs. Routinely implement and practice emergency plans. Coordinate with local emergency medical services (EMS) to ensure the safety of the members.

- *Amenity versus profit center.* The club operator in cooperation with the aquatic director must determine which programs will be offered as amenities to club membership and which programs will incur an additional fee.

- *Rental of space to community programs.* Consider renting space or time slots to local community programs to enhance the position of the club in the community and provide a revenue opportunity for the club. Physical therapy centers may be interested in conducting rehabilitation in the pool and the local high school swim team may need additional practice facilities.

- *Scheduling for optimal use of pool.* The pool should be active from open to close. Use creativity in class scheduling to ensure all possible programs have a regular time slot. Organize programming to use 100 percent of the pool. Hold children's swim lessons at one end of the pool while conducting a group exercise class or personal training session at the other end.

- *Using and purchasing aquatic exercise equipment.* The recent proliferation of equipment specifically designed to enhance water exercise makes programming opportunities more diverse. Equipment ranging from water treadmills to toning boots, belts, and gloves makes water exercise demanding and entertaining. Be sure to use equipment specifically designed for water activities.

- *Create diversity in programming.* The age old complaint that water exercise is boring should never be heard in a well-organized aquatic program. Create programming that involves all ages and fitness levels to create an exciting fitness opportunity.

- *Encourage social interaction.* Social interaction is one dynamic that appeals to many water exercise enthusiasts. Pay special attention to introducing class participants and encouraging social interaction throughout the class or lesson. Often this social interaction will keep members participating when the desire to exercise diminishes.

- *Marketing strategy.* Marketing creatively allows the club operator to reach people who typically may not be first in line to purchase a club membership. Overweight individuals, older adults, sedentary people, and physically challenged individuals all may find aquatics a comfortable way to begin a regular exercise regimen.

- *Pool maintenance and temperature.* For programs to be successful, the pool must be expertly maintained. Employ a pool maintenance specialist or train a member of the maintenance team as a certified pool operator. The temperature of the pool will be a point of constant dispute. Lap swimmers and intense exercisers prefer a cooler pool (80 to 83 degrees), whereas group exercise participants, children, and those recovering or rehabilitating an injury or suffering from arthritis will prefer a warmer pool (approximately 84 to 86 degrees). Find a temperature that is acceptable to all groups and maintain that temperature.

For more information regarding aquatics programs and certifications contact the following:

(continued)

YMCAs—check local listings for the office in your area.

The American Red Cross—check local listings for the office in your area.

United States Water Fitness Association (USWFA) 407-732-9908.

Aquatic Exercise Association (AEA) 813-483-8600.

RACQUET SPORTS PROGRAMMING

The decline in popularity of racquet sports in the 1980s has been well documented. Tennis hit its peak in popularity during the 1970s and declined through the 1980s with recent data showing a possible resurgence. Racquetball hit its height in popularity during the 1980s. In 1978 the Tennis Industry Association (Lustigman 1994) estimated there were more than 35 million tennis players. Recent surveys by the National Sporting Goods Association (Connor 1995; NSGA 1995) estimate the number of tennis players dropped to 14.2 million in 1993 and 11.6 million in 1994, yet a slight growth of 3.1 percent in 1995 over 1994 shows some promise. Recent data in the 1997 IHRSA state of the industry report (IHRSA 1997) cited tennis as one area of recreational sports that is beginning to rebound citing an impressive 21% increase in racquet sales during 1996 over 1995 sales. The American Amateur Racquetball Association estimates the number of active racquetball players in the United States continues to decline (Lustigman 1994). Recent data from the National Sporting Goods Manufacturers Association details an 8.2 percent decline in the number of racquetball players from 1994 to 1995 (Handley 1995). This continues the trend shown in the same 1994 study that detailed a 4-million player drop in the number of players from 1984 to 1994. See figures 9.2 and 9.3 for levels of tennis and racquetball participation.

The drop in participants is also reflected in the precipitous drop in racquet sport equipment sales.

With programming trends moving toward more individual sports that refresh body, mind, and soul and away from competitive activities, the future of racquet sports is in the balance. Although recent trends indicate a potential resurgence in some racquet sports, tennis and squash in particular, creative programming is the key to revitalize these programs in facilities willing to dedicate the time and energy required to be successful. The goal is to continually introduce new players to the sport, encourage frequent play from enthusiasts, and reactivate former players.

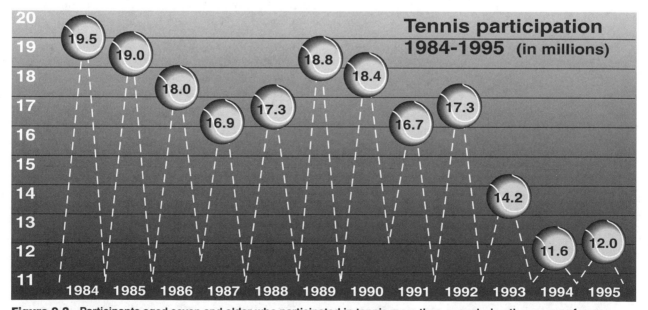

Figure 9.2 Participants aged seven and older who participated in tennis more than once during the course of one year.

Reprinted, by permission, from A. Lustigman, 1994, "Reviving racquet sports," *Club Industry* (October): 26; and data from National Sporting Goods Association, 1995, *Sports participation survey* (Mt. Prospect, IL: NSGA).

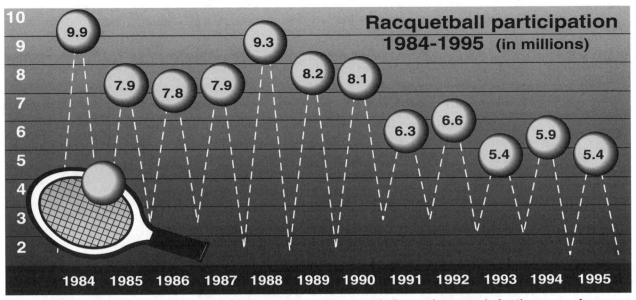

Figure 9.3 Participants aged seven and older who participated in racquetball more than once during the course of one year.

Reprinted, by permission, from A. Lustigman, 1994, "Reviving racquet sports," *Club Industry* (October): 28; and data from National Sporting Goods Association, 1995, *Sports participation survey* (Mt. Prospect, IL: NSGA).

Developing a Racquet Sports Program

Hiring a qualified club professional or director is the first step toward developing a quality program. The club pro nurtures the program by involving people in the social aspects of the sport, encouraging their skill development, and developing programs to keep the sport interesting and entertaining. Some examples of programming opportunities that may enhance the image of racquet sports in health club facilities include the following:

- *Setting up leagues.* Leagues are a wonderful way to get people involved and keep them active in the sport. By rating players according to their ability, this program enables persons of relatively equal abilities to be paired for competitive matches. Establish leagues within the club, locally with other tennis facilities, regionally, and nationally. The U.S. Tennis Association (USTA) recreational league tennis program provides an example of their success, with more than 175,000 adult participants.

- *Clinics.* Offering free clinics to beginner, intermediate, and advanced players is a good way to introduce new players to the techniques of the sport and to continue the skill development of enthusiasts. Clinics typically offer intensive skill-development coaching and drill practice to incorporate those skills

into the game. Bringing in a guest pro or celebrity will enhance the participation in the clinic. Offer league sign-ups and special events at clinics to capture enthusiasm.

- *Tournaments.* Competitive tournaments give players the opportunity to test their skills against another player of similar skill. Tournaments can be highly competitive or social and fun. Creative planning is key to gaining registrants. Some examples of tournaments include club championships, father and son, battle of the sexes, interclub championships, and firecracker Fourth of July tournaments. The possible themes are endless. Tournament types include round-robin, single elimination and double elimination, and many other creative formats.

- *Team tennis.* Team tennis emphasizes the social, yet competitive, aspects of the sport. Arrange teams and typically include both men and women. Teams play each other in a series of matches, including singles, doubles, and mixed doubles.

- *Junior programs.* Junior programs are the future of racquet sports. Junior tennis, racquetball, and squash programs offer lessons, clinics, and competitive opportunities similar to adult programs. These programs foster lifetime racquet sport enthusiasts. The USTA

(continued)

National Junior Tennis program assists clubs with junior development programs (see the following contact information).

- *Seniors programs.* Programs designed to match older adult players on a social and competitive basis are gaining popularity. These programs emphasize the social aspect of a match as much as the physical fitness benefits. Plan these programs during nonprime time to expand racquet memberships without causing further congestion on the courts during peak playing times.

- *Special events with a social emphasis.* Mixed doubles tournaments are an excellent example of special events centered on a social event. Plan a fun tournament followed by a mixer or social event designed to introduce players to potential playing partners.

- *Celebrity appearances.* With assistance from racquet sport equipment vendors or other sources, plan celebrity appearances in conjunction with a clinic or tournament. Celebrity visits cause excitement in the racquet programs and encourage new member sign-ups and adherence by regular players.

- *Women's leagues.* Similar to seniors activities, special events and leagues for women enhance

racquet sport participation through social interaction. You can often schedule these leagues and tournaments, as with seniors, during nonprime time, either midmorning or late evening.

- *Matchmaking services.* One primary reason members are not active in racquet sports is the inability to locate a suitable playing partner. Develop programs and player groups within the club to supply players with a list of potential playing partners. Introduce players to each other and encourage them to get together. Whether the system is formal or informal, this is one of the most important responsibilities of a club pro or program director.

For more information regarding racquet sports programming contact the following:

American Amateur Racquetball Association (AARA) 719-635-5396

U.S. Tennis Association (USTA) 718-592-8000

International Health, Racquet and Sportsclub Association (IHRSA) 617-951-0055

U.S. Professional Tennis Association (USPTA) 713-525-2010

United States Squash Racquets Association 610-667-4006

AGE GROUP PROGRAMMING

As the graying of America continues and the concerns of active older adults become vital to the success of the health club industry, attention to programming to meet the needs of particular age groups grows. These aging baby boomers committed to a healthier lifestyle demand programs not only for themselves, but also for their children.

Active Older Adult Programming

As stated earlier, the number of active older adults is growing at a much greater pace than any other age group. It is estimated that by the year 2000, 35 million people, or 13 percent of the U.S. population, will be 65 years of age or older. During the next 30 years the number of people over the age of 50 years will increase by 74 percent, while those under 50 years will grow by only one percent.

Club operators have known of this demographic trend for years, but is the industry prepared? According to the National Sporting Goods Manufacturers Association 1995 participation study (NSGA

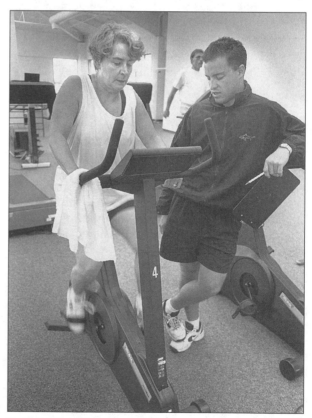

© Mary Langenfeld

1995), fitness participation grew 17 percent for Americans 65 years and older, followed closely by the 55 to 64 age group with a 15 percent increase in participation. The 1997 IHRSA state of the industry report (IHRSA 1997) cited a 669% growth in commercial club memberships held by persons 65 years and older from 1987 through 1995. The statistics for 1995 show that this population now comprises a full 10% of commercial health club memberships. Programming trends recognize the aging of the American population. Many facilities offer an active older adult program, that emphasizes activities such as low-impact group exercise, mind-body wellness, and exercise programs with a social component. If facilities are to survive, they must realize that the primary market for the health club industry of the future will be the active older adult.

The various systems of the body begin a gradual and irreversible physiological decline after the age of 50 years. However, evidence strongly indicates the pace of this decline can be slowed through regular exercise. Research on active older adults indicates that regular exercise slows the biological aging process by regulating blood sugars, controlling hypertension and blood pressure, increasing mental functioning, increasing lung capacity, decreasing the incidence of back pain, decreasing arthritis pain, increasing sexual interest and satisfaction, increasing heart function, maintaining bone density, and improving attitudes and sociability. Developing a program that enhances the physiological functioning of the body and improves the self-esteem and outlook of older adults will no doubt meet the needs of this aging population.

Developing Active Older Adult Programming

Developing a program to attract and retain active older adults must be well planned and implemented. Evaluate continuous feedback from participants to continue the growth and improvement of the programming. Issues to consider when planning active older adult programming include the following:

- *Create programs that overcome barriers to exercise.* Older adults often are hesitant to initiate exercise programs because they fear they will overdo it, they fear they are too old to exercise, they lack self-esteem, and they find a lack of programming opportunities. Create programs specifically for the senior population that start slowly and build the active older adult both physically and mentally. Water exercises are an excellent example of successful programs implemented for the active older adult. The water eases fears of falling while offering a medium of resistance that helps build the physical stamina of the participant.

- *Create diverse programming.* An active older adult is often considered to be anyone 40 years and older. Programming for those adults who have retired and have a substantial amount of leisure time must be dramatically different from programs for the highly stressed executive who has little time to spare. Incorporate social opportunities for those members who crave social interaction and time-conscious

programs for those who are still working. Avoid stereotyping this population through program offerings. Not all older adults are overweight and arthritic. Create diverse opportunities for all fitness levels.

- *Create exercise prescriptions.* Exercise programming for the active older adult must be individually determined by a professional trained to look at all aspects of exercise for the older adult. Prescriptions for the long-term exerciser will be dramatically different from the exercise routine for the beginner. Both populations, however, should be carefully screened, encouraged to visit their physicians before initiating an exercise program, and given an exercise level that begins well within their tolerance level and gradually increases. Emphasize the safety of the program.

- *Create a friendly environment.* Strive to create a friendly environment for the active older adult. Train the staff to recognize and respond to the needs of this population; be sure that the facility's layout is easily negotiated, that the signage and directions throughout the facility are easy to read, that the operating instructions for exercise equipment are magnified, if necessary, and that the equipment is available to increase workloads by small increments.

- *Hire appropriate staff.* Staff members should be certified to establish credibility for the program

(continued)

and older if possible to serve as role models. Train the staff to work with the older and deconditioned population.

- *Determine the target market and advertise appropriately.* As stated, the older adult population is quite diverse. Specify the target market appropriate for the available programming or create new programming opportunities. Develop advertising that welcomes the older adult. Use older people in the ads who show vitality and confidence.

- *Develop appropriate membership structures.* The active older adult will not respond to the high-pressure sales tactics used in some clubs. Instead, create membership programs that encourage the older adult to use the club during nonprime time. With the availability of time and social programming that attracts

the older adult, nonprime time memberships may create a win-win situation for both the member and the club.

- *Discounting or not?* Many clubs offer senior citizen discount programs for their older adult population. Discuss and determine your facility's philosophy. Some argue that this population needs discounted memberships and incidentals to maintain their membership, whereas others point to statistics that state that 80 percent of all U.S. savings are controlled by persons over the age of 50 years. Decisions regarding discounts must be determined for each club operation.

For information regarding the active older adult, contact the National Institute on Aging at 301-496-1752.

Children's Programming

Quality children's programming offers a facility much more than a way to preoccupy children while their parents exercise. On the contrary, a quality children's program can be a powerful tool in both membership sales and retention. A children's facility that offers fun and entertaining creative play opportunities can be attractive to working parents concerned about their child's physical development. Moreover, as society becomes increasingly dangerous and the days of roaming the neighborhood on a bicycle disappear, parents are searching for a safe outlet for their children. Clubs who develop or purchase a program designed for children will find themselves with more satisfied members.

Statistics today regarding the activity and fitness level of America's youth do not present an optimistic picture. Statistics from the Surgeon General's Report on Physical Activity and Health cited in the 1997 IHRSA state of the health club industry report detail the precipitous decline in physical activity as age or grade level increases. These statistics show that nearly half of young people aged 12 to 21 are not vigorously active on a regular basis. High school physical education class enrollment is down 17 percent to only 25 percent from 1991 to 1995 and sadly only 19 percent of these young people are physically active for 20 minutes or more during these classes every day of the school week. Clearly these young people are not experiencing the increased incidence of regular exercise that the baby-boomer generation is. The number of overweight

children and adolescents in the United States more than doubled, from 5 to 11 percent in 6 to 17 year olds from 1985 to 1995. This is due in large part to the

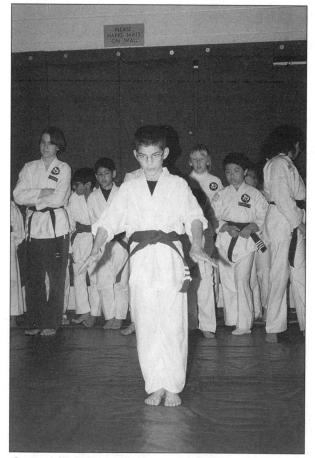

Courtesy of Dallas Texins Association

decrease in activity mentioned. It is important to note, however, that the number of active children still significantly outnumbers adults. Common sense tells us that children who are physically active grow up to be more active adults than their inactive peers. Thus participation in lifelong activities such as racquet sports and swimming may form a lifetime habit of healthy activity.

Developing Children's Programming

Developing programming for children is much more involved than throwing a ball into an open racquetball court. Quality programming takes careful planning, selective hiring, and continuous evaluation. Issues to consider when developing a children's program include the following:

- *In-house or outside contractor.* Clubs who recognize the need for children's programs but do not have the resources or staff needed should consider an outside vendor. Many companies are now marketed to assist the club operator with this specialty program offering. Working parents who realize the need for creative play outlets for their children are willing to pay for these services. Consider an outside vendor if you cannot accommodate the following issues in developing an in-house program.

- *Coordinate efforts with local schools.* Contact the local school system to inquire about the need for a cooperative arrangement to assist parents with after-school care. This could create a win-win situation in the community and introduce community members to your club.

- *Staffing.* Staffing a children's center should be a club operator's number one concern. Qualified, energetic, creative, positive, and experienced personnel are necessary for a successful program. Club operators should conduct complete background checks on all staff working with children. Thoroughly research all job references and criminal background history.

- *Profit center or amenity?* Determine the financial standing of the children's program. Will the facility charge entry or activity fees, or will it serve strictly as an amenity to the facility? Club operators should consider the current membership dues rates for families as well as attrition and retention rates to determine the most profitable way to offer children's programs.

- *Year round or summer only?* Will the children's programming be offered year round in conjunction with programs aimed at families, or will the intense offering of children's programs be only during the summer?

- *Dedicated space.* To offer quality programming, a dedicated space for children is necessary. Designated space for a children's center shows commitment to the program, giving members confidence in the long-term offering of the program. Allow enough space to section off areas for creative play, cribs, quiet time, and crafts.

- *Create a safe environment.* Carefully plan the dedicated space to eliminate any potential dangers. Be sure toys are designed specifically for the age of the children using the center, eliminate sharp edges or protruding corners, use additional padding under carpet to cushion falls, eliminate any small toys or objects that can cause choking, and offer enough supervision to continually observe the children's activities.

- *Create activity programs that encourage play.* Children are not interested in the concept of fitness. They are, however, always interested in fun and entertaining activities. Create programs that offer opportunities to develop aerobic fitness, balance, gross and fine motor skills, social skills, and imagination in the activities offered. Constantly change activities, as a child's attention span is short. Study children and their games to create activities that build on what they enjoy.

- *Create a plan to handle discipline.* In any gathering of children, the potential exists for an unruly child. Create systems for discipline that are acceptable to the parent, yet effective for the child. Consider convening a panel of parents to develop a disciplinary policy.

- *Coordinate children's and adults' activities.* Plan special events or games for the children at the same time the club is offering a special adult function or popular class. The children will enjoy spending time with other kids and the parent can have a carefree workout.

(continued)

- *Develop an emergency plan.* Collect medical information on every child. Develop and regularly practice the emergency plan. Be sure all staff members are certified in first aid and CPR.
- *Parents on property.* Determine rules and regulations regarding whether the parent must remain in the facility while their child is in the children's center.

For information on children's programs, contact the International Kids' Fitness Association at 804-360-4285 or your local YMCA or YWCA.

TRENDS IN PROGRAMMING

It is often difficult to determine if current trends in activity are simply flashes in the pan or are programs sure to become staples in our health club program offerings. The following programs are currently experiencing a great deal of popularity and managers should consider them for inclusion in future programming calendars.

In-Line Skating

The popularity of in-line skating is indisputable. According to American Sports Data and the National Sporting Goods Association, the sport has grown from 20,000 skaters in 1984 to more than 19 million in 1994 (Nottingham 1994a). A 1995 study from the National Sporting Goods Manufacturers Association recorded a substantial one-year participation increase of 20 percent from 1994 levels to 1995 (Connor 1995). In-line skate equipment sales have been the single most successful product launch in sporting goods industry history, selling in excess of $600 million in 1994. Studies show that although 64.5 percent of skaters are under the age of 17 years, 46 percent are women and 37 percent have average household incomes higher than $50,000 per year (Nottingham 1994a). A survey of retailers and manufacturers conducted by Kurt Salmon Associates predicts that in-line skating will be the fastest growing sport during the years of 1995 to 2001. There is no question in-line skating is here to stay and managers should incorporate it into the programming calendar.

Developing an In-Line Skating Program

Developing an in-line skating program is an excellent way to interest some club members that traditional programming may not reach. In-line skating is fun, it can be done outdoors, it is appropriate for all fitness levels, and if done properly is safe. The following are some issues to consider when offering in-line skating programs.

- *Locate a skate school to work with.* Finding a resource that can assist with equipment rental, certified instructors, and expertise is crucial to program safety and success. Check references looking for a safe track record.
- *Review insurance policies.* The initial thought that in-line skating programs are too risky is not necessarily the case. Demonstrate to the carrier that the program is taught by International In-Line Skating Association (IISA)-certified instructors and that safety gear is required. Explain where the classes will take place, the number of participants per instructor, and that participants are required to sign a waiver.
- *Use only IISA-certified instructors.* The IISA trains instructors internationally. The IISA sets requirements for safety and education

through a standardized format for instruction (see the following contact information).

- *Designate a skating location.* The location for the skating activities should have a smooth surface. An underused parking lot, basketball court, or tennis court works well.
- *Offer lessons and clinics.* Offer introductory lessons and clinics to raise interest in the in-line skating program. The local skate shop will provide equipment for use or rental. Offer these clinics on a complimentary basis and encourage participants to bring a friend. Skating should be a fun and social activity.
- *Safety is the number one lesson.* Allow all participants to have a successful and safe experience with in-line skating. Protective gear must be worn. Classes must move at a comfortable pace and never ask participants to do any skill they are not comfortable with.

For information on in-line skating contact the International In-Line Skating Association (IISA) at 404-728-9707. For certification call the IISA at 305-672-6714.

Mind-Body Programs

The pace of living races out of control. Physiologically, the demands are overwhelming. Statistics indicate that 70 percent of all physician office visits are related to stress, which exacerbates disease states such as heart disease, hypertension, depression, and cancer. As fitness centers position themselves as wellness centers, increasing energy and programming to reduce the negative effects of stress are emerging. Programs designed to assist members with relaxation, recovery, and stress reduction are growing. These mind-body programs focus energy on developing not only the physical aspect of the individual, but also the mental and spiritual aspects. For wellness to occur, participants must address all components of self and locate a facility that will assist them in that effort.

As baby boomers age and seek methods to regain balance, reduce stress, and enhance self-concept through their health and wellness centers, they are being introduced to nontraditional mind-body techniques as well as conventional exercise modalities. Mindless activities, such as weight training and cardiovascular training, are losing the popularity battle to activities that force the mind and spirit to concentrate while the body is working. Mind-body offerings such as yoga, neuromuscular integrative action (NIA), tai chi, meditation, guided imagery, body balance, breathing techniques, Pilates, Alexander, and martial arts (see the following for details of these) are growing at a rapid pace. These programs encourage participants to halt the mind chatter and relax totally. This relaxation and focused breathing returns the body to its resting state, lowering blood pressure, heart rate, body temperature, and metabolic rate. This relaxation reaction is the opposite of the stress response, that many maintain in a chronic state. This total relaxation assists in counteracting the negative health effects of stress.

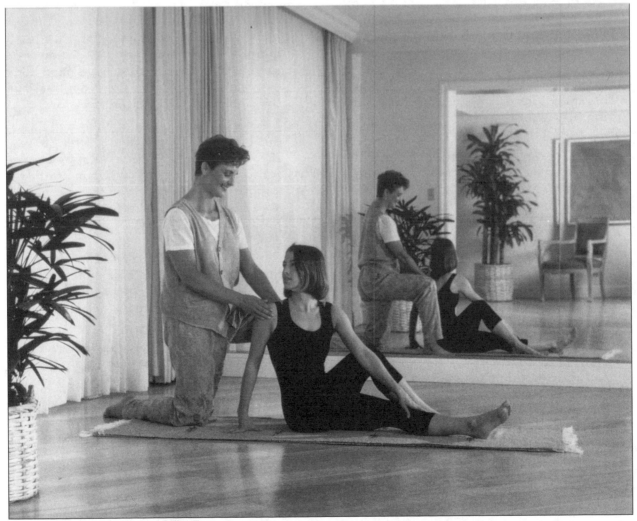

Courtesy of The Spa at the Crescent, Dallas, Texas.

Developing Mind-Body Programs

The consumer today is bombarded with mind-body information. Information regarding methods to reduce stress and rebalance life is available at every turn. Educated consumers expect more from their health and wellness facility than conventional cardiovascular and resistance training. In fact, many consumers who would not typically be prospects for health club memberships are joining due to mind-body programs. In response to this growing demand, many facilities are incorporating programs such as tai chi, NIA, yoga, and Pilates into their programming calendar. Facilities considering adding mind-body techniques should look at the following.

- *Instructors.* Instructors for mind-body programs have been rigorously trained. Locating a qualified instructor who will blend with the staff and member population is often the most difficult task in implementing these programs. National organizations often can assist in recruiting instructors.

- *Environment.* For the class to effectively reduce the stress level of participants, the environment must be strictly controlled. Designate a quiet space and equip it with a sound system, proper flooring, and low lighting. The temperature of the room should be slightly warmer than conventional exercise space. Keep noise pollution to a minimum. A typical aerobic room will work well if you adjust the temperature upward, dim the lights, and eliminate noise pollution.

- *Equipment.* Equipment to implement many of the mind-body classes is minimal. You can implement yoga, tai chi, and Pilates mat classes with little equipment. Mats and music are mandatory. Optional equipment includes yoga blocks, straps, towels, a Universal Reformer for Pilates, and much more. Most equipment does not need to be immediately available to begin the program. Test the waters with the membership and purchase equipment to expand the offerings when demand warrants.

- *Marketing.* Marketing mind-body programs must be done carefully. When offering programming in this area, do not stray too far from the beaten path. Market using terminology the membership is looking for. Terminology such as stress reduction, body balance, and flexibility training might be effective in some facilities. Slowly introduce programming and terminology and build a level of education and enthusiasm.

- *Amenity or for-fee class?* Club operators can expect to incur an instructor fee ranging from $25 to $100 per class to offer mind-body programming. A review of current membership dues levels, member demand, and attrition levels will assist the club operator with this decision.

- *Scheduling.* Removing a popular step class during evening prime time to offer a yoga class may not make members happy. Carefully consider scheduling when offering mind-body programs. Tai chi and yoga are often taught before the workday to relax and energize participants or at the conclusion of the day to decrease stress. Consider offering these programs later in the evening or during nonprime time so the class does not compete with the high activity and noise inherent during prime time.

- *Dress comfortably.* Encourage instructors and members to dress comfortably. Loose clothing not only will enhance participation and ease of movement, but also will encourage members not comfortable with the spandex set to explore these opportunities.

Mind-Body Exercise Methods

Yoga. Developed in India, yoga means union, the blending of mind and body in movement. B.K.S. Iyengar Yoga National Association of the United States 800-889-YOGA.

Tai chi. Tai means grand, chi means energy or life force. Tai chi combines a form of meditation in motion with a style of martial arts.

Pilates. Pilates emphasizes slow, controlled movements developing mind and body. Pilates is typically done on a Universal Reformer—an adjustable platform or bed equipped with straps and springs for resistance. Contact the Pilates Studio 800-474-5283 or the PhysicalMind Institute 508-988-1990.

Alexander technique. A method of learning to use body and mind more efficiently and freely. Contact the American Center for the Alexander Technique (ACAT) 212-799-1468 or the North American Society of Teachers of the Alexander Technique 800-473-0620.

Meditation. It emphasizes freeing the mind and body of tension through focused breathing and concentration on a fixed image or object.

Martial arts. Many styles, such as karate, tae kwon do, and judo, are included. Martial arts improve concentration, confidence, and physical condition of participants.

NIA technique. Neuromuscular integrative action (NIA) is a technique founded on the work of Debbie and Carlos Rosas. It is a cardiovascular movement class that draws on the elements and wisdom of the ancient disciplines such as yoga, tai chi, and tae kwon do, as well as contemporary influences of dance and fitness. Contact Neuromuscular Integrative Action (NIA) 800-762-5762.

IN CLOSING

In this chapter we have looked at the reasons behind popular programming, the benefits they offer your members, and issues to consider when planning and implementing these programs. We have reviewed time-tested programming, such as fitness assessments and current programming trends, such as in-line skating. Not all programs discussed in this chapter will work in every setting. Careful assessment of needs, planning, implementation, and evaluation as we discussed in this chapter will help program managers determine the programs most appropriate for their setting. Use the contact organizations and information in this chapter to ease the effort in gathering additional information.

KEY TERMS

Achievable age

Lifestyle management

Mind-body programs

Risk age

Weight control

Wellness education

RECOMMENDED READINGS

American College of Sports Medicine. 1995. *ACSM's guidelines for exercise testing and prescription.* 5th ed. Baltimore: Williams & Wilkins.

Broderick, A. 1994. Heartbeat of success. *Fitness Management* (May): 32-34.

Bryant, C.X., J.A. Peterson, and R.J. Hagen. 1994. Weight loss: Unfolding the truth. *Fitness Management* (May): 42-44.

Connor, D. 1995. Walking, swimming top list of favorite fitness activities. *Club Industry* (June): 9.

Fitnews. 1995. Industry may hinge on kids' exercising. *Fitness Management* (September): 12.

Gerson, V. 1995. Water program trends and tips. *Fitness Management* (April): 32-34.

Handley, A. 1995. How to improve your racquetball program. *Club Industry* (April): 30.

Hauss, D.S. 1995. Never say diet. *Club Industry* (June): 19-26.

Herbert, W.G., and P.M. Ribisi. 1995. Exercise Lite meaning and implications. *Fitness Management* (April): 44-45.

Hoeger, W.W.K. 1995. Is water aerobics aerobic? *Fitness Management* (April): 29-30, 43.

International Health, Racquet and Sportsclub Association. 1994. *The 1994 IHRSA report on the state of the health club industry.* Boston: IHRSA.

————. 1995. *The 1995 IHRSA report on the state of the health club industry.* Boston: IHRSA.

————. 1997. *The 1997 IHRSA report on the state of the health club industry.* Boston: IHRSA.

Keeny, B.A. 1994. Kids. *Club Business International* (March): 65-70.

Loyle, D. 1994. Take aim at the 40-plus market. *Club Industry* (November): 17-21.

————. 1995a. Feeling well prompts exercise as much as looking good. *Club Industry* (June): 9.

————. 1995b. In-line fitness? *Club Industry* (September): 9.

Lustigman, A. 1994. Reviving racquet sports. *Club Industry* (October): 24-31.

Management Notebook. 1995. How to develop an over-40 program. *Club Industry* (July): 72, 74.

Morris, B.A. 1994. Make a splash. *Club Industry* (November): 26-30.

————. 1995. Measure up your members. *Club Industry* (October): 35-42.

National Sporting Goods Association. 1995. *Sports participation survey.* Mt. Prospect, IL: NSGA.

Nottingham, S. 1994a. Are you in-line for profits? *Fitness Management* (May): 36-40.

————. 1994b. Juggling the learning curve. *Fitness Management* (August): 40-42.

Outlook. 1995. Basketball, in-line skating top list of popular youth activities. *Club Industry* (October): 18.

Pessin, F. 1995. Getting in touch with the mind/body market. *Fitness Management* (October): 40, 45.

Peterson, J.A., and C.X. Bryant. 1990. Young at heart after 50. *Fitness Management* (August): 30-31.

Pinhoster, G. 1995. Far out fitness. *Club Industry* (July): 29-32.

Wilder, M., and D. Wilder. 1993. Come play with us. *Club Industry* (September): 34-37.

Winters, C. 1995a. Pump it up. *Club Industry* (February): 31-40.

————. 1995b. Should you outsource your aerobics program? *Club Industry* (September): 61-62.

Yacenda, J. 1990. Older exercisers can train intensively, too! *Fitness Management* (August): 14-16.

CHAPTER 10

Profit Center Programs

Profit centers offer opportunities to enhance the profitability of the organization. We can consider several programs and operations potential profit centers. In this chapter we review the operation of four common profit centers seen in all health fitness settings, including pro shops, food and beverage outlets, child care, and spa services (see figure 10.1). Is your facility optimizing the profitability of the organization by including profit centers in the operation? Would your membership support a new profit center? What is the process involved in implementing a profit center? How can you avoid the common mistakes many club operators make when implementing profit center programs? Find out the answers to these questions in this chapter.

Managing a health fitness facility in any setting has become a highly complex and demanding position. No longer can club operators simply open the doors and expect initiation fees and dues revenue to guarantee success. Within each facility lies the opportunity and financial necessity to create additional programming and services to generate profit.

These profit centers will not guarantee financial success, but if run properly they can assist in generating a positive bottom line result. For example, IHRSA's 1995 state of the industry recap (IHRSA 1995b) reported that clubs with the highest percentage of nondues revenue grew twice as fast in terms of both revenue and profitability than clubs with lower percentages of nondues revenue. IHRSA's *Profiles of Success* (1995a) report further explained the growing importance of profit centers by saying, "Clubs generated a greater percentage of their revenues than before from profit centers and programs." This demanding trend is sure to continue into the 21st century. In the IHRSA state of the industry report (IHRSA 1994), Charlie Swayne, owner of Valley View Fitness and Racquet Club and marketing professor at the University of Wisconsin, LaCrosse, confirms the importance of profit centers:

> *Once a club approaches market saturation, membership growth tends to decline. When that happens, in order to further grow the business, it is imperative to grow and establish revenue-generating programs and profit centers.*

DEVELOPING AND ORGANIZING PROFIT CENTERS

Profit centers are programs or services offered within the boundaries of the club operation that provide additional revenue and profit to the bottom line of an organization. Financially, these profit centers are often run as separate entities within the global profit and loss statement of the facility. Operation-

ally, most profit centers are run as separate departments within the scope of the organization. It is without question that profit centers are vital to the financial success of the organization. The IHRSA *Profiles of Success* (1995) survey found that clubs that were the most successful in generating nondues revenues had lower attrition rates than the average industry figures, 32 percent versus 36 percent, respectively. The survey stressed the importance of profit centers and it identified their development as one of the three main areas operators should address to remain competitive. *The* 1996 IHRSA *Profiles of Success* report indicates many organizations are heeding this advice. According to the published data, the clubs in the study saw a 7.1 percent increase in total revenues and "steady revenue-per-member figures in spite of a lower net membership growth of 5.7 percent. Fitness-only clubs, which are typically the most dependent upon membership sales for growth, generate, on average, almost 27 percent of their revenues from non-dues sources, as opposed to just 20 percent in 1994." This higher percentage of revenue from sources other than dues indicates more involvement in club activities by the membership, thus higher retention rates and improved profitability. See table 10.1 for profit center performance data.

> *No doubt, the ability of the facility manager to plan and organize a variety of businesses within the global organizational mission will contribute to the financial success of the operation.*

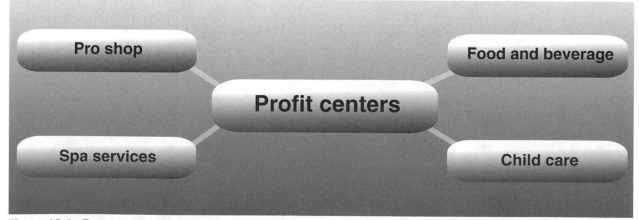

Figure 10.1 Examples of profit centers in a health fitness setting.

Table 10.1 Profit Center Performance Comparisons

	Restaurant	Pro shop	Child care
Size (sq. ft.)	2,343	325	904
Total revenues	$141,845	$87,526	$18,099
Revenue/square foot	$61	$269	$20
Profit	–$1,644	$16,565	–$14,341

Developing and operating successful profit centers is a demanding aspect of the facility manager's responsibility. The type of business and the daily operation of each profit center vary greatly, not only from each other but also from the general operation of a health fitness facility. Few academic preparatory programs for the health fitness industry teach the basics in managing and operating food and beverage outlets, retail merchandising, child development, or spa services. In most cases, the services of an experienced consultant are necessary to develop a realistic business plan and operating strategy for each profit center. The expense incurred hiring a consultant is money well spent when you consider the time, effort, and initial financial commitment of a less than successful venture.

The steps necessary to initiate a profit center are in many ways similar to the steps you take to plan and develop a fitness center but on a much smaller scale (see table 10.2). First, determine the purpose of the profit center. Will this profit center exist to generate a predetermined flow-through profit, or will it exist as a value-added service that breaks even in profitability yet enhances the value of the membership, thereby improving sales and retention? Once you make this decision, determine specific, measurable goals and objectives for the operation. After researching issues such as competition, market demand, consumer interest, income, and price considerations (see also chapter 5), develop a marketing plan with an identified target market, typically the existing membership and local community. Often an informal member survey can provide a great deal of information for this aspect of the business plan.

Developing a detailed business plan that defines the purpose of the profit center and includes a market analysis, goals and objectives statement, marketing plan, management plan, and financial pro forma is vital for a successful venture.

A management plan that considers issues such as staffing, space allocation and design, equipment needs, vendor management, operating procedures, and cash and point of sales procedures is the next logical step. Finally, develop a financial pro forma evaluating the capital investment needs, operating expenses, tax and insurance considerations, bookkeeping procedures, documentation, and potential profitability. With this information in hand, the club operator has a road map for developing a successful profit center.

Before the start-up of a profit center, a club operator selects a member of the existing staff or hires a qualified individual to oversee the development and operation of the endeavor. Identifying an individual with a background and interest in the venture relieves much of the start-up burden from the already busy club manager. The individual selected should have direct

Table 10.2 Business Planning for Health Fitness Profit Centers

Step 1	Statement of purpose
Step 2	Market analysis
Step 3	Marketing plan development
Step 4	Management plan development
Step 5	Preparation of financial pro forma
Step 6	Successful profit center

access to the club manager and business plan for continued advice and direction. Link the individual's compensation to the successful launch and operation of the profit center. This individual should also be responsible for making the existence of this new service or product evident to the membership. Use the marketing and advertising strategies identified in the marketing plan to assist in this effort.

Selecting a qualified and motivated profit center manager will enhance the potential for success.

Contractual Service Providers

Many facilities may not have the expertise, interest, or personnel available to develop and operate a profit center. Fortunately for these facilities, many vendors exist who can develop and operate the profit center on behalf of the club for a large percentage of the profit. We discussed using a vendor or contractual service provider in detail in chapters 8 and 9 as it relates to programming. Many advantages and disadvantages discussed in these earlier chapters also apply to profit center operations. The primary benefit for the club operator in hiring a contractual service is removing the burden of start-up and daily management, both financially and operationally. The disadvantages for the club operator include loss of control issues and reduction in the profitability potential. Each organization must determine whether using an outside vendor to manage and operate profit centers is a wise decision. Consider the following issues when looking at vendor resources:

- *Purpose of profit center*. As mentioned previously, the purpose of the profit center is either to generate a direct profit or offer an additional member service, thus enhancing the value of the membership. If generating a direct profit is the goal, using an outside vendor significantly hinders the potential profitability. However, if the purpose is to offer an additional member service, an outside vendor is a valuable resource.

- *Club commitment*. The start-up and daily operation of a profit center can be overwhelming. If the operator of the club is not fully committed, both financially and operationally, to the start-up and successful management of the venture, we advise strong consideration of an outside vendor.

- *Vendor selection*. Many vendors exist in the health fitness industry to manage and operate leased vendor profit centers. This vendor will be a constant reflection of the club; therefore, the vendor selected must be reputable and fit the image of the organization. Carefully investigate the vendor qualifications and reference list. If you cannot find suitable vendors, the club has no choice but to retain the operation of the profit center.

- *Availability of resources*. You need many resources to successfully launch and operate a profit center. Significant capital investments are not uncommon when adding a profit center such as a restaurant or pro shop. Additionally, a great deal of operational commitment is necessary. Staff time, management time, interruptions in daily business flow, marketing, and advertising commitments may present overwhelming burdens on existing club operations. If resources are not available to meet the commitment needed for success, consider an outside vendor who can assume these responsibilities.

- *The lease contract*. The manager should outline many issues detailing the extent of involvement by the club in the vendor lease contract. Include issues such as a description of the leased space, length of lease, the rental fee or percentage of revenues or profit terms, payment of utilities, repair and maintenance fees, insurance considerations, and any club employee discounts. Legal review of any contracts is warranted.

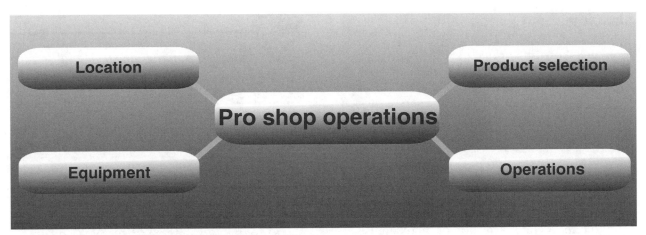

Figure 10.2 Issues to address in pro shop implementation.

PRO SHOP OPERATIONS

A pro shop is the retail merchandising of consumer goods that relate to the activities of the participants in a facility (see figure 10.2). The long-term success of a pro shop is often determined during the initial planning stages when issues such as location, daily management strategies, inventory control, point of sale procedures, pricing, and advertising are determined. The result of a well-planned pro shop is a financially sound profit center that provides significant contributions to the revenues of the organization.

According to the IHRSA *Profiles of Success* (1996) industry report, 58.3 percent of the fitness centers in the sample offered pro shops in their facility, generating an average of $269 per square foot. Almost half of the clubs with pro shops listed their shops as one of their top five profit centers. For those pro shops owned by the club, many produced significant income for the organization. Industry analysts believe this revenue potential promises to increase. An analysis by industry experts found that club operators expect pro shop sales to contribute a larger percentage of total revenues in the year 2000 (6.2 percent) than in 1994 (5.5 percent). A sound business plan, experienced merchandising, quality product selection, and high-level member service will help ensure this trend.

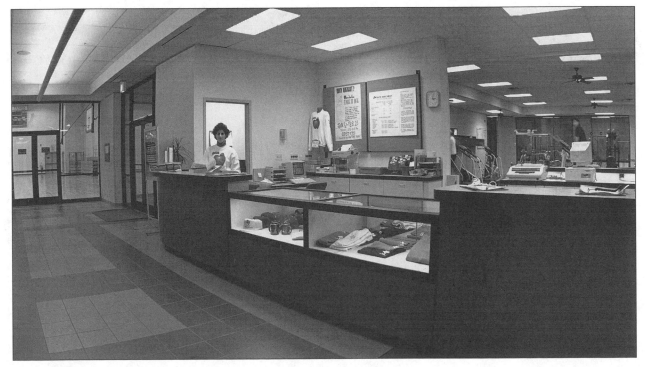

Courtesy of Dallas Texins Association

Location

Most pro shops are located near the main entrance of the facility so daily traffic patterns expose the membership to the merchandise it offers. Most pro shops are either located behind the service desk or in a space close to or adjacent to the service desk. Facilities that position their pro shop behind the service desk use service desk personnel to assist customers with purchases, maintain control of the inventory, and to merchandise the products. Other facilities build separate pro shop areas and staff their shop with designated personnel. These shops tend to offer a wider selection of merchandise because of the increased staffing commitment by the club, the additional space allocation, and the availability in many cases of designated storage areas for merchandise. The benefits of a free-standing pro shop include improved security of merchandise, increased display and merchandising space, additional storage space, and typically higher revenues. The downside, however, is increased overhead for both staffing and operational costs. The purpose of the pro shop, profit or member amenity, as well as desired total revenues, will assist the club operator in determining the size of the pro shop space.

Products

The diversity of fitness and health products in the marketplace provides the club operators with a variety to meet the needs of their target markets. The pro shop can sell apparel, fitness accessories such as weight training belts and gloves, convenience items such as socks and toiletries, and specialty items such as exercise watches and nutritional products. See table 10.3 for samples of pro shop products.

Although apparel continues to be the primary source of income in most pro shops, innovative merchandising of accessories and other products has increased the level of revenue generation and member satisfaction.

The availability and type of product is key to the success of the pro shop profit center. Members expect a variety of the latest styles and colors in apparel to meet their various size requirements. The merchandise must be accessible to the browsing member. Although shoplifting is always a concern, the accessibility of the product is necessary to yield greater sales. Many pro shops find success in offering styles and brand names that are hard to find in local department stores. Private label or logo items also offer a unique product not available elsewhere and advertise the club when worn in public. The savvy pro shop manager will observe what members wear to exercise and stock the shop with items reflecting current trends in exercise clothing and accessories. A special order option should also be available to members as an additional service.

The products the pro shop offers must meet the needs and expectations of the membership.

Table 10.3	Pro Shop Inventory Items		
Apparel	**Fitness supplies**	**Racquet sport supplies**	**Spa products**
Logo wear	Weight belts	Racquet strings	Shampoo
Socks	Swim goggles	Racquet grips	Massage oil
Swim suits	Weight gloves	Balls	Body scrub
Sweats	Nutritional supplements	Goggles	Body sponges
Shorts	Personal radio	Racquet shoes	Sunscreen
Leotards	Exercise bands	Racquets	Facial products
Tights	Exercise tapes	Hats	Body lotion

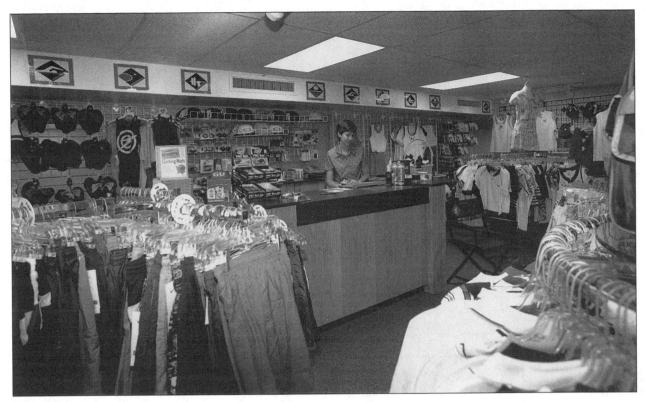

© Tom Wallace

The member who is paying monthly dues expects top-quality merchandise at reasonable prices. Although the convenience factor is an issue, clubs should be careful not to price merchandise beyond what the market will bear. The pricing of items in the pro shop must compete with comparable items found locally in department or sporting goods stores. The average markup on pro shop items ranges from 30 to 100 percent depending on the type of item. Clothing and soft goods are typically at the higher range of the markup scale (i.e., 80 to 100 percent), whereas hard goods are on the lower end (i.e., 30 to 60 percent). Often the vendor of the product can be a valuable source in percentage of markup. The vendor, when providing a suggested retail price, can help to ensure you mark your items at a price competitive in the general marketplace.

> *The merchandising of the pro shop inventory is often critical to the success of the profit center.*

Creative displays, continual refreshing of the displays, and staff members who wear items sold in the shop are examples of profitable merchandising. Many creative pro shop managers place displays in key areas throughout the facility. Using planned sales and discounts will also bring customers to the shop. These customers, while browsing for sale items, might also purchase new items at full price. Merchandising to meet the needs of the membership is a primary task of the pro shop manager.

Equipment

An initial equipment investment is necessary in the start-up of a pro shop. Slat walls and grid systems are versatile solutions for wall displays. Display racks and shelving may also be necessary depending on the size of the pro shop. Many equipment vendors will design display systems to fit the layout of the pro shop. Additional equipment includes a point of sale system or cash register. A point of sale system that integrates with the club's accounting computer systems is the optimal approach. Also, consider lighting when developing a pro shop. Track lighting is effective in highlighting the constantly changing displays.

Operations

The general operation of a pro shop is often similar to that of club operations, yet on a much smaller scale. Delegation, motivation, and accountability for results remain the backbone for success. Carefully selected, qualified personnel with experience in retail will help ensure success. Details of other issues to address in operating a successful pro shop follow.

Cost of Sales and Profitability

The *cost of goods sold* is the cost of merchandise sold or services performed.

> *The cost of sales is typically expressed as the percentage of the amount spent to purchase the item (wholesale purchase price) versus the amount the item is sold for (retail price).*

For example, if the club purchases a T-shirt for $5.00 and sells it for $10.00, the cost of sales is 50 percent. The mathematical expression to determine cost of sales using this example is as follows:

$$\frac{\text{wholesale purchase price (\$5.00)}}{\text{retail selling price (\$10.00)}} \times 100 = 50 \text{ percent}$$

Conversely, the *markup* of an item is defined as the percentage of the difference in retail and wholesale prices divided by the wholesale purchase price. The mathematical expression to determine the markup of an item using this example is as follows:

$$\frac{\text{retail sales price (\$10.00) -}}{\text{wholesale purchase price (\$5.00)}} \times 100 = 100 \text{ percent}$$

Cost of sales is an important determinant in the overall profitability of the pro shop. The lower the cost of sales, the greater the opportunity for profit. If the average cost of sales for all items in the pro shop is too high, the margin for profitability decreases. Items that are discounted or placed on sale can have a dramatic negative effect on the cost of sales. Using the T-shirt example discussed earlier, the T-shirt was purchased for resale for $5.00, with an intended retail price of $10.00, or a cost of sales of 50 percent. If this T-shirt is discounted to $7.50 retail,

the cost of sales increases to 66 percent. In other words, the profit is significantly decreased because an additional 16% was now spent to offer that product. A great deal of such discounting can dramatically reduce profits.

Careful inventory control is necessary to avoid having a stock of items that will not bear retail prices. Maintaining an inventory through careful ordering practices and creative merchandising will decrease the need to reduce excess inventory, or dead stock, through sales and discount offers.

A trend now often seen in health fitness pro shops is the co-op plan. In this plan members pay a monthly fee in exchange for discounted prices (usually 15 percent over cost) on all merchandise purchased. For example, an item that cost $50.00 would sell for $100 to the general membership; however, the co-op members pays $58.00 for their purchase. Co-op membership fees range from $6.00 to $10.00 per month and are straight profit for the club. The inventory turnover is three times faster in a co-op than a regular pro shop operation.

The successful pro shop will show a profit margin of 15 to 40 percent after you have subtracted cost of sales, labor and benefits, and expenses, depending on the size of the shop, the types of items sold, merchandising and promotional techniques, sales staff, product variety, pricing structure, and employee discounting policies. The average profit margin for pro shops in 1994 was 24 percent (IHRSA 1995).

Staffing

The staffing of the pro shop can affect the amount of revenue generated. A pro shop staff excited about their inventory and their contribution to the bottom line will actively pursue the membership for sales. The motivated staff will continually refresh and change displays to create an excitement in the pro shop and will offer members the personal service they deserve. As discussed throughout this text, personal service is important to the dues-paying member. The staff of the pro shop who know members personally, know their style and color preferences, and work closely with them to obtain the items they want can increase sales. Members are motivated to purchase from staff who are knowledgeable about all aspects of offered merchandise. The staff can create proactive sales by calling repeat customers when new items have arrived for the shop. This high level of personalized service in concert with the convenience factor will make the pro shop an attractive alternative to local department stores.

Compensation packages for pro shop managers and staff vary greatly. As mentioned earlier, it is always wise to tie a portion of the compensation package to the overall performance of the pro shop, not only for the manager but for staff as well. Incentives, bonuses, or percentages are powerful motivation for the sales-minded individual. The IHRSA state of the industry report (IHRSA 1995) stated that the average compensation for a pro shop manager was approximately $16,500 per year, with a range in salaries of $8,730 to $23,750. Hourly staff were paid an average of $6.00 per hour for full time and $5.75 for part time. The size, level of profitability, and geographic location of the club will assist in determining fair pay rates.

Vendor Management

Undertake the start-up of any pro shop cautiously. Work closely with vendors to purchase small quantities of items in which the membership has expressed interest. If vendors are reluctant to supply small quantities, it is wise to work with a distributor who may provide several lines in small quantities. When selecting vendors, stay away from those that sell goods to local merchants at a discounted price. Practices such as this prevent pro shop managers from being able to set competitive prices, thereby reducing the profit potential. Merchandise purchased directly from the manufacturer usually yields the lowest purchase price, whereas higher prices come from the distributor. A combination of sales representatives, catalogs, and trade shows provides good selections of merchandise. Whether the pro shop arranges to purchase directly from the manufacturer or through a distributor, consistently high-quality products and on-time delivery should be expected and provided.

Vendor payment for merchandise is handled by prepayment, cash on delivery (COD), or credit, typically 30-day terms. To protect the cash flow of the pro shops, many facilities establish a line of credit, which varies from manufacturer to distributor, depending on the length of time as a customer, the volume of purchase, and the billing history.

Inventory Control

Inventory maintenance and control is an important responsibility of the pro shop manager. The inventory must be trendy, stylish, and constantly turning to reflect changing styles and seasons. Turning the inventory refers to the constant cycling of new merchandise into the retail display as older merchandise is purchased or stored until the season cycles back around. Inventory typically is turned two to three times a year. Starting cautiously when ordering merchandise is a safe plan. The inventory should be enough to encourage browsing, yet not so much that it will not sell at retail prices. To maintain the level of merchandise in inventory, determine when to reorder by setting par levels, or levels that indicate when reorder is necessary. For example, the monthly par for racquetballs might be one dozen cans. The month-end inventory reveals there are six cans of racquetballs in the shop, therefore you should order six additional cans. The par level is influenced by the projected sales of the item and the time necessary to obtain delivery. Although ordering more inventory than you can sell will negatively affect the financial results, items that are sold out and on order for extended periods can be a negative factor with the members. Open lines of communication with the manufacturer or the distributor will help prevent sporadic supply.

Advertising and Promotion

An advertising and promotion plan is a necessity if a pro shop is to be successful. First determine whether the pro shop will cater to the general public or confine sales to members and guests. If the general public is the target population, then use traditional advertising methods. If the pro shop sales are restricted to members and guests, then do most of the advertising in the facility. Design all sales areas to lure members and guests, and change displays regularly. Various sales promotions range from monthly sales; using the staff as models for selected attire; and providing gift certificates, discount coupons, two-for-one offers, and holiday specials. Another option involves the vendors in your promotional efforts. For example, in-house fashion shows are an excellent opportunity for members to preview next season's line before its arrival in the shop.

Point of Sale

A point of sale system and written accounting procedures are important in determining profitability. A system that accounts for all sales and produces daily sales figures can assist the pro shop manager in discovering the success of particular advertising and promotional efforts. See figure 10.3 for a sample of a point of sale ticket or receipt. Daily sales reports are also important for the accounting and financial record-keeping personnel who must ensure all tax laws are adhered to. The point of sale system may assist with inventory control by automatically removing an item from

```
ABC CLUB
1234 MAIN ST.
DALLAS, TX

PHONE 214 555-5555
DRAWER 2
CLIENT: SMITH KIMBERLY
        Date: 08/23/97      17:22:59
Invoice#: 0000022652
Cashier: ROD
     1 *FACIALS                      68.00
     1 *50 MIN MASSAGE               68.00
                                    ========
        Total Purchases    $        136.00
            State Tax       $          0.00
                                    ========
        Total Invoice       $        136.00

Method of Payment    PAID   $        136.00
       AMEX     $   136.00
    Number:  5111 1111 1111 111
  Expires:           9/99

              CHANGE        $          0.00

* Indicates Gift Certificate

Signature  Kimberly Smith
          _____

THANK YOU for letting ABC Club serve your
needs.
```

Figure 10.3   Point of sale ticket or receipt.

stock when purchased. Written procedures determined by the pro shop manager in cooperation with the club accountant will place strict guidelines on opening and closing procedures, cash handling, and member billing. Record-keeping procedures for items such as total sales, cost of sales, total income before expenses, sales by individual, and expenses will assist in determining the pro shop profitability.

FOOD AND BEVERAGE OUTLETS

Food and beverage outlets can range from a small vending machine operation to a full-scale restaurant. In many cases the issues important for these outlets' success are similar no matter the scope of the food, beverage, and service delivery (see figure 10.4).

Food and beverage, or F&B, outlets offer the club operator the potential for significant profits. You must consider many factors, however, when contemplating the addition of food and beverage services to the club operation.

- Will the members support a food and beverage operation?
- What type of cuisine should you offer?
- What space allocation is necessary?
- Will you serve alcohol?
- What staffing will you require?
- Will the food and beverage operation consist of a sit-down restaurant or a fast food or buffet concept?

Formalize these basic decisions in a concept development proposal and business plan. As mentioned previously, the services of an experienced consultant may be a wise consideration.

Type of Outlets

Several types of food and beverage outlets are commonly found in health fitness settings. The scope of these outlets demonstrates the anticipated level of membership need or the commitment level of the organization. Food and beverage options primarily

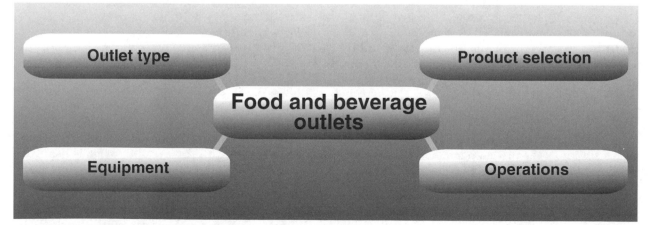

Figure 10.4   Issues to address in food and beverage outlet implementation.

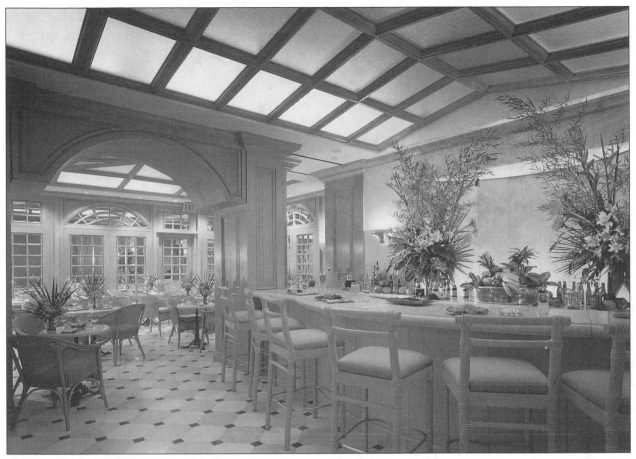

Courtesy of The Spa at the Crescent, Dallas, Texas

offered through vending machines reflect a low anticipated need or a low level of commitment on behalf of
the organization. Conversely, a full-service restaurant
reflects a high level of anticipated member need and a
significant financial and operational commitment on
behalf of the organization. Several intermediate levels
of need and commitment are viable options.

Recent industry data (IHRSA 1995) reflect the many
levels of need and commitment offered in fitness facilities across the country. According to this report,
approximately half of all fitness clubs offer a snack bar
or cafeteria outlet to their members. A cocktail lounge
or bar facility is also popular. Full-service restaurant
facilities are available in approximately 23 percent of
clubs, generating approximately $61 per square foot.

*Whatever the scope of the operation,
the club operator should anticipate a 10 to 20
percent bottom line profit from a well-managed food and beverage outlet.*

Products

The type of food and beverages you offer will vary
depending on several factors, such as the scope of
the outlet; the availability of kitchen equipment,
refrigeration, and food preparation space; the anticipated member demands and desires; the tastes and
trends in the geographic region; and the creativity of
the chef and his or her staff. It is without question
that there is a high level of demand for healthy
dining alternatives. The club operator who can define the product offerings to fit the needs and desires
of the membership; present the product in an appealing way; and provide outgoing, efficient, and
friendly service will see strong financial results.

The consumer looking for healthy dining alternatives often equates healthy with a fresh product or
produce. Food that is not processed or prepack-
aged often places additional strain on the kitchen
and the chef. Fresh foods and produce require
careful handling, more refrigeration, and greater
preparation time as they must be prepared daily.
Determine the kitchen configuration and staffing
guides accordingly.

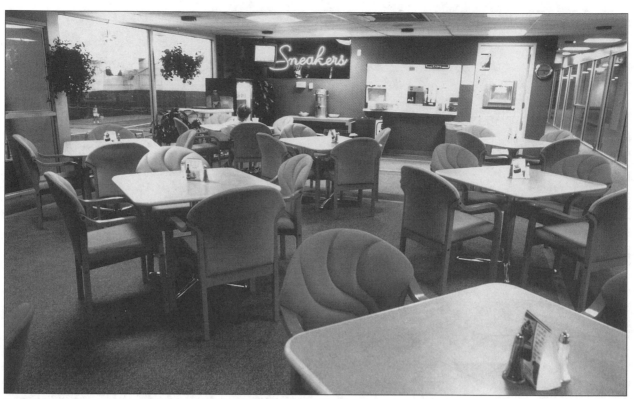

© Tom Wallace

Present the product in a way that is appealing to the consumer. The variety of colors and textures found in fresh fruits, vegetables, and grains provide the creative chef with an excellent foundation from which to work. No longer must consumers consider healthy foods poor tasting and of minuscule portions. Consumers across the country are now able to easily find beautifully presented, filling, healthy alternatives to high-fat, high-calorie fast food in their own club.

Equipment

A significant financial investment is often required when initiating a food and beverage operation. Determining the scope of the product offerings is a prerequisite to determining equipment specifications. A vending machine operation may require only refrigeration, running water, and food preparation space, whereas a full-service restaurant will require a much larger equipment commitment. A small prep kitchen can cost from $5,000 to $15,000 to equip, and a full-service kitchen can run from $50,000 to $100,000. The services of a kitchen consultant or an experienced kitchen equipment vendor who can assist with equipment specifications and kitchen layout is an invaluable investment.

Operations

Operational details often spell fantastic success or overwhelming failure for a food and beverage operation, regardless of the quality of food offered. Deal proactively with operational details to ensure success of the outlet.

Cost of Sales and Profitability

As in pro shop operations, cost of goods sold is a major determinant in bottom line profitability. The cost of raw food materials and beverages must be tightly controlled to ensure success of the profit center. The well-trained chef will create menus that control portion sizes, particularly of high-cost food items such as seafood, meats, or poultry; use regional food specialties or produce currently in season, that you can acquire inexpensively; and include plenty of low-cost fruits, vegetables, pastas, and grains in the dishes offered. Although the cost of sales is partially determined by retail food prices, the experienced food and beverage operator will maintain food costs in the 25 to 40 percent range and alcohol or beverage costs in the 25 to 35 percent range. Maintaining these food costs, the operation has the opportunity to produce a profit. One way to look at food costs is to consider that for an outlet with a 35 percent food cost, for every dollar of revenue, 35¢ immediately pays for raw food materials. Consider now that, of the remaining 65¢, staff wages and benefits and restaurant operating supplies, such as silver, china, glass, and disposable cups, platters, and so on must be paid. A well-run restaurant should have between 10¢ and 20¢ of each dollar remaining after cost of sales, labor and benefits, and operational expenses have been paid. This is not an easy task.

Staffing

The second major determinant in food and beverage outlet profitability is labor costs. Improper staffing can have disastrous results. Food and beverage outlets that are understaffed offer poor service to time-conscious consumers. Overstaffed outlets rob potential profits from the bottom line. Careful management of labor and benefit spending will enhance the probability for success.

> *The experienced food and beverage outlet manager will allocate 30 to 40 percent of total food and beverage revenues to wages and benefits.*

According to the IHRSA 1995 state of the industry report (IHRSA 1995b), the average food and beverage outlet manager is paid $20,000 per year with the range of $15,000 to $30,000. The median hourly wage for full-time service staff was $6.50 per hour, and part-time staff were paid an average of $5.00 per hour. You must carefully review and implement these salary averages, considering geographic region, demand for food and beverage personnel, and economic growth of the area since the time of this survey.

Other key personnel include the chef and the registered dietitian. The chef is an important part of the public relations and promotional effort for the club restaurant. His or her ability to prepare dishes that meet the needs of the membership is key to the restaurant's success. Continually refreshing the menu with new items is necessary to keep the daily consumer interested. The chef should continuously seek member feedback by circulating through the restaurant at peak times.

The registered dietitian works closely with the chef to ensure the health statements regarding fat and calorie content are accurate. The registered dietitian may be a member of the staff or a contracted vendor who assists with menu development, recipe analysis, and personalized menu planning or presents educational nutritional lectures. The level of nutrition services demanded by the membership will help the club operator determine the level of involvement by the registered dietitian.

Hours of Operation

Another primary consideration when optimizing profitability is determining the hours of operation. Business levels must be sufficient to cover all overhead expenses. Careful tracking of revenues by mealtime throughout the seasons of the year will provide the club operator or food and beverage manager with valuable information regarding profitable hours of operation. Flexibility in operation hours over the seasons can greatly enhance profitability. Give careful thought to changing food and beverage outlet hours of operation. Any change in hours should be publicized via the newsletter, posters, fliers, and word of mouth so customer dissatisfaction does not result.

Vendor and Inventory Management

Vendor and inventory management is critical to the success of the food and beverage outlet. Locating reliable vendors who supply consistently high-quality products and produce on time is a difficult yet worthwhile task. Often these high-quality vendors can demand and receive elevated prices for their merchandise. If the goal of the food and beverage outlet is to deliver a high-quality product, give careful consideration to paying premium wholesale prices.

A well-planned control system to maintain inventory levels and proper food rotation can play a big role in profitability. Carefully maintain inventory to avoid having an important item out of stock, thus frustrating a potential customer. Conversely, do not overstock items, and properly rotate food to ensure spoilage does not occur. The chef should implement a detailed inventory system, which includes regular item counts, comparison against predetermined par levels, and a checks and balances system that compares inventory consumed with revenues. A sample food inventory sheet is shown in figure 10.5.

Daily Market List							Week of:						
Item	**BID**			**Order**			**Item**	**BID**			**Order**		
Artichoke 24 ct							Leeks, Bunch						
Asparagus STD 15#							Onions, Green 24ct						
Beans, French 5#							Onions, Yellow Jumbo						
Beans, Round 10#							Onions, Red Med. 25#						
Beans, Yellow Wax 10#							New Potato, Creamer						
Beets, Red w/Tops							Potato, Idaho 70ct						
Broccoli 14ct							Potato, Sweet 50#						
Brussel Sprouts 10#							Potato, Yukon Gold						
Bok Choy 10#							Peppers, Red Bell						
Cauliflower							Peppers, Yellow Bell						
Cabbage, Green							Peppers, Green Bell						
Cabbage, Red							Peppers, Serrano						
Cabbage, Napa							Peppers, Jalapeno						
Carrots Bulk 25# Med.							Peppers, Poblano						
Celery, Stalk							Peppers, Other Specify						
Corn, Sweet							Mushrooms Med.						
Cucumber, English							Mushrooms, Large						
Daikon							Mushrooms, Shiitake						
Eggplant 18ct							Mushrooms, Oyster						
Eggplant, Japanese							Mushrooms, Portabello						
Endive, Belgian							Mushrooms, Other Specify						
Fennel w/Tops 12ct							Tomatoes, Roma						
Garlic, Peeled 5#							Tomatoes, 5 x 6/Home Grown						
Ginger Root, Hawaiian							Tomatoes, Cherry Red						
Horseradish Root							Tomatoes, Yellow Pear						
Italian Parsley 12ct							Tomatillos 5#						
Lettuce, Tx Bibb							Turnips						
Lettuce, Red Leaf							Parsnips						
Lettuce, Romaine							Lemons, 200ct Sunkist						
Lettuce, Frisee							Avocado, Breaking						
Lettuce, Tatsoi							Apples, Specify						
Lettuce, Other							Apples, Granny Smith XFancy						
Watercress 12ct							Bananas 5#						
Radicchio							Grapes, Red Seedless						
Spinach, Bunch							Grapes, Black Seedless						
Cilantro 12ct							Grapes, Green Seedless						
Sprouts, Daikon							Jicama 5#						
Snow Peas							Kiwi, Flat						
Sugar Snap Peas							Cherries						
Fava Beans							Grapefruit, Ruby 27ct						
Green Peas, Shelled 1#							Orange, 88ct Sunkist						
Peas/Beans/Other							Lemons, 200ct Sunkist						
Squash, Yellow XFancy							Limes, Pony						
Squash, Zucchini 1#							Tangerines						
Squash, Spaghetti							Melons, Cantaloupe 18ct						
Squash, Acorn							Melons, Honeydew 6ct						
Squash, Butternut							Melon, Other Specify						
Squash, Sunburst							Pineapple 6ct						
Shallots, Peeled 5#							Mango 12-14ct						

Figure 10.5 Using a food inventory sheet will assist you in planning and maintaining inventory levels.

Daily Market List	BID			Order			Item	BID			Order		
Item													
Papaya 9-12ct							Lamb, Rack, Aussie Frenched						
Plums, Specify							Venison, Rack NZ						
Nectarines							Venison, Loin						
Peaches							Venison, Stew Meat						
Pears, Red Bartlett							Pork Loin, Boneless #414						
Pears, Specify							Pork Tenderloin CC						
Starfruit							Pork, Rack Crown Roast						
Strawberries							Ham, Nueskes						
Raspberries							Ham, Specify						
Blueberries							Salami, Genoa						
Blackberries							Sausage, Italian Hot						
							Sausage, Chix Apple						
Golden Circle							Sausage, Specify						
Spring Mix 2# Bag							Bacon, Sliced Nueskes						
Arugula 1#							Turkey Breast Raw						
							Turkey Breast Golden						
Herbs							Duck, Whole						
Basil							Foie Gras Sonoma 'A'						
Chervil							Duck Breast						
Chives							Duck Legs						
Dill							Quail						
Lavender							Quail Legs						
Marjoram							Pickle Whole, Vienna						
Oregano							Chicken, AWOG						
Rosemary							Breast, Random/BLess/SkLess						
Sage							Airline 10-12 oz.						
Tarragon							Smoked Salmon						
Thyme							Whole						
Savory							Sliced						
M.M. Marigold													
Mint (Pepper)							**Seafood**						
							Sword CC 3-5" eye						
Meat							Snapper 6-8 Skin or Scaled						
Beef, Tender CH. PSMO 6 up							Salmon, Norw. 8-10						
Rib Choice 109							Scallops, Sea 10-20						
Brisket							Bay Scallops						
Beef, Ground 85-15							Tuna 3-5"						
Strip 1 x 1							Trout 8oz. Boned						
B3R - Flank #2							Sole, Specify						
Veal Butt Tenders							Black Drum, 6-8 Skin On Scaled						
Veal Bones 50#							Lobster Culls						
Veal, Flank							Mahi Mahi						
Veal, Rack Split Chine Of							Grouper						
Veal, Loin							Sturgeon						
Lamb, Loin, Aussie, Stosilver							Shrimp 16-20						
Lamb, Leg Bone-in							Green Headless						
Lamb, Rack Chine Off							Ocean Garden or Compass						

(continued)

Daily Market List							Week of:							
Item	BID		Order				**Item**	BID		Order				
Shrimp, P&D 90-110							Asiago, Black Wax							
Crabmeat							Feta, Greek							
King Crab 60/40							Stilton							
Crawfish Tailmeat							Manchego							
Crab Claws							Brie, 50% 1 kg							
Mussels, Specify														
Clams, Specify							**Mozz Co.**							
Oysters, Specify							Mozz Tubes 7#							
Catfish							Goat Cheese							
							Creme Fraiche 5#							
Cheeses							Mascarpone 5#							
Cheddar Yellow Sharp, 10#							Queso Fresco 3#							
Mont. Jack 10#							Cacciotta							
Maytag, Blue 4#														

Food Service Regulations

Many cities and states enforce regulations regarding food service. Food storage, preparation, and handling are all carefully regulated. Food service workers must also be regularly certified in food handling and preparation techniques and regularly tested for potentially harmful communicable diseases. Contact local and state agencies to determine the food service regulations that apply, and ensure these regulations are met. Disregard for the seriousness of these regulations and for the vigor in which they are enforced may result in closure of the restaurant and negative publicity for the club.

Service Quality

As in every other area of the club, the quality of service offered in a food and beverage outlet can often determine the success of the operation. The most delicious, beautifully presented food will go unnoticed if the service is poor. Offer and continually reinforce extensive training in the fine points of food and beverage service. The food and beverage outlet manager must ensure all food service workers are efficient and friendly in their duties.

Pricing

The members expect quality, convenience, and value for their dollar. Pricing of food and beverages in a club should consider these expectations. The expected bottom line profit, the type of clients and their income, the initiation fees and dues structure, the participant volume, and local competition should all be regularly monitored and reflected in pricing efforts.

Common Food and Beverage Mistakes

Small management errors can greatly impact food and beverage outlet profitability. Review these common errors regularly to ensure optimal profitability.

- Foods costs too high
- Excessive labor spending
- Insufficient purchasing procedures
- Attempts to satisfy everyone's tastes
- Exotic menu selection
- Poor service
- Insufficient facilities or equipment

SPA SERVICES

The term *spa* has long been a point of confusion for the fitness industry. The word spa often describes both the wet facility, also known as the whirlpool, and the growing profit center in which relaxing and healing services such as massage and facials take place. Historically spas evolved around natural mineral or hot springs. People would travel many miles to bathe and drink the medicinal waters for their healing powers. Over the years a spa has come to mean a place of healing and relaxation, that may or may not be centered around water or a natural mineral spring. Many health and wellness centers are now incorporating spa services, such as massages and facials, into the operation of the facility to provide the member with a place of relaxation and stress

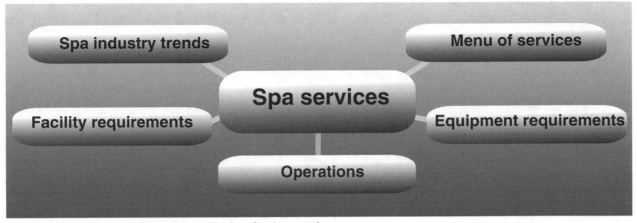

Figure 10.6 Issues to consider in spa services implementation.

reduction and to provide the operation with a profit center opportunity (see figure 10.6).

Spa Industry Trends

Long thought to be for only the rich and famous, spa services are becoming an integral part of the well person's lifestyle because of the relaxation and stress-reduction benefits these services provide.

> *The spa industry has been the fortunate benefactor of the enhanced concern for many regarding total fitness and wellness and the desire of baby boomers to slow the signs of aging.*

Resort and destination spas, once considered fat farms, are now the chosen vacation for many individuals and families seeking a healthy vacation or getaway. The emergence of day spas offers urban consumers the opportunity to escape their hectic surroundings and relax and rejuvenate for an hour or a day without having to leave home. Many of the growing number of day spas are located within the walls of existing health and fitness centers, beauty salons, or luxury hotels. According the 1995 IHRSA state of the industry report (IHRSA 1995b), 60 percent of health clubs offer massage services. Cornell University in cooperation with I/SPA, the International Spa and Fitness Association, recently published an extensive study of the trends that impact the spa industry (I/SPA 1995). Their study found that approximately 5 million people use spa services each year and that number is growing. Although most spa participants currently are women, the number of men is increasing. Their study indicates that the future of the spa industry is bright. The holistic approach to health taught at spas across the world is an attractive health care alternative and disease prevention tool for the highly stressed, overworked corporate businessperson. As the consumer becomes better educated regarding the therapeutic physical, mental, and emotional benefits of spa services, the number of individuals regularly using these services will increase. The result is a positive professional image of the facility offering total wellness and a strong bottom line opportunity for health fitness facilities.

Menu of Services

The list of possible services a fitness or wellness center could offer their members is restricted only by the amount of space, facilities, and creativity available. The list of possible services for both skin care and body care is extensive. Examples of skin care services include aromatherapy facials; glycolic peel facials; moisturizing facials; cleansing facials; waxing services for the lip, brow, back, bikini area, legs; and so on. The list of body care services includes Swedish, sport, aromatherapy, and shiatsu massage, as well as reflexology, herbal wraps, loofah scrubs, thallasotherapy, and fango treatments, to name a few. In addition, many salon services, such as hair care and nail care, are now being offered. (Refer to table 10.4 for descriptions of skin, body, hair, and nail care services.) Facilities that venture into skin care and hair care services make a larger financial and spatial commitment to the spa concept and provide themselves with the opportunity to reap the financial benefits of these services growing in popularity.

Table 10.4　Spa Service Descriptions

Body therapies

Swedish massage	The classical European massage technique of gentle manipulation of the muscles using massage oils. Used to improve circulation, ease muscle aches and tension, improve flexibility, and create relaxation. This is the most commom form of massage performed in the United States.
Sports massage	Performed with or without oil , this massage uses similiar strokes as the Swedish massage, yet typically with much deeper pressure. This massage enhances circulation and reduces preexercise muscle tightness or postexercise muscle soreness.
Aromatherapy massage	Combining the sense of smell with touch, this light, rhythmic massage uses essential oils to balance and restore energy levels. Different types of essential oils produce different results (i.e., relaxation versus stimulation).
Reflexology	Ancient Chinese technique using pressure point massage, usually on the feet, but sometimes on the hands and ears, to restore the flow of energy throughout the body.
Shiatsu massage	This traditional Japanese massage is typically performed on a *tatomi* (floor mat) with no oil. This acupressure massage technique applies pressure to specific points in the body to stimulate and unblock *meridians* or pathways in the body through which life energy flows.
Thallasotherapy	Treatments using the therapeutic benefits of the sea and seawater products. Seaweed and algae wraps, and seawater hydrotherapy treatments are common.
Fango	The Italian word for mud. Used in treatments, a highly mineralized mud may be mixed with oil or water and applied over the body as a heat pack to detoxify, soothe the muscles, and stimulate circulation.
Loofah scrub	A full body scrub with a loofah sponge, used to exfoliate the skin and stimulate circulation.
Herbal wrap	A body wrap using strips of cloth that are soaked in a heated herbal solution and wrapped around the body, followed by a period of rest. Used to eliminate impurities and detoxify, as well as for relaxation.
Hydrotherapy	This includes using underwater jet massage, showers, jet sprays, and mineral baths.
Salt glow	The body is rubbed with a course salt, sometimes in combination with fragrant oils, to remove the outer layer of dead skin and stimulate circulation.

Skin care therapies

Aromatherapy facial	The use of essential oils to moisturize, cleanse, and increase the circulation to the face. Fragrant essential oils enhance relaxation.
Glycolic peel facial	The use of low-level glycolic acids to remove the outer layer of dead facial skin, cleanse, and moisturize the skin of the face. Typically done in a series of 6 to 10 treatments.
Moisturizing facial	This facial is ideal for those who suffer from dry skin or those who are exposed to harsh enviromental conditions. Uses masques, massage, and cleansing to rehydrate the skin and enhance circulation.

Facility Requirements

Most health fitness facilities contemplating adding spa services to their operation will initiate their effort by offering massage services. Whether the health fitness facility offers massage only or a menu of body, skin, and salon services, the facility requirements are crucial to the success of the operation. The environment must create a sensory refuge from the hustle and bustle of everyday life.

> *Massage is an ideal way to enter the spa arena as it is simple and inexpensive to initiate, not difficult to hire qualified staff, a service the member or consumer is familiar and comfortable with, and has significant flow-through profitability.*

Spa services should offer the member a luxury experience in a quiet and relaxing atmosphere. Carefully consider renovating existing space for spa services. Although you won't require a great deal of space to add services such as massage, the location of the space is crucial. The ideal spa treatment room must be located in a quiet area away from the normal traffic patterns of the club. The rooms must be relatively accessible from the locker rooms or provide convenient dressing or locker facilities close by. The decor and lighting of the spa treatment rooms and surrounding areas should be soft and indirect to create an ambiance of relaxation and stillness. Equip the treatment rooms with a sink and electrical outlets. Play relaxing music in the treatment rooms and surrounding areas. The ventilation of the treatment areas is crucial. Although the treatment room is typically kept warmer (70 to 76 degrees F) than the health club environment, the room must never feel stuffy or hot. The space requirement for each treatment room is approximately 120 square feet. Creating a private, luxurious treatment room and surroundings will enhance the relaxation of the service, project a positive image for the facility, and encourage repeat business.

Equipment Requirements

The equipment requirements for spa services vary depending on the type of services the club offers and the personal preferences of the technicians hired to perform the services. Equipping a massage room will cost the club operator approximately $1,500 to $3,000. Additional operating supplies such as linens, oils, towels, and so on will cost approximately $500 to $1,000, depending on the volume of traffic anticipated and the quality of the supplies provided. Facial rooms will cost the organization approximately $7,000 to $10,000 to equip. Operating supplies will necessitate an additional investment of $500 to $1,500. Retail sale of facial products en-

hances the profitability of the spa by providing revenue with little overhead. An initial investment in this retail inventory can range from $500 to several thousand dollars. You can equip nail care stations for $1,000 to $5,000, depending on the types of equipment you purchase. A listing of the necessary equipment for each spa treatment room is listed in table 10.5. (Table 10.5 is intended to be thorough, but not exhaustive. The preferences of the therapist you hire should determine the equipment and supplies you order.) Depending on the type of treatment room, it is important to purchase the highest quality equipment available. The equipment used in most services will dramatically affect the overall service delivery. Use a spa consultant or ask the service provider you have hired before selecting and purchasing any spa equipment.

Operations

The operation of a spa facility is much different than that of a health fitness facility. The types of products needed and the services delivered differ dramatically from health fitness operations. The club operator should explore using an experienced spa consultant or hire experienced treatment professionals to enhance the probability for success.

Marketing

Marketing spa services within the health fitness operation can enhance the professional image of the wellness facility. Careful consideration of the marketing aspects of the spa services can improve member retention and enhance the profile of the facility within the community.

Before offering spa services, the club operator should perform a market survey to analyze the need and desire for the services to be offered; determine the target market for the services; evaluate the competition and their pricing structures; and review all local, state, and federal codes involving spa service delivery. The increasing demand for spa services nationwide should provide the club operator with a reasonable sense of security in offering these services. Local examination of the demand for these services, however, is always warranted. Determining the target market is an interesting consideration for the club operator. Will services be available to members only or will the local community have access to these services? If the community is invited to enjoy the services, how will you determine pricing? Will members receive discounts on products and services? Will you allow community members who frequent the spa to join the fitness facility at discounted prices? Several opportunities exist for creative marketing. The club operator should review what competition exists in the community for these services, keeping in mind that many people enjoy these services only if they are convenient. Pricing for the services should be competitive, with dues-paying members receiving discounts on services and products. Review local and state codes and regulations as they relate to the physical treatment room, the treatment provider, and the facility offering spa treatments.

> *An innovative marketing staff can use the spa facilities to enhance the image of the organization, to increase member satisfaction and retention, and as a powerful recruiting tool.*

Once you have researched and made decisions on these issues, the marketing personnel should put together a collateral piece explaining the benefits of spa services, a brief description of the services, the rates for each service, the types of services offered, the qualifications of the treatment providers, the cancellation policy, and how to schedule an appointment. Additionally, we recommend that you print information regarding the service itself. Many first-time spa goers are apprehensive about the service. In this brochure answer questions regarding modesty, where to go, how to pay, and how to communicate with the therapist in this brochure. The enjoyment of the service will be heightened if the client knows what to expect and can totally relax and enjoy the service.

A final marketing issue deserving discussion is gift certificates. Many individuals receive their first spa experience as a result of a gift certificate. Provide gift certificates for a massage for tournament prizes, charity donations, or new member gifts. Gift certificates for spa services are popular gift items. The likelihood that someone will spend money on a spa service for someone they care about before they would spend the money on themselves is great. Positioning gift certificates for spa services, particularly during the Valentine's Day, Mother's Day, Father's Day, and Christmas holiday periods, will serve the spa well in generating strong revenues year round.

Staffing

The staffing of the spa facility is crucial to its success. The treatment providers must be qualified and experienced to offer the type of luxury service the club is marketing. Staff for spa services are often either hired by the facility and work as employees or are contracted as laborers who work for a percentage of the revenue. If the goal of the facility is to provide the organization with a profit position, hiring the treatment providers as staff members and paying an hourly wage plus commission is desirable. If the spa services are only an amenity to enhance the professional image of the facility and profitability is not crucial, using outside contractors is worth considering. Typically, treatment providers hired as staff members are paid an hourly wage for the hours they are scheduled to be available plus a commission for each hour of service they provide. This commission gives the treatment professional a vested interest in building a regular clientele. Gratuities are customary. The gratuity can be at the discretion of the client, or you can apply a service charge to the service and include it in the service price. Competitive compensation for treatment providers will range from $15.00 to $40.00 per hour of service. Benefits are an optional incentive the club can offer a treatment provider who demonstrates a commitment to the profitability of the spa. Although the treatment provider may be able to earn more per hour in a private practice, the benefit of working for an organization that pays all overhead, purchases all supplies, markets aggressively for clients, and may or may not offer a benefit package cannot be overestimated.

Staff members who perform services are typically required by local and state regulations to maintain a current license or registration. Maintain proof of these licenses and registrations in the human resources files of the organization. Regular training and continuing education classes are recommended for treatment providers to stay abreast of current standards of practice in the industry. Maintaining membership in the American Massage Therapy Association (AMTA) or other governing body will help in the continuing education process.

Any facility employing more than five treatment providers should consider appointing a department head or senior treatment provider. In addition to being an experienced technician, this individual should possess business, communication, and supervisory skills that will allow her to handle all scheduling; commissions and gratuity reconciliation; product and supply ordering; and all hiring, training, and discipline of staff. This

Table 10.5   Spa Equipment and Operational Supply Lists

Massage room equipment

Massage table	Face cradle
Rolling chair or stool	Towel/sheet storage cabinet
Hydrocollator	Clock
Roll cushions/supports	Floor and room heater

Facial equipment

Facial bed with arm set	Heating pad
Three tiered trolley w/drawer	Wet sterilizer kit
Steamer with ozone and stand	Facial chair with back support
Champion Lucas spray	Magnifying lamp w/stand
Galvanic machine, high frequency machine, brush and suction machine (all in one)	Hot towel cabinet
	Therafin wax unit
Double pot wax melter	Electric terry booties
Electric terry mitts	UV sterilizer (dry)

Manicure equipment

Manicure table	Manicurist's chair
Client chair	

Pedicure equipment

Pedicure tub (requires water hookup and drain)	Pedicurist's accessory cart
Pedicurist's chair	

Nail care miscellaneous equipment

Hand polish dryer	Foot polish dryer
Therafin wax unit—foot	Therafin wax unit—hand
Nail polish rack	Finger bowls
Locking cabinets and drawers	Magnifying lamps
Terry foot mitts	Cotton dish for pedi station
Terry hand mitts	Large sanitizer jar

individual should work closely with the marketing and professional staff of the club to ensure all staff understand the benefits of spa services and to assist in marketing.

Legal Considerations

As mentioned, a variety of local and state regulations exist regarding the operation of spa facilities.

Treatment providers in many states must maintain current registration and licensure. Additionally, the facility or salon itself must be registered or licensed by the state. Particular treatment practices, such as those that deal with implement sterilization and cleanliness and draping or covering a client during the service, are also regulated in many states. Be sure to check with the state department of health or human services that oversees the operation of spa or salon facilities.

In addition to state registration and licensure, each therapist must be covered by a professional liability and malpractice insurance policy with a minimum of one million dollars coverage. This insurance policy is available to the treatment professional through membership in professional organizations such as the AMTA.

Profitability

For those facilities that have waded through the maze of renovation, organization, licensure, and registration and have opened a spa facility, the potential profits are significant. Massage services typically produce a 40-to-55 percent profit after all wages, benefits, and operational expenses are paid. Facial and nail care services typically generate a 30-to-50 percent profit when revenues from both treatments and retail skin care product sales are considered. Maintaining a tight control on operational spending, wages, and benefits can yield the club operator a successful profit center.

Maintenance

The spa area should receive normal custodial cleaning, with special attention to the floors around the treatment table, the doorknobs, light switches, and cabinet doors. These areas should be sterilized as part of a daily cleaning schedule. Linens should be changed following each service, including pillowcases and any draping material. These linens should be washed separately from other club linen as they may contain oils, muds, facial products, wax, and so on. The table surface should be cleaned with alcohol between each service. All implements used in a facial or nail service, such as nail nippers or facial tweezers, must be sterilized between each use. The therapists must be required to wash their hands following each service and anytime before working on the client's face. Alcohol can be used if water is not easily available. These sanitation rules are established to prevent the transference of any skin infection or communicable disease from one client to another.

Check with local and state officials for specific rules and regulations in your area.

Professional Organizations and Resources

Professional organizations exist to assist the club operator in developing spa facilities and treatments. You may contact the following organizations for assistance with local and state regulations and locating potential staff.

American Massage Therapy Association (AMTA)—check local listings or contact a local massage therapy school.

International Spa and Fitness Association (I/SPA) 202-789-5920

Health and Human Services department of your state government.

CHILD CARE

Child care facilities are rarely profitable as individual entities and may actually be a cost department when viewing them superficially. Child care is often considered a headache to operate, yet may mean the difference between an individual joining your club or a competitive club. To combat this potential financial drain on club profitability, many leading health fitness facilities are expanding their child care offerings to include creative play centers. These centers not only provide a wonderful amenity for club members, but also can generate additional revenue. (See children's programming information in chapter 9.) These creative play centers provide the children with a wonderful outlet that they look forward to and a powerful sales and retention tool. In today's market a child care center is a necessary ingredient for providing a full-service health fitness facility (see figure 10.7).

Despite the difficulties that child care centers are experiencing, their popularity is high among members of health fitness facilities. More than 66 percent of clubs polled in the IHRSA *Profiles of Success* report (1996) offer child care facilities. The increasing number of members with infants and children and the ongoing need to attract new members make child care centers a necessity for today's health fitness facilities.

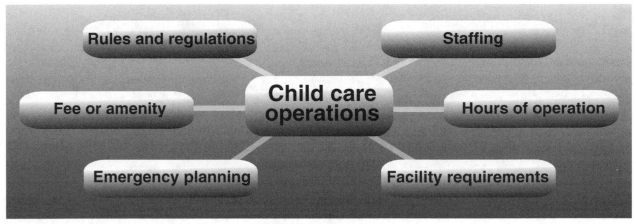

Figure 10.7   Issues to consider in child care operations implementation.

Rules and Regulations

The operation of an on-site child care facility has become a complicated matter. Ongoing litigation of child care centers has caused federal and local government agencies to reevaluate licensing standards for all child care facilities. The confusion that exists with health fitness centers that have child care centers is the difference between a complete day care center and a nursery or drop-in care center.

The complaint among club owners is that the type of care offered in a health fitness facility is different from that offered by a full-time day care facility. The parents of the children are on the premises and available in case of an emergency. The length of time that a child is left at a health fitness facility averages between 1 and 2 hours, compared with the 8 to 10 hours a child spends at a full-time nursery.

As a result, a wide variation of child care regulations exists from state to state. Before including a child care facility in the operation, contact city or state officials for clarification of the code requirements. For example, some states require ratios for the number of square feet per child and a child-to-staff ratio depending on the age of the child. You can prevent costly mistakes when you conduct thorough research and planning before you implement a child care service.

Staffing

The staffing of a child care area depends on whether the facility must meet licensing standards. The staff requirements of a drop-in care center are established by the city or state governments. Prerequisites for employment include age, education, and experience. The most widely used child care employees are young mothers who have their own children and want to supplement their incomes, or university students studying child development or primary education who want experience working with children. According to a recent IHRSA state of the industry report (IHRSA 1995), child care center managers have a median income of $15,000 per year.

Those individuals who apply for the child care center positions must be carefully screened and interviewed; have all references checked; and show competency, good judgment, and self-control in working with children. Child care workers must be energetic and excited about working with children. Some health fitness center directors even ask for character references so they can obtain further insight into how these individuals handle themselves around children and pay for complete criminal background checks to ensure the candidates are appropriate to work with children.

Hours of Operation

The peak hours of health fitness centers dictate the child care center's hours of operation. Facilities that have a constant flow of participants leave the nursery open 10 to 12 hours a day. If the participant usage is sporadic, a split schedule is used based on the high-volume hours. To accommodate the long hours of some nursery operations, management dictates shifts that last three to four hours to limit the stress of child care. Other clubs restrict the number of children that are allowed at one time and limit the age requirements to children older than six months or one year. A maximum time limit for child care is also recommended to prevent parents from taking advantage of the service.

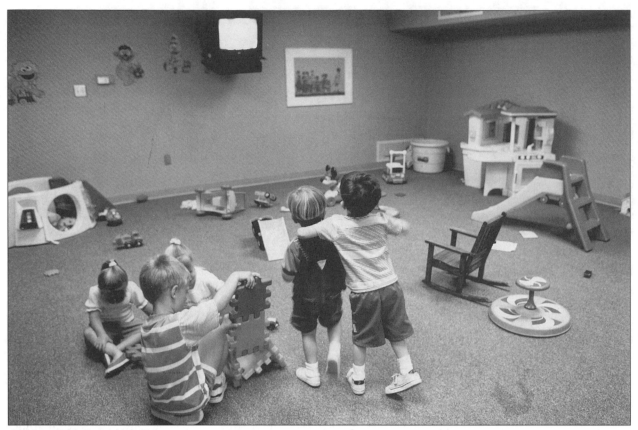

Courtesy of Little Rock Athletic Club

Program directors should coordinate the hours of operation of the child care center with the adult programming in the club. Late evening social events, for example, may not be an option to members with children unless the child care center is open for operation. Creative child care directors may offer a children's Halloween costume party while the club offers a similar party for the adults. Coordination in programming special events allows both groups to participate.

Fee for Service or Amenity

Fees for child care service range from a free service to $1 to $5 per hour per child. The fees are generally adjusted to a minimum level because the nursery is offered as a benefit to the patrons. Many clubs also offer a descending fee scale for families with more than one child. The average hourly rates for child care workers are from $5.50 to $6.00 per hour, depending on factors such as the size and location of the club, the part-time or full-time status of the individual, the number of children being supervised, and the child development programs offered by the club. Using a reservation system requiring members to call in advance to make a reservation for the child can assist the center manager with appropriate staffing levels to ensure quality care. This system can also inform the child care manager when additional staff is required to care for a higher than anticipated number of children. Conversely, a day with fewer children can be staffed appropriately.

Facility Requirements

Child care centers built in health fitness centers are currently constructed in rooms from 500 to 800 square feet and placed away from fitness-related areas close to the main entrance of the facility. A bathroom is built into the room, or an existing bathroom close to the center is made available for the children's use and equipped appropriately. Activity areas in the child care center should be divided. Provide an area for infants or quiet rest, creative learning, and play. This segmentation makes supervision of the children easier. Some fitness centers have nurseries with access to an outdoor play area. Outdoor play must be carefully considered because research indicates most injuries children experience in child care settings occur outdoors. Everything in the child care center should be up to professional safety standards, including covered electrical sockets, daily maintenance requirements, extra padding under carpets and in play areas, and toys that are safe for children's use. Wherever the child care facility is located, it must offer a safe environment for energetic play. A one-way mirror or observational window is an additional item that parents like so they can periodically monitor their children.

Emergency Plan

Events such as choking, poisoning, or serious falls may not be a consideration in the adult areas, but must be considered by the child care center manager. Rethink contents of the first aid kit when considering children. Meticulously keep individual health, physician, and guardian records detailing any special medical conditions for the child. Each child should have a detailed registration and medical history card immediately available in case of an emergency.

> *Just as the activity areas have a set and practiced procedure in the event of an emergency, so must the child care center. The types of emergencies will differ from the adult areas and therefore require unique procedures.*

Plan and regularly practice procedures to immediately notify the parent in addition to activating the emergency response plan in the facility. Many facilities provide a beeper to the parent of a child in the center so immediate notification is possible. It may be necessary to mobilize other members of the fitness center staff to assist if evacuation is necessary. Special considerations exist for the children's area that you must think out and practice. See chapter 13, Health and Safety Guidelines, for additional information regarding emergency planning.

Security

Security in the child care area must be of utmost concern for the program manager. In addition to medical emergencies in the child care area, analyze and reanalyze the security of the children to ensure their safety. In today's age of difficult divorces, the health fitness manager and organization must ensure that only the correct parent or guardian drops off or picks up the child. Detailed records including signatures and photographs of the parent or guardian should be available for immediate comparison. Strictly enforce check-in and check-out procedures. Some clubs now put a color- and number-coded bracelet on the parent dropping off the child and only that parent is authorized to pick up the child. It is prudent to consult with a safety and security expert to ensure that procedures in place do not allow any room for errors in judgment.

> *The philosophy for operating the child care area should be such that occasional inconveniences may occur for the parent in order to provide safety and security for the child.*

IN CLOSING

Profit centers must exist for clubs to remain competitive and profitable in the future. The profit centers discussed in this chapter—pro shops, food and beverage, spa services, and child care—are examples of popular profit centers found in all types of health fitness settings. In this chapter we have discussed the important factors regarding the planning, implementation, and operation of these profit centers. You can apply these strategies and practices to many different profit centers currently in demand by consumers. Review and implementation of these strategies and practices can assist the health fitness manager in operating successful profit centers.

KEY TERMS

Cost of goods sold (or cost of sales)

Markup

Profit centers

Spa

RECOMMENDED READINGS

Handley, A. 1995. Setting up new profit centers. *Club Industry* (January): 41-42.

Harp, G. 1989. Mining the fashion gold. *Fitness Management* (December): 22-25.

Hartsough, C. 1994. Spa cuisine—Healthy profits. *Spa Management* (Spring): 22.

Hildreth, S. 1994. Super profitable amenities. *Club Business International* (June): 16-17, 46-49.

International Health, Racquet and Sportsclub Association. 1994. *The IHRSA report on the state of the health club industry.* Boston: IHRSA

———. 1995a. *Profiles of success.* Boston: IHRSA.

———. 1995b. *The IHRSA report on the state of the health club industry.* Boston: IHRSA

———. 1996. *Profiles of success.* Boston: IHRSA.

International Spa and Fitness Association (I/SPA). 1995. *Cornell study on the spa industry.* Washington, DC.

Lustigman, A. 1994. Sweat shops. *Club Industry* (January): 24-30.

Management Notebook. 1993. Nursery notes. *Club Industry* (September): 41-42.

Moffat, T. 1996. Hot profit centers: Pro shops. *Club Industry* (January): 48.

Nixon, T. 1989. Make money with massage. *Fitness Management* (September): 40-42.

Patton, R.W., W.C. Grantham, R.F. Gerson, and L.R. Gettman. 1989. *Developing and managing health/fitness facilities.* Champaign, IL: Human Kinetics.

Tucker, R. 1989. Are spa services in your profit future? *Fitness Management* (September): 32-35.

Yacenda, J. 1985. Sportswear boutiques. *Fitness Management* (October): 37, 41.

Zill, R. 1995. Creating a great massage room. *Spa Management* (Spring): 13.

CHAPTER 1

Staff Selection and Development

Exciting features of a well-designed facility, along with its equipment and programs, are important contributors to the success of a health fitness enterprise. However, these features pale in importance compared with the staff members who operate the facility, initiate and maintain member contact, and implement the programs. The world's most lavish facility will falter if it does not have the staff to tie it together and breathe life into the programs while stimulating the membership.

A successful operation is, ultimately, based on selecting a qualified staff, then training and developing them to be contributing members of a dynamic and effective team of professionals.

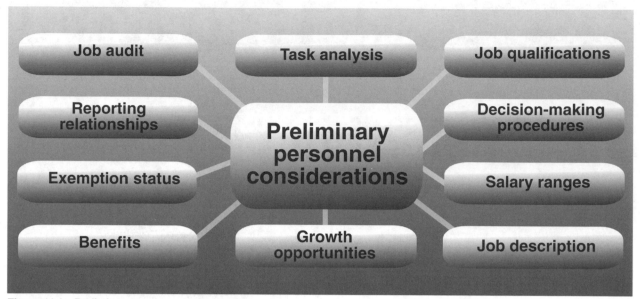

Figure 11.1 Preliminary personnel considerations.

In this chapter, we describe the preliminary considerations for identifying staff needs. We identify the tangible and intangible qualifications needed for most personnel. We then focus on the process of effective staff recruitment, selection, and development. We discuss methods of recruiting and interviewing candidates. We finally illustrate ways to orient staff members once you hire them and identify training and development programs that you can use to enhance the organizational development and program delivery of health fitness programs.

PRELIMINARY CONSIDERATIONS

There are many things to consider before beginning the hiring process. It is important to constantly appraise the line and staff personnel to determine the minimal human resources needs to fulfill the mission of the organization (see figure 11.1). This assessment includes a job audit and task analysis. Once you determine that a position is needed, you must have a detailed *job description* before interviewing candidates.

Job Audit

The first step in selecting staff members is to perform a *job audit* to determine the minimum number

of people you need to accomplish the mission of your organization. You will want to provide adequate coverage for the essential services in all areas of the facility throughout the daily operating period. Once you determine this, establish the position titles and their associated job descriptions. To better understand these issues let's look at some industrywide data.

The average health fitness commercial enterprise operates in a 25-thousand-square-foot multipurpose facility with fitness, aerobics, aquatics, and racquet spaces and requires approximately 40 employees to maintain the facility and deliver its programs and services. In this average organization, there are approximately 10 full-time employees—1 for each 200 members. Approximately 30 percent of these full-time employees are managers supervising at least 2 other full-time employees and 10 part-time employees. Interestingly, there are more part-time staff than full-time staff in most health fitness programs. There are approximately 30 part-time employees—1 for each 50 members in a program. Bear in mind that these are only averages for the industry. Smaller multipurpose facilities, for example, have only 1 full-time employee for each 250 members. Larger full-service facilities that include labor-intensive programs such as spa services have 1 full-time employee for each 150 members. Comparing your existing personnel data with those in table 11.1 provides some guidelines for determining your overall staffing needs.

Table 11.1   Average Health Fitness Industry Data on Employees

	Number	Members per employee	Employees per manager	Annual turnover
Full-time employees	10	200	3	15%
Part-time employees	30	50	10	30%

Reprinted, by permission, from IHRSA 1994.

Another job audit consideration is the turnover rate among staff members. The health fitness industry turnover rate for full-time employees is about 15 percent per year; for part-time employees it is about 30 percent per year. There is a significant correlation between the turnover rate in the part-time staff and that of the membership attrition (IHRSA 1994). It seems that job longevity of part-time staff, such as the exercise leaders who have direct contact with members, clearly affects the loss of members in programs. Although this correlation may not impact the number of part-time personnel you want on the payroll, it certainly defines their importance in the mission of the organization. It also underscores the need for hiring and retaining high-quality part-time staff for integrity and continuity of programs, especially if you are concerned with high member turnover rates. Therefore, seeking long-term employment with part-time staff is important. Hiring individuals desiring permanent part-time work, such as retirees, and job-sharing candidates, such as homebound spouses, are good examples; establishing good internship programs with local colleges and universities is another vehicle assuring quality part-time staff. Although interns' length of stay is short, their enrichment to the program with current knowledge and enthusiasm offsets this disadvantage.

Another point to consider with a job audit is the overall cost of employees. Is the cost of your payroll within the bounds of industry standards? Payroll in the commercial setting is approximately 35 to 40 percent of operating budget. The clinical setting requires a slightly higher payroll, owing to the greater legal requirements of staff credentials. Corporate and community programs usually fall somewhere between the commercial and clinical ranges. Benefits will also be a consideration because taxes, vacations, insurance, and other overhead account for 25 to 50 percent of the full-time staff's payroll. Approximately 50 percent of full-time employees in the health fitness industry presently receive full benefits. Approximately 95 percent of full-time staff get free club membership; only 25 percent get pension or retirement plans. Regardless of the perks offered to full-time staff, benefits are expensive to provide. If you presently have higher than industry averages for full-time staff enjoying full benefits, consider increasing the part-time payroll, expanding internship programs, or contract labor, that requires less in the form of benefits. This process of getting lean is clearly an industry trend.

The job audit should address the prospect of contract labor, for which benefits and other overhead such as office space and personnel bookkeeping are not a consideration (see chapter 16). At any rate, perform the job audit to learn where your organization stands with respect to the industry, your competition, and how closely you meet the member's expressed and implied needs for programs and services. If you are out of line, then you may need to rethink your position on staffing.

Familiarization with employment laws is also important in the job audit. In the corporate or governmental setting it becomes especially important that you maintain compliance with hiring mandates. We include detailed discussions of legal matters in chapter 17.

Consider *succession planning* for the organization when crafting the job descriptions for new positions. Are you planning for a successor in each manager's position? Is one of the competent managers, not presently identified for advancement in her present department, capable of retooling for a major need elsewhere within the organization? Can you rearrange existing staff structures to meet new personnel needs without undertaking the time and expense of recruiting, interviewing, hiring, and training new people? This would obviously be the most cost-effective approach to filling personnel vacancies.

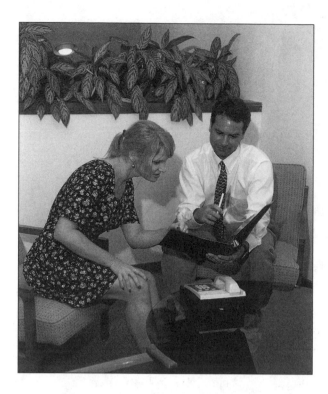

The job audit is a dynamic and ongoing process that managers and decision makers must constantly undertake. The ever-changing nature of our industry requires that you be a nimble-minded decision maker, constantly tweaking the organizational structure and addressing the changing mission of the organization, that is foisted upon you by a changing marketplace.

Task Analysis

Once you have completed the job audit and you determine a need exists for a position within your organization, identify the type of tasks needed to perform the job. If the job audit indicates that you need to fill a previous position, interview an incumbent in the job or related job area to begin gathering ideas about what tasks and job skills are needed.

Incumbent Interview

When the job identified exists and is presently filled, it is helpful to get an idea what job skills are needed for the position. A detailed list of routine tasks performed in the job is revealing. Often, many more tasks are performed in a position than supervisors think or intend. Observe the job being performed on several occasions and at different times of day. Many staff members perform different tasks at different times of day and on different days of the week. A midmanager who normally supervises the fitness instructors, for example, may use a complex computer program to schedule his staff only once a month. Yet, these computer skills may be an essential part of the job. When conducting an *incumbent interview* address these considerations and leave some open-ended responses for the incumbent to identify tasks that could better meet the program's goals and objectives.

Clarifying Tasks

Develop a complete list of tasks for the identified position. Temper and modify this list with input from other managers and staff. Also consider how trends in the industry, competitors' programs, and new equipment in the marketplace affect tasks for the proposed job. Once you have listed the tasks required for the job to the satisfaction of all concerned, you will be able to establish the qualifications necessary to successfully perform the job. You can find examples of specific tasks for personnel in chapters 7 (Service Desk Management) and 14 (Facility Maintenance Management).

Job Qualifications

Once the task analysis is complete, identify clear and appropriate qualifications for the job. It is important not to set qualifications too high, because you cannot legally hire someone who fails to meet advertised qualifications. There may be a candidate lacking in one area of identified qualifications that offsets this deficiency with extraordinary skills or abilities in other areas. Carefully word the job description to allow room to choose the candidate who best combines the concrete as well as the intangible requirements for the job. Some ideas for wording job qualifications include the following:

- Demonstrated ability to _____ required.
- In-depth knowledge of _____ required.
- Extensive experience in _____ required.
- Proven ability to _____ required.
- Proven track record of _____ needed.
- Familiarity with _____ would be ideal.
- Degree relevant to _____ preferred.
- Advanced degree in relevant field is a plus.
- An equivalent combination of formal training and successful experience desired.

These sample phrases provide the latitude to select someone who may be lacking in one area but compensates with exceptional abilities in another area. Using such phrases does not mean that hiring standards are compromised; it means that you have more flexibility in hiring without undue justification or fear of legal reprisal. We will discuss legal considerations in more detail in chapter 17.

Intangible Characteristics

We have mentioned intangible criteria and how they can help balance the lack of specific educational or experiential requirements. Intangible factors might include the following:

Attitude	Management style
Interpersonal skills	Initiative
Creativity	Self-confidence
Personality	Temperament
Appearance	Maturity
Assertiveness	

As mentioned, these intangible characteristics may be more critical to the success of the job performance (e.g., front service desk) than the more easily measured tangible characteristics.

Educational Background

Education is important for almost any position in the health fitness industry. Reading skill is a must for any job in this industry; yet, it is not a given that applicants can read even if they have educational diplomas. You can check for literacy for walk-in applicants by insisting that they fill out application forms on the spot.

Health fitness staff spend a great deal of time with the members and frequently communicate with them on matters related and unrelated to health and fitness. It is always helpful to have staff members who are conversant on matters beyond their professional competencies.

The current club member is frequently an avid reader of health-related literature. It is critical that your staff be well educated in health fitness areas and remain abreast of the information explosion in this industry.

Finally, computer literacy is becoming a necessary skill for success in this industry. Almost everyone must now have word processing and spreadsheet skills.

Education is important for effective program delivery, and it enhances the credibility of the staff in the eyes of the members. Although industrywide licensure requirements in this country do not exist, educational requirements are necessary substitutes, and serve as leveling tools, for *screening* for professional competence. However, schools differ in their excellence as well as their focus. This is especially true of colleges and universities. Evaluate schools by curriculum and faculty when possible. Some smaller universities and community colleges frequently have practitioner-oriented programs, whereas many larger research institutions do not.

It is vital that any applicant you consider for a professional or managerial position have training in as many of the following course areas as possible:

Accounting	Human motivation
Adult fitness	Basic nutrition
Athletic facilities and management	Stress management
Athletic training	Human movement theory
Behavior modification	Fitness internship
CPR and first aid	Kinesiology
Exercise leadership	Marketing management
Exercise physiology	
Financial management	Organization and administration
Health behaviors and psychology	Personnel management
Health tests and measurements	Public relations
Health promotion and wellness	Sport psychology
Human anatomy and physiology	Exercise testing and prescription

Professional Certification

Professional certification programs can supplement educational requirements and serve as an additional leveling tool for evaluating and screening candidates. A candidate who holds a certification has an implicit body of knowledge or set of skills in a particular health fitness area. Most certifications are now national in scope and have reliable levels of expectation, as well as current content, on examinations.

Historically, certification programs were often activity specific and tested for areas such as aerobics or strength training. The American College of Sports Medicine, however, has traditionally offered a generalized health fitness certification with a tiered approach for professionals at different levels within the industry. The lower levels are designed for entry-level professionals and the upper levels are designed for managers. There are two different tracks identified by ACSM: clinical, and health and fitness. Both tracks require a written and practical examination. This organization seems to be used as the gold standard for those states exploring legislative actions for licensure for health fitness professionals. Today, however, many organizations, such as the Aerobics and Fitness Association of America (AFAA), the International Association of Fitness Professionals (IDEA) and its affiliate the American Council on Exercise (ACE), National Strength and Conditioning Association (NSCA), and the YMCA, have begun offering more broadly developed certifications in the health fitness field. In fact, more than 50 professional organizations now claim to offer some type of certification. You are wise to familiarize yourself with these certifications as there is a difference in rigor, quality, and orientation for the many credentialing groups in this industry.

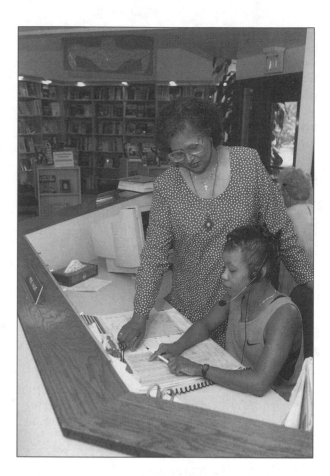

Experience

The entry-level positions within the organization require little experience. In-house staff training and development can bring a good candidate up to pace quickly. Yet, candidates with direct or related experiences will always be at an advantage in the job market. For example, students who have had part-time experiences or internships are more desirable for filling positions than those without any direct experience.

Midmanagement and upper management positions normally require several years management experience in the health fitness industry. Staff positions, such as office personnel and maintenance personnel, also have requirements of related experience and attendant clerical and computer skills.

Reporting Relationships

Be sure the lines of communication are clearly understood by all concerned before the interview stage. It is also important during an interview that you discuss the job as a position within the organization instead of as a person. This removes personalities from considerations pertaining to the job and re-

moves the perception of permanence for those presently filling positions. Consider the following regarding reporting relationships:

- What position does this job report to, both directly and indirectly?
- Where does this job appear on the organizational chart?
- What position, if any, reports to the job?
- What is the relationship between this job and other jobs in the organization?

It is important to determine what position within the organization will be dealing with the new employee regarding critical decisions, such as salary advancement, promotion, and retention.

Decision-Making Processes

It is important to understand the department's or organization's decision-making process for two reasons: It gives a more complete picture of the available position and prepares the interviewer to answer questions applicants are likely to ask. Consider which positions in the organization are responsible for personnel decisions regarding the following:

Salary increases

Promotions

Training

Performance appraisals

Transfers to other positions

Disciplinary actions

Vacations

Leaves of absence

Exemption Status Determination

It is important that the job being developed is evaluated for exemption status. As defined by the Fair Labor Standards Act, the term exempt literally means exempt from overtime compensation; that is, an employer is not required to pay exempt employees for time worked beyond their regularly scheduled work week. All managers in the health fitness industry are normally exempt personnel. Accordingly, it is not uncommon for managers with set salary schedules to work far more than a normal 40-hour week. Indeed, most individuals in this industry would be delighted to have such a work schedule. Problems can arise when disparities in compensation occur between exempt and nonexempt personnel. For example, nonexempt personnel, such as part-time personal trainers, can easily exceed the compensation of exempt staff by providing personal training for extra compensation during their off-clock periods. Resolve and clarify these issues before employing new hires to minimize morale problems among existing staff.

Salary Ranges

The next aspect of familiarization with a position concerns salary ranges. It is a matter of choice whether the salary is disclosed during interviews, but the initial interviewer needs to know what the salary range is to determine whether the candidate warrants further consideration. If, for example, there is an opening for a Fitness Program Director paying an annual salary from $40 to $55,000 and the applicant is currently earning an annual salary of $54,500, there is a problem with salary advancement for the prospective candidate. This makes hiring this individual unfair to both parties because of limited potential for salary advancement. It is important to know salary ranges for the position before the interview to avoid unnecessary and troublesome problems with screening and selecting candidates.

Benefits

Approximately 50 percent of the health fitness programs in the commercial setting offer a benefit program for full-time employees; most of the programs in the corporate, clinical, and community settings offer comprehensive benefit packages for full-time employees. These benefits might include a combination of health, dental, profit sharing, retirement, social security, unemployment insurance and compensation, disability, vacation, tuition reimbursement, leaves, and holidays, to mention a few. Understand these benefit programs before the interview process because they serve as an excellent selling point to prospective candidates. Some programs offer free lockers, workout privileges, reduced cost for food and beverages, or discounts in the retail outlet. Some programs, especially in the corporate and clinical settings, provide tuition reimbursement benefits.

It is a good policy to prepare a written list and description of the benefits offered to clarify the package and sell the benefits to prospective employees.

Growth Opportunities

Another aspect of the preliminary process of hiring is understanding what growth opportunities are afforded employees. Most professionals are interested in knowing whether they will be able to attend conventions, conferences, seminars, certifications, and workshops to continue their professional development. If the organization provides release time, travel expenses, or registration fees, it is a good selling point to share this information with prospective candidates. In-house professional development opportunities are important selling points as well. The YMCA's in-house programs for professional growth are excellent and serve as motivational tools for employees seeking advancement within the organization.

Writing the Job Description

The job description is a tool that succinctly provides the information acquired during the familiarization stages of the hiring process. It is a tool to use in every aspect of the recruitment, interviewing, selection, hiring, training, and development process. It also serves well as a reference when evaluating disciplinary actions and promotional reviews.

The job description preparation begins with the task analysis—gathering data regarding the job performance. The job description evolves from this analysis and you can develop it in two different formats: generic and specific. Generic job descriptions are written in general terms and are good approaches to take for describing similar positions in different areas within the organization. The fitness instructor position is an excellent example of a position that you could write in such broad terms and use for various areas within a large facility environment. Specific job descriptions, on the other hand, define the duties and tasks of one particular position. They are written when a position requires the performance of unique or distinct responsibilities, thereby separating it from the other jobs. The aerobics coordinator or the front office secretary would be examples of specific job descriptions found in most settings. The following are some specific guidelines for writing effective job descriptions:

- Arrange duties and responsibilities in a logical and sequential order.

- State separate duties clearly and concisely.

- Avoid ambiguous words and generalizations.

- Don't list every task.

- Include specific examples of major duties where possible.

- Use nontechnical language.

- Indicate frequency of occurrence of duties.

- Refer to titles and positions regarding reporting channels.

- Use present tense.

- Be objective and accurate in describing the job.

- Be sure that all job requirements are job related.

- Use action words such as organizes, coordinates, administers, and prepares.

Publishing the Job Description

The exact job description will be dictated by the specific environment and needs of an organization. What follows provides the basic categories of job information required for most positions:

Date

Job title

Division or department

Reporting relationship

Location of the job

Exemption status

Salary grade and range

Work schedule

Job summary

Duties and responsibilities, including extent of authority and degree of independent judgment required

Job requirements, including education, prior work experience, certifications, and skills

Physical environment and working conditions

Equipment and machinery to be used in work

Other relevant factors, such as member contact or access to financial data

Sample job descriptions are provided at the end of this chapter. Once you complete the preliminary stages of the personnel development you can begin the hiring process. Figure 11.2 illustrates these steps.

RECRUITING CANDIDATES

Once you have developed the job description, you can begin the recruiting process. Recruiting enough candidates to have a pool to draw from is extremely important. The changing demographics of our country create challenges for employers in the health fitness industry. Historically, the manager had difficulty with staffing only during the peak seasons surrounding the first quarter boom period for the fitness business. In the 1980s, the workforce was growing at three percent annually; but a mere one percent growth in workforce is predicted for the year 2000. Moreover, there has been a significant reduction in available college graduates, which may remain until the baby boomlets, children of the baby

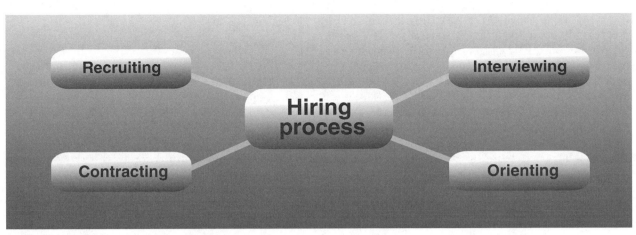

Figure 11.2 Stages in the hiring processes.

boomer generation, start graduating from college at the turn of the century. Because most hiring in the health fitness industry comes at the entry and junior management levels, the recruitment process becomes critical. This is especially true when considering the importance of the well-educated and trained part-time staff discussed earlier.

Take several factors into account before embarking on a recruitment campaign:

Budget—available money to recruit candidates. Professional search firms frequently charge as much as 20 to 25 percent of the candidate's negotiated annual salary.

Yield—number of qualified candidates for time and money spent.

Job level—entry-level employees versus mid- or upper management.

Affirmative action—certain sources, such as government agencies, can help meet goals. We will address this topic further in chapter 17 on legal issues.

Recruiting Sources

There are several sources for recruiting good employees. Table 11.2 illustrates the more important sources to recruit qualified candidates for the various exempt and nonexempt staffing positions you may need. Using as many sources as possible to recruit candidates will have a high yield in developing a good staff. It is much easier and enjoyable to front-load your work in seeking out good candidates than it is to back-load it and deal with underproductive and inadequate hires that were hastily employed.

Screening Candidates

Once you have advertised the position, resumes and letters of application will start arriving. The phones will start ringing, and applicants will walk in seeking interviews. Keep the resumes where you can access them, but assure confidentiality. Keep an active file of resumes from previous searches that you can blend with the new ones arriving from the recruitment campaign. Active file status is usually limited to a six-month period. Moreover, handle the job posting from in-house recruitment as if you considered an in-house applicant one of the short-list candidates. It is a good morale booster to include even the remotely qualified in-house applicants in the pool for interviewing. Screening candidates is an important process. This screening process should be performed by the individual to whom the candidate will report or by a search and selection committee. The processing involves comparing all the resumes with the job qualifications identified in the job description. You can accomplish this by using a checklist or a linear rating system from 1 to 10 regarding each job qualification. You can use any number of methods as long as they achieve the desired goal—reducing the resume list to the top three to five candidates, commonly called the *short list*.

Telephone Screening

Although it may not be applicable to screen all candidates by telephone (e.g., in-house candidates), you should do it with as many applicants as possible to have a common frame of reference during the screening process. The telephone interview serves two major purposes: it establishes continued interest in a job candidate, and it helps to validate the candidate's qualifications for the job. However, it is no substitute for a face-to-face interview; it is simply a preliminary screening tool. Please note that the phone interview is best achieved when you make a preliminary phone call to schedule the interview. Once the phone interview is started, the line of questions should be similar for all candidates to make an adequate comparison of the short-listed candidates. The line of questions for exempt positions, however, differs from nonexempt positions. The following is a list of examples for each type of position.

Sample Questions for Nonexempt Position Applicants

- Why they are leaving their present (or last) employer
- What they do (or did) in a typical day
- What they like (or liked) most and least about the job
- Why they are applying for this particular position

Table 11.2   Advantages and Disadvantages of Various Recruitment Sources

Recruitment sources	Advantages	Disadvantages	Job level
In-house job posting.	Creates openings at lower levels. Saves time and money. Boosts employee morale. Reveals hidden talents.	Managers feel they no longer have free choice. Time may be lost in replacements.	Nonexempt and exempt.
Professional referrals.	Inexpensive. Expeditious.	May result in discrimination.	Nonexempt and exempt.
Print advertising.	Reaches wide audience. Can target market.	Can be costly. Can delay filling job.	Nonexempt and exempt.
Internet advertising.	Reaches wide market.	Difficult to target. Expensive to screen.	Nonexempt and exempt.
Employment agencies and search firms.	Access to large labor pool. Can help fill job quickly.	Can be costly. Can refer unqualified applicants.	Employment agencies, nonexempt. Search firms, exempt.
School internships and recruiting.	Opportunities to groom future managers. Opportunities to select top graduates.	Must evaluate potential as opposed to concrete work experience.	Nonexempt and exempt.
Walk-ins, call-ins, write-ins.	Low costs. Good public relations.	Time consuming. Poorly monitored.	Nonexempt and exempt.
Computerized systems.	Extensive database. Can help quickly.	Can be costly. Requires specific hardware.	Exempt.
Professional associations.	Cost effective. Can get many good resumes quickly.	Can be expensive. Can get broad range of abilities, experiences.	Nonexempt and exempt.

> **Sample Questions for Exempt Position Applicants**
>
> - Why they are leaving their present (or last) employer
> - What they know about your organization
> - What they have contributed in past positions
> - What they feel they can contribute to your organization
> - What they expect from your organization
> - How this position fits into their long-range goals

Based on these preliminary questions and others that spontaneously occur during the telephone interview, you can make decisions regarding the merit of pursuing a face-to-face interview with the candidate. The objective is to verify that the candidate qualifies for the position by the conclusion of the interview.

Reviewing Credentials

Always review the applicant's resume and application before the interview. By doing so you will become familiar with the person's credentials, background, and qualifications. Indeed, professionals in the human resources industry are increasingly appalled at the amount of inaccuracy and the number of falsehoods they find on resume and job application information. By doing this homework you will be better able to ask relevant questions of the candidate during an interview.

> *Errors or false credentials can be found on as many as 25 percent of resumes.*

The following are some areas to consider when reviewing credentials:

Overall appearance of the resume and job application

Omissions to questions on the application

Work history gaps, overlaps, or inconsistencies

Frequency of job changes

Salary history

Skills and abilities related to present job

Reasons for leaving prior employment

Verifying References

The third step in staff selection is to verify references and previous employment. This responsibility can be handled by the department head, the selection committee, or, if the company is large enough, by the human resources department. This step is vitally important and should not be glossed over. However, most reference checks result in positive recommendations for the candidate. This is becoming even more true as former employers of candidates may inflate the recommendations and mask deficiencies of their former employees for fear of legal repercussions. Accordingly, one must work hard to get good and accurate references on prospective employees by seeking out as many sources of information as possible.

> *Accurate checking of references and unreferenced work on the candidate's resume can provide insights about the candidate that are not readily apparent from the resume.*

INTERVIEWING CANDIDATES

Interviewing candidates for positions is an important aspect of the hiring process. It requires considerable time, skill, and experience on the part of the interviewer to be successful in getting the best candidates for the jobs available.

Scheduling Interviews

Schedule the formal interview at a time mutually convenient for the candidate and the interviewer. Usually, the candidate arranges personal schedules to meet the interviewer's time frame, but both parties should remain flexible. Once the interview is scheduled, company policy determines if the candidate is to be reimbursed for travel expenses, if any, to the site. There is also the question of lodging and meals. Some other expense items to consider are reimbursements for second and third interviews, and relocation expenses if needed. It is wise for an organization to have clear guidelines concerning these policies before interviewing for a position.

Unclear policies can create unnecessary obstacles between a potential employee and the employer. Therefore, make all your interviewees aware of the company's policy on expense reimbursement.

Conducting Interviews

The candidate should always be interviewed by the person to whom she will report and by the human resources department, if one exists. In fact, in corporate and clinical settings the human resources department will probably handle all personnel issues until the interview process begins. However, we recommend that several people from within the department and from other departments that the position would have contact with, along with at least one person from senior management, also interview the candidate. Interviewers may wish to use some questions in table 11.3. Each interviewer can provide a different perspective on the candidate. You can then take these suggestions into account when making the hiring decision. One way to coordinate different interview perspectives is to have each interviewer complete a rating sheet, such as the Employee Interview Checklist (see table 11.4) on every candidate. Then, you can correlate the ratings before making the hiring decision.

During the interview, a rule of thumb is that the interviewer should be speaking no more than 30 percent of the time; the remainder should be spent in active listening and taking notes. Most people think at a rate of 400 words per minute; most people speak at 125 words per minute. Therefore, the interviewer can use the majority of the time the applicant is speaking to

- analyze what the applicant is saying,
- correlate present statements with earlier comments,
- craft out the next line of questions,
- glance at the application to verify information,
- study body language of the applicant,
- evaluate how well this applicant fills the job requirements,
- evaluate how well this applicant suits the corporate culture, and
- take notes.

According to Dr. Tom Collingwood, former director at the Cooper Institute for Aerobics Research (Patton et al. 1986), regardless of the stage of the employment process, interviewers should look for the following characteristics in their professional health fitness personnel:

1. *Good role model.* The applicant displays a positive image of good health and fitness, is a nonsmoker, and has a high level of physical activity.

2. *Physically fit.* The applicant scores better than average on all fitness tests.

3. *Positive attitude.* The applicant is creative, enthusiastic, adaptable, and highly motivated in

---

Table 11.3   Structured Interview Questions

1. How did you originally get your job with your present employer?
2. How long have you been employed by them?
3. Briefly describe your present job responsibilities.
4. What are some of the most enjoyable aspects of your job?
5. What are some of the things that you enjoy least?
6. In what way has your job changed since you began?
7. Why do you want to leave your present position?
8. How would your colleagues and your present supervisor describe you?
9. Was there anything you did not like about your employer?
10. How long have you known you were going to leave your present position?
11. What would be some advantages to you if you joined our company?
12. What would be some advantages we would receive by hiring you?
13. How does the position you are applying for fit in with your personal and professional goals?
14. What can you do for us that someone else could not do?
15. What are the three best reasons to hire you?

Table 11.4   Employee Interview Checklist

Applicant name _____ Date _____

Position applied for _____

Salary range _____ Salary requested _____

Category

Education (degree _____)

Certification (type _____)

Experience (years _____)

Rating:	1	2	3	4	5
	poor	fair	good	very good	excellent
Appearance					
Alertness					
Knowledge					
Enthusiasm					
Communication skills					
References					
Overall comments					

	Yes	No
Candidate is qualified to fill the position.	( )	( )

delivering programs, plus has the ability to motivate others.

4. *Dependable and trustworthy.* The applicant shows a history of job loyalty and commitment and is able to maintain client confidentiality.

5. *Desires professional growth.* The applicant is active in professional organizations, shows interest in publishing and performing research, and has well-defined career goals.

6. *Exercises leadership.* The applicant can supervise and teach a variety of exercise programs, including aerobics, weight training, water classes, and flexibility. This would not be a criterion for some personnel such as support staff.

7. *Good communication skills.* The applicant demonstrates good people skills and computer skills.

Avoiding Legal Problems

There are several areas that you must avoid during an interview; these are detailed in chapter 17 regarding legal issues. However, some common examples of problem areas during the interview are identified here.

Health Issues

Discussion of past injuries is illegal, but asking about present limitations is legal. Let's say you are interviewing for an aerobics instructor and you're wondering if the applicant has had any back or knee problems. It is illegal to ask such questions. What you need to say is, "Do you have any present limitations that may restrict or limit you from performing the job as an aerobics instructor?"

Day Care Issues

You may suspect that an interviewee needs extensive day care services; however, you must restrict your discussion to the job. Simply inform the candidate of the required hours for the job, including any overtime that is anticipated, and ask if that presents any problem. Don't raise the issue of children.

Gender Issues

Perhaps you are trying to achieve a better gender balance among your personal trainers. Be careful to avoid biasing your recruiting and interview scheduling along these lines. Gender only becomes an occupational qualification for positions such as locker-room attendants where work tasks could be compromising. You may make your desires for gender balance a long-term goal, but must avoid the issue on a specific search.

Height and Weight Issues

Height and weight cannot be factors in the hiring process. Personal grooming is a legitimate business factor, particularly in high-level contact with fitness members. You should always address concerns about grooming; however, avoid height and weight issues.

Age Issues

Age discrimination is an area that will undoubtedly become a greater issue in the health fitness industry because of the historical focus on youth. It is in everyone's best interest to begin refocusing on an older workforce because of their increasing availability, especially on a part-time basis, and because members are getting older and may be better able to relate to an older staff member.

Making the Short List

Once you have concluded the interview rounds, it should be possible to reduce the list to a short list of qualified candidates. Indeed, it may be that one candidate stands head and shoulders above the remaining candidates, and you may want to proceed with the hiring process. However, it is most common to determine a short list after a second look at the best of the remaining candidate pool.

Follow-Up

Once you have completed the winnowing process, one or more of the candidates will emerge as more desirable than the remainder of the applicants. If there is only one candidate who seems to be superior to the others, you usually make a job offer at this point. However, the more common occurrence is that there are two or three viable candidates remaining and you plan a second interview round. This second interview round usually takes on a more specific and job-related flavor. The mid- and upper-management candidates, for example, are frequently put into a stress interview in which situational management scenarios are presented to see how the candidates handle the various situations. You may ask them how they would reduce operating expenses or how they would start a campaign for increasing membership. You might ask entry- or junior-level professional staff candidates to teach an aerobics class or perform a personal training session with one of the supervisors. Such active interviewing usually gives the decision makers another dimension from which to view the prospective candidates.

Additionally, there is usually a social element to the second interview round to determine if the candidate matches well with the existing staff and the corporate culture of the organization. If the position being recruited is a senior position within the organization, it is wise to consider an on-site inspection of the manager at work. Obviously, there are travel expenses associated with such an undertaking; however, you can obtain invaluable information from a visit to the candidate's work environment. You can get a sense of management style, organizational abilities, facility management, and member management, to mention a few. This on-site visit is critical if you are seeking upper-management positions within the organization. After the second round of interviewing and possible site visits, there frequently emerges a candidate who is offered the job.

HIRING A CANDIDATE

Before the candidate becomes employed the terms of the employment must be negotiated, and frequently the employment is contingent on passing health screening tests.

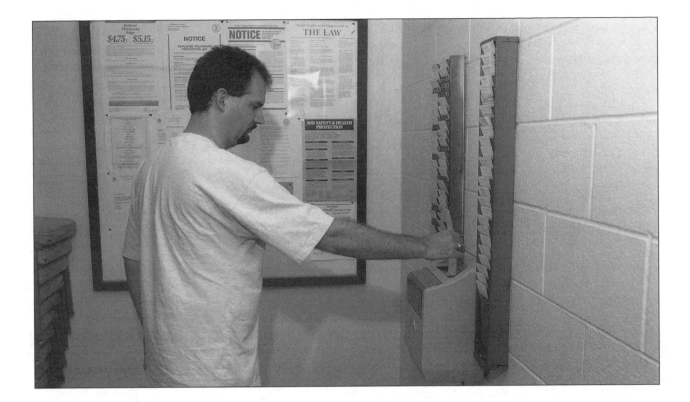

Negotiating Terms

We discuss negotiating contract terms and the legal implications of contracts in chapter 17; however, we don't want to understate the importance of the contractual process. The prospective employee sets the stage for career development during this crucial process; salary and job titles are set and career paths launched or stunted based on the parameters of the negotiated employment terms. Likewise, the employer must balance available resources with the candidate's perceived abilities during negotiation, or the employer will unbalance resources, rewards, and incentives for future negotiations with existing or subsequently hired employees. The terms of employment agreed upon do not always cement the deal; successful employment is frequently contingent on passing preemployment screening.

Preemployment Testing

The testing of prospective employees (*preemployment testing*) before the hiring processing is not uncommon in the health fitness industry. The amount of testing varies widely across the settings. There is more testing in the corporate and clinical settings where the potential for corporate image issues or patient litigation is greater than in the commercial

or community setting. There are many work environments that engage in testing, including written tests of job knowledge, psychomotor tests, and personality tests. There are also physical exams, drug tests, AIDS testing, and polygraph tests, to mention a few. The most common testing done before hire in the health fitness industry is that of drug screening. Once any testing has been successfully completed, the job offer is made, and, assuming it is taken, orientation begins.

ORIENTING NEW EMPLOYEES

Starting the new hire off on the right foot is extremely important. An orientation program sets the stage for a short learning curve about your policies, procedures, culture, and programs.

Probationary Period

Probationary periods usually last from 30 to 180 days, depending on the work environment and circumstances. During this period, you can terminate employment at will under most employ- ment arrangements. Although this may seem tenuous to new employees, most employers expect mistakes and performance variances while employees become familiar with the work environment. However, excessive underperformance gives the supervisor an opportunity to terminate the employee and seek new hires more capable of fulfilling the job requirements.

The human resources department in large organizations usually handles inducting new employees into the company; however, smaller organizations may have someone, say in the business office, handle most of the induction process. Table 11.5 is a checklist that covers most of the bases during this process.

Employee Handbook Orientation

Orientation procedures familiarize the new hire with the employee handbook. The employee handbook usually includes a discussion of the company, the facility itself, its hours and procedures of operation, equipment, programs, and other personnel. Orientation also includes learning company policies, available fringe benefits, accepted behaviors and dress codes, job responsibilities of others, chain of command, and accepted reporting procedures. Some companies provide more information during their orientation process than others; generally the smaller the program, the less information is available in written form. The main purpose is for the new employee to learn how the company and the facility operate and exactly what is expected in his or her new position.

TRAINING

Although many new employees will come to the job with numerous skills and abilities, it is important that they learn and adopt standards of practice within your organization.

Employee Expectations

Once you have completed the orientation of an employee, you can usually begin the training process immediately. Couch the employee training within the framework of both the employee and the organization. The employee usually has some basic expectations for employment, including the following:

1. *Fair wages.* Wages should be high enough to enable employees to possess the essentials of life and should bear some relationship to their contribution to the organization.

2. *Reasonable hours.* Even employees who are willing to work long hours want reasonable assignments. Eliminating split shifts, providing flextime schedules where possible, and accommodating personal needs, such as family and school, go a long way to making employees content.

3. *Good working conditions.* Providing a safe and pleasant work environment is important. Providing professional staff uniforms, access to an employee cafeteria, opportunity to work out in the facility during off hours, and other perks do wonders to the esprit de corps of the staff.

4. *Sense of improving status.* Employees expect to improve their status with the organization over time. Status can come from increased responsibility, promotions, raises, or simply a new title.

5. *Feeling of contribution.* Staff feel the need to contribute to the program. This can be accomplished with praise, opportunities for continued growth, and advancements within the organization.

6. *Respect for management.* Employees are much happier and productive when they respect the management of their program and think that they are competent, fair, and appreciative of their contributions. Good communication can go a long way in this regard.

Wage issues would have been handled before employee training. Employers should make every effort to satisfy working environment needs whenever possible. In the health fitness industry, most employees are part-time personnel with high rates of turnover. We discussed earlier the importance of minimizing the turnover of part-time employees, and this should serve as an extra incentive for management to accommodate staff needs and expectations whenever possible.

Basic Training—On the Job

The first consideration when setting up a training program is to provide employees the big picture with regard to the program, facilities, and operations. The training program should be comprehensive. One way to start the training program for the professional staff member is to have him or her role play as a new member being introduced to the facility and services. In this way, the employee gets to see the program from the eyes of the member. Include new member orientations, fitness and

Table 11.5 Checklist for Inducting a New Employee

Name of employee_____ Name of supervisor _____

Department _____ Hire date _____

Supervisor — Indicate information discussed with new employee. Return this form to personnel immediately after completing.

Employee records	Date	By whom (initial)
Application and personal history		
Tax withholding W-4		
Identification card		
Insurance card		
Employee Information		
Duties		
Working hours		
Rate of pay		
Probationary period		
Employee Benefits		
Group insurance		
Holiday pay		
Pension		
Vacation pay		
Uniforms		
Club use		
Child care		
Meals		
Leave of absence		
Credit union		
Miscellaneous information		
Parking		
Bulletin boards		

(continued)

Table 11.5 *(continued)*		
Miscellaneous information *(continued)*	**Date**	**By whom (initial)**
Safety programs		
Where to put personal effects		
Fellow employees (introduction)		
Exact working hours		
Lunch and rest periods		
Smoking rules		
About leaving the job		
When and where to report accidents		
Reporting lateness or absence		
Reporting address change		
Fitness facility and locker room use		
Use of telephone		
Organizational chart		
Policy regarding pay raises		
Housekeeping		
Care and use of equipment and supplies		

wellness evaluations, introductory personal training sessions, samplings of available food and beverages, and so on.

Once the new member completes the role playing, begin the basic training in all program areas. This serves two purposes: it gives new employees a comprehensive understanding of the program, and it cross trains them so they might fill in for absentee colleagues during emergencies. Make an effort to expose new employees to all program areas during the basic training. Develop and use a checklist of experiences and skills required in each program area to ensure that employees are fully introduced

and trained in all aspects of each program area. This means that the new employee shadows a midmanager in charge of a particular program area for a time to become familiar with the operations in the manager's areas. Exclude back-of-the-house operations such as accounting and housekeeping from this training rotation.

Start the exposure to each program area with the big picture; then break it down into its smaller elements. Give employees a chance to experience some early successes on the job. Teach them about things they know first, such as exercise testing for the fitness staff or service desk operations for

Table 11.6	Training Topics
Emergency management	Cardiopulmonary resuscitation First aid Emergency procedures
Emergency documentation	Medical clearance Informed consent Injury reports Bloodborne pathogens
Member management	Meeting and greeting members Telephone protocols Service standards Suggestion/complaint protocol Services/billing procedures Conflict resolution techniques
Facility management	Equipment maintenance Work order Chemical control Sound system operation Environmental control Purchasing procedures
Financial management	Time card procedures Payroll procedures Budget adherence
Program management	Special event orders Member assessments Opening/closing procedures

Delivery Methods and Situations in Employee Training

Lecture—explain large amount of information to large group

Group—stimulate thinking with little new information

One on one—explain information to someone when immediate feedback and reinforcement are essential

STAFF DEVELOPMENT

The staff training programs in most settings are designed to teach the skills required to perform a specific job and to facilitate the delivery of seamless, safe, and high-quality service to members. Staff training is intended for all employees. On the other hand, you can design staff development programs for all employees or for a few specific employees. Initiate the development programs for all employees when conditions warrant a review of standards and guidelines for the organization. The following conditions might warrant general development programs:

- High member attrition
- Increased absenteeism
- Increased employee turnover
- Introduction to new equipment or technology
- Orientation to new program being developed
- Too many accidents
- Certification renewals (e.g., CPR)

Specific development programs most often focus on management skills needed to achieve broader organizational objectives. You would usually design these programs to groom those who are distinguishing themselves in their job performance for positions with greater responsibility. The following are some examples of these development activities.

Cross-Training

Select individuals who are prospects for advancement within the organization for *cross-training*. This means that you would train an employee to perform the duties of other employees, especially those at

the facility staff. Your new staff members will feel comfortable with this as a first venture; then the other aspects of the training program will not seem so difficult to learn. Also, keep communication lines open, talk to the trainees, and, more importantly, listen to what they have to say. Some generic training is also important. This would include, but are not be limited to, topics found in table 11.6.

The delivery of these training procedures depends on the type of setting involved. Corporate and clinical settings usually have a human resources department to handle much of the generic training, with the health fitness department handling most of the specific training. Commercial and community settings frequently have to handle most if not all the training within the health fitness program. Regardless of who handles the training, the appropriate and efficient methods of delivery for different situations are detailed here. Lecture formats are common in large organizations where new hires need to be trained on a topic common to all employees, such as emergency procedures during a fire. Small groups or individual training is the best format for training in which staff needs skill development such as CPR training.

the same level within the organizational chart. This does not cause the organization to suffer because the individuals selected for this activity are usually over-achievers willing to make up lost time and overcome potential compromise to assigned duty areas. The cross-training serves the dual purpose of having emergency replacement for absentee staff and develops understanding in prospective managers of the programs they will manage once they reach a management level, from which they will train all staff.

Continuing Education

Many organizations provide staff development through continuing education. Tuition reimbursement programs for employees enrolled in academic degree programs are commonplace in corporate and clinical settings, but less common in commercial and community settings. Travel expenses and conference registration expenses also provide continuing education for employees seeking advancement. Where the employer does not pay expenses for continuing education, sometimes release from duties with pay is available and stimulates employees to seek further education. Some professional associations require a certain number of continuing education experiences for maintaining active status within the organization. Continuing education credits are usually awarded for such experiences and serve as a means of encouraging employees to remain abreast of their specializations through ongoing professional development.

Certifications

Employers frequently use the *certification* programs we discussed earlier in this chapter as a means of continuing education and professional development for employees. Club Corporation of America, for example, uses the American College of Sports Medicine's health fitness instructor certification as a staff development tool and expects this certification for continued employment and advancement within their organization. Release time or expense reimbursement for certification programs is becoming increasingly popular.

Professional Organizations

There are numerous professional organizations in the health fitness industry, each serving a different purpose and audience. A comprehensive list of such organizations would be difficult to achieve in the space available, but some major organizations include the following:

Aerobics and Fitness Association of America (AFAA)

American Alliance for Health, Physical Education, Recreation and Dance (AAHPERD)

American Association for Cardiovascular and Pulmonary Rehabilitation (AACVPR)

American College of Sports Medicine (ACSM)

American Council on Exercise (ACE)

Association for Worksite Health Promotion (AWHP)

International Association of Fitness Professionals (IDEA)

International Health, Racquet and Sportsclub Association (IHRSA)

Wellness Councils of America (WELCOA)

Y Programs (e.g., YMCA, YWCA)

Arguably, these organizations represent the mainstream professional associations in the health fitness industry. Certainly, we could make a case to include others in this list; however, most others serve a limited audience. At any rate, participation in professional organizations enriches both the employee and the program because of staff revitalization and program offering as a consequence of the professional organization.

ORGANIZATIONAL DEVELOPMENT

The organizational development of a health fitness entity is highly variable and relates to the setting in which the program is functioning. Corporate, clinical, and franchised commercial programs are frequently embedded within the larger organizational structure and corporate culture, limiting one's freedom to exercise independent management style and organizational structure. Smaller organizations, such as sole proprietorships in the commercial environments or community programs, provide more freedom for differing management styles and structures. Still, leadership development is important in any setting.

Management Training

Many organizations include generalized management training in staff development programs. They frequently make specialized experiences in financial, human resources, and general management training programs available to fast-track employees. Personal development programs are also available in some settings and include the following:

- *Stress management*—designed to assist in coping with all types of stressors.

- *Time management*—designed to increase job efficiency.

- *Sensitivity training*—designed to improve interpersonal relations.

- *Conflict resolution*—designed to minimize difficulties in communications.

- *Application*—all of these directed to work and home environments to ultimately improve job performance.

Team Building

Because most staff are reasonably well educated, motivated, and have a diverse set of tasks to perform, they exercise considerable freedom in the work environment. Although the employer expects staff to maintain service standards, there remain certain latitudes regarding program delivery. Accordingly, a cohesive and well-bonded team of professionals harnessing a host of creative spirits is extremely important to most health fitness programs. This process requires team building among staff and managers. This can only be accomplished with excellent leadership. Some techniques that encourage team building are the following:

- *Retreats*—designed to reevaluate mission, scope, or policies.

- *Departmental competitions*—designed to appreciate differential roles in the organization.

- *Company projects*—designed to break down interdepartmental barriers or provide community service.

- *Social outings*—designed to break down barriers for communication within and between departments.

Provide these activities as needed. Retreats could be an annual event, social outings a monthly event, and company projects could be on no planned schedule.

Alternative work arrangements for employees can also be a great morale booster and team builder. Approximately 14 percent of American companies now offer sabbaticals during which long-standing but overworked employees may take several months off to rejuvenate themselves, develop a new skill, or simply take a break.

> *Top down communications do not work well in the health fitness industry.*

Flextime is a popular tool to accommodate busy people with many commitments that overlap during the workday. Work sharing, in which two or more people combine to fill a single job, is now becoming popular. The manager who accommodates the staff when possible and without compromise to the organization's mission will find that his or her team of professional staff is happier and more productive.

Mentoring

Formal business planning and implementation usually take place in a routine and impersonal manner while focusing on task-oriented objectives. Although this method is efficient, there is little opportunity for nurturing staff development during such activities. *Mentoring* is an excellent method of enriching the organizational development of health fitness professionals interested in career development. Mentoring programs are usually developed when a senior manager and a junior manager (or a prospective junior manager) agree to a mentoring relationship. The senior manager then arranges more personal meetings as needed. The senior partner in this mentoring relationship coaches and counsels the junior partner. The coaching aspect of mentoring focuses on developing job skills and knowledge, and the counseling is concerned with problems of attitude and motivation or difficulties with interpersonal relationships that might hamper job performance. The coaching and counseling help the junior manager engage in self-analysis and job clarification. This process combines the manager's insights and knowledge to produce mutually acceptable goals for the subordinate. These goals are usually measurable and the mentor develops action plans for achieving them. These sessions are frequently confidential and can be helpful in preempting stunted career paths or premature terminations.

Succession Planning

Succession planning is a process of developing a plan to determine who replaces whom when a vacancy within an organization occurs. It may mean that an outsider needs to come aboard if there is no talent pool currently capable of handling a vacancy. However, it may also mean that with adequate staff development, managers within an organization may enjoy upward career mobility. This is a real morale booster. Ideally, you should strive for two or more individuals as potential replacement candidates for major positions within the organization. This creates healthy competition and improves productivity. It also provides upper management with an action plan for existing staff if some unexpected personnel action such as relocation or termination occurs.

OTHER HUMAN RESOURCES

There are numerous opportunities for using other human resources to implement successful programs. Hire part-time contractors with special skills and abilities not found in abundance among full-time personnel. Part-time employees save in the organization's benefits costs and office space. *Interns* and volunteers can also enrich a program with new perspectives and unique abilities without additional payroll expenses in many cases. These individuals can add immeasurably to a program.

Outside Contractors

Independent contractors are self-employed workers in a variety of fields in both exempt and nonexempt capacities. Health fitness enterprises may employ independent contractors for short- or long-term assignments, without any commitments or obligations normally expected in an employer-employee relationship. Some outside contractors contract for the entire operation of corporate health fitness programs. Other contractors may simply provide a single service, such as temporary secretarial or aerobics instruction assistance.

Interns

Interns are an excellent resource for any health fitness program. They infuse the program with new blood and ideas brought straight from their academic institution. They are usually infectiously enthusiastic, and this spills over to the other staff, breathing new life into the program. Most interns know quite a bit but need help applying their knowledge in the programming context. Interns do require supervision and expect to learn from the internship experience. They frequently are hoping for employment following their internship. Accordingly, such a program gives the employer a free look at a significant talent pool. However, like entry-level employees, interns need strong direction and regular feedback as well as ongoing evaluation. Because most internships in the health fitness industry are noncompensated, there is a significant financial incentive for managers to develop a strong internship program. Always weigh the costs of staff time in the training process against the obvious benefits of an internship program.

Volunteers

Volunteers can be extremely important to a program. The volunteers can come from agencies such as the American Heart Association or American Cancer Society and can deliver entire programs such as smoking cessation. These agencies can be invaluable for enriching programs that need an occasional boost for the membership. Volunteers can also be helpful when additional personnel is needed to deliver special event programs. Putting on a fun run or some other charitable event will require and garner volunteers. Many of the YMCA program activities are conducted by volunteers that originate both from within and outside the Y's organization. Most settings can benefit from using these volunteers.

Many programs use volunteers in the form of advisory boards to their organization. Advisory boards are a group of volunteers, frequently composed of members or influential people in the community or workplace who advise decision makers, but have no right to depose management. The advisory board can be helpful in defusing discontent among members by serving as a buffer between members and management, serving as marketing tools for new members, assisting with suppliers and vendors, and providing input on community resources otherwise unavailable to management.

Consultants

Consultants are needed by most health fitness programs at some time. Consultants are specialists who can provide unique information and services in such areas as general management, facility development, programming, personnel, marketing, purchasing, and special events. You can hire consultants for one day or for several weeks or months. Some consultants are hired on a permanent retainer basis and can even evolve into employee relationships. In an ever-changing world with a knowledge explosion facing us, it is wise to look for specialized expertise when the need arises.

Job Model—Fitness Manager, Aerobics Coordinator

The fitness facility, staff, and programming constitute a significant opportunity to provide additional value for all members and guests. The Fitness Department is unique in that it is the only department within the organization that is accessible to all members and guests. Therefore, the quality each area in the Fitness Department achieves has a direct impact on member satisfaction, usage, enrollment, attrition, and revenues of the organization. The Aerobics Coordinator must be able to recruit, hire, orient, and train all aerobics personnel and manage all aerobics facilities effectively if we are to achieve the mission of the organization.

Purpose

The Aerobics Coordinator is responsible for scheduling and implementing the exercise and aerobics class programming in the aerobics and aquatics areas and for supervising all part-time and contract labor in these program areas. The Aerobics Coordinator also provides essential leadership in formalizing membership communications pertinent to the aerobics program through newsletters, bulletin boards, and announcements.

Reporting Line

The Aerobics Coordinator reports to and takes day-to-day direction from the Fitness Director.

Role Definition

The Aerobics Coordinator's job is divided into primary tasks, then into specific accountabilities and responsibilities. The Aerobics Coordinator needs certain skills and personal traits to perform these tasks and responsibilities effectively.

Primary Tasks

The Aerobics Coordinator is hired to do the following:

1. Design and coordinate the implementation and scheduling of quality exercise and aerobics class programming in the aerobics room and aquatics areas for the members.

2. Ensure that all exercise and aerobics staff understand that they are to meet members' needs through personal recognition and by providing quality service and exercise and aerobics programming.

3. Ensure that exercise and aerobics programming and classes of all assigned instructors meet operating standards.

4. Recognize and act on sales opportunities with members in recommending other services and programs.

5. Recruit, screen, interview, audition, and select qualified instructors in compliance with industry and governmental standards.

6. Train, develop, and evaluate exercise and aerobics staff through formal programs, materials, and communication systems to ensure successful program and service delivery. Examples include the following:

   a. Staff training manuals.

(continued)

   b. Current music tape library system.

   c. Aerobics and fitness update seminars.

   d. Continuing education series.

   e. Staff evaluation system.

   f. Master class workshops.

7. Actively participate as an instructor, working with members in exercise and aerobics classes and evaluating exercise and aerobics programming.

8. Ensure that all exercise and aerobics teaching stations are properly maintained, equipped, and adequately stocked with supplies.

9. Review time cards for accuracy in completing weekly payroll reporting, and ensure that exercise and aerobics staff follow all administrative procedures and guidelines.

10. Maintain effective membership communications through coordinating newsletter, flyer development, bulletin board, and poster announcements regarding fitness department activities, classes, and special events.

11. Maintain operating expenses of the exercise and aerobics programs within budgeted allocations.

12. Market the exercise and aerobics program through special events, workshops, written articles, and presentations to both the professional and lay communities.

13. Serve as a member of the management team for the Fitness Department at all times.

14. Assume a leadership role as a professional in the area of exercise and aerobics.

15. Actively participate as a Fitness Department employee in working with members in fitness programs and special events.

16. Assume any other duties deemed necessary by the Fitness Director.

Necessary Skills

To be an effective Aerobics Coordinator, certain skills need to be developed or acquired before assuming the position. These skills include the following:

1. Administrative
   a. Time cards and sheets
   b. Reports

2. Employee development
   a. Recruiting, interviewing, and hiring
   b. Training and development
   c. Evaluation
   d. Counseling, discipline, and termination

3. Fitness programming
   a. Instructional development
   b. Equipment development
   c. Operations management

4. Marketing
   a. Membership services
   b. Program promotion

5. Sales
   a. Personal selling
   b. Program selling

6. Supervisory
   a. Interpersonal communications
   b. Delegation
   c. Leadership
   d. Organization
   e. Planning
   f. Scheduling
   g. Team building
   h. Time management

Responsibilities

The Aerobics Coordinator must assume many responsibilities to be successful. These responsibilities include the following:

Personal

1. Understanding the reasons for and requirements of policies and procedures.
2. Visibly supporting and implementing policies and procedures by actively functioning as a member of the organization's management team.
3. Behaving as a role model for a fit and healthy person.
4. Understanding the role and contribution of each employee in the Fitness Department to the mission of the organization.
5. Seeking opportunities for personal growth.
6. Leading and motivating others.
7. Managing time effectively.
8. Taking initiative to solve problems.
9. Dressing professionally as required.
10. Attending meetings and seminars as scheduled.
11. Working additional hours when necessary.
12. Maintaining professional certifications in IDEA, ACSM, and appropriate agency for CPR.
13. Keeping a positive attitude and smiling face in working with members and staff.
14. Attending staff meetings and member functions as needed.

General Professional

1. Assisting the Fitness Director in developing an annual business plan for the exercise and aerobics programs to generate revenue for the Fitness Department.
2. Controlling operational expenses for the aerobics programs in accordance with budget allotments identified in the business plan.
3. Monitoring aerobics program operational expenses weekly according to plan and budget and assisting the Fitness Director in making appropriate decisions and changes as needed to keep revenue ahead of plan and budget.
4. Completing all required financial work, reporting, and audits accurately and on time.
5. Ensuring that all aerobics program employees know the contribution of their assigned area to the overall mission of the club.

Member Services

1. Monitoring exercise and aerobics staff interactions with members to ensure that all members receive the level of attention and service as stated in the operating standards.
2. Anticipating the exercise and aerobics needs and interests of members in developing appropriate aerobics programs and activities operations.
3. Handling member complaints and concerns quickly and effectively regarding operational matters.
4. Assuring that the aerobics staff maintain a service environment through appearance and attitude.
5. Encouraging members to reach their fitness and wellness goals.
6. Assisting members in monitoring their exercise programs.

(continued)

Employee Relations

1. Knowing the names, positions, and hours of all aerobics program employees.

2. Monitoring aerobics staff scheduling.

3. Assisting the Fitness Director in recruiting, interviewing, and selecting aerobics staff in compliance with our standards.

4. Assisting the Associate Director in the employee orientation, training, and development for his or her specific position; supplementing any appropriate training for job-specific responsibilities.

5. Monitoring staff performance in aerobics programming and recommending corrective action to instructional staff as needed.

6. Providing regular job performance feedback through informal and formal evaluations, and helping the aerobics instructor complete corrective or additional development.

7. Serving as a mentor for subordinate instructors.

Marketing and Sales

1. Identifying and pursuing realistic marketing and sales opportunities in and outside the club.

2. Serving as a role model in applying successful personal selling for fitness and club services and programs.

3. Recognizing and acting on opportunities for members to take advantage of other club services and programs.

4. Assisting the Fitness Director and other managers throughout the Fitness Department in staying updated and supporting fitness programs and membership sales.

5. Being familiar with the competition within the market and recommending changes for aerobics programming and services in line with current market trends and competition.

Operations

1. Ensuring that daily operations in the aerobics program areas adhere to all standards within the following areas.
   a. Service standards
   b. Staffing standards
   c. Equipment operations
   d. Facility operations

2. Providing consistent supervision of exercise and aerobics areas.

3. Ensuring that all operational administrative work and reporting pertaining to the aerobics program area are completed accurately and on time. Areas include the following:
   a. Maintenance
   b. Service
   c. Staffing
   d. Scheduling

4. Assisting the Fitness Director in maintaining an effective member feedback and communication system.

5. Maintaining active contact as an exercise and aerobics instructor with members.

6. Assisting with supervision of the club through manager on duty assignments as requested by the Fitness Director.

7. Performing any other duty as needed.

Expectations

Work Experience

1. 18 months as a full-time professional in the fitness industry
2. 12 months as an aerobics instructor
3. 3 months experience in a supervisory role

Personal Interests

1. Sports, dance, gymnastics, and fitness
2. Continuing education
3. Personal growth

Education

1. Master's degree in health and fitness or related field
2. ACSM health fitness instructor's certification
3. ACSM health fitness director certification eligible
4. CPR instructor's certification
5. IDEA or AFAA certification

Required Training Time

1. Internal = 60 to 90 days
2. External = 90 to 120 days

Anticipated Tenure

1. One to three years

Evaluation

Rate the following attributes on a five-point scale, with five being the highest, three average, and one poor. This is a generic evaluation and you should supplement it with a detailed evaluation of the employee's specific job skills.

Personal

1. _____ **Appearance**
   Well groomed
   Dresses appropriately
   Displays high energy level

2. _____ **Initiative**
   Displays initiative in conversation
   Works on own initiative
   Has good follow-through

3. _____ **Integrity**
   Admits mistakes
   Keeps word
   Stands up for principles

4. _____ **Commitment**
   Accepts responsibility
   Is dependable
   Is persevering with detail

5. _____ **Confidence**
   Takes reasonable risks
   Has good eye contact in conversation
   Speaks with authority

(continued)

6. _____ **Intelligence**

Arrives at good solutions

Displays quick-witted behavior

Applies creativity to problem solving

7. _____ **Attitude**

Displays a good work ethic

Is usually an optimist

Likes people

8. _____ **Stability**

Displays emotional balance

Is calm during emergencies

Doesn't get easily frustrated

9. _____ **Flexibility**

Willing to learn and take on
challenge

Is a good team player

Looks for creative alternatives

10. _____ **Humor**

Smiles easily

Makes people smile

Is characterized as a happy person

Performance

1. _____ **Communication**

Articulates ideas easily

Gets support on controversial issues

Handles personnel problems easily

2. _____ **Knowledge of duties**

Knows all policies and procedures

Understands basis of policies and
procedures

Understands principles behind
policies

3. _____ **Knowledge of professional field**

Knows principles of fitness

Knows assessment procedures

Knows programming procedures

4. _____ **Punctuality**

Is on time for meetings

Turns in assignments on time

Rarely misses work assignments

5. _____ **Leadership skills**

People are willing to follow his or
her lead

Is frequently asked for his or her
opinion

His or her opinion is accepted and
followed

6. _____ **Time-management skills**

Gets things done

Appears organized

Makes lists

7. _____ **Financial management**

Forecasts budgets well

Controls expenses well

Creates revenues effectively

8. _____ **Program management**

Develops creative programs

Implements programs effectively

Evaluates programs routinely

9. _____ **Personnel management**

Trains subordinates well

Supervises personnel effectively

Is sought as a mentor

10. _____ **Operations management**

Things work smoothly for him or her

Is quick to deal with problems

Is a good planner

Total points = _____

Scoring

Excellent   =   80 to 100

Average   =   65 to 79

Below average   =   below 65

Evaluation Report

Employee's name _____

Title _____ Department _____

Evaluator's name _____

Title _____ Department _____

Date _____

Type of evaluation

____ Scheduled performance review   ____ Corrective

____ Probationary   ____ Exit

____ Other _____

Evaluator comments

_____

_____

_____

_____

_____

Employee comments

_____

_____

_____

_____

_____

Follow-up date _____

Evaluator signature _____

Employee signature _____

SAMPLE JOB MODEL AND EVALUATION

Club Corporation of America has developed a system of job modeling that creates a detailed job description but also adds other elements to the model. This model helps in the hiring process. It places some expectation on the tenure at each position within the organization. It facilitates in the evaluation process by providing a built-in evaluation instrument for each job within the organization, and it helps career planning for employees because each job model builds on the next career step for the successful employee. The following is an example of Club Corporation of America's job model.

SAMPLE JOB DESCRIPTIONS

The following are examples of job descriptions for typical positions within a health fitness organization. These descriptions are not as elaborate as job models detailing specific tasks and evaluation techniques. However, the job descriptions provide a perspective on the types of qualifications and responsibilities seen in various jobs in the health fitness industry.

Management Position

Position   **Executive Director, clinical or corporate setting**

Qualifications

1. Doctoral degree (PhD or EdD) or MS in physical education, exercise physiology, or related field with evidence of publication.

2. Minimum of two to five years experience as director (manager, supervisor) of a spa, health club, or fitness facility.

3. Knowledge and experience in developing and implementing health promotion programs.

4. Knowledge of budget preparation, revenue projection, financial review, and personnel management.

5. American College of Sports Medicine certification as program director or health and fitness director.

Responsibilities

1. Report directly to vice president.

2. Develop and supervise all operations and programs, and hire and train personnel.

3. Provide staff for all health promotion, wellness, and fitness programs.

4. Develop yearly budget.

5. Conduct monthly and annual financial reviews.

6. Develop public relations, advertising, and marketing strategies.

7. Conduct ongoing training workshops for the staff.

8. Conduct departmental staff meetings.

9. Conduct employee evaluation interviews.

10. Develop departmental performance standards.

Supervisor Position

Position   **Fitness Supervisor**

Qualifications

1. Master's degree in physical education, exercise physiology, or related field.

2. Minimum one year supervisory experience of a fitness staff in community, commercial, corporate, or clinical fitness facility.

3. Knowledge of administrative procedures and personnel management.

4. Background in health promotion, specifically stress management, nutritional awareness, and lifetime fitness.

5. American College of Sports Medicine certification for health and fitness instructor or exercise specialist.

Responsibilities

1. Report to executive director.

2. Supervise operations of fitness center.

3. Supervise all department heads.

4. Develop fitness evaluation tests and protocols.

5. Develop exercise prescriptions and programs.

6. Develop counseling procedures.

7. Hire and train fitness staff.

8. Conduct departmental meetings.

9. Conduct employee evaluation interviews.

10. Conduct ongoing training workshops for staff.

Entry-Level Professional Position

Position **Exercise Physiologist and Fitness Instructor**

Qualifications

1. Bachelor's degree in physical education, exercise physiology, or related field. Master's degree preferred.

2. Minimum one year experience as an instructor in a community, corporate, commercial, or clinical health and fitness facility.

3. American College of Sports Medicine certification for health and fitness instructor preferred.

Responsibilities

1. Report directly to fitness supervisor.

2. Conduct client interviews.

3. Perform fitness tests.

4. Develop exercise prescriptions and program.

Sales Management Position

Position **Sales Director**

Qualifications

1. Minimum one to three years sales experience, preferably in a health club.

2. Previous health club operations experience helpful.

3. Good communication skills.

4. Ability to work variable hours.

Responsibilities

1. Supervise membership sales staff.

2. Conduct personal sales of memberships.

3. Prepare weekly, monthly, and annual sales projections and reports.

4. Assist operations manager with running the facility.

Operations Manager

Position **Operations Manager**

Qualifications

1. Minimum two to three years health club experience.

2. One year supervisory experience.

3. Knowledge of facility operations, including front desk, programming, scheduling, and membership sales.

4. Bachelor's degree in physical education or business helpful.

5. International Racquet Sport Association management training.

Responsibilities

1. Report to general manager.

2. Supervise all facility operations staff.

3. Schedule work hours, programs, and special events.

4. Provide member services.

5. Prepare monthly financial reports.

IN CLOSING

In this chapter we have provided some guidelines for planning your staff needs, recruiting prospects, interviewing candidates, and hiring preferred candidates. We recommended some strategies for orienting new employees and gave some pointers on how to effectively train the new staff member regarding the details of the job and the work environment. We concluded the chapter with a discussion of the importance of creating management development programs for those staff members with advancement potential within your organization. Strategies for maximizing this development included team building, mentoring, and succession planning. Finally we discussed the benefits and disadvantages of using other personnel, such as outside contractors, interns, and volunteers.

KEY TERMS

Certification

Cross-training

Incumbent interview

Interns

Job audit

Job description

Mentoring

Preemployment testing

Probationary period

Screening

Short list

Succession planning

RECOMMENDED READINGS

Anderson, R.L., and J.S. Dunkelberg. 1993. *Managing small businesses*. St. Paul: West.

Arthur, D. 1991. *Recruiting, interviewing, selecting, and orienting new employees*. New York: AMACOM.

International Health, Racquet and Sportsclub Association. 1994. *Profiles of success: The 1994 IHRSA/Gallup industry data survey of the health and fitness club industry*. Boston: IHRSA.

Lynton, R. 1990. *Training for development*. West Hartford, CT: Kumarian Press.

Mitchell, G. 1987. *The trainer's handbook: The AMA guide to effective training*. New York: AMACOM.

Patton, R.W., J.M. Corry, L.R. Gettman, and J.S. Graf. 1986. *Implementing health/fitness programs*. Champaign, IL: Human Kinetics.

Patton, R.W., W.C. Grantham, R.F. Gerson, and L.R. Gettman. 1989. *Developing and managing health/fitness facilities*. Champaign, IL: Human Kinetics.

Wilson, B.R.A., and T.E. Glaros. 1994. *Managing health promotion programs*. Champaign, IL: Human Kinetics.

CHAPTER 12

Health Fitness Equipment Considerations

The selection, purchase, maintenance, and operation of exercise equipment are all part of an important process in the health fitness industry. Each represents a significant investment of time and money, and any poor decisions made during the process can haunt you later. There is a wide selection of products in varied price ranges on the market that you can choose from. In this chapter, we provide the potential buyer of exercise equipment with some criteria for selecting equipment, as well as some ideas about purchasing, maintaining, and operating it. In addition, we offer some insight into other health and fitness industry equipment considerations. Many facilities have laundry equipment as well as water treatment systems for aquatics and supportive equipment for racquet sports. We offer some guidelines for these areas as well.

Table 12.1 Type and Number of Members per Equipment Items

Type of equipment	Avg. total pieces	Avg. no. of members per equipment piece
Cardiovascular	31	77
Free weights	81	30
Resistance stations	27	88

Reprinted, by permission, from IHRSA, 1994, *Profiles of success* (Boston: IHRSA).

SELECTING HEALTH FITNESS EQUIPMENT

Selecting health fitness equipment is a baffling process for the average buyer because of the many vendors and types of products on the market. Canvassing classified advertisements in trade journals and visiting exhibits at trade shows can certainly confuse all but a few professionals who spend most of their time dealing with such matters. Indeed the potential buyer must use certain criteria to make a good decision. We present the following information on selecting equipment without regard to priorities because each buyer has different priorities depending on the situation.

Function

A piece of exercise equipment is normally designed for a particular function or purpose. For example, a bicycle ergometer is designed to function as an exercise station for cardiovascular endurance development; free-weight bars and the attached plates are designed primarily to develop muscle strength and endurance. However, you can use most equipment to accomplish secondary functions. For instance, you can use the free-weight equipment with low resistance to accommodate a high number of exercise repetitions for achieving cardiovascular endurance. Thus, determining which functions a piece of equipment will serve is one of the first decisions you must make. When determining what kind of programming spaces a facility requires, you have to make arbitrary decisions about the need for strength development equipment, cardiovascular development equipment, and diagnostic and testing equipment, as well as support equipment such as laundry, computers, and office equipment. The focus of this chapter is on exercise equipment.

Table 12.1 illustrates the different types and numbers of members for each equipment item found in a sample of commercial fitness centers during 1994. These data give some perspective as to the relative importance placed on each type of equipment. Cardiovascular equipment included step machines, exercise bicycles, treadmills, and rowing machines

Table 12.2 Average Number of Cardiovascular Equipment Pieces in Inventory

Cardiovascular equipment	% of clubs	Average number of pieces
Step machines	98%	8
Exercise bicycles	97%	8
Computerized	95%	7
Noncomputerized	70%	3
Recumbent	72%	2
Treadmills	83%	5
Rowing machines	62%	3
Computerized	59%	2
Noncomputerized	48%	2
Cross-country ski simulators	57%	1
Upper body ergometers	22%	1
Downhill ski simulators	5%	1

Reprinted, by permission, from IHRSA, 1994, *Profiles of success* (Boston: IHRSA).

Table 12.3 ° Average Number of Free-Weight Equipment Pieces in Inventory

Free-weight equipment	% of clubs	Average number of pieces
Benches	98%	10
Squat racks	88%	2
Bars	94%	10
Dumbbells	95%	50
Plate loaded machines	87%	4
Other	93%	5

Reprinted, by permission, from IHRSA, 1994, *Profiles of success* (Boston: IHRSA).

as the main categories. Free weights included benches, racks, bars, dumbbells, and plate loaded machines. Resistance stations included selectorized weight stack machines, hydraulic, pneumatic, and electronic units. Some industry numbers can be ascribed to the ratio of equipment types and the number of members using a particular type of equipment.

The selection of equipment should match the marketing image you want to project. The hard-core power studio is probably dominated by free-weight equipment, whereas the executive fitness center probably has more selectorized, weight-stacked equipment. Thus, the basic questions to ask in the early stages of decision making include the following:

1. What kind of image do you want to project?

2. Who will be using the equipment?

3. What is the basic purpose of the equipment?

4. Will there be an emphasis on strength or endurance equipment?

You can only answer these questions if you have defined a clear mission and conducted solid market research. Tables 12.2, 12.3, and 12.4 illustrate the average number of pieces of equipment in a large sample of health fitness centers (excluding corporate and clinical settings) during 1993. This gives an idea as to the emphasis and relative importance placed on each type of equipment within a fitness equipment category. Bear in mind that new equipment has been introduced since this study and that the average facility in the United States is approximately 25,000 square feet. If a facility is considerably larger or smaller than average, factor adjustments in the numbers into the situation.

Cost

Also consider the cost when selecting exercise equipment. The price of a single piece of exercise equipment can range from a few dollars to several thousand dollars. For example, you can use a dumbbell to assess or develop forearm strength and endurance at a cost of only a few dollars, and you can accomplish the same type of assessment or development by a high-tech computer product line for several thousand dollars. The difference, of course, is the degree of sophistication involved in the equipment. Most sophisticated equipment interfaces with a computer system for

Table 12.4   Average Number of Resistance Equipment Pieces in Inventory

Resistance equipment	% of clubs	Average number of pieces
Selectorized weight stacks	97%	25
Hydraulic	16%	5
Pneumatic	20%	9
Electronic/computerized	20%	8

Reprinted, by permission, from IHRSA, 1994, *Profiles of success* (Boston: IHRSA).

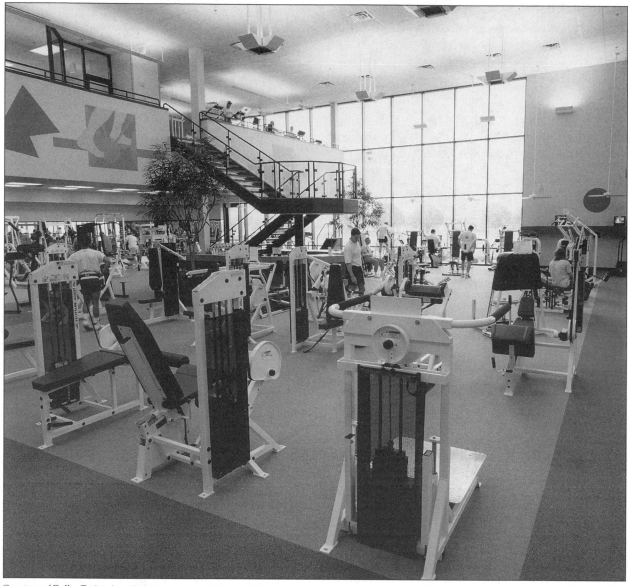

Courtesy of Dallas Texins Association

analysis, logging, or tracking purposes. There is a similar cost contrast between bicycle ergometers and treadmills in the cardiovascular area. Exercise caution when selecting equipment. There is often a point of diminishing returns when upgrading older equipment lines for newer products, and the cost of equipment can easily place a program in financial difficulty. Moreover, expensive equipment can place such a burden on the budget that other important areas of the program, such as personnel, might suffer. Still, equipment is a highly visible marketing tool, especially in the early stages of program development. Personnel, on the other hand, become critical in member adherence and renewals. A balance of expenditures is essential.

A guide to scale equipment costs against other expenses is that equipment should not represent more than three percent to five percent of the total start-up costs for a facility. A typical start-up facility in 1997 spent approximately $75,000 at a minimum to initiate a fitness program.

Paying for exercise equipment is usually required before or at the time of delivery. Although delivery dates frequently extend to eight weeks or longer, large expenditures of money over short periods can be burdensome. Consider alternatives to purchasing new equipment outright if you are already under the pressure of heavy expenditures.

One alternative to purchasing new exercise equipment is to buy used equipment. A series of phone calls to the equipment manufacturer you are interested in may provide you with contacts for trade-in equipment. Many vendors are a good source for used equipment because they frequently have trade-in agreements with their customers. The second-hand equipment market is becoming an affordable option for equipment. Many of these vendors refurbish the equipment to nearly new condition before resale. You may also choose to recondition your own used equipment. Various companies now can restore your old equipment to a nearly new condition and save you about 30 percent of the cost of new equipment.

A combination of used and new equipment is also an option during the start-up period. If the new equipment is made more visible to the members, the general impression will be that you have purchased all new equipment for the facility. Although this arrangement is less than ideal, it can frequently be a necessary compromise when investors are seeking an early break-even period and a quick return on their investment. A lease or a lease-purchase arrangement is another possibility. Again, these arrangements can be favorable to impatient investors and owners seeking early returns on their investments.

Several companies are now emerging as vendors of used and rental exercise equipment. You can obtain locations for these companies through trade journals or even local classified advertisements. There are also leasing companies now that advertise repossessed equipment with creditworthy clients for lease-purchase contracts. The purchase price on this equipment is discounted to as little as 10 percent of its original price. Several other businesses offer similar services and products to the resourceful consumer.

Expect to receive about 35 to 65 cents on the dollar when trading in used exercise equipment.

Depreciation and salvage value of exercise equipment after its usable life is another cost consideration. From an accounting perspective, the usable life of most exercise equipment is about five years; however, the life expectancy and the salvage value of some equipment is better than others. Generally, brand name equipment is superior in this regard and offsets some of the extra expense during the initial purchase.

Finally, consider the operational expense of equipment. Electronic equipment, for example, is more expensive to operate than mechanical equipment. Electronic part replacements and ongoing electricity costs can become a major expense.

Space

The amount of space needed or available often determines the type or amount of equipment selected in a health fitness facility. This accounts for circulation of participants and the average space needed for larger items such as treadmills and smaller items such as bicycle ergometers, as well as large free-weight racks and single-station selectorized equipment. If your facility is planned for nothing but multistation selectorized equipment, then these assumptions are invalid and you should consult the vendor. Note that most exercise equipment manufacturers offer space-planning services that are invaluable, especially if you are planning to use only one brand of equipment. Figures 12.1 and 12.2 illustrate two typical equipment layouts.

A rule of thumb for designing exercise spaces is that one station of exercise equipment occupies approximately 46 square feet of floor space.

To optimize the space use, plan for as many exercise patterns in one space as possible. For example, arrange a circuit on selectorized weight equipment around a group of ergometers to accommodate a super circuit if a member wants to cross train for strength and endurance during the same workout period. Patton et al. (1989) have excellent discussions regarding space planning for exercise equipment that remain relevant today.

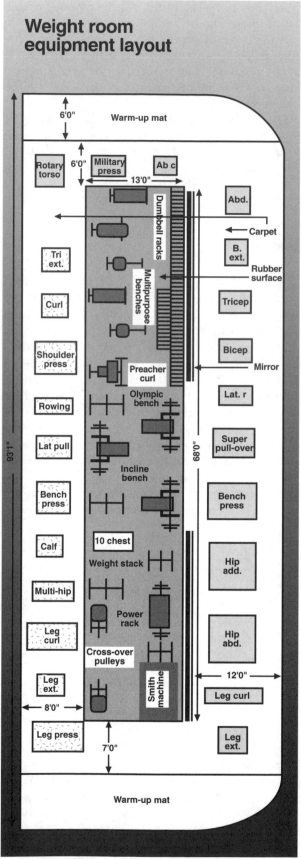

Figure 12.1 Weight room equipment layout.

Durability

Durability is an important consideration when selecting exercise equipment. There is no ironclad way to calculate the useful life expectancy of a piece of exercise equipment. Equipment of a particular type enjoys more use in some settings than it does in others. Also, the user is fickle; he or she may drift from one type of exercise equipment to another in search of one that yields large gains with the least pain. Some trendy equipment will experience intense periods of heavy use for short times, followed by periods of little or no use. However, we offer some guidelines for determining probable durability of a given type of equipment.

- *Joints.* Welds should be sturdy, and top-quality equipment will have the welds ground smooth. Bolted joints are useful where equipment must be disassembled to move or to remove or replace connecting parts.

- *Chassis.* Moving parts should be enclosed to reduce cleaning and maintenance.

- *Padding.* Double stitching should be standard on the front and back of pads. No staples are used on quality pads. Closed cell foam should be used in heavy wear areas; softer material is used in support areas.

- *Bearings.* Bearings should be suited to their use; delrin or nylon on weight stacks, self-lubricating brass bushings on pivots, and roller or pillow-block bearings on linear movements.

- *Chains, cables, belts.* Chains, aircraft cable, and belts are usual choices for connecting user to weight stacks. Cables and belts are quieter, and belts are thought to be more durable than cables.

- *Electronics.* Electrical components and moisture are not well suited for one another. Take care to avoid sweating onto display boards of equipment and secure water bottle holders on equipment at a level well below and away from any circuitry.

The warranty on equipment serves as a rough indicator of its life expectancy. For example, manufacturers of selectorized strength equipment frequently warranty the structural frame for life, the moving parts for a year, and the upholstery for 90 days. Each material obviously has a different projected life span. Read the small print in a warranty that promises a lifetime guarantee; little in this world is guaranteed for life, especially in the realm of exercise equipment. The manufacturers are careful to extend a warranty to customers that requires low repair activity at their expense. Therefore, assume that expected deterioration rates of equipment under normal conditions will exceed the warranty period advertised by the manufacturer.

Another indicator of durability is your competitors' experiences with the equipment. A canvassing of other programs in your area that are similar in size and clientele can give you a good idea about the durability of a type of equipment. This evaluation, coupled with trade journal commentary, will assist you in making the right decision about exercise product durability.

Safety

The safety of intended users should be your first consideration when making decisions about exercise equipment. Formal law and legal precedent dictate that agencies and administrators of health fitness programs have a responsibility to provide a

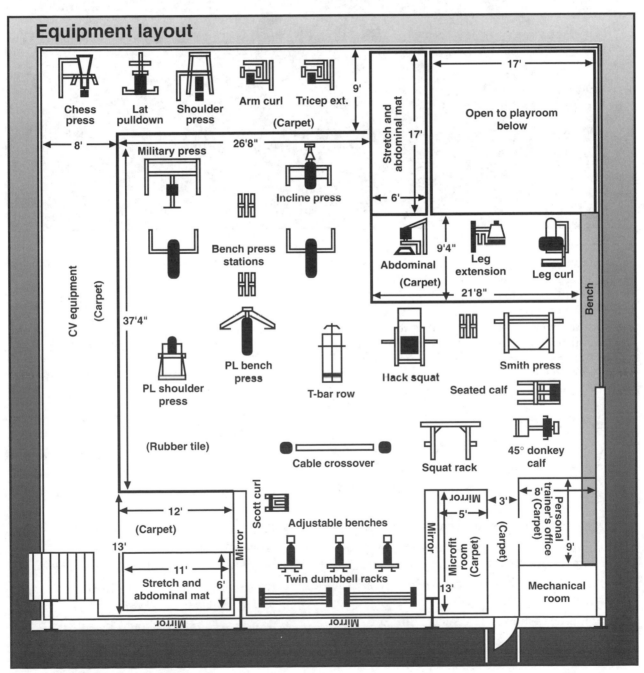

Figure 12.2 Typical equipment layout.

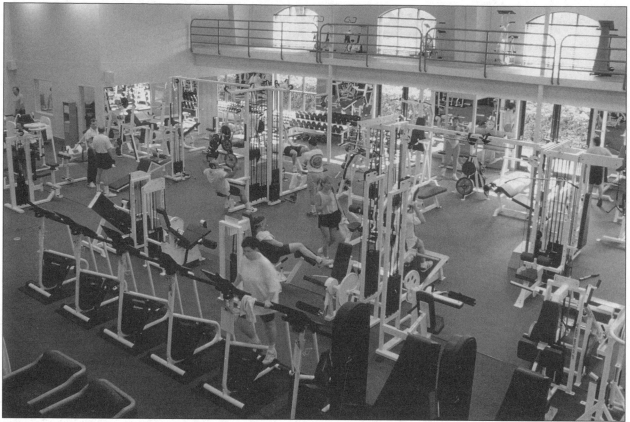

Courtesy of the Four Seasons Resort and Clubs at Las Colinas, Irving, Texas

reasonably hazard-free environment for exercise experiences. *Safe place statutes* in some states, which entitle the users to safe environments, place an extra burden of care on activity providers. In any event, it is important that the equipment you purchase is as safe as possible for the intended users. Use the following suggestions to avoid some trouble spots for exercise equipment on the market.

Weight Machines

- Cable systems should have plastic-coated cables, which are less likely to fray.

- Movable attachments should not have soft metal pulleys.

- Movable parts should be easily lubricated.

- Frames should have the capacity to be anchored to the floor or wall.

- Frames should have several welding marks at junctions.

- Equipment should be coated with corrosion-resistant paint.

- Safety stops in selectorized machines should be aligned.

- Cotter pins should not be difficult to place in stack.

- Nonslip surfaces should surround lifting area.

- Lifting area should be free of clutter.

- Floor surface should be of high-density, shock-absorbing material.

- Plates, bars, and collars should be stored after each use.

- Appropriate fasteners of free weights should be available.

- Sleeves for bars should not be bent or frayed at the ends.

- Preset barbells and dumbbells should be welded in place.

- Benches should be sturdy enough to support anticipated loads.

- Bench bolts and nuts should be welded in place.

- Bench surfaces should be padded to avoid splinters and the like.

- Selectorized stacks should be shrouded with protective covering.

- Safety stops preventing a crushing injury should be designed into equipment.

Always assign a professional staff member to exercise areas where exercise equipment is available to members.

Cardiovascular Equipment

- Electrical plugs should be grounded. Ground-fault interrupters should be on the power source.
- Treadmills should have an emergency stop button on handrail.
- Spotter's platform should be available on treadmills that elevate.
- Cycles and rowers with turbines should have protective guards.
- Countdown timers should automatically stop equipment.
- Treadmills should have guardrails on three sides.
- Instructions for safe use should be permanently mounted on unit.
- Preventive maintenance should be easily accomplished (e.g., lubrication).
- Climbing walls should have belaying systems.

Staff supervision of the areas where participants use equipment is extremely important. The following is a checklist of supervision guidelines and standards of care in equipment areas:

1. Include safety instruction and demonstration of safe and appropriate training techniques, including, but not limited to, warm-up and stretching progression, lifting and spotting techniques, exercise and workout progression, and any other daily training activities.

2. Supervise proper exercise technique and educate the participant in understanding the training effects of both appropriate and inappropriate exercise technique.

3. Post safety instructions and illustrations for proper technique in appropriate areas.

4. Instruct participants on the safe use of equipment, and warn against known dangers or defects.

5. Ensure that the extent of all warnings is sufficient to enable the average person to understand the probability and magnitude of the risk.

6. Be able to administer first aid and CPR, and know which procedures to follow in case of accident or injury.

7. Document all emergency care and keep it on file for review.

8. Develop training programs to each participant's fitness level. Monitor and supervise individual training, and adjust the training program to meet participant needs. Do not allow the participants to exercise beyond their capacity.

9. Teach the proper sequence of exercise selection for participant skill level, and define and require suitable conduct at all times.

10. Document and file each participant's training program. Also document instruction, supervision, and participant competence to verify that all participants received the appropriate standard of care.

11. Involve and inform parents when working with children so they are aware of the measures you take to ensure their children's safety and development.

Versatility

Look for versatility when purchasing health fitness equipment. Each piece must be able to perform more than one function. For example, the equipment should be capable of diagnosing ability, rehabilitating injury, or training the injury-free member in a club. In addition, it should be reliable so you obtain the same information on the same subject in repeated tests. It should also be accurate in that it truly measures what you intended in the test (e.g., treadmills may best measure running ability). Finally, the equipment should provide objectivity; the same results should be achieved when two different people test a member.

The equipment should be somewhat portable. Frequently, a piece of equipment must be moved from one location to another in the club, which is facilitated if the unit is on casters or rollers. Although you may see portability as an unnecessary extra, it could become a significant factor when equipment emergencies arise.

> *A major consideration for any equipment purchase is the ability to modify the equipment for different populations.*

Can children, women, and large men use the same piece of equipment effectively? If not, then you might want to seek alternative product lines. Some vendors offer products that can accommodate a wide range of body sizes and types. Unfortunately, many manufacturers have developed their equipment for the standard man or woman. Such equipment cannot comfortably accommodate different populations with unusual sizes and shapes without using pads, pillows, and other devices to adjust the user to the equipment design. The versatility of product design should weigh heavily in your decision making.

User Appeal

The intended user must find the equipment appealing if it is to be successful in the club setting. Several factors are involved in making a piece of equipment appealing. For instance, name recognition is one important appeal factor. Cybex, Body Masters, Quinton, StairMaster, and Life Fitness equipment, for example, have instant credibility and appeal among many users. A buyer seeking selectorized equipment would probably have high acceptance with any Cybex equipment brought into a facility. Indeed, some buyers purchase a few Cybex units and supplement the remainder of the equipment with other product lines to appease the customers' demand for Cybex.

Free weights have recently enjoyed a groundswell of support. Although no particular product line has emerged as a consumer leader, sturdy and massive-looking equipment is desired by many devotees of the power-lifting circles. This appeal is consistent with the concern for function in preference to appearance. Most free weight users are more concerned with results than with convenience and appearance of the equipment. Harried club members, in contrast, may be concerned with getting a quick but effective workout by using the selectorized equipment that doesn't require a spotter and that they can accomplish with minimal time and fuss. Time-urgent users will be concerned about efficiency as much as power lifters are concerned about

the effectiveness of the equipment available. Deal with all these considerations when selecting exercise equipment.

Maintenance Contracts

Some manufacturers offer service contracts at the time of purchase. This is an important consideration for those buyers who don't have access to maintenance and repair personnel. Typically, the maintenance contract dovetails with the warranty, and the fees are associated with the amount of equipment to be serviced. An average facility with a full complement of resistive and cardiovascular equipment should plan on spending about $100 to $500 per month for external maintenance contracts. Although this removes many headaches for the club, it places an extra burden on the budget. If the buyer has access to good maintenance personnel, the maintenance contract will not be a significant consideration in the decision-making process. This is especially true if a large inventory of spare parts is possible. We strongly recommend that you investigate the availability of parts and service before purchasing any equipment. A regional service center located nearby should place that vendor at an advantage over competing product lines of equal price and quality but farther from the club.

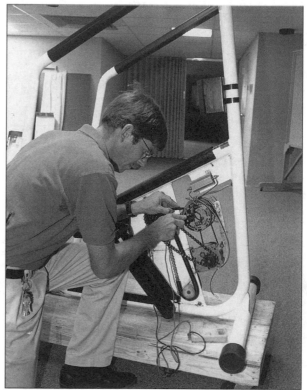

© Tom Wallace

Table 12.5	Sample Format for Equipment in Inventory			
Equipment items	Good	Average	Poor
Treadmill, no. 1	X		
Treadmill, no. 2	X		
Treadmill, no. 3			X
Cycle ergometer, no. 1		X	
Cycle ergometer, no. 2		X	
Cycle ergometer, no. 3			X
Rower	X		
Minitrampoline		X	
Stair climber			X
Ski trainer, downhill		X	
Ski trainer, cross-country	X		
Recumbent trainer		X	
Quadrupedal climber			X

Adapted, by permission, from R.W. Patton, W.C. Grantham, R.F. Gerson and L.R. Gettman, 1989, *Developing and managing health/fitness facilities.* (Champaign, Il.: Human Kinetics), 229.

PURCHASING HEALTH FITNESS EQUIPMENT

Purchasing equipment is a complex process influenced greatly by the setting. The procedures you employ to secure the type and amount of equipment you need vary depending on whether the facility is corporate, community, clinical, or commercial. Government agencies, for example, may have a purchasing department governed by state or federal laws. Hospitals may have corporate purchasing guidelines if they are members of a large group of hospitals. A community hospital, in contrast, may have more latitude in the purchasing process. Commercial fitness centers may be similar to hospitals, in that chain fitness centers often have centralized purchasing to enjoy the economics of scale in large-volume buying. Smaller, sole-proprietorship programs may have greater latitude in decision-making and procedural processes regarding equipment purchases. Thus, it is difficult to generalize about purchasing procedures. This difficulty is compounded when one considers the geographic setting (concentration of indoor versus outdoor equipment), the intended user market (upscale, single-station units versus downscale, multistation units), the desired image (lavish versus spartan), and a variety of other factors that clearly influence the decision-making processes when purchasing equipment. To assist you in your

purchasing decisions, the relative appeal of various equipment and activities in health club settings is illustrated in figure 12.3. Notwithstanding these limitations, let's examine some broad concerns that most programs will need to address when purchasing equipment.

Taking Inventory

Unless you are opening a new facility and purchasing new equipment, it is important to begin the purchasing process with an *inventory* of current equipment. It is equally important to determine the condition of each inventory item. A complete list of equipment and its condition tells you not only what you need at the moment, but also what you will need later. It is important to plan ahead when purchasing equipment for many reasons, including member needs, tax planning, program planning, and budget planning. Table 12.5 illustrates a sample format for taking inventory of equipment that is adaptable to most settings.

Consider replacing an item in the poor category of the equipment inventory when planning next year's budget. Red flag the average category for ordering replacement parts to repair pads, cables, motors, and other repair-prone equipment. This inventory keeps track of equipment condition, assures quality control of equipment condition, and permits a good system for equipment budget planning.

Reviewing the Equipment Market

Taking stock of the available equipment on the market is no small task. It seems as if half the products at trade shows are computerized to operate a myriad of bells and whistles. One approach to avoiding purchasing errors in such a high-tech field is to hire an equipment consultant. A one-hour consultation fee is money well spent to avoid costly mistakes, such as buying inappropriate, obsolete, or high-maintenance equipment. You can find consultants in the professional journals advertising products, services, and consultants. Networking with colleagues in similar settings is usually a good referral source for consultants as well.

A second approach is to contact vendors who represent a large variety of product lines and who can offer comparative opinions about available equipment. It is wise, however, to get a second vendor's opinion in this regard to account for the potential bias created by different profit margin

Popular equipment and activities in health fitness facilities

Equipment/Activity	Value
Resistance machines	9.359
Free weights	7.72
Treadmills	7.43
Stationary bikes	7.363
Stairclimbers	6.396
Aerobics (step)	3.475
Rowing machines	2.547
Swimming (laps)	2.5
Aerobics (high-impact)	2.449
Aerobics (low-impact)	2.272
Racquetball	1.767
Nordic ski machines	0.696
Aerobic rider	0.692
Tennis	0.585

Figure 12.3 **Health fitness facility members' use of equipment and participation in activities in 1996.**
Reprinted, by permission, from IHRSA, 1997, *Profiles of success* (Boston: IHRSA).

agreements between manufacturers and vendors. A third approach is to study the equipment on the market personally by spending time at trade shows and reading the journals in which the equipment is advertised. Many facility managers and owners take interest and pride in having expertise regarding exercise equipment. A better approach for the internal surveillance of equipment on the market might be to assign your staff members various areas of responsibility and get input from them before you make final decisions on equipment purchases. A final approach is the trial method. Today, vendors are frequently willing to place a piece of their equipment in your facility for a short trial period.

Writing Specifications

Once you have determined what kind of equipment you want in your facility, it is important that you write down clear *specifications* to assure that you get exactly what you want. Equally important, you want to get the equipment for the least amount of capital expenditure. If you use a bidding system to purchase equipment items, then clear and precise specifications are essential. The inability to develop good specifications is often the greatest source of purchasing mistakes; avoid these mistakes by following the suggestions described here.

The first step in writing good specifications is to get as much information about the desired equipment as possible. This can be your best defense against demanding club members, owners, and purchasing agents. Armed with the details of the equipment features and construction, you can write lockout specifications for the equipment type and model you want to purchase. Lockout specifications are prepared in such a way and detail that you are assured of getting a bid only on the product that you have decided is best for your needs. On a bid sheet, it is not sufficient to state merely that you want "Brand X, Model B, or equivalent." Substitutions are commonplace among purchasing agents trying to save precious dollars. You may also be deceived by a lower bid and buy what turns out to be an undesirable piece of equipment. Be specific! State the previous information, but be careful to add the size, color, materials, design, and performance characteristics that are necessary. This lessens your chance of disappointment, but does not always guarantee satisfaction. To guarantee satisfaction, provide all necessary information and indicate that no substitutions or alternate models are acceptable. Unfortunately, this is not permissible in many purchasing environments unless the equipment is an accessory to a previously purchased item that needs an attachment. In addition, it is helpful to contact the manufacturers of the equipment you want, because they can help prepare the specifications.

There is a trend toward listing not only the brand, model, and detailed characteristics of a piece of equipment, but also two or three acceptable brand names and models that meet the specifications. For example, you may list Nautilus single-station exercise leg-extension equipment in the description, but include Body Masters and Cybex as acceptable brands with models to serve as substitutes or alternatives that meet the specifications. This gives the bidder the flexibility to offer competitive *bids* on acceptable equipment items.

The detailed specification of equipment can also have the effect of intimidating potential bidders. If you write absolutely lock-out specifications, without providing alternative brands and models, there will be little variability and competitiveness in the bid returns. Indeed, such tight specifications deny you the opportunity to learn of legitimate alternatives to the product identified as acceptable. One approach to take when a good price on an alternative item comes in well under the price of the originally identified item, but meets the specifications, is to ask for a nonreturnable sample that the staff and club members can field-test before the final decision for equipment purchase is made. Many manufacturers will accommodate serious requests for field-testing a new product or product line. In fact, strategically placed products in prestigious facilities are frequently viewed by vendors and manufacturers as inexpensive advertising.

Getting Bids

Getting bids is not a simple process. It is important to issue bids far enough in advance to attract responsible bidders. Cut-rate vendors, eager to submit alternative and frequently unacceptable equipment bids, can often respond on a moment's notice.

> *The responsible bidder requires enough time to evaluate adequately the specifications, service, and warranty requirements of the bid. To deal with this issue, develop a bidder list.*

The bidder list is important to the purchasing process. It effectively defines the competition you want involved in providing the needed equipment and sometimes the follow-up service of warranty performances. The list of criteria for suitable bidders should include history on delivery and service, dependability, size of inventory, financial stability, and promptness in financial matters. The bidder list is further reduced if you insist that the bidder assist in installation and provide on-site repair, backup parts in stock, and a two-year warranty period. All these requirements add to the cost of the equipment; therefore, you should not impose them in the specifications unless they are necessary to the operation of your program. It is handy to put the bidder lists on a computer where a database management system can update your list with minimum effort. You may wish to notify the bidders on your list that you are accepting bids by using a form similar to the Notice to Bidders form (see figure 12.4).

There is, in some situations, a distinction between informal and formal bidding processes. The informal bidding process frequently involves several phone calls to bidder list vendors, and this process can get down to repeated calls to negotiate the final price. Such arbitration is effective in many situations, if permitted. The sole proprietorship uses this process to the maximum, as large-volume purchasing is not possible. The formal approach necessitates that a bid sheet be developed and distributed to a number of the vendors on the bidder list. Many large programs and institutional settings require that you assure competitive bidding by having a minimum of three bidders. Even in a formal bidding process, it is customary to invoke an informal communication at the end to maximize the competition between close bids. This assures that you receive the lowest bid, and leads to the letting of the bid.

The lowest bidder usually gets the contract to supply the equipment. After all, the competitive process was established to get the lowest price for tightly specified equipment. Often, the lowest bidders will have cut their profit margin to get your bid, and thus they will be less likely to overwhelm you with follow-up service calls if there is little profit in the offing. This is one reason why service is frequently built into the bidding process.

Another factor that influences the selection of the lowest bid is the proximity and history of the bidders. A local bidder with whom you have had a good relationship over the years might justifiably be selected over an outsider with whom you have

The Board of Education of _____ School District

No. _____ of the town(s) of _____ popularly

known as _____, (in accordance with Section 103 of

Article 5-A of the General Municipal Law) hereby invites the submission of sealed bids on

_____ for use in the schools of the district. Bids will be

received until _____ on the _____ day of _____, _____,
         (hour)   (date)   (month)   (year)

at _____ at which time and place all bids will be
          (place of bid opening)

publicly opened. Specifications and bid form may be obtained at the same office. The Board of Education

reserves the right to reject all bids. Any bid submitted will be binding for _____ days

subsequent to the date of bid opening.

Board of Education _____ School District No. _____

of the Town(s) of _____ County(ies) of _____

By _____   _____
      (Purchasing agent)   (Date)

Figure 12.4 Notice to bidders form.

never done business. However, exceptions to accepting anything but low bids are rare, and you should apprise your local vendor of being underbid. If you ever get in the habit of buying from one vendor, you can forget competitive bidding. Temper your decisions about letting bids go to the low bidder only with good judgment. One last comment regarding the letting of bids is that if everything is equal, stay with a standardized equipment line. The more equipment you have from a single manufacturer or vendor, the better.

Purchasing the Equipment

The purchase of the equipment is straightforward, depending on your fitness setting. For institutions that must adhere to legal procedures and policies the process becomes more complicated than the simple phone call from the sole proprietor of a local fitness center. In any event, the purchasing process should begin well in advance of the need for the equipment. It should follow a consistent order of procedures. The following procedures are tailored to a medium-sized institutional setting, but they are applicable to all settings:

1. *Initiation.* A request is made to the manager to fulfill, augment, supplement, or improve the program.

2. *Request review.* The manager or central office approves or rejects the request after careful consideration of needs and budget.

3. *Budget review.* The manager reviews the request and, if approved, assigns a code number to the equipment item in the budget category identified.

4. *Specifications prepared.* Prepare detailed specifications and make them available to vendors.

5. *Bid evaluation.* Evaluate bids to assure quality requirements and examine the lower bids to make recommendations for purchase.

6. *Purchase order development.* Develop *purchase orders* and send to the vendor.

7. *Payment.* Cut check and mail it on delivery and performance of contract.

8. *Payment schedule.* General rule is 50 percent down and 50 percent on receipt of equipment. Sometimes you can arrange COD. Plan on freight, installation, and taxes being added to cost. Withhold 10 percent of payment for 30 days to encourage prompt, effective installation.

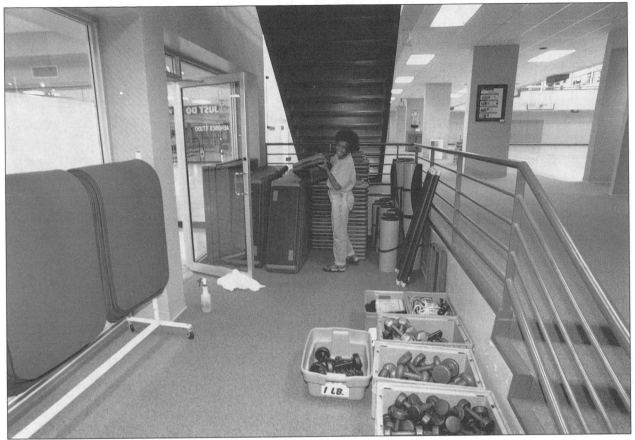

© Tom Wallace

MAINTAINING HEALTH FITNESS EQUIPMENT

Once you have purchased the equipment, the endless process of maintenance begins. The stress of 500 to 1,000 users per day on the equipment in a facility is considerable. The life span of equipment parts and materials can be short if you do not employ proper maintenance procedures periodically.

Internal Maintenance

The day-to-day maintenance of equipment is considered internal maintenance. Establish external maintenance through contractual agreements with vendors and professional service companies that maintain exercise equipment in a given service area. The internal maintenance of equipment is extremely important because it limits the amount of external service needed and preempts or delays costly breakdowns. Moreover, many internal maintenance procedures are also considered cleaning procedures. Cleanliness is imperative in the health

fitness business and cannot be overemphasized. Therefore, internal maintenance must be a highly organized and ongoing process. Although we discuss this further in chapter 14, table 12.6 provides a checklist of equipment maintenance guidelines, and schedules where appropriate, to follow when internally maintaining equipment.

Note that some vendors assist buyers with maintenance of exercise equipment. For example, in-service training is available from many vendors to train staff in the care and service of their products. Some vendors provide national hotlines to address maintenance or emergency parts issues. A few vendors notify buyers when warranty periods are about to expire and offer extended maintenance contracts.

External Maintenance

Consider the first aspect of external maintenance before the purchase: Don't buy anything you can't get repaired. If the equipment is mechanical, anticipate problems in advance and plan on breakdowns. Pay attention to warranty conditions and durations

Table 12.6 Checklist for Internal Maintenance of Exercise Program

Equipment frames

_____ Tighten all nuts and bolts.
_____ Use chrome polish on chrome as glass cleaner shows fingerprints.
_____ Use car polish on painted surfaces.
_____ Use fine steel wool to remove rust; then use nonabrasive polish.

Upholstery

_____ Clean daily with upholstery cleaner. Wipe clean frequently with warm water and mild soap.
_____ Remove pad for repair at first sign of hairline crack.
_____ Have backup pads available for high-use equipment.
_____ Wax upholstery monthly with hard floor wax.
_____ Rotate cushions if possible.
_____ Remove chewing gum by carefully scraping and wiping with kerosene.
_____ Remove ball point ink with rubbing alcohol. Remove shoe polish or paint with kerosene or turpentine and rinse.

Pulley systems

_____ Inspect all parts and connections regularly.
_____ Replace damaged pulleys and frayed cables immediately.
_____ Adjust cables and chains regularly for proper tension.
_____ Watch for and correct slack developing in pulley systems.
_____ Wipe chains and cables regularly with oiled cloth.
_____ Don't spray system with oil as it will drip onto floor or soil clothes.

Treadmills

_____ Adjust rear drums to ensure proper belt tracking.
_____ Put dance wax between belt and platform bed periodically.
_____ Lubricate all moving parts regularly, except sealed bearings.
_____ Mount control panel away from moving parts if possible, as vibrations are major cause of control panel repairs.
_____ Clean treadmill belt regularly with mild soap and water.
_____ Inspect electrical cords and plugs regularly; replace as needed.
_____ Locate equipment near electrical outlets to avoid injury to members and damage to equipment.

Bicycle ergometers

_____ Keep gears lightly lubricated.
_____ Replace worn belts and chains as needed.
_____ Clean upholstery and frames daily with mild soap and water.
_____ Wax upholstery periodically with a hard wax.
_____ Polish painted surfaces periodically with car wax.

and the location of the nearest service center. Warranty conditions are calculated by taking the average amount of maintenance-free service for a given product; therefore, expect service demands to increase about the time the warranty period expires. Location of service centers in the immediate area is a favorable factor when buying a product or product line.

Another external maintenance consideration is the service contract. In large metropolitan areas, start-up companies are emerging to meet the equipment service needs of the health fitness profession. You can contract any equipment services, including many internal maintenance procedures identified earlier. The fees vary, depending on the degree and amount of services required. Typically, a service contract ranges from $100 to $500 per month for a medium-sized club with an average amount of new equipment. Table 12.1 illustrates that the average club has approximately 31 cardiovascular units, 81 free-weight items, and 27 resistance stations.

OTHER SPECIALIZED EQUIPMENT

There are numerous other items of equipment that most health fitness facilities must have to operate their programs—laundry equipment, office equipment, fitness testing equipment, health promotion items, and various sports and games apparatus, to mention a few.

Laundry

Most health fitness programs need equipment to launder and dry uniforms and towels. Although some settings, such as hospital-based facilities, can farm out their laundry services to other departments within the organization, most health fitness settings perform their laundry function in-house. Larger operations are now using washer-extractors. These units are heavy-duty washer-extractors taking up to 125 pounds and capable of almost completely drying the materials by spinning down the loads at 300 Gs. Moreover, most newer units have advanced programmable microprocessors that simplify operations and expand their capabilities. The net effect of this process is that each laundry load can be quite large and handled efficiently, and the materials come out of a spin cycle damp, but not wet. This reduces the amount of drying time and, consequently, the need for as many dryers. Although washer-extractors are more expensive than traditional washing machines, they have been proven cost effective in that they are durable, require about half the total number of washers and dryers needed in a traditional laundry room, and conserve energy costs. The space recommendation of 150 to 300 square feet in the laundry area is reduced by more than half the previous needs when standard washers and dryers were used. Consequently, with building and maintenance costs rising, the trend is toward smaller, more compact laundry areas with more efficient and durable equipment.

Office Equipment

Most health fitness programs have business office areas of varying sizes. Once again, corporate and clinical programs may defer some office functions to other places within their organization. Commercial programs dealing with most of the business issues will normally require more office equipment than most other settings. Some equipment to support office functions includes the following:

Telephone systems

Desks and chairs

Computers

Postage meters

Fax modems

Card readers

Printers

Pager systems

Answering systems

Lounge furniture

Scanners

Copiers

Certainly, as business and communication technology inevitably expands, so will the needs for increased business office equipment.

Locker-Room Equipment

The locker room should provide approximately 15 to 25 square feet of space per person expected to use the locker room at any time. This range is due to the different locker configurations and equipment that is used in the environment. In most instances, no more than 15 percent of a program's membership will be occupying the

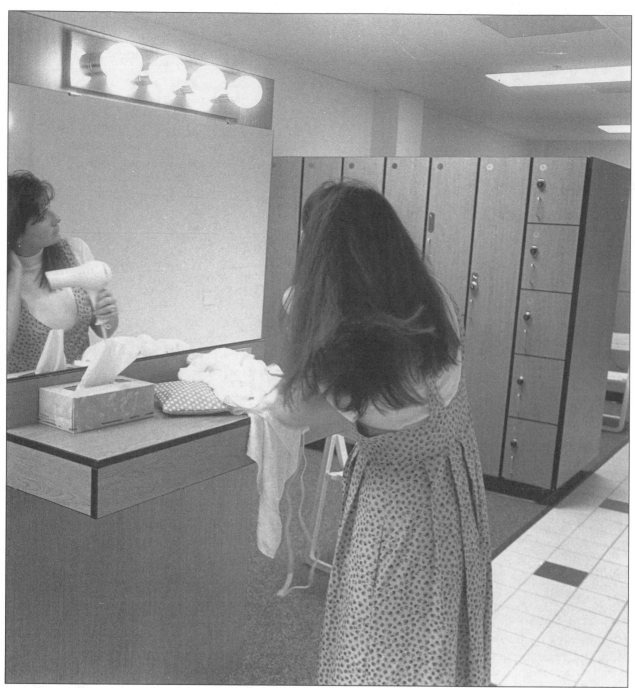

© Mary Langenfeld

locker room at any one time; therefore, there should be enough lockers to accommodate this load with a partial, full, or some kind of locker configuration. If the facility provides permanent rental lockers, then there should be enough lockers to handle 70 to 85 percent of the users, with some additional daily use lockers to handle other members and guests. Usually, the square footage allocated to the locker rooms will be about 25 to 35 percent of a facility's total square footage.

Health fitness facilities should provide an adequate number of showers in the locker room to handle expected usage; a shower total of approximately one percent of the total membership is usually adequate. For example, for 2,000 members there should be a total number of 20 showers. Most facilities have abandoned gang shower arrangements in the men's areas in preference to single-stall setups. Other equipment, such as hair dryers and grooming accessories, are frequently provided in locker rooms as well. For detailed discussions of these issues, see Patton et al. (1989).

Fitness Testing, Health Promotion, and Wellness

For certain programs, the availability of space can be classified as an equipment consideration. Allocate the fitness testing, health promotion, and wellness areas enough space and equipment to perform their expected functions. Table 12.7 gives some guidelines about the type and amount of space as well as the equipment requirements for fitness testing, health promotion, and wellness programs.

Gymnasium

A gymnasium is frequently provided in health fitness facilities. The minimum space needed for a gymnasium would be a full-sized basketball court of 50 by 84 feet with at least 5 feet of unobstructed area around the court. Consider overlapping markings for basketball, volleyball, and badminton along with appropriate equipment for each sport. Also consider wall clocks and scoreboards. Ceiling heights of at least 22 feet are minimum in these spaces. If you provide spectator seating, you need three square feet per spectator; portable bleachers can be a solution to spectator seating. You would need a variety of equipment to accommodate the activities in this area.

There are a host of other equipment issues that we could address for health fitness programs. However, we address equipment needs in areas such as the spa, child care, and aquatics elsewhere in the book.

IN CLOSING

This chapter provided some guidelines for selecting, purchasing, and maintaining exercise equipment and other specialized equipment. Selecting the right equipment is critical to the success of programs, and we presented important criteria to assist in this decision-making process. The rate of change in the industry is such that an outside consultant may be helpful in the selection and bidding processes. Once the equipment is purchased and installed in your facility, the ongoing process of maintenance begins. Internal maintenance procedures must take place on a day-to-day basis, and external maintenance considerations are equally important. Without good equipment that is well suited to the membership and properly maintained and serviced, a club cannot function effectively.

Table 12.7   Space and Equipment Needs for Fitness Testing, Health Promotion, and Wellness Programs

Type of space	Amount of space	Equipment needed in space
Fitness testing	120-180 sq. ft.	Bicycle ergometer or treadmill, skinfold caliper, anthropometric tapes, sit-and-reach bench or goniometers, tensiometers or strength equipment, blood pressure equipment, scales
Counseling room	90-120 sq. ft.	Office furniture
Seminar room	20 sq. ft./person	Audiovisual equipment, tables, chairs

KEY TERMS

Bids

Inventory

Purchase orders

Safe place statutes

Specifications

RECOMMENDED READINGS

American College of Sports Medicine. 1996. *ACSM's health/fitness facility standards and guidelines*. Champaign, IL: Human Kinetics.

International Health, Racquet and Sportsclub Association. 1994. *Profiles of success: Industry data survey of the health and fitness club industry*. Boston: IHRSA.

————. 1997. *Health club trend report*. Boston: IHRSA.

Patton, R.W., W.C. Grantham, R.F. Gerson, and L.R. Gettman. 1989. *Developing and managing health/fitness facilities*. Champaign, IL: Human Kinetics.

PART

III

BACK-OF-THE-HOUSE MANAGEMENT

Health and Safety Guidelines

As the examination of the back-of-the-house issues facing the health fitness manager begins, health and safety of the members is the highest priority. What actions do you take each day in the club to ensure member safety? How often do you hold emergency drills to ensure the staff is properly trained? Is the club in compliance with local, state, and federal health and safety codes, including the bloodborne pathogen standard? What emergency and safety documentation should you maintain? What safety and first aid supplies should every club have on hand? Use the information in this chapter as a guideline, keeping local and state regulations in mind as you prepare safety plans for your facility.

A prudent fitness center manager knows it is not if an incident or medical emergency will occur, but when.

Accidents and injuries are inevitable in an environment in which people are moving at a rapid pace, pushing their physical limits, and competing against themselves or others. How you handle these unexpected, unavoidable events, however, can literally mean life or death. Not only the possible life or death of the person(s) involved, but the financial health of the organization following a poorly handled emergency. Well-organized safety procedures and emergency plans allow the trained and practiced staff to respond with confidence rather than react with anxiety to potential danger. In this chapter we evaluate the components of thorough safety and emergency plans (see figure 13.1). We analyze various dangers that exist in different health fitness programs and discuss the necessary emergency plan modifications for these settings. We review health and safety codes and standards to ensure staff is properly qualified and prepared. We provide sample documents to protect the organization in the event of an emergency and lists of supplies that all health fitness settings should have on hand.

CREATING SAFE ENVIRONMENTS

A safe club environment for exercising members should be a given. Although many clubs place the highest priority on safety, some do not incorporate even basic health and safety practices into daily operations. Compounding this issue is the irresponsible or ignorant actions of careless members. The best intentioned policies and procedures implemented to ensure member safety are often ignored by careless members. Only an aware and educated staff and a well-planned and maintained facility can

overcome the obstacles to a safe exercise environment. Ongoing training of staff and immediate correction of potentially dangerous situations must be a consistent practice in all health fitness settings.

Facility

Implementing health and safety practices and procedures assists the health fitness manager in maintaining a safe club environment. Facility development and design techniques as well as city, state, and federal health codes implementation can build a foundation for a safe environment. Evaluate the club for safety while the physical structure is in design stages to eliminate many potential problems long before the first member enters the club. Consistent staff training and practice of health codes and standards can also assist.

Signage

Health codes are unique in each city and state. Therefore, communicating health and safety information protects the member or guest from injury and the organization from frivolous legal action. Use appropriate signage throughout the facility to assist staff in providing important information to the facility user.

Use signage to provide direction, indicate points of entry or exit, provide instructional or safety information, and communicate the events occurring in the club. For signage to be effective, however, it must clearly and concisely present the intended message, be easily read, and be properly located in the facility. Local, state, or federal guidelines may specify details regarding message, design, or placement of signage, licenses, or certifications. We rec-

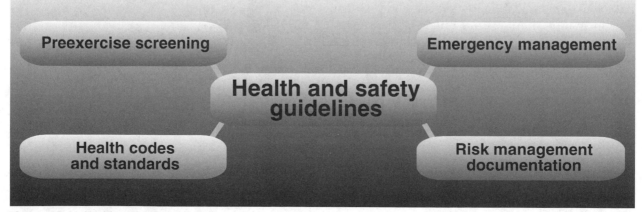

Figure 13.1 Health and safety overview.

ommend consulting proper organizations before design and purchase of club signage. Additional recommendations for signage include the following:

- *Use basic terminology.* The use of layman's terms will be better understood by the general member population. Use terminology for the target audience.

- *Use signs that can be easily read.* Select type styles that are easily read from a distance of 10 to 15 feet and place the sign 5 to 7 feet from the ground.

- *Determine the message.* Predetermine the message using as few words and symbols as possible. Show this wording to several individuals to test the accuracy of the message you want to convey.

Bloodborne Pathogen Standard

Bloodborne pathogens offer a new challenge to the health fitness manager. Bloodborne viruses that are of primary concern to the health fitness industry include HIV or AIDS and hepatitis B. The facility manager is responsible for understanding the threat inherent with regular fitness center operations, the potential dangers for exposure to staff or members, and the necessary prevention techniques.

> *Published guidelines by the* Occupational Safety and Health Administration (OSHA) *provide health fitness managers with ample information regarding the required training and record-keeping procedures related to the bloodborne pathogens standard.*

To adequately protect staff and members, it is important that facility managers know

- what bloodborne pathogens are,

- what occupational exposure to a bloodborne pathogen means,

- what the potential infectious materials are and how to prevent exposure,

- what the possible methods of transmission are and how to control them, and

- what protective equipment is required to protect the first responder to an emergency situation.

This information and much more is available from OSHA. Regional offices for this organization are located throughout the country to assist you with this task. Additionally, IHRSA has prepared a briefing paper for health fitness facilities regarding the OSHA bloodborne pathogens standard. This information is provided here.

IHRSA Briefing Paper

OSHA Bloodborne Pathogen Standard

HIV and Hepatitis B Regulatory Alert

OSHA Bloodborne Pathogen Standards

Club Action Required

What is the purpose of the bloodborne pathogens standard?

OSHA, Occupational Safety and Health Administration, has issued standards to reduce occupational exposure to blood and other potentially infectious materials that could lead to disease or death in the workplace.

Bloodborne pathogens are microorganisms in human blood that can cause disease in humans, that include the hepatitis B virus (HBV) and the human immunodeficiency virus (HIV).

Who is covered by the standards?

The standards apply to employers with employees who may be reasonably anticipated to come in contact with human blood and other potentially infectious materials to perform their job.

Are health clubs covered by the standards?

Yes, because it is likely clubs have employees that may be reasonably anticipated to come in contact with human blood or other infectious fluids, such as

- any club personnel responsible for first aid;

- housekeeping/laundry staff who could handle bloody towels, razors, or other potentially infectious waste;

- fitness staff who have close contact with members or sharp objects or equipment that could be bloody; and

- personal service workers whose jobs involve close personal contact with clients or members, such as hairdressers, barbers, and massage therapists.

What are the other potentially infectious materials besides blood?

Potentially infectious materials include semen, vaginal secretions, cerebrospinal fluid, synovial fluid, pleural fluid, pericardial fluid, peritoneal fluid, amniotic fluid, saliva in dental procedures, and any body fluid visibly contaminated with blood.

What does the standard require employers to do?

The standard requires an employer to establish a written exposure control plan and other procedures for reducing the risk of disease or death from bloodborne pathogens. The written plan must

1. identify the tasks, procedures, and job classifications where occupational exposure to blood occurs;

2. set forth a schedule for implementing the provisions of the plan; and

3. specify the means to protect and train those employees.

Procedures that employers are required to perform include the following:

1. Use engineering controls where appropriate (i.e., controls that isolate or remove the bloodborne pathogens from the workplace, such as puncture-resistant containers for used needles).

2. Introduce work practices to reduce contamination, such as providing hand-washing facilities that are readily accessible to employees.

3. Provide, at no cost to the employee, appropriate personal protective equipment, such as gowns and gloves.

4. Introduce requirements for housekeeping decontamination procedures, a written sched-

ule for cleaning and handling regulated waste, and specific procedures for handling contaminated laundry.

5. Offer, at the employer's expense, voluntary hepatitis B vaccinations to all employees with occupational exposure, and prescribe appropriate medical follow-up and counseling after an exposure incident.

6. Train workers, initially then annually thereafter, to alert them to the risks posed by bloodborne pathogens.

7. Provide appropriate labels and maintain records of exposure incidents, postexposure follow-up, hepatitis B vaccinations, and employee training.

When did this regulation become effective?

In most states, covered employers were required to have an exposure control plan by May 5, 1992. Information and training requirements and record keeping were required by June 4, 1992. All other provisions took effect on July 6, 1992.

Although it is important to take steps to comply with this standard immediately, OSHA is currently focusing its enforcement on the medical and dental community.

What is the penalty for failure to comply with bloodborne pathogens standard?

The violation of an OSHA standard can involve potential criminal liability or civil liability and fines. The severity of the penalty is directly related to the seriousness and willfulness of the violation.

Where can we get more information on the bloodborne pathogens standard?

Check your phone book under the US Government, Department of Labor, Occupational Safety and Health Administration (OSHA). Ask your local OSHA office to send you the Prototype Bloodborne Exposure Control Plan.

You may also want to contact local medical providers or local medical societies to see if they will share their plan with you. In addition, there are some private companies that will assist you in meeting the requirements of the regulations.

Personnel

Properly training health fitness center personnel ensures a safe exercise environment. Personnel should be constantly aware of potentially dangerous situations and empowered with the responsibility and accountability to immediately correct dangerous conditions. Management must also strongly encourage cardiopulmonary resuscitation and first aid training as an integral part of the ongoing training and awareness programs. Highly qualified personnel who are not hesitant to implement and enforce safety standards are the key to safety in an exercise setting.

Cardiopulmonary Resuscitation and First Aid Certification

Maintaining adequate health and safety certifications among the staff is an important responsibility of the facility manager. Require all fitness, activity, and child care staff and encourage the remaining staff to maintain current CPR certification. Although this requirement may be difficult in facilities that experience high turnover rates, setting a guideline that all new staff members be CPR certified within the first month of employment places this certification at a high level of importance. Certifying a long-term staff member or manager as a CPR instructor is an easy way to offer continuing education classes not only for new staff but for members as well.

Although not as essential as CPR certification for all staff members, you should offer first aid certification to staff regularly. Whether a manager is certified to teach first aid or you arrange a cooperative program with the local chapter of the American Red Cross, find a method to expose staff to this important information. Have all managers and long-term staff trained in first aid techniques to increase the probability that a certified staff member will be available to assist in the event of an emergency.

Emergency Training

Educate new and existing staff about their personal responsibilities in the event of an emergency. This training should be a priority of the supervising manager, should begin with employee orientation, and should never cease. The training must encompass all types of emergencies including medical, fire, aquatic, or disaster. The training must consist of written documents to review as well as hands-on practice drills in which staff members simulate an emergency event. Training must be ongoing, offering the staff a level of confidence in their practiced

emergency response. We discuss many potential emergency situations in this chapter. A planned, practiced, and refined emergency response should be the standard to create and maintain a safe exercise environment.

Emergency preparedness should be a part of the ongoing training program from orientation to termination.

PREEXERCISE SCREENING

In any health fitness program, pay careful attention to the procedures for screening clients and handling those clients as a result of that screening. The present *standard of care* requires that preparticipation screening procedures be in place and practiced.

Screen individuals before activity so you can identify and recommend more advanced screening or refer to a medically based exercise program those with disease or significant risk factors. This will reduce the incidence of cardiovascular problems during physical activity by nearly 50 percent (ACSM 1992).

When developing your club's policies and procedures, consider the safety of the participants. The American College of Sports Medicine (ACSM) identifies four primary purposes of preparticipation health screening. These purposes are

- identifying and excluding individuals with medical contraindications to exercise,

- identifying individuals with disease symptoms and risk factors for disease development who should receive medical evaluation before starting an exercise program,

- identifying persons with clinically significant disease considerations who should participate in a medically supervised exercise program, and

- identifying individuals with other special needs.

The ACSM (ACSM 1995) and a joint task force of the American College of Cardiology and the American Heart Association have published guidelines for exercise testing and prescription. We have combined recommendations from these two sources and present a medical management model for handling clients in figure 13.2.

In this medical management model, participants are identified through marketing efforts, then screened via a health questionnaire or risk factor analysis. The Health Screen Form used by the YMCA of the USA (see figure 13.3) or the Physical Activity Readiness Questionnaire (PAR-Q) (see chapter 7) are good examples of health screening tools. Both address the major factors involved in potential cardiovascular problems. Whether a screening tool is selected from existing references or developed by a facility, the tool must be cost effective, time efficient, and valid according to the medical director or consultant. In some settings, such as corporate where medical evidence of a stress-related disorder such

as high blood pressure might mean exclusion from a potential promotion, you must address careful review of a screening tool and its confidentiality. Discuss such issues with a legal representative.

> *Implement a screening tool as a minimal standard for entry into a moderate intensity exercise program.*

Medical Clearance

In the medical management model, results of the health screening are examined to see if the participant is apparently healthy, with low or average risk for disease, or if the participant is high risk. ACSM classifies risk into three strata:

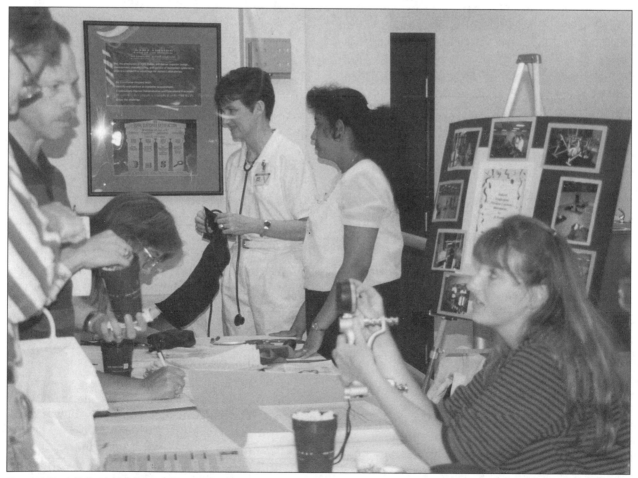

Courtesy North Dallas Athletic Club, Dallas, Texas

- *Apparently healthy*—individuals who are asymptomatic and apparently healthy with no more than one major coronary risk factor

- *Increased risk*—individuals who have signs or symptoms suggestive of possible cardiopulmonary or metabolic disease or have two or more coronary risk factors

- *Known disease*—individuals with known cardiovascular, pulmonary, or metabolic disease

See the ACSM's *Guidelines for Exercise Testing and Prescription*, 5th ed., for more detailed information regarding risk stratification and coronary risk factor classification.

Individuals deemed high risk or any person identified through screening to have potential health problems should see a physician and obtain medical clearance before undertaking any fitness testing or exercise program. Figure 13.4 provides an example of a physician release for activity form. Every health fitness organization should either have a medical director or medical consultant who provides medical clearance for the participants or directs participants to their personal physician for medical clearance. With your medical director and legal counsel, establish an exact procedure for identifying high-risk individuals, their risk stratification, and physician release for activity procedures.

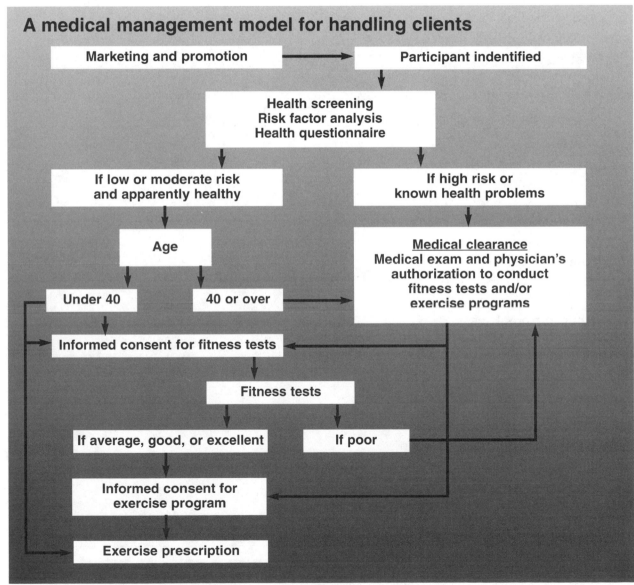

Figure 13.2 A medical management model for handling clients.
Adapted, by permission, from R.W. Patton et al. (1989).

Name: _____   Date: _____

Male: _____   Female: _____   Age: _____   Height: _____   Weight: _____

This form is intended to obtain relevant information about your health that will assist the staff in helping you with your program. Please answer all questions to the best of your knowledge.

1. **Weight:** According to the attached recommended weight chart, is your current body weight
   _____ underweight (more than 5 pounds under ideal)?
   _____ normal (within 5 pounds of ideal)?
   _____ 5 to 19 pounds overweight?
   _____ more than 20 pounds overweight?

2. **Blood pressure**
   Do you have high blood pressure?   Yes   No
   Have you had high blood pressure in the past?   Yes   No
   Are you on medication for high blood pressure?   Yes   No

3. **Smoking**
   Do you smoke?   Yes   No
   Are you a former smoker?   Yes   No

   If yes, give the date you quit. _____

4. **Diabetes**
   Do you have diabetes?   Yes   No

5. **Heart problems**
   Have you ever had a heart attack?   Yes   No
   Heart surgery?   Yes   No
   Angina?   Yes   No

6. **Family history**
   Have any of your blood relatives had heart disease, heart surgery,
   or angina?   Yes   No

7. **Orthopedic problems**
   Do you have any serious problems that would prevent you
   from exercising?   Yes   No

   If yes, explain: _____

8. **Other problems**
   Do you have any reason to believe you should not exercise?   Yes   No

   If yes, explain: _____

9. **Emergency**
   Please list a relative we may contact in case of an emergency:

   Name: _____   Telephone: _____

   Relation: _____

Note: The law varies from state to state. No form should be adopted or used by any program without individualized legal advice.

Figure 13.3   Health screen form.
Adapted from *Health enhancement for America's work force: Program guide* with permission of the YMCA of the USA, 101 N. Wacker Drive, Chicago, IL 60606.

Physician Release for Activity

Dear Dr. _____:

The following individual has indicated that you are his/her primary physician. This individual has shown interest in beginning a moderate activity/exercise program at ABC Fitness Center. Please provide us with your recommendation regarding activity for this individual and any restrictions and/or limitations you suggest for his/her activity program. Should you have any questions or concerns, please do not hesitate to contact me at the number below. Thank you.

Participant/patient:

_____

_____

Physician recommendation:

_____ Patient may participate in unrestricted physical activity.

_____ Patient may participate in light to moderate activities only.

_____ Patient should not participate in activity at this time.

_____ Other: please specify.

_____

Please specify any restrictions or limitations you feel appropriate:

_____

Physician: _____ Telephone: _____

Signature: _____

ABC Fitness Center contact person: _____

Telephone: _____

Figure 13.4   Physician release for activity.

Health History Questionnaire

A health history questionnaire is an excellent tool to gather and maintain detailed health status information on a large group of participants. Use the health history questionnaire form as the primary health screening device to determine risk stratification or as an adjunct document to another health screening tool. However you use the questionnaire, the information it contains will be valuable to the club's programming staff faced with the responsibility of preparing and directing a safe and effective exercise program for the participant. See figure 13.5 for a sample health history questionnaire form.

You need a systematic approach to ensure the information contained in the health history questionnaire is accurate, current, and readily available in case of an emergency.

> *Require a completed health history questionnaire on file before finalizing any membership agreement.*

Require a completed health history questionnaire on file before finalizing any membership agreement. By including the completion of this form in

Health History Questionnaire

General information: Date: _____

Name: (Last) _____ (First) _____ (MI) _____

Address: (Street) _____ (Apt #) _____

(City) _____ (State) _____ (Zip) _____

Birthdate: _____/_____/_____   Age: _____ Gender: Male   Female

Height: _____ inches   Weight: _____ lb

Personal medical history:

Do you have a recent or past history or has any physician ever told you that you have any of the following?

_____ heart disease/cardiac surgery   _____ peripheral vascular disease

_____ irregular heart beats   _____ hypertension

_____ defective heart valve(s)   _____ cancer

_____ heart murmurs   type: _____

_____ angina   _____ back pain

_____ heart attack (MI)   _____ joint pain: _____

_____ pulmonary disease   _____ migraine headaches

_____ stroke   _____ asthma

_____ diabetes   exercise induced? _____

_____ epilepsy   _____ arthritis

_____ high cholesterol levels   _____ lightheadedness/fainting

last measured level: _____   _____ allergies

specify: _____   _____ fatigue

Do you currently smoke cigarettes? _____ Yes _____ No If yes, how many per day? _____

   If you previously smoked, when did you quit? _____

   How many cigarettes did you smoke per day prior to stopping? _____

   Cigars per day: _____   Pipes per day: _____

Circle the most appropriate description of the amount of stress you feel daily:

   No stress   Occasional mild stress   Frequent moderate stress

              Frequent high stress   Constant high stress

Females only: Is there a possibility you could be pregnant?   _____ Yes _____ No

Please list any surgeries you have had and the date each surgery took place: _____

_____

Please list any medications you are currently taking, the reason you are taking them, and the dosage
   (including birth control). _____

_____

_____

Are you allergic to any medications? _____ Yes _____ No   If yes, please list: _____

_____

Figure 13.5 Health history questionnaire.

Do you have any medical limitations that would restrict your participation in activity? _____ Yes _____ No

    If yes, please specify: _____

Physician's name: _____ Telephone: _____

Emergency contact: _____ Relationship: _____

Telephone: (Home) _____ (Work) _____

Family medical history:

    Has anyone in your immediate family (parents and/or siblings) had heart disease or a heart attack

    prior to the age of 50 years? _____ Yes _____ No

    If yes, please specify: _____

    Is there a history of any of the following conditions in your blood relatives?

    _____ diabetes   _____ high blood pressure

    _____ high cholesterol levels   _____ stroke

Exercise/activity:

    Do you currently exercise on a regular basis? _____ Yes _____ No

    If yes, please specify what you do regularly on a weekly basis: _____

    _____

    Please check the total minutes of aerobic activity you do on a weekly basis:

    _____ < 40 minutes   _____ 81-100 minutes

    _____ 40-60 minutes   _____ > 100 minutes

    _____ 61-80 minutes

What are your goals in beginning an exercise program? (Please indicate all that apply.)

    _____ to lose weight   _____ to reduce stress

    _____ to improve cardiovascular fitness   _____ to stop cigarette smoking

    _____ to improve flexibility   _____ to lower cholesterol

    _____ to improve muscular conditioning   _____ to improve nutrition habits

    _____ to reduce low back pain   _____ to feel better overall

    _____ to gain weight/muscle   _____ to tone/firm

    _____ to increase energy level   _____ to rehabilitate injury

    _____ Other: please specify: _____

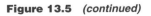

Figure 13.5 *(continued)*

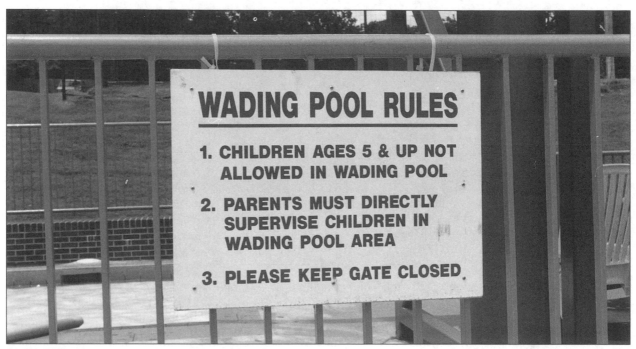

© Tom Wallace

the introductory process of membership, the club is ensured that documents are complete and available on all members of the facility and that review of the document for potential risk is complete before finalizing the membership agreement.

The information contained in the health history forms is valuable only if it can be retrieved. A poor filing and control system renders the information useless and the organization in a less than optimal legal position. Maintain the information in a computer database that allows the club to track the existence, age, and the entirety of the information. Maintaining the data on computer also ensures only authorized individuals have access to the information and that the data is available quickly in the event of an incident or injury. If a computer system is not available, use a manual filing system that prevents creating duplicate filing systems and the potential for lost forms. Set a standard that all health history questionnaires, and any other personal health information, be maintained at all times either in the individual's membership file or in a filing system maintained by the fitness director. Implement a process to regularly review the information to ensure data is complete and current.

Health-Related Physical Fitness Assessments

Many health fitness settings perform fitness evaluations routinely to determine health-related physi-

cal fitness capacity or fitness as it pertains to disease prevention and health promotion. Proper procedures to identify and test only appropriate individuals is as important as preparticipation screening. Individuals undergo voluntary fitness-related physical assessments for several reasons. ACSM identifies the following purposes of fitness testing:

- Provide data helpful in developing an exercise prescription.
- Collect baseline and follow-up data allowing the evaluation of progress by the exercise program participant.
- Motivate the participant by establishing reasonable and attainable fitness goals.
- Educate the participant about concepts of physical fitness and individual fitness status.
- Stratify risk.

Regardless of the individual reasons for a fitness assessment, it is imperative that the fitness professional be well trained and qualified to administer all components of the assessment safely. The law varies from state to state regarding the fitness evaluator's required qualifications. Review local and state laws to identify specific requirements. The test technician must be able to determine the most appropriate testing protocols for all individuals based on their age, physical condition, health status, and current physical activity level. Any individual administering fitness assessments should be certified by the

American College of Sports Medicine or other reputable certifying agency or organization.

Similar to preparticipation screening, develop, adopt, and adhere to a pretest procedure. To reduce the already minimal risk of incident during a submaximal fitness assessment, the participant should complete a comprehensive medical history form and be well prepared regarding the testing procedure before test administration. Information covered in the medical history should include any medical diagnosis of disease; previous physical examination findings; history of symptoms; recent illnesses, hospitalizations, or surgeries; orthopedic problems; use or allergies to medications; and other habits, including, but not limited to, caffeine intake, cigarette smoking, work history, exercise history, and family medical history. Following the completion of the medical history information and before administering the assessment, the test technician should explain the purpose and inherent benefits of the assessment as well as the potential risks involved and ask the participant to sign an informed consent for testing form. Consult the American College of Sports Medicine's *ACSM's Guidelines for Exercise Testing and Prescription*, 5th ed. (1995), for additional information regarding informed consent. The test technician should carefully review this information before proceeding with the assessment. Should either the client or the test technician feel that testing is not appropriate, or at any point request to stop the test, the fitness assessment process should cease immediately. For a detailed discussion regarding both clinical and health-related fitness testing, consult the *ACSM's Guidelines for Exercise Testing and Prescription*, 5th ed. (1995).

Guest Screening

A constant challenge facing most health fitness settings is the registration and screening procedures for guests using the facility.

Regardless of whether the guest is accompanied by an existing member; participating in a special event; or sponsored through a cooperative arrangement with a local hotel, business, or organization, the club must recognize that the standard of care regarding preparticipation screening is still in effect.

The club must prepare and practice a registration and screening regimen that provides the facility with a level of confidence that every guest is apparently healthy and that he or she knowingly assumes all risks related to participation in physical activity in the facility. Additionally, the facility staff should provide the guest with a brief orientation to the activity areas and equipment. The registration and screening procedure should also obtain basic information regarding the guest in the event of an incident or emergency, such as the identity of the individual, basic demographic information, and a signature on a waiver or assumption of risk statement. Many facilities also use guest registration forms as sales tools to identify prospective members. Most facilities use a two-part guest registration, the PAR-Q or a similar instrument for screening with a form asking for the guest's name, address, phone number(s), an emergency contact name and phone number, and a signature. Work with your legal counsel to determine a registration and screening procedure, identify appropriate information to gather, and select the content of the waiver or assumption of risk statement. Figure 13.6 provides an example of a guest registration and screening form.

The general manager must oversee a comprehensive emergency plan with department managers assuming roles of responsibility in their particular areas.

EMERGENCY MANAGEMENT

The term *emergency* is defined as an unforeseen combination of circumstances and the resulting state that calls for immediate action. Emergency preparedness is the responsibility of every health fitness center. Facility management and staff should be trained and practiced in handling any conceivable emergency situation—life-threatening medical emergencies, accidents, sudden illness, fire, weather conditions, natural disasters, or bomb threats. Emergencies can occur in any area of the facility, the cardiovascular area, weight-training area, the pool, the racquet courts, in a restaurant, or a child care setting. Prepare an emergency plan that addresses these possible incidents.

It is an accepted standard of care in the health fitness industry that prompt and effective aid be provided to members and guests in the event of an emergency. Is your facility prepared? Is each staff member appropriately trained? Was a drill to test the emergency response held in the past three months? Has your emergency plan been tested and refined? If the answer to these questions or others like them is not a resounding yes, review the following sections regarding emergency plan development and evaluation. We owe it to our members and guests to be organized, trained, and prepared to respond to any emergency situation.

Emergency Plan Development

Where does one begin when developing an important procedure such as an emergency plan? If the club is located in a large development such as a resort, office tower, or shopping complex, contact the building supervisor or the security department to review existing emergency plans that you can modify to fit the club. Large facilities and smaller, free-standing facilities should contact city resource departments, such as the police or fire departments, advisory physicians, legal

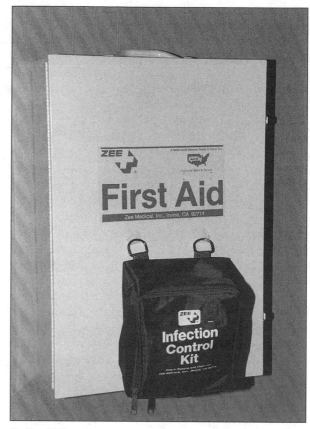

© Tom Wallace

Please complete the Physical Activity Readiness Questionnaire (PAR-Q) and the information below prior to initiating activity.

Name: _____   Date: _____

Address: _____

_____

Telephone: (Home) _____   (Work) _____

Emergency contact: (Name) _____   (Telephone) _____

Have you visited ABC Club before? _____ Yes _____ No If yes, when? _____

I understand and acknowledge that there are inherent risks associated with exercise and use of exercise equipment and facilities, such as those available at ABC Club, and I agree that all exercise and activities that I engage in at ABC Club will be done at my own risk. I waive my right to any claims against ABC Club (or any affiliated agent) which may arise out of any activity, event, use of ABC Club equipment or facilities, or my presence on the premises, including personal injury, theft, and all property damage, even if caused by the negligence of any of these persons. However, I am not waiving any claims to the extent it may be based upon gross negligence or willful misconduct.

Signature: _____   Date: _____

Figure 13.6   Guest registration form.

consultants or counsel, or local safety consulting companies for assistance. Although this chapter provides issues to consider when developing an emergency plan and ideas currently in use in many health fitness settings, no emergency plan will fit all facilities.

Tailor a specific plan and associated documentation to handle anything from medical emergencies to the evacuation of the club, considering the location of the club, its physical layout, staff coverage, location of emergency supplies and medical information files, as well as the location of all doors and emergency exits.

Involve all club personnel in developing the emergency plan to ensure it is appropriate for each area of the club. Reinforce that all club personnel be well versed in the procedures, and remind all staff members of the consequence of their ongoing training in order to act prudently in the event of an accident or incident.

Emergency plans must be detailed, but not overly complicated. The plan should be logical and written in concise terms that are easily understood by staff and members. Modify emergency procedures to fit not only the type of emergency, but also the location of the emergency. For example, the procedures for response to a life-threatening medical emergency will differ from the plan for fire evacu-

ation. A medical emergency on the fitness floor should be handled differently than a medical incident in the swimming pool or child care center. Fortunately, emergency plans need not be memorized in their entirety. However, every staff member should memorize the code or phone number that sets the plan in motion. Beyond that, post specific emergency plans next to every telephone in each area of the club for quick reference. Make available follow-up emergency documentation to the department managers and manager on duty for immediate distribution following an event. Figure 13.7 provides a sample medical emergency plan for a free-standing facility.

Carefully review the completed emergency plan with local fire and police departments. Maintaining contact with these city resource departments through regular practice sessions will ensure they are aware of the specific needs of the facility.

Emergency Plan Contents

As mentioned, you need to develop an emergency plan for the specific needs of each facility. The following list of plan components assists in developing or refining an emergency plan. See figure 13.8 for a sample emergency plan for a large resort facility.

Medical Emergency Procedures

1. Activate the emergency system by dialing "99" on the phone. This will notify the manager on duty and all professional staff of the location of the emergency.

2. Get the closest first aid kit and first responder kit. Kits are located in all activity areas, both locker rooms, and at the service desk.

3. If you are told to call for help:

    a. For ambulance, police, or fire, dial 911.

    b. For poison control, dial 555-5555.

    c. If directed to do so, page the club for a doctor.

4. Go to the main entrance, wait for the emergency team to arrive, and lead them to the scene.

(See detailed procedures on opposite side.)

(continued)

Figure 13.7 Medical emergency plan (free-standing facility).

(Back of page)

Detailed Medical Emergency Procedures

Staff who witness or are informed of a medical emergency in the club should follow these procedures:

1. The first responder should stay with the victim, leaving only to make the call to activate the emergency system which will locate and notify the general manager, manager on duty, and all professional staff to proceed to the location of the emergency.

2. Designate a staff member, if available, to retrieve the first aid kit and first responder kit. If help is not available, leave the victim to retrieve these supplies. If blood or bodily fluids are involved, do not render aid without first putting on *all* first responder kit protection barriers.

3. The general manager or manager on duty should assess the situation. Personnel trained in first aid and CPR should administer aid per training. If the medical emergency is severe, page the club for a doctor or medically trained personnel and give the location of the incident.

4. The general manager or manager on duty will designate someone to call 911. If you are told to call 911, proceed to the nearest phone located at _____, and do as follows:

   a. Call 911 (For poison control call _____.)

   b. Speak calmly and clearly: "We have a medical emergency at ABC Club. The individual appears to have (provide the suspected condition). Please send an ambulance/paramedic team to the ABC Club, 1234 Main Street (provide any specific directional information that may be helpful). Enter the club through the main entrance, I will meet you at the main entrance to the club."

   c. Obtain an estimated time of arrival (ETA). Have someone relay the ETA to the manager on duty at the scene. Give them your name and the number from which you are calling. Stay on the line until they hang up. Do not hang up first.

   d. Proceed to the main entrance and wait for the paramedics. Be sure all doorways are unlocked and open to speed the entry of the medical team. Lead the paramedics to the location of the accident.

5. Ask the paramedics which hospital they will be taking the victim to.

Follow-Up

1. Restrict all access to the scene of the incident if blood or bodily fluids are present.

2. Ensure staff members trained in biohazard spill clean-up are properly attired prior to beginning clean-up efforts.

3. Clean all spill areas with a solution of water and household bleach. Only staff members trained in spill clean-up should assist with clean-up.

4. Make sure all staff members involved immediately wash their hands with soap and water.

5. Make sure any exposed linens and first aid supplies are disposed of per OSHA guidelines.

6. Direct all staff members involved to go to a quiet place and write their account of exactly what happened, who was present, what was done, etc.

7. The manager on duty should complete an incident report, gather all other staff documents, and provide the information to the general manager.

8. The manager on duty or general manager should contact the family or "emergency contact" for the individual, notifying them of the incident and the name of the hospital.

9. Contact the hospital to check on the condition of the victim.

10. Take inventory of the first aid kit, first responder kit, and biohazard spill kit and reorder any necessary supplies.

11. Meet with all staff to debrief them regarding the incident, to evaluate the activation of the emergency plan, and to modify the plan as necessary.

12. Perform a staff training for all staff members regarding the incident and modifications in the emergency plan.

Figure 13.7 *(continued)*

We recommend a two-page emergency plan. The first page simply states the vital procedures a first responder should follow. The detailed information and directions are located on the back for quick reference by the manager on duty or assisting staff members.

• *Activation code.* Activating the emergency plan is the most essential component. Select a method to discretely notify staff and management in the event of an emergency. You can do this by announcing a code over a public address system, sending a code over a group paging system, or setting a prearranged sequence of telephone calls in motion. Direct all professional staff and managers to immediately proceed to the location of the incident.

• *Telephone numbers.* Make sure several telephone numbers are readily accessible. Although

---

Medical Emergency Procedures

1. Activate the emergency system by calling the emergency number "99". This number will ring the emergency phone of the on-site operator.

   Tell him/her:

   What the problem is (heart attack, seizure, fainting).

   The number of persons involved.

   What you need (police, fire, ambulance).

   Your specific location.

   Location of the nearest phone.

   (Do *not* call 911 directly—call the operator who will ensure the paramedics are met at the entrance to the property and escorted to you.)

2. Retrieve the closest first aid and first responder kits—or send someone to retrieve them. (See back for locations of kits.)

3. Return to the victim and do not leave him/her until EMS arrives.

4. Perform any first aid or CPR you are trained to provide. If blood or bodily fluids are present—do not render aid without first putting on *all* barriers in the first responder kit.

(Detailed emergency plan directions are on the back of this page.)

(Back of page)

Detailed Medical Emergency Plan

1. Dial "99" to call the on-site operator emergency phone.

   Note: Code 99 should be used only in life-threatening emergencies. Otherwise, call the operator by dialing 0 and tell them the information in step 2.

2. Speak calmly and clearly and tell him/her:

   What the problem is (heart attack, seizure, fainting).

   What you need: (ambulance, police).

   The number of persons needing help.

   Your exact location (aerobics room, indoor pool, locker room).

3. Retrieve the nearest first aid kit and first responder kit, or send someone to retrieve them. The kits are located: behind service desk, in restaurant, fitness desk, child care, outdoor pool, locker room supply room.

4. Return to the victim and stay with him/her until EMS arrives. The on-site operator will make all necessary telephone calls and notify all parties.

5. Render any first aid or CPR you are trained to provide. If blood or bodily fluids are present, put on all barriers in the first responder kit prior to rendering aid.

(continued)

Figure 13.8 Medical emergency plan (facility in large complex).

6. The on-site operator will notify the following:

911—The operator should relay the following information:

"We have a medical emergency at ABC Club, 1234 Main Street. The individual appears to have (name condition). Please send an ambulance to the main entrance of the property off of Main Street. Security officers will be waiting and will lead the emergency team to the scene."

Poison control—555-5555

Security—An officer will be dispatched to the scene with emergency supplies. A second officer will be dispatched to the main entrance of the property to meet and escort the paramedics to the scene. A third officer will be dispatched to unlock all gates, doorways, and elevators to speed the entry of the ambulance.

General manager and department heads—A group page will be sent indicating the location of the emergency.

Obtain an estimated time of arrival (ETA) and relay it back to the manager on duty at the scene.

STAY ON THE LINE UNTIL THE DISPATCHER HANGS UP—DO NOT HANG UP FIRST.

7. The manager on duty after arriving at the scene will do the following:

Assess the scene.

Delegate a staff member to retrieve the closest cordless emergency phone.

Ask the operator to make a public address announcement requesting the assistance of any medically trained members.

Delegate a staff member to retrieve the victim's medical information file.

Delegate a staff member to control the crowd.

Delegate a staff member to locate the parent if it is a child that is involved.

Ask the paramedics which hospital the victim will be transported to.

Initiate Follow-Up Procedures.

8. Follow-up.

a. Restrict all access to the scene of the incident if blood or bodily fluids are present.

b. Ensure staff members trained in biohazard spill clean-up are properly attired prior to beginning clean-up efforts.

c. Clean all spill areas with a solution of water and household bleach. Only staff members trained in spill clean-up should assist with clean-up.

d. Make sure all staff members involved immediately wash their hands with soap and water.

e. Make sure any exposed linens and first aid supplies are disposed of per OSHA guidelines.

f. Direct all staff members involved to go to a quiet place and write their account of exactly what happened, who was present, what was done, etc.

g. The manager on duty should complete an incident report, gather all other staff documents, and provide the information to the general manager.

h. The manager on duty or the general manager should contact the family or "emergency contact" for the individual and notify them of the incident and the name of the hospital.

i. Contact the hospital to check on the condition of the victim.

j. Take inventory of the first aid kit, first responder kit, and biohazard spill kit and reorder any necessary supplies.

k. Meet with all staff to debrief them regarding the incident, to evaluate the activation of the emergency plan, and to modify the plan as necessary.

l. Schedule a staff training for all staff members regarding the incident and modifications in the emergency plan.

Figure 13.8 *(continued)*

most cities in the United States use the 911 emergency system, some cities may not have this service, or their plan may direct them to call an in-house emergency department who then activates the 911 system. Keep telephone numbers for emergency assistance, poison control, general manager's home number or pager number, and other management phone numbers posted by every telephone.

> *Keep available a secondary or backup communication system, such as cellular phones or radios, to use if the telephone system is not functional.*

• *Location of nearest telephone.* Detail the exact location of the nearest telephone if there is not a telephone in an activity area.

• *Location.* Post an emergency plan with detailed instructions regarding the location and quickest way to this area in each area of the club. The printed location on the emergency plan should direct emergency medical services (EMS) to the closest point of building entry. In many larger facilities, you can contact an internal department such as security or an operator. These internal departments have the responsibility to activate 911, meet EMS as they enter the property, and direct them to the emergency site.

• *Locked doors or gates.* If the possibility exists that a door or gate will prevent the prompt entry of EMS, note the location of the door or gate and the location of the key.

• *Location of emergency supplies.* Provide a detailed explanation of the location of the nearest first aid kit, first responder bloodborne pathogen kit, and bloodborne cleanup kit. Recommended contents of each kit are listed respectively in table 13.1.

• *Information to share.* When calling for assistance, be prepared to relay who you are, where you are (post the club address on the emergency plan), the number you are calling from, the type of emergency, what has happened, how many people need assistance, their gender and approximate ages, what is currently being done to assist them, and the estimated time of arrival of emergency support. Teach staff members to stay calm and to stay on the line until emergency assistance tells you to hang up.

• *Directions for personnel responsibilities.* The plan should designate the first responder to direct the incident until a manager arrives and can assume responsibility and control. The first responder should stay with the injured party, leaving only to activate the emergency plan or call for assistance. The first responder or manager should then delegate a communication staff member who will call 911 or another predetermined resource and provide incident data listed in the previous directions for information to share. Delegate additional staff members to assume crowd control responsibilities, retrieve any health history information that may be on file, meet and direct EMS to the scene, or record the names of individuals who are present and who may have witnessed the incident.

• *Call for member assistance.* Many organizations include in their medical emergency plan a call for any medically trained members (i.e., doctors or nurses who may be in the facility exercising) to proceed to the location of the incident for assistance.

• *Incident and accident reports.* Immediately following the removal of the victim by emergency personnel, the manager on duty should direct the staff to go to a quiet place and write down everything they can remember about the incident and the care provided, including time lines if possible, names of witnesses, care administered, and so on. During this time, the manager on duty should complete an incident or accident report. A sample of this form is illustrated in figure 13.9.

Additional Suggestions

• Designate a cellular phone to use in the event of an emergency. This cellular phone allows the manager to make phone calls while moving throughout the club.

• Keep a flashlight in all first aid kits as well as designated areas throughout the club in the event of a power outage.

Fire and Evacuation Plan

During any emergency situation, the health and safety of the members and guests is the highest priority for management and staff of the facility. The ability to calmly and systematically notify members of an emergency that requires evacuation and clear the building quickly is important. Establishing a fire and evacuation plan that specifies

Date of incident/accident: _____ Time of incident: _____ A.M./P.M.

Injured member/guest: _____ Age: _____

Membership number: _____

Address: _____

_____

Telephone: (Home) _____ (Work) _____

Location of incident: _____

_____

Describe in full how incident occurred and what actions were taken by staff.

(Write everything you can remember no matter how insignificant it may seem.)

_____

_____

_____

Describe the injury in detail and indicate the body part(s) affected:

_____

Did any medically trained members (doctors, nurses) assist?

_____

Staff members present: _____

Witnesses: _____

_____

Was the emergency plan activated? _____ Was EMS called? _____

Was the individual taken to the hospital? _____ Yes _____ No

If yes, what hospital? _____

If no, did he/she refuse medical attention? _____

Was the family notified? _____ Who? _____

On the back of this page, please document any observations or comments regarding this incident you feel important.

Signed by: _____ Date: _____ Time: _____

MOD/dept. head: _____ Date: _____

Follow-up notes:

Contact made by: _____ Date: _____

Condition of member: _____

Figure 13.9   Incident and accident report form.

procedures to effectively and efficiently evacuate the building is the responsibility of management. Similar to the medical emergency plan, obtain assistance in preparing this procedure by contacting on-site security personnel or building managers, or local resource departments, such as police or fire departments. A sample fire and evacuation plan can be reviewed in figure 13.10.

> *Review and practice your completed fire and evacuation plan in cooperation with local emergency services.*

Fire Emergency Procedures

Staff members who locate smoke or flames should do the following:

1. Go to the nearest phone, dial "99" to activate the emergency system or go to the nearest fire pull station and pull the alarm.
2. Retrieve the nearest fire extinguisher. Fire extinguishers are located at the service desk, the locker room storage area, laundry, the kitchen, child care, the mechanical room, and the fitness desk.
3. Return to the site of the fire.

   Rescue anyone in immediate danger, and direct persons to nearest exit.

   Confine fire by closing all doors in the area.

   If the fire is small, try to contain it using the fire extinguisher.

   If the fire is large or there is a great deal of smoke, begin the evacuation procedure.

Evacuation Procedure

In the event of a fire alarm, the staff will execute the following evacuation plan.

General manager or manager on duty:

1. Report to the fire control panel located behind the service desk. This panel will indicate the location of the potential fire.
2. Immediately proceed or send someone to the location to determine whether the fire exists or if it is a false alarm. The person dispatched to the location should carry an emergency use cordless telephone or radio to expedite communication with the general manager or manager on duty.
3. If a fire does exist, call 911 from the fire control panel telephone.

   Provide the following information to the fire department dispatcher:

Your name:	John Doe
Club name:	ABC Club
Club address:	1234 Main Street
Club telephone:	222-222-2222
Location of the fire:	In the laundry room

   Advise them someone will meet them at the club's main entrance.

   Obtain an estimated time of arrival (ETA).

   Stay on the line until the dispatcher hangs up or you must evacuate.

   If it's a false alarm, the manager will sound the "all clear" alarm signaling that it is safe to reenter the building and reset the fire alarm system.
4. Make the following announcement on the Public Address System:

   "Attention members and guests: Please proceed to the nearest exit and leave the building. (Repeat three times.) Thank you." Repeat periodically during evacuation.
5. Dispatch a staff member to the main entrance to meet and lead the fire department to the fire.
6. Make final sweep of club, as possible, to ensure all persons have evacuated.

Department heads, managers, and fire wardens:

1. Department heads, managers, and trained fire wardens should proceed immediately to their stations when the fire alarm sounds to begin evacuation of the area. Execute the following responsibilities:
   a. Know all possible evacuation routes.

(continued)

Figure 13.10 Fire and evacuation plan.

b. Calmly direct members, guests, and staff to the nearest accessible exit.

Note: Elevators will not work. Be sure elevators are clear and direct to the nearest exit.

c. Delegate staff members to assist in evacuating the child care area. (Be aware that mothers and fathers may come to this area during the evacuation.)

d. Make a sweep of your assigned area to ensure all have evacuated.

e. Gather any and all records that may assist in ensuring all persons are accounted for: member and guest sign-in sheets, appointment books, staff schedules, etc.

f. Leave area closing all doors behind you.

g. Direct all persons to a predetermined area. Do not allow anyone to leave or reenter the building.

h. Report to the manager on duty that your area is all clear.

i. Begin process of accounting for all members, staff, and children.

Fire Safety Tips	
Heavy smoke	—Stay close to the ground and take small breaths.
Closed doors	—Before opening any closed doors, feel the door to see if it is hot. If it is hot, do *not* open the door.
Elevators	—The elevators will not work if the fire alarm has sounded.
Handicapped persons	—Delegate a staff member to assist handicapped persons.

Figure 13.10   *(continued)*

Aquatic Emergencies

A medical emergency in the aquatic facilities requires special considerations. Trained and certified Water Safety Instructors (WSI) or lifeguards typically handle aquatic emergencies until emergency personnel arrive. Specific aquatic emergency guidelines include the following:

- If the victim is unconscious, suspect a neck injury.

- Possible neck injury—Do not remove the victim from the water. Ensure all vital signs are stable. Stabilize the victim's head and body and await the arrival of emergency personnel. Use only the tools and techniques in which you are trained and well practiced.

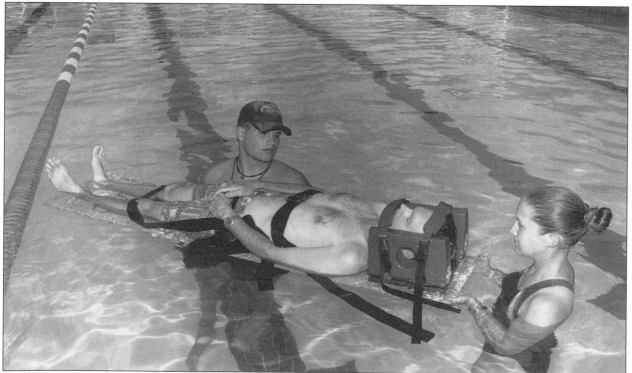

© Tom Wallace

- Possible drowning—Remove the victim from the pool. Turn victim on side to allow water to drain. Check vital signs and begin CPR or mouth-to-mouth resuscitation as necessary.

- Activate emergency procedure.

Aquatic emergency equipment and guidelines are required at all public pools. Check with local and state regulatory agencies for a complete listing of required aquatic safety and emergency equipment and guidelines. Samples of safety guidelines and emergency equipment include the following:

Safety signs—pool rules and so on

First aid kits

Life ring and buoys

First responder kits

Shepherd's crook

Backboard

Cervical ring

Megaphone

Clear depth markers on side of pool

Pool gates secured and locked when pool is closed

Emergencies Involving Children

The child care facility in every club should emphasize safety as a part of the daily operation. Even carefully supervised children will have accidents. Establish and practice safety procedures in the child care area. The following are some guidelines to ensure a safe play environment:

- Obtain a medical history on all children.

- Obtain a signed parental directive and emergency medical authorization form. (Seek advice of legal counsel in preparing this form.)

- Set rules requiring the parent or guardian to remain on property at all times.

- Create a safe play environment by covering all electrical outlets, removing or padding all sharp corners, installing padded carpet to protect against falls, and purchasing only child-safe toys and equipment.

- Maintain strict rules to ensure direct staff supervision at all times.

- Practice emergency procedures monthly.

- Conduct weekly safety inspections of indoor and outdoor play areas.

Disaster Plan

Disasters can come in many forms: earthquakes in California, hurricanes on the East Coast, terrorist acts in New York City and Oklahoma, and floods in the Midwest. Whether it is a violent weather storm, a flood, a shooting, or an act of terrorism, all endanger lives and create a costly disruption or perhaps financial ruin for the organization. As with medical emergencies, these problems are difficult (if not impossible) to prevent. However, being prepared when faced with a disaster situation could ensure the safety of the member, minimize liability, and control the extent of damage. Minimize the impact of a disaster with sound emergency and evacuation procedures that are practiced; complete insurance coverage evaluated annually (see chapter 18); a solid risk-management program; and strong communication channels with members, local business associates, and reciprocal clubs.

Weather Emergencies

Natural weather emergencies often strike with minimal warning. The geographic region where the facility is located will assist in predetermining the types of weather systems that may pose a threat. Preparation of emergency procedures when facing a tornado, hurricane, or flood will minimize liability and control damage. Points to consider when preparing a threatening weather plan include the following:

- Weather advisory television channels, radio stations, or telephone numbers.

- An outdoor activity (playgrounds, pools, athletic fields, etc.) evacuation plan.

- A communication plan and script for member communications.

- A predetermined evacuation zone or shelter and procedures to evacuate all members to this area.

- Definitions of commonly used watch and warning systems in the community.

- Specific procedures for member behavior depending on the type of threatening weather—tornado, lightning, hurricane, and so on.

Bomb Threat

It is unfortunate that this type of procedure is necessary for health fitness organizations. Although many of these threats turn out to be false alarms, they should never be taken lightly. Specific procedures for gathering information from the caller and prompt evacuation and follow-through procedures are necessary to

---

Information

Staff members receiving a bomb threat phone call should ask the following questions and complete this report. If you do not understand what the caller is saying, ask him/her to repeat.

1. When is the bomb going to explode?
2. Where is the bomb going to explode?
3. What does the bomb look like?
4. What will cause the bomb to explode?
5. Why did you place the bomb?
6. What is your name?
7. Where are you calling from?

What exactly did the caller say? _____

_____

Caller characteristics:

_____ male or female   _____ length of call

_____ approximate age   _____ race

_____ time of call   _____ extension call was received on

Voice characteristics (circle all appropriate responses):

serious   joking   anxious   very sure   unsure

Accent: what kind: _____   Familiar: who: _____

Background noises (circle all that apply):

street noises   restaurant/bar

voices   PA system

music   office sounds

machinery   animals

quiet   other: _____

_____

Time caller hung up: _____   Your name: _____

Procedures

Staff member receiving call:

1. Keep caller on the line as long as possible.
2. Contact general manager or MOD immediately.
3. Complete information checklist.

General manager/MOD

1. Contact local police department/bomb squad.
2. Contact building management.
3. Make decision regarding club evacuation.
4. Evacuate building using evacuation plan and script as follows:

   "Please cease exercise, gather your personal belongings and exit the building and proceed to (a predetermined location). This is not a drill."

5. If there is time, initiate search of immediate area or area indicated for any unusual objects. Do not touch any items found.
6. Await all clear signal from authorities.

Figure 13.11 Bomb threat information and procedures.

ensure the safety of the membership. Figure 13.11 shows an example of bomb threat procedures.

Nonlife-Threatening Emergencies

Nuisance emergencies, such as power outages or accidental fire sprinkler system activation, can create havoc in a facility in which the staff is not prepared. The facility manager or chief engineer should train staff members to respond quickly when faced with such an emergency.

Power Outage

Power outages occur frequently in many facilities. However, for those facilities in which a power outage is not routine, loss of power can frighten members if the staff does not confidently respond. Ensuring the safety of the membership is necessary to properly handle this type of situation. The following information may be helpful in creating a power outage response plan:

- Ensure no one has been hurt as a result of the sudden stoppage of equipment.
- Confidently communicate that someone is looking into the problem.
- Confidently request all members remain where they are until emergency generator lighting or flashlights are available to assist them in moving around the club.
- The director of maintenance or chief engineer should clearly label all breaker boxes in the electrical room so that trained personnel can locate a breaker that has switched off resulting in an isolated power outage.
- In the event of a complete power outage, ask members and staff to wait patiently for a few minutes to see if power is restored. If it is not restored quickly, ensure emergency lighting is working in all areas and assist members as necessary to exit the building.
- Once power is restored, check the calibration on all exercise equipment, reset time clocks and cash registers, reboot computers, and so on.

Accidental Activation of Fire Sprinkler System

Accidental activation of the fire sprinkler system can result in a great deal of water damage to the facility. Flooding of a facility can ruin expensive

National Health Club Association Safety Checklist

- Train staff to handle accidents that occur at your club. Have an incident report form that acting managers and witnesses can fill out.
- Have a regular maintenance schedule for all equipment and document it.
- Acquaint all new members with proper usage of exercise equipment.
- Make sure your membership agreement contains a release form outlining the inherent dangers involved in working out. Attach a hold-harmless statement to both the membership agreement and guest passes.
- If a piece of equipment is damaged or broken, render it inoperable and place a "do not use" sign securely on the unit.
- Train your staff in CPR and first aid. Require all instructors to be certified.
- Your wet area flooring should contain non-skid tile or similar surface.
- Conduct periodic staff meetings that deal exclusively with the safety of your club.
- Develop procedures regarding children under age 18 years and obtain written parental permission.
- If you sponsor events (i.e., bike races, marathons, weightlifting contests) that occur on your premises, be sure your insurance carrier is aware of these events.
- Have proper spacing of your exercise equipment stations. Be sure your members can move freely from station to station without bumping into other members during their exercise.
- Check all cables on your cable equipment for fraying. Also check to see if any snap shackles need replacing.
- Check barbells and dumbbells. Make sure the fixed weight ends are secure and tight.
- Secure all electrical cords between cardiovascular pieces so that members will not trip over them.
- Make sure that all temperature settings and timing devices on your Jacuzzi, steam room, and sauna are working properly. Have warning signs in this area of the club that deal with the use of these amenities and recommended time limits.

specialty wood flooring, such as a group exercise floor or racquet court. To prevent the accidental activation of the fire sprinkler system, incorporate the following suggestions into a regular maintenance checklist:

• Ensure all sprinkler heads are recessed or protected. Most instances of accidental activation occur when the exposed sprinkler head is knocked off or bumped loose. You can prevent this by ensuring heads are completely recessed or by placing a cage over exposed sprinkler heads.

• The maintenance director should train key personnel on the location and procedure to shut off this system.

Emergency Plan Evaluation

As stated throughout this section, an emergency plan is only effective if it is efficiently and effectively practiced and activated. For a facility with a high rate of staff turnover, we recommend monthly practice sessions. For facilities with a more stable staff who have repeatedly trained on these procedures, quarterly practice sessions may be adequate. Closely observe and document the response by management to each practice session.

However, practicing the emergency response system is not enough. Perhaps during a practice session an alarm or announcement was not audible in a particular area of the club, a staff member responded inappropriately, or a form was incomplete and needs modification. You can address all these issues during a vital debriefing session after each drill. Involve building management, maintenance, and local city resource departments in all emergency drills. These trained individuals may offer additional information or ideas that better prepare the staff to respond. Evaluating an emergency response plays a large part in the ongoing training of staff and should not be overlooked.

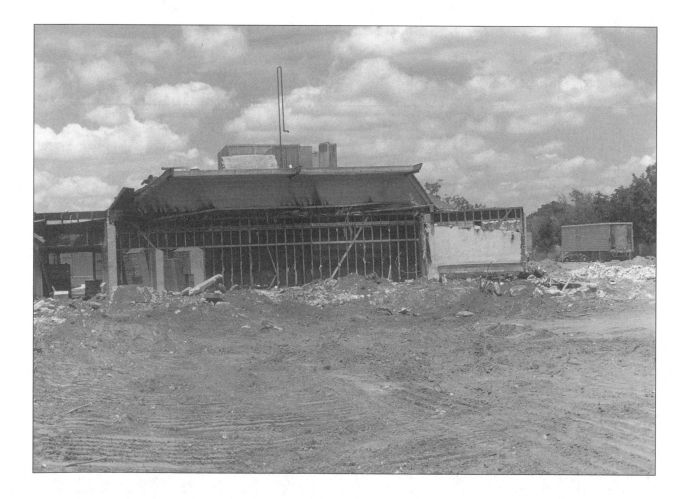

Following each practice session, require managers and staff to complete all paperwork, including incident reports and so on for the mock session. Finally, hold a staff debriefing session following each mock or actual activation of any part of the emergency system to discuss and refine all aspects of the response system.

RISK-MANAGEMENT DOCUMENTATION

Documentation is an important part of *risk management*. Maintaining complete records, including medical history, informed consent, physician release and parental consent forms, maintenance checklists, and safety surveys are invaluable in the event of an accident. Many of these forms and checklists have been presented throughout this text for your review. We recommend that each organization's legal counsel and medical director review these or any forms or checklists.

Maintenance Records and Safety Checklists

Regular maintenance inspections are important in preventing incidents or accidents. Maintenance inspections of exercise equipment, wet facilities, mechanical equipment, and the facility grounds will assist in identifying potential accident or injury situations. We presented extensive information regarding proper selection, installation, and maintenance of exercise equipment in chapter 12. We recommend preparation of an equipment history card and maintenance checklist for the specific equipment layout of the club. Chapter 14 includes samples

Task	Initials

Membership director:
  1. All new members complete health history questionnaire. Forms forwarded to fitness director for review.
  2. PAR-Q and guest registration completed on all guests.
  3. All reviewed health history and related forms filed properly.
	_____
	_____
	_____

Fitness director:
  1. All health history questionnaires reviewed by FD. Medical clearance forms requested where necessary.
  2. Equipment maintenance review and checklist complete.
  3. Maintenance requests written as necessary.
  4. CPR certifications current on all fitness staff.
  5. Emergency plan posted by all phones.
  6. Monthly emergency plan practice session complete.
  7. Aquatic emergency supplies in proper location.
	_____
	_____
	_____
	_____
	_____
	_____
	_____

Maintenance director/chief engineer:
  1. Mechanical system review and checklist complete.
  2. Fire warning system tested monthly.
  3. First aid and first responder kits fully stocked.
  4. Monthly test of emergency public address system complete.
  5. Weekly safety review and checklist of grounds complete.
  6. All sprinkler heads protected (recessed or cages).
	_____
	_____
	_____
	_____
	_____
	_____

Child care director:
  1. CPR certifications current on all child care staff.
  2. Outdoor equipment safety review and checklist complete.
  3. Parental consent forms current.
  4. Monthly emergency evacuation practice complete.
	_____
	_____
	_____
	_____

To be reviewed at weekly department head meetings.	

Figure 13.12 General manager's safety overview and checklist.

of this form as well as general facility and mechanical maintenance information and checklists. Proper maintenance of all club equipment and facilities provides a safer environment for the member. Proper documentation of regular maintenance practices provides the organization with a means of defense in the event of legal action. The National Health Club Association Safety Checklist is provided here.

Manager's Safety Checklist

Management of health and safety issues in a health fitness facility can demand a great deal of valuable time if not managed properly. You must insist on the awareness and action of all departmental managers and staff in this effort to offer a safe and productive environment. Appointing specific individuals who you can hold accountable for regular health and safety tasks (e.g., a safety ranger or chief) will assist in this large task. Weekly review of task completion and issues demanding a proactive

remedy will enable even the busiest general manager to be aware of health and safety issues in the facility. A reference checklist for general manager review can simplify this task. Figure 13.12 provides a basic checklist that you can modify to incorporate aspects of each individual facility.

SAFETY SUPPLIES

Safety supplies are essential to appropriately respond to an emergency. First aid kits that are completely stocked provide the necessary items to assist a member in the event of a minor cut or a life-threatening event. First responder kits provide the staff with all the OSHA required and suggested protective barriers necessary to respond to a medical emergency in which the potential for contamination exists. Biohazard spill cleanup kits package nicely all the personal protective devices and necessary cleaning supplies to reduce the risk of secondary

---

Table 13.1   First Aid Kit, First Responder Kit, and Biohazard Spill Kit Contents

First aid kit supplies

Ace elastic bandages	Cotton balls	Paper and pen
Alcohol pads	Cotton swabs	Plastic bags
Ammonia capsule	CPR protective mask	Prewrap
Antibiotic cream	Eye drops	Quarters
Antiseptic	Eye pads	Safety pins
Aspirin	First aid guidebook	Saline solution
Athletic tape	Flashlights	Scissors
Bandage—triangular	Gauze	Sterile pads
Band-Aids	Hydrogen peroxide	Telfa pads
Blister pads	Ibuprofen	Thermometer
Burn cream	Insect repellent	Tweezers
Cleansing towelettes	Instant cold packs	Tylenol
	Latex gloves	

First responder kit supplies

Apron (fluid proof)	Latex gloves	Safety glasses
CPR protective mask	Masks	Shoe covers
Face shield	Resuscitation bag	

Biohazard spill cleanup kit supplies

Biohazard materials bag	Disposable towels	Face shield
Bleach	Eye protection	Latex gloves

contamination following an incident in which possible infectious conditions exist. The contents of these important safety kits are listed in table 13.1.

Additional safety equipment that you should keep on hand are flashlights and *sharps containers*. Flashlights can assist during a medical emergency in which vision may be difficult without additional light and during power outages. OSHA requires the sharps containers for the proper disposal of any sharp items that may potentially cause a biohazard risk. Sharps containers prevent the accidental incision or puncture of a staff member by containing these items in a solid waste container. OSHA requires proper disposal of full sharps containers or any biohazard waste.

IN CLOSING

This chapter reviewed health and safety guidelines for all areas of the facility. We provided specific preexercise screening guidelines and samples of appropriate forms. Review your facility's safety plan quarterly to ensure proper accounting of all necessary practices. Refine specific health and safety policies and procedures in concert with the medical director and legal counsel.

KEY TERMS

Bloodborne pathogens

Emergency

Occupational Safety and Health Administration (OSHA)

Risk management

Sharps containers

Standard of care

RECOMMENDED READINGS

American Coaching Effectiveness Program. 1989. *Sports injuries, Level 2*. Champaign, IL: Human Kinetics.

American College of Sports Medicine. 1992. *ACSM's health/ fitness facility standards and guidelines*. Champaign, IL: Human Kinetics.

American College of Sports Medicine. 1995. *ACSM's guidelines for exercise testing and prescription*. 5th ed. Boston: Williams & Wilkins.

Arnheim, D. 1995. *Essentials of athletic training*. New York: Mosby.

Herbert, D. 1993. Emergency response may be a requirement. *Fitness Management* (November): 52.

————. 1994. Equipment related risk management. *Fitness Management* (May): 48.

International Health, Racquet and Sportsclub Association. 1995. *OSHA bloodborne pathogens standard briefing paper*. Boston: IHRSA.

Jacobs, P. 1994. Brace yourself. *Club Industry* (January): 16-18, 20-22.

National Health Club Association Safety Checklist. Denver, Colorado.

Occupational Safety and Health Administration Pamphlets. Pamphlets available through the Government Printing Office, Washington, DC, 202-219-9187.

> Protecting yourself against serious bloodborne infections on the job.

> Occupational exposure to bloodborne pathogens.

> Occupational exposure to bloodborne pathogens: Precautions for emergency responders.

Patton, R.W., W.C. Grantham, R.F. Gerson, and L.R. Gettman. 1989. *Developing and managing health/fitness facilities*. Champaign, IL: Human Kinetics.

CHAPTER 14

Facility Maintenance Management

Establishing a maintenance management program best suited for a health fitness organization is an important but arduous task. Realizing the positive impact that a clean, well-maintained facility has on prospective members and current member adherence; taking the necessary time to identify maintenance needs; developing and implementing a plan; and regularly evaluating the plan are essential for an organization's survival. In today's competitive market, operators must place a high priority on such areas as housekeeping, general maintenance, equipment repairs, renovation improvements, and preventive maintenance.

This chapter addresses the organizational steps involved in creating a maintenance program for the corporate, clinical, community, and commercial health fitness sectors. We discuss a four-step strategic planning process that incorporates a needs assessment, program planning, implementation, and evaluation. The chapter also discusses the various labor options available in different fitness settings, and concludes with how to organize and initiate a preventive maintenance program. The intent of the chapter is to present a guide for fitness professionals to follow in organizing and implementing a well-designed maintenance program.

The importance of keeping a clean and well-maintained facility cannot be emphasized enough. Today's consumer is more aware of the areas to evaluate when choosing a quality health fitness facility. Checklists established as guidelines for rating health fitness settings now classify facility convenience as number one, followed by maintenance and equipment upkeep, qualified staff, program variety, and organizational management. Otherwise said, in the eyes of a prospective member, having a clean facility ranks second in value when considering the purchase of a health fitness membership.

Maintaining a clean, well-kept facility is equally important to existing members. The results of annual member surveys have shown facility cleanliness ranks first in the areas members like most about a facility. For example, a recent survey conducted on 2,500 members of the Little Rock Athletic Club revealed that the three things members liked most about the club were the following:

1. Cleanliness of the facility—49 percent
2. Quality of the staff—34 percent
3. Facilities and atmosphere of the club—17 percent

The proper maintenance of a health fitness facility is easy to define and evaluate. However, achieving an acceptable, consistent level of maintenance is difficult. Generally, if everything is working properly and cleanliness is up to par, members are happy, and a facility manager should feel a sense of pride and accomplishment. Unfortunately, the dynamics of being in the health fitness business do not always provide this luxury.

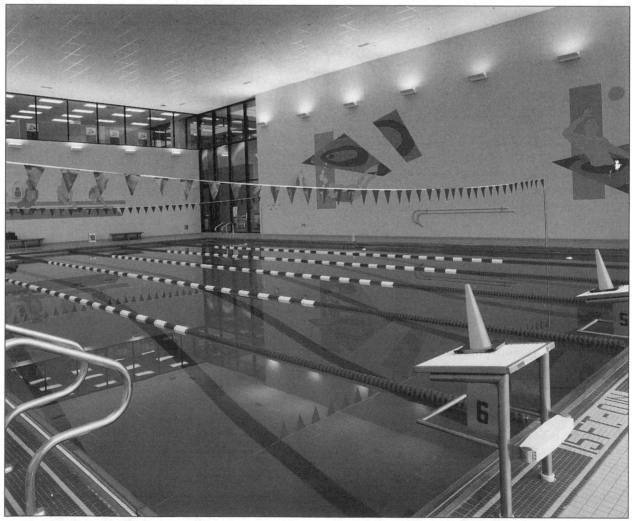

Courtesy of Dallas Texins Association

> *Often facility managers become jugglers, weighing the options of maintenance, repair, and replacement costs against profit, budget, and staffing priorities.*

We can define facility maintenance management as the set of work-ordered activities that, when properly managed, allow for continued operation of a facility. These activities include decisions, work orders, and actions taken by maintenance employees. The coordinated effort between management, employees, and other members of the maintenance team can make or break a facility.

FOUR AREAS OF MAINTENANCE MANAGEMENT

When discussing maintenance management there are four areas managers should focus on to ensure successful facility operation:

1. *Quality.* The difference between quality facilities and lesser facilities is noticeable. Consider all features of the facility from the ground up—floor surface, carpet, heating, ventilation, air-conditioning–*HVAC systems* equipment, wall surface, lighting, and so on. Today's health fitness facilities must not only look good, but be durable to withstand the test of time. The old adage, "You get what you pay for," is true where quality is considered.

2. *Safety.* All equipment in the facility must always be in top working order. In today's lawsuit-oriented society, club operators cannot afford to take risks when member's safety is involved. Strictly observe and evaluate potential liability areas (i.e., wet areas, weight rooms, swimming pools, day care, and restaurants). Preventive maintenance is the preferred method for enhancing member safety. Waiting until after an accident occurs to address a problem is too late and too expensive.

3. *Cleanliness.* The daily maintenance of a club must be thorough and consistent. A facility maintenance program should take into account such things as after-hours cleaning, locker-room maintenance, prime time cleaning, special events, parties, and outdoor maintenance. Each area has its unique need for workers, maintenance regimen, and supplies.

The goal of any maintenance program should be to transform qualitative care into quantitative care. In other words, become specific with the desired maintenance needs and communicate these needs to corresponding staff members.

4. *Amenities.* The extras included to service the member's needs are considered amenities. These items include such things as towels, swimsuit plastic bags, hangers in lockers, and personal toiletries (shampoo, conditioner, shaving cream, deodorant, body lotion, hair spray, etc.). Understanding your member's needs will determine the level of amenities and the most cost-effective way to provide them. Member's perception of quality is often dictated by the details. A smart operator never downplays the importance of the little things. Often these differences provide the touches necessary to separate an organization from the competition.

Use each of the following as an indicator for assessing and evaluating a facility, regardless of the setting. Continuous review of these four areas ensures that you always maintain a level of excellence.

DETERMINING MAINTENANCE NEEDS

Establishing and refining an organized facility maintenance program should be a goal of every manager. Because few fitness facilities have similar design, the scope of maintenance needs varies. The facility requirements for a full-service, multirecreational fitness facility are significantly different from those of a corporate club in an office building. Facilities encompassing 10,000 square feet do not have the same maintenance needs as a facility of 75,000 square feet. For example, operators of large multipurpose facilities allocate approximately seven percent of their total expenses for maintenance and repairs, whereas smaller facilities budget half of that amount. Larger facilities generally have both indoor and outdoor maintenance considerations, compared to predominately indoor needs for smaller facilities. Due to the increased complex size, larger facilities use both contract and in-house employees, and smaller facilities incorporate primarily in-house personnel.

Although many differences apply to settings with such size variances, you can apply the process you use for determining the required maintenance

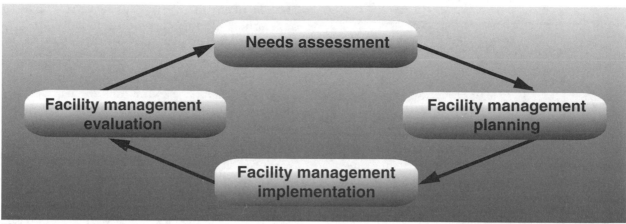

Figure 14.1 Facility management planning process.

to any setting, whether it be commercial, corporate, community, or clinical.

Developing a maintenance management program must start with a *strategic plan*. Everyone agrees that a maintenance program is necessary, but to what degree will you implement the program? How much money will it cost? Will you use additional personnel or contract labor? Should maintenance be performed after hours or only during the workday? These are questions that you must address during the early stages of organizing a maintenance program. Consider workforce, payroll, supplies, facility scheduling, and insurance risks. A sound strategic plan provides the direction to follow once you have established the profile of an organization.

Patton et al. (1989) found that a strategic management plan is a four-step, iterative process that involves

- assessing needs and interests,
- planning the program,
- implementing, and
- evaluating the program to ensure that goals are being met.

The cycling or *iterative process* is what makes this plan so effective. For example, as you implement and evaluate a maintenance program in the third and fourth stages, you collect information on how to improve for future planning. This cycling phase allows you to use information obtained from an initial program to design a new and improved model of maintenance. The manager then continues through the four stages on the follow-up program and so on. The four-stage management process is illustrated in figure 14.1.

NEEDS ASSESSMENT

The first stage in developing a facility maintenance program is to perform a *needs assessment* to evaluate the new or existing facility. You need a clear understanding of the size and scope of the organization to adequately assess maintenance needs.

The information phase of the I-formation model is when you can conduct surveys to obtain, evaluate, and analyze data for developing recommendations.

Perform a comprehensive facility evaluation that obtains answers to the following questions:

1. What is the overall size of the facility and grounds?
   - Determine the overall size of the facility by measuring each room and activity area to obtain total square footage or refer to construction plans.
   - If outdoor maintenance is required, establish the acreage or square footage of the grounds, and determine the specific uses for the area.
   - Note if the facility is totally enclosed in one building or separated into multiple complexes.

2. What are the hours of operation?
   - List the number of days per week the facility is open and the operating hours.
   - How is holiday scheduling handled?
   - Identify the best times of the day to perform maintenance.
   - What times per day do you consider prime time?
3. What is the operating budget for maintenance?
   - The various settings (corporate, commercial, clinical, or community) generally dictate the availability of funds.
   - If performing in-house maintenance, consider payroll, payroll taxes, supplies, and capital costs (equipment).
   - If contracting an outside service, obtain bids and determine a monthly charge for the service.
   - Weigh the costs of including a mix of contract labor and in-house personnel.
4. How many members are you serving daily?
   - What is the average number of members who use the facility daily?
   - Which days of the week are the busiest?
   - Are weekends a slower time for usage than weekdays?
5. What is the availability of staff?
   - Is in-house staff available to perform maintenance needs?
   - How will you divide the daytime and evening maintenance?
   - Can maintenance tasks coincide with other job responsibilities?
   - Is contracting for outside services a possibility?
6. What are the mechanical aspects of the facility?
   - Become familiar with the following areas in a plant:
     Pools—mechanical areas (filters, heaters, pumps, chlorinators, etc.)
     Spas—mechanical areas (filters, heaters, pumps, chlorinators, etc.)
     HVAC systems—heating, ventilation, and air-conditioning
     Boilers—steam rooms
     Water control systems and shut-off valves
     Electrical panel placement
     Lighting systems throughout the facility
     Security and energy management systems
     Emergency sprinkler systems

Whether considering in-house personnel or contracting with an outside cleaning service, the next step in the needs assessment process is to establish itemized cleaning and maintenance specifications for each room and activity area. Outline a detailed description of the nightly, daily, and weekly tasks for the complex. Give additional consideration to special use areas that require specific maintenance and cleaning treatments. For example, in a locker room the various cabinet finishes and floor surfaces used, such as carpet, tile, and marble, all have certain requirements for proper cleaning. Address each area before contract labor or in-house employees begin a regular maintenance schedule. Figure 14.2 provides a sample cleaning task list.

After compiling a facility cleaning task list, if you are considering in-house maintenance, develop a list of supplies, vendors, and equipment (carpet cleaners, pool vacuum systems, automatic scrubbers, etc.). This step allows operators the opportunity to become familiar with the various types of chemicals available, how they should be applied, and their corresponding interactions with other chemicals. Managers will also be introduced to working with vendors and learning the supply and cost side of the business.

After completing the needs assessment, perform data analysis to define where the organization is currently and where it wants to be in the future. The answers you obtain from the needs assessment provide a road map to follow while presenting ways to implement the program. The analysis provides answers to such questions as the following: Is the facility large enough to justify the cost of contracting for maintenance services or should in-house personnel be used? Does the number of members served daily support both a daytime and evening housekeeping crew? Does the number of mechanical and electrical systems validate the need for a full-time operations manager? Is the operating budget large enough to support the maintenance needs of the organization?

During the needs assessment phase, managers must keep in mind that every facility is unique. Factors such as the existing facility layout, equipment placement, wall partitions and barriers, types of furniture and fixtures, and local and state regulatory statutes are some areas to consider when establishing a maintenance program. Collectively, these factors play an important role in determining which direction to follow when assessing the various cleaning and maintenance options available.

Supervisor Work Assignment

SHIFT: 1, 2   Date: _____/_____/_____   Supervisor: _____

General duties: Supervisors are responsible for seeing that all shift personnel are in proper uniform, and that the uniforms are clean and worn neatly. Also, supervisors will review daily the accuracy and integrity of staff time cards.

Position	Duties	Freq/time
Laundry	1. All equipment is clean and operating properly.	[ ] Hourly
	2. Load each washer to no more that 3/4 full.	[ ] Hourly
	3. Load each dryer to bottom of dryer window.	[ ] Hourly
	4. Towels are folded and stacked with round ends together.	[ ] Hourly
	5. Room is clean and neat.	[ ] Hourly
	6. Lint traps are cleaned.	[ ] Hourly
	7. Washers and dryers are never left unattended during operation.	[ ] Every 2 hours
Locker rooms	1. Shelves are stacked with clean towels.	[ ] Hourly
	2. Soiled towels are in bins for return to the laundry.	[ ] Every 1/2 hr
	3. Vanity toiletries have been stocked; sink tops, bowls, and drains have been cleaned.	[ ] Every 1/2 hr
	4. Soap/shampoo dispensers have been cleaned and filled and are working.	[ ] Hourly
	5. All mirrors have been cleaned; light bulbs are working.	[ ] Every 2 hours
	6. Large and small wastebaskets are not filled more than 2/3 full.	[ ] Hourly
	7. Carpets have been swept or vacuumed.	[ ] As needed
	8. Saunas and whirlpools have clean towels, papers, cups, etc. Check for proper temperature.	[ ] Hourly
	9. All hair dryers are clean and working.	[ ] Hourly
Housekeeping	1. Large and small wastebaskets in lounge and bar have been emptied.	[ ] Hourly
	2. Vacuum club manager's and accountant's offices; trash has been emptied.	[ ] Before 9 A.M.
	3. Exterior property is free of all trash.	[ ] Before 9 A.M. and 4 P.M.
	4. Public bathrooms are clean and neat; supplies have been filled.	[ ] Hourly
	5. Fourth floor locker rooms are maintained (cf. steps 1-6 in L/R).	[ ] Hourly
	6. All vinyl floor surfaces are spot cleaned as needed.	[ ] Hourly
	7. Lounge area is free of paper, cups; carpet is spot cleaned as needed.	[ ] Hourly
	8. Stairways and walls are spot cleaned as needed.	[ ] Hourly
	9. Nursery trash has been emptied and toilet cleaned.	[ ] Before end of shift

Figure 14.2 Supervisor work assignment—cleaning task list.

FACILITY MAINTENANCE PLANNING

Facility maintenance planning uses the information derived from the needs assessment and applies that data toward the management plan. Having a clear understanding of the scope of cleaning and maintenance requirements for the facility plan allows management the opportunity to choose a format best suited for the club. Without incorporating the needs assessment it is difficult to establish goals and objectives for the maintenance division.

Maintenance goals vary considerably, depending on the intended use of the facility. Some typical maintenance goals include the following:

Maintenance Goals and Objectives

Overall Maintenance Goal

To provide economical maintenance and housekeeping services allowing the facility to be used for its intended purpose.

Specific Maintenance Objectives

- Perform daily housekeeping and cleaning to maintain a presentable facility.
- Promptly respond to and repair minor deficiencies in the facility or equipment.
- Develop and implement a system of regularly scheduled maintenance to prevent premature failure of the facility, its systems, and equipment.
- Operate the facility utilities in the most economical manner while providing necessary reliability.
- Provide easy and complete reporting and identification of necessary repairs and maintenance work.
- Maintain proper level of materials and spare parts to support timely repairs.
- Accurately track the costs of all maintenance work.
- Perform cost bidding to ensure lowest cost solutions to maintenance problems.
- Monitor the progress of all maintenance work.
- Maintain historical data concerning the facility, mechanical systems, and exercise equipment.

The goal statement defines the emphasis or direction for the maintenance effort and should indicate the intensity of effort required. For example, if a goal states that the locker rooms are to consistently meet the maintenance standards established by management, then this should be emphasized to the person(s) responsible for cleaning that area. For goals to be effective they must be enforced with specific objectives. These objectives should address the various components of the entire maintenance program.

Components of daily maintenance work include activities that maintain and restore the function of the facility. This category is divided into the following subdivisions: housekeeping, general maintenance, preventive maintenance, repair, replacement, improvement, and utilities. Place each maintenance task in one of these categories. Although the names of these categories are likely to vary from setting to setting, the basic elements, as listed, are present in every facility maintenance program.

Housekeeping

Housekeeping is the group of daily tasks—basic cleaning, emptying trash receptacles, replacing towels and toilet paper, sweeping, mopping, and dusting—that make the facility presentable and functional for member and guests. A sample objective for the housekeeping function is the following:

Ensure that all locker-room facilities are cleaned at least once every 20 minutes.

General Maintenance

General maintenance might also be referred to as infrequent housekeeping. General maintenance often requires trained personnel to use specialized equipment. Typical general maintenance activities include steam-cleaning carpets, painting walls, stripping and rewaxing wood floors, changing filters on heating and air-conditioning equipment, and sweeping parking lots. General maintenance improves and preserves the appearance of a facility and is performed at regular intervals based on seasonal considerations and aesthetic preferences. An objective for general maintenance is the following:

Promptly respond to and repair any discrepancies or deficiencies in facility operations.

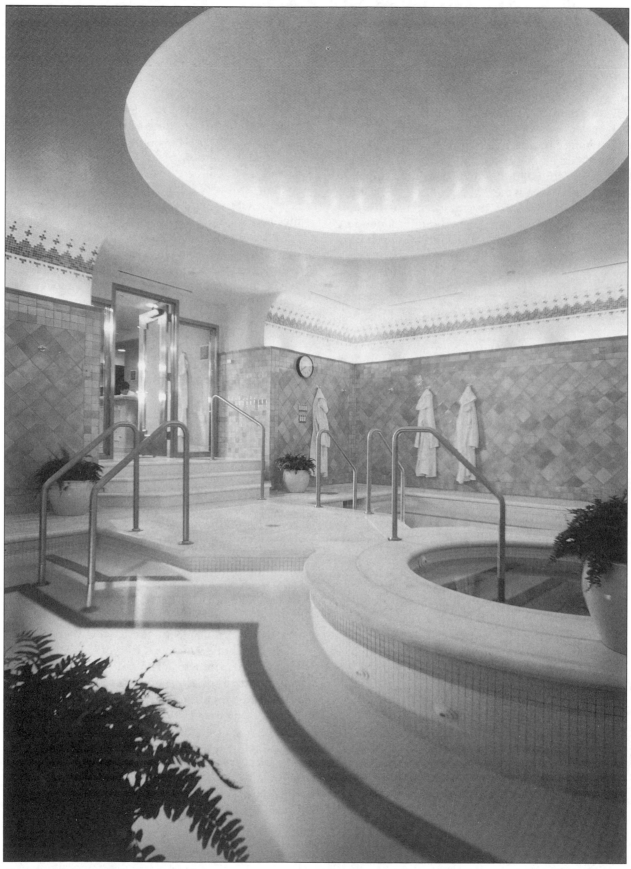

Courtesy of The Spa at the Crescent, Dallas, Texas

Preventive Maintenance

Preventive maintenance comprises a major portion of the maintenance effort in a health fitness facility. These tasks are intended to ensure the continuous operation of all areas within the facility. Preventive maintenance programs are performed at regular intervals, usually by a skilled employee.

The difference between preventive maintenance and general maintenance is that the preventive maintenance tasks are established by manufacturer's recommendations and should be followed to maintain the life of the equipment.

When preventive maintenance is neglected, dramatic, costly, and potentially dangerous failures often occur. For this reason, consider a formal preventive maintenance program a high priority. A preventive maintenance objective is the following:

Establish a program of routine inspection and service of exercise equipment to prevent premature failures.

Repairs

Repair work involves restoring to operation some component or piece of equipment after it has failed. Unfortunately, failures do not occur at convenient times and must be dealt with immediately, usually at the expense of other scheduled maintenance. In establishing objectives for completing repairs, it is often necessary to set priorities based on the importance of need for repair. These priorities set the maximum time required to complete repairs. Therefore, as problems occur, the repair is classified by priority and workload. Repairs that are not immediately required (low priority) are often reclassified for future scheduling. A typical objective for repair work is the following:

Complete 90 percent of all repair work within a designated time (i.e., within one to three weeks of notification, depending on the nature of the repair).

Replacement

Replacement, as a facility management element, is confined to a program of planned replacement of facility components. It may include such things as air-conditioning compressors, furnaces or water heaters, or steam room generators. Replacement is performed when the equipment has reached the end of its useful life—when it can no longer perform due to internal damage or its repair is no longer cost effective.

Although the decision to replace a piece of equipment is generally inevitable, it is not without a variety of options. Accordingly, a program of planned replacement should revolve around the costs of the equipment, installation, and maintenance. Considering these factors, a maintenance manager has an opportunity to analyze the impact of using a different model that is perhaps more expensive initially, but requires less repair or energy to operate and is not replaced as often. The replacement objective for a facility is the following:

Establish a program of planned replacement of facility components that replaces failing equipment with new or rebuilt components.

Improvements

Improvement projects enhance the proper operation and can possibly reduce the operating costs for a facility. These projects may include installing an energy management system to conserve electricity, upgrading an existing pool filter system to improve water clarity, or providing security cameras for members' safety. Each improvement positively affects the overall efficiency of operating and managing a complex.

The age of the facility or the equipment already in place dictates other maintenance projects, but improvement projects are often initiated by the operations manager or general manager. Although the initial cost of an improvement project may appear high, the long-range results should always reflect a cost savings to the facility or an increased perceived value to the member. An improvement objective is the following:

Identify and conduct any improvement project that will provide a payback of the initial investment in three years or less.

Utilities

The maintenance areas previously discussed have generally required on-site labor. However, utilities work calls for skilled laborers from the utility companies or independent electrical or plumbing contractors. Utilities work includes furnishing electrical power, water, gas, collection and disposal of sewage and other wastes, as well as disposal of storm water.

Local municipal utility companies usually provide utilities for small health fitness settings (smaller than 34,000 square feet). In this instance, the involvement of a maintenance manager is minimal. For most small to midsize facilities, the utility responsibilities are limited to verifying monthly bills and calling the utility company when service is interrupted or repairs are required.

However, in larger settings (greater than 85,000 square feet) the involvement of a full-time operations manager is a necessity. Some facilities have full electrical generating equipment, boilers for heat distribution, and even a small sewage treatment plant. Such systems become minifacilities within themselves, requiring around the clock attention. These systems are a large investment and contribute substantially to the operating cost of a facility. An objective for utilities is the following:

To regularly maintain and immediately respond to any and all utility problems or repairs.

EVALUATING STAFFING OPTIONS

A principal function of the maintenance planning process is to list the primary categories of facility management and match those categories to a respective setting. In some cases, the operating manager is responsible for all facets of the facility; in others, there is a shared responsibility involving outside vendors or contract personnel.

For example, in a corporate fitness setting, the housekeeping and repair work could be the responsibility of the landlord of the building or the corporation. In a commercial setting the operations manager may be in charge of all the subdivision areas. Despite the setting, define each maintenance category and identify responsibilities before evaluating staff options or establishing job descriptions.

Out of the needs assessment and program planning phase emerges a maintenance organization of a particular size and scope necessary to meet the goals and objectives of the facility. In IHRSA's 1994 annual industry data survey, *Profiles of Success*,

facility standards have been established for different sizes of commercial fitness facilities. For the purpose of describing the relationship between management and the maintenance organization, three classes of organizations are used:

Large facility—85,000 square feet and more

Midsize facility—34,000 to 85,000 square feet

Small facility—34,000 square feet or less

Large Facility Maintenance

Large health fitness centers often have several layers of divisions and use full-time maintenance personnel, the number of which depends on the facility size. The operations director or facility manager is generally a skilled person with a mechanical background and previous experience in facility management. The facility manager answers directly to the manager of the club and has a support staff available for both daytime and evening maintenance. The facility manager's overall responsibility is to coordinate the direct effort of the maintenance division. Internal personnel, often referred to as locker-room attendants, handle daytime housekeeping responsibilities. Primary duties of a locker-room attendant

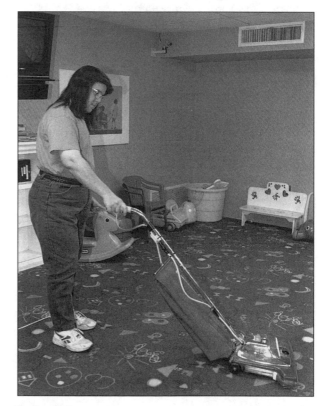

© Tom Wallace

include maintaining a clean and sanitized locker room, providing general facility maintenance, and performing laundry tasks. Either a contract maintenance service or an in-house staff with a supervisor usually conduct evening housekeeping. In some cases, independent contract services are hired on retainer to maintain HVAC, boiler, or pool systems.

Maintenance personnel in a large setting generally have regularly assigned duties and have the workforce to perform preventive maintenance. As a result, they can prevent or quickly repair many mechanical problems. This benefit is not always available to midsize and small clubs, which end up spending most of their days putting out fires. A sample organizational chart for a large fitness organization is shown in figure 14.3

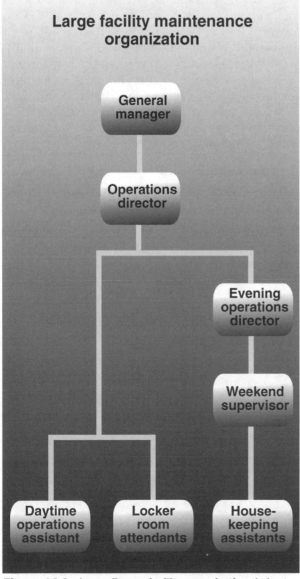

Figure 14.3   Large fitness facility organizational chart.

Midsize Facility Maintenance

Although in a midsize setting the maintenance needs are reduced, the basic elements of control and execution that apply to a large facility also exist. Overall maintenance responsibilities usually belong to a multitalented maintenance supervisor who has knowledge of a variety of mechanical systems. The maintenance supervisor is sometimes assisted by either a part-time or full-time employee who performs minor repairs and equipment upkeep. Because housekeeping is a major portion of the work, locker-room attendants or service desk personnel are regularly scheduled to complete pre-assigned tasks around the high usage areas of the facility. Evening housekeeping is performed by either a contract maintenance service or an in-house crew with a supervisor. Service contractors are brought in to perform major repairs, such as plumbing, HVAC, and electrical work.

Operations in a midsize maintenance organization are less structured than those of a large organization. More time is spent in emergency responses and repairing minor equipment problems than modifying and improving the facility. Communication is a primary consideration for the midsize maintenance organization. Consequently, key members of the maintenance staff usually carry walkie-talkies or pagers to alert staff of problems in a timely fashion. Figure 14.4 illustrates the structure of a midsize maintenance organization.

Small Facility Maintenance

Generally in small health fitness organizations, only one or two people are involved in maintenance. In such a setting, the maintenance worker, a jack-of-all-trades, works directly for the general manager and is responsible for all maintenance duties. Housekeeping is handled internally with all levels of personnel involved in the daytime cleaning. In the evening, housekeeping duties are performed by staff before closing or designated employees assigned to complete more rigorous cleaning tasks. A small setting uses contract services more than a midsize facility. In small facilities, the major system components (plumbing, heating, air-conditioning, electrical) are repaired almost exclusively by service contractors. A sample organizational chart for a small club setting is shown in figure 14.5.

You can adapt the three classes of maintenance management (large, midsize, and small) to fit most health fitness facility needs. The reasons for

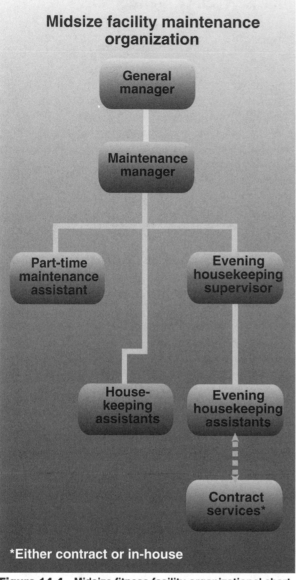

Figure 14.4 Midsize fitness facility organizational chart.

choosing to conduct maintenance internally are plentiful—better control, scheduling flexibility, hiring individuals with requisite skills, ability to define specific duties, and quick response to emergency maintenance tasks. However, if conditions are not favorable for hiring an internal staff, consider contracting for maintenance services.

Contracting for Maintenance Services

In the commercial health fitness industry, *contract maintenance* usually refers to such services as evening housekeeping, general repair and preventive maintenance of equipment (both exercise and mechanical), lawn care, and computer and pool maintenance. Although these services are used as needed, rarely does a facility manager contract all maintenance work to an outside service. Consequently, it is not uncommon to have a mix of in-house and contracted services to obtain the quality of maintenance services required. Analyzing the needs assessment and cost comparisons between each option suggests the best direction to follow. There are, however, several factors that may allow an independent contractor to provide services at a lower cost than in-house employees:

- Specialization allows higher productivity.
- Specialization allows the purchase of expensive servicing and diagnostic equipment.
- Spare parts inventory can ensure quicker repair time.
- Employee benefits can be varied with greater flexibility.

Make the choice between hiring in-house employees and contracting for services based on several factors:

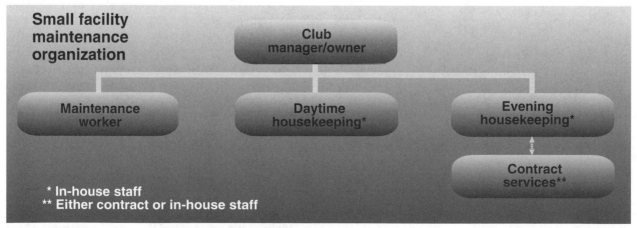

Figure 14.5 Small fitness facility organizational chart.

- *Frequency of need.* Certain maintenance actions are necessary only infrequently or seasonally. For example, the routine inspection and preventive maintenance for heating and air-conditioning systems requires a skilled technician, yet few health fitness facilities have the number of HVAC systems to justify a full-time worker. You may reduce or control maintenance costs by identifying these infrequent maintenance activities and considering the cost of contracted services.

- *Inadequate in-house personnel.* Depending on the complexity of an organization's mechanical equipment, having qualified personnel may be essential. The sophistication of some systems may require the contract services of specialists. State and local regulations may require a particular level of qualification and licensing for certain work. If in-house personnel do not possess or cannot obtain such certifications, you should provide contracted services.

- *Workload and staff balancing.* A dilemma occurs when some maintenance work can be performed by in-house personnel, but there is only enough to justify part-time employment. It may be possible to combine several of these tasks to justify a single maintenance person. Creating a full-time job by combining work tasks provides the desired flexibility and responsiveness for emergency maintenance needs. However, you should cover overflow work by a contract service or through authorized overtime rather than adding a potentially underused employee to the payroll.

- *Other cost considerations.* Adding a maintenance employee to an organization's payroll requires assuming the employee benefits costs of an additional employee. These benefits commonly include health care insurance, workers' compensation insurance, retirement plans, bonuses, paid vacations, and several other benefits. Even if there is justification to use in-house maintenance personnel, the added cost of providing full benefits may be too expensive. In the unskilled trades (housekeeping, security, child care), the cost of contracted services is often less than the total cost of wages and benefits combined.

In a corporate fitness setting, maintenance is generally contracted through a service provided by either the building landlord or the corporation. Because the fitness facility is housed on company grounds this maintenance arrangement is usually the only option available. Unfortunately, this method does not always ensure a well-maintained and clean atmosphere. The maintenance standards for a fitness facility are much higher than for an office building. Regular facility usage by clients through-out the day necessitates continued housekeeping and maintenance repair. Periodic cleaning by a building maintenance crew is both impractical and inefficient. Consider identifying the areas that need emphasis and renegotiating with the company for additional maintenance services.

The maintenance arrangement for a clinical setting is similar to a corporate fitness facility. If the facility is on the hospital campus, the wellness or fitness center usually contracts with the hospital maintenance staff for housekeeping and general repair. Because the cleaning standards and consistent housekeeping requirements for a hospital are much higher, this system has proven to be more effective than in the corporate setting. Those facilities that are off the hospital campus have the option of entering into a contractual arrangement with an outside service or hiring personnel for maintenance and housekeeping needs.

Community fitness facilities have the same options available as commercial settings. They may choose to enter a contractual arrangement with an outside cleaning service, hire their own maintenance and housekeeping personnel, or use a combination of both options. Some community settings can contract cleaning services already being used by that city to perform evening cleaning duties. During the day most community centers use a limited maintenance staff and in-house personnel to accomplish all maintenance and housekeeping needs.

If given the option, health fitness managers should choose to have on-site, qualified maintenance staff available. There is great security in knowing that quick response time is available for any maintenance problem. However, smaller facilities might find that financial limitations dictate that fitness staff or service desk attendants may have to assist with maintenance responsibilities. Although not preferred, if supervised and scheduled properly, this approach can accomplish the necessary housekeeping goals. This option should always be weighed against the possible negative effect on customer service and the maintenance standards established for the facility.

IMPLEMENTING A MAINTENANCE PROGRAM

Patton et al. (1986) reported that implementing any program involves five steps:

1. Reviewing the planned objectives for the program
2. Reviewing the planned tasks for the staff

3. Delegating the tasks to the staff

4. Scheduling the tasks for action

5. Supervising the program implementation to ensure tasks are accomplished

This model assumes that the needs assessment has been analyzed, goals and objectives identified, staff or contract labor hired, and the maintenance plan is ready to be implemented.

The I-formation management model (chapter 4) defines this area of management as an implementation phase, taking into account maintaining operations, diagnosing problem areas, identifying efficiencies, and monitoring results. This phase establishes whether the implementation of the maintenance program will meet the requirements of the needs assessment.

In addition to the steps mentioned, an integral part of implementing a maintenance program is to identify functions that facilitate the maintenance work performed. These functions assist in identifying and coordinating the daily tasks and ensure the proper level of maintenance is being sustained. Such functions include

- work identification;
- scheduling;
- purchasing, supplies, and inventory control;
- cost controls;
- equipment and mechanical histories; and
- work tracking and monitoring.

These functions are inclusive and may not be present in every health fitness setting. Depending on size and scope, some managers may choose to implement only a few of the functions, and others may fully integrate all the functions mentioned. Despite the setting, we recommend that management personnel are familiar with and understand how to implement each function if deemed necessary.

Work Identification

All maintenance work has a point of origin. Preventive maintenance, for example, is a planned activity scheduled to prevent equipment breakdown or to meet seasonal needs, such as switching from heat to air-conditioning. Housekeeping is a regularly scheduled activity. However, general maintenance and repair work are not scheduled until someone notices a problem and reports it to the maintenance staff. In the case of preventive maintenance and the daily rounds of equipment checks, the staff should log any problems they notice for repair. Implement a formal reporting system to identify needed repairs. In addition to using maintenance personnel, club operators depend on staff and member input for obtaining work orders. Many facilities have found that adopting a work order request form successfully allows staff and members to report maintenance or equipment problems. A sample work order request form is shown in figure 14.6 and is discussed in detail later in this chapter.

Request for Maintenance Services		
Description of requested services		
Location	**Work requested by**	**Phone**
Date submitted	**Request priority (please circe one)**	A - Immediate attention B - Urgent attention C - Routine attention
Below portion to be completed by Maintenance Division		
Special instructions		
Date completed	**Completed by**	**Time to complete**
Remarks		
Repair costs		

Figure 14.6   Request for maintenance services.

Scheduling

Because maintenance work elements are both planned (preventive maintenance and housekeeping) and unplanned (repairs), the maintenance manager or general manager must be able to schedule accordingly. Typically, in the health fitness business it is necessary to provide scheduled staff for the jobs planned while maintaining flexibility for unforeseen problems that frequently occur. Develop fixed schedules to cover such areas as preventive maintenance and housekeeping. Identify tasks with a corresponding time goal for completion. Anticipate time intervals for the unexpected repair work as well. Developing historical data for the time it takes to perform various tasks is the only way to prepare a realistic schedule. Depending on the size of the facility, some managers incorporate daily time logs to track work completion. Figure 14.7 provides a sample maintenance schedule.

Purchasing, Supplies, and Inventory Control

As maintenance work is routinely carried out, there is a constant need for materials and supplies to sustain the work being performed. This necessitates a system for predicting needs, purchasing, and inventorying materials and supplies. According to *Cleaning Maintenance Management Magazine* (Williams 1994), when preparing an annual maintenance budget, two factors help predict total supplies needed and proper inventory levels for a year: frequency of need and the impact of not having a sufficient supply on hand. Routine preventive maintenance tasks require a predictable type and quantity of materials. Repairs, being unpredictable, may cause interruptions to facility operations if parts are not readily available.

A common procedure for ordering supplies and materials is through a *purchase order system*. The

	Tuesday evening cleaning shift **Assigned to housekeeping supervisor**
Time	**Facility area**
6:00 P.M. – 6:30 P.M.	Clean administrative offices, tennis entry and walk, and lower hallway.
6:30 P.M. – 8:00 P.M.	Continuously walk through facility correcting problem areas; provide special attention to rear hallways, employee entrance, and rear stairways.
8:00 P.M. – 9:00 P.M.	Clean aerobic studio and transition area.
9:00 P.M. – 9:30 P.M.	Clean day care.
9:30 P.M. – 10:00 P.M.	Lunch break.
10:00 P.M. – 10:30 P.M.	Clean fitness and membership offices. ***Place vacuum in pool.**
10:30 P.M. – 12:30 P.M.	Sweep designated indoor tennis courts (see schedule).
12:30 P.M. – 1:00 A.M.	Empty trash cans on all tennis courts and pick up loose trash around courts.
1:00 A.M. – 2:00 A.M.	Clean gymnasium floor, floor molding, backboards, and water fountains. Spot clean all racquetball courts, clean glass, and dust mop all wood floors. ***Remove vacuum from pool.**
2:00 A.M. – 2:15 A.M.	Walk through the entire facility for problem areas; check and lock all entry doors; set security alarm.
	Housekeeping assistant evening schedule
8:00 P.M. – 11:00 P.M.	Clean assigned areas per housekeeping guideline.
11:00 P.M. – 11:30 P.M.	Break time.
11:30 P.M. – 2:30 A.M.	Clean assigned areas per housekeeping guideline.
	Laundry assistant evening schedule
10:30 P.M. – 2:30 A.M.	Launder all soiled towels and member laundry. Return clean laundry to the front desk.

Figure 14.7 Sample maintenance schedule.

purpose of a purchase order system is to internally account for all maintenance items ordered and received. A purchase order describes what specific supplies you need to order, the estimated cost, what vendor you are using, bids from various vendors, who is ordering the supplies, and management authorization. Figure 14.8 provides a sample purchase order form. Each order is given a number and filled out in duplicate with a copy given to the employee who initiated the order and the bookkeeper or accounting department. If the amount of the order is higher than a prearranged limit, approval must be obtained through management before initiating the order. When the supplies arrive, the purchase order and vendor invoice are matched before acceptance. Only a system of this nature can provide accountability against cost overruns and unnecessary supplies being ordered.

The level of the inventory control depends on the size and control of the inventory. In most health fitness settings the maintenance workforce is small, the facility systems are simple, and the number of renovation projects are minimal. Consequently, the facility manager or maintenance person can keep the supplies and spare parts inventory mentally. If the complexity of the facility increases (through renovations or expanded sites), you must formalize a system for monitoring the level of consumables (toilet paper, Kleenex, paper towels, etc.). You can do this manually or through a computer system. Manually, inventories are usually maintained on index cards in a file. When an order is received, the quantity of new materials is added to the index card. When products are expended, the quantity used is subtracted from the card. If you regularly update this system and there is sufficient security on the stored materials, you can rely on a manual system to depict the inventory status. Have one person be responsible for issuing purchasing orders, maintaining the number entry, and verifying management's approval of the purchase. You can set up a computer inventory system to automatically generate purchase orders for inventory items when the stock level reaches a designated low point.

Purchase Order

Date: _____   Date needed: _____

Name: _____   Dept.: _____

Vendor: _____

Item	Item #	Qty	Price	Page
_____	_____	_____	_____	_____
_____	_____	_____	_____	_____
_____	_____	_____	_____	_____
_____	_____	_____	_____	_____
_____	_____	_____	_____	_____
_____	_____	_____	_____	_____

Purpose or event: _____
_____
_____

For Office Use Only

Date ordered: _____   PO #: _____

Vendor #: _____   Invoice #: _____

Amount	G/L code	G/L #
_____	_____	_____
_____	_____	_____

Obtained from general supplies: Yes _____   No _____

If yes, which ones? _____

Figure 14.8   Purchase order form.

Cost Controls

Although most health fitness organizations have an accounting system that monitors accounts payables and receivables (see chapter 15), it is the ultimate responsibility of the maintenance manager to identify and code all supplies and materials used. Without this interaction between accounting and maintenance it would be difficult to control the cost breakdowns between divisions (i.e., fitness, tennis, day care, pro shop, restaurant, etc.). Despite the scope of the setting, maintenance managers must have a system (manual or computer) to provide feedback for the maintenance transactions that occurred that day.

The purpose of cost accounting is to measure the ongoing and historical costs of each maintenance activity. From this measurement, the maintenance manager can make decisions to redirect or reallocate resources to reduce possible cost overruns. For example, excessive overtime costs might lead to hiring or reassigning additional full-time personnel. The maintenance manager also has the ability to frequently monitor and manage the annual budget to meet financial goals. Consequently, the timeliness of reporting ongoing costs is an essential factor.

Equipment and Mechanical Histories

To properly predict and adjust the maintenance program, the manager must have a thorough understanding of the life of the particular facility and the components within the facility. Only with a total building history can you make proper decisions regarding the best course of maintenance for a given problem. Keep accurate documentation of all construction and renovation plans. Track major and recurring minor repairs. Record periodic inspections by the health department, OSHA, and fire department and update them for future reference. Accurate facility records enable immediate troubleshooting and repairs.

A proper equipment history should include the make and model of the equipment, date of installation, all major repairs, any preventive maintenance, and parts replaced. You can use a regularly maintained equipment history to predict the need for eventual replacement or rebuilding of a unit, or when trying to diagnose an unexpected problem, which you can often trace to a recent repair. Figure 14.9 provides a sample equipment history form.

Equipment History Card		
Equipment name		
Manufacturer		**Model No.**
Equipment location		**Specific installation area**
Date of original installation		**Installed by**
Equipment Repair History		
Data	**Description**	**Repair costs**

Figure 14.9 Equipment history form.

Work Tracking and Monitoring

In addition to monitoring the cost of all the maintenance work performed, it is important to ensure that all work is completed in a timely manner.

> *Because forgotten preventive maintenance or neglected repair work can frequently lead to costly repairs, facility downtime, or potential injury of an employee or member, we recommend a system for tracking the source, assignment, and accomplishment of all work.*

Establish internal procedures to alert management or operations personnel of all maintenance problems. Follow this with a corresponding system to ensure quick turnaround of all repairs and to inform the member of expected completion time. If you do not accomplish member-identified minor repairs in a reasonable amount of time, the member may decide that it is useless to report minor problems. If minor problems are not reported, they could lead to major problems. Consequently, the work tracking system must be timely and complete.

Most health fitness facilities use a work request form (see figure 14.6) to track member-identified repairs or problem areas. The work request form should provide space for the following information:

• *What*—a concise statement of the problem. There is sometimes the tendency to request specific actions or solutions rather than stating the problem.

• *Where*—the location of the problem. Depending on the size of the facility, this may include the name of the specific area where the problem has occurred or any other necessary information to enable the maintenance worker to locate the problem.

• *Who*—the name and phone number of the member or employee making the request. The maintenance staff uses this to obtain further information on the problem or to let the member know when work has been completed.

• *When*—the date and time that the request was made. Include follow-up information regarding when the repairs were made, who completed the repairs, and how long it took to fix. Also include estimated or actual repair costs for parts to assist bookkeeping in tracking overall repair charges.

These forms are usually placed at strategic points (check-in desk, membership office, locker rooms) around a facility where members or employees may quickly and conveniently report any repair work needed. Once the work is completed, the work request forms are recorded and filed for future reference.

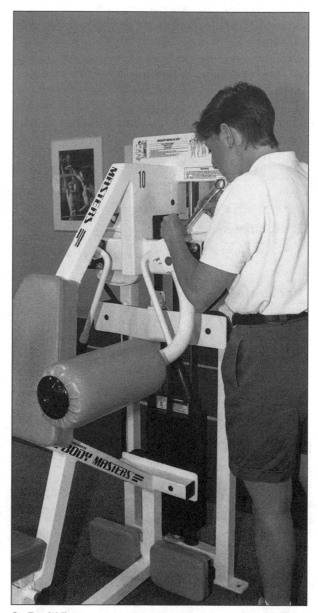

© Tom Wallace

EVALUATING FACILITY MAINTENANCE

The implementation phase ensures that the system established for overall maintenance care is well organized, properly staffed, and contained within the financial parameters authorized by management. The only way to assure this is through an internally developed set of goals and objectives as discussed previously in this chapter. By regularly reviewing and updating these goals and objectives, a facility manager will always be able to assess whether the maintenance program is producing the intended results.

Once the implementation phase is initiated, the ongoing evaluation process begins. Patton et al. (1989) include two steps in an evaluation phase: process evaluation and outcome evaluation (you can find additional information on process and outcome evaluation in chapter 20). Essentially, these evaluations involve analyzing the implementation tasks that were assigned to the staff to determine (a) if maintenance tasks are being accomplished (process evaluation), and (b) if objectives of the maintenance program are being met (outcome evaluation). Figure 14.10 summarizes process and evaluation techniques.

> *Evaluating a maintenance program is different from evaluating a scheduled activity program that has a beginning and ending point. Facility maintenance is dynamic and continuous and must be reviewed at regular intervals. Perform any changes or modifications to an existing maintenance program daily rather than waiting for an "appropriate time."*

Schedule periodic meetings with personnel to review the maintenance process. Staff should maintain careful work order records detailing when the work was completed, how long it took to complete, what materials were used, and who performed the work. Maintenance software programs are now available to tabulate work order data and assist in

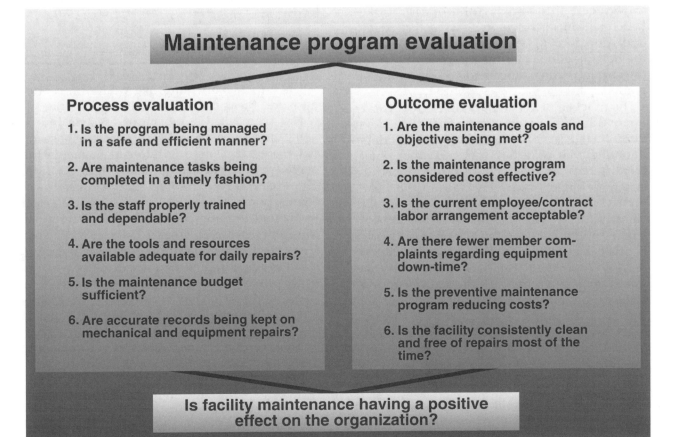

Maintenance program evaluation

Process evaluation

1. Is the program being managed in a safe and efficient manner?

2. Are maintenance tasks being completed in a timely fashion?

3. Is the staff properly trained and dependable?

4. Are the tools and resources available adequate for daily repairs?

5. Is the maintenance budget sufficient?

6. Are accurate records being kept on mechanical and equipment repairs?

Outcome evaluation

1. Are the maintenance goals and objectives being met?

2. Is the maintenance program considered cost effective?

3. Is the current employee/contract labor arrangement acceptable?

4. Are there fewer member complaints regarding equipment down-time?

5. Is the preventive maintenance program reducing costs?

6. Is the facility consistently clean and free of repairs most of the time?

Is facility maintenance having a positive effect on the organization?

Figure 14.10   Maintenance process and outcome techniques.

inventory management. More information on maintenance software vendors can be found in chapter 19.

> The third category of the I-formation management model is innovation. Incorporating new and creative changes into facility maintenance management will always be a challenge for club operators.

However, an example of a new and innovative program called *benchmarking* has recently been introduced into the health fitness market. Basically, benchmarking is the process of measuring services, supplies, and practices against competitors, similar facilities, or industry standards. Although this practice began in 1980 as a means to improve worker performance and productivity in large corporations such as Xerox, Eastman Kodak, and L.L. Bean, only recently has it been introduced into the health fitness market. Benchmarking involves reviewing the existing operation, looking at other operations, selecting the best practices, and incorporating them into the current maintenance and housekeeping operations.

The practice of benchmarking begins with an internal analysis of the existing facility and identifying what areas to benchmark. Second, determine the data collection methods, and, finally, identify comparative clubs or facilities. Because benchmarking is relatively new to the health fitness business, no industry standards exist specifically for health fitness facility maintenance. However, there are national standards reported annually by *Cleaning & Maintenance Management Magazine* and the Cleaning Management Institute (Publishers Survey 1995; Rice 1995) for all facility types nationwide (hospitals, schools, hotels, etc.). You can use a number of categories from this survey to compare the average health fitness facility to an existing setting. Some areas to consider benchmarking might include the following:

- *Estimated annual cleaning costs per square foot*—annual cleaning budget divided by average interior facility square feet.

- *Wage rates*—average hourly rates for shift supervisors, average cleaning worker, and starting cleaning worker.

- *Maintenance spending per facility*—estimated costs for chemicals, paper products, powered cleaning equipment, nonpowered equipment (mops, brooms, etc.).

- *Staff time allotment for common tasks*—percent of total annual cleaning work hours spent by staff in such areas as floor care, vacuuming, locker-room care, trash collection, dusting (nonfloor), carpet cleaning (other than vacuuming), and other miscellaneous tasks.

- *Compare total annual cleaning budget*—total cleaning budget compared with similar fitness settings of same approximate size.

Examples of some of the national maintenance management benchmarks mentioned previously are listed in table 14.1, *a*, *b*, *c*, and *d*.

> Benchmarking assists managers and maintenance personnel in justifying and evaluating overall performance.

It is impossible to improve what you cannot measure. Measuring productivity does not always have to entail a sophisticated system. In fact, you can establish categories to provide baseline parameters that communicate to management the overall performance of the maintenance division. These categories could include weekly towel counts, numbers of work orders completed each week, and the number of emergency response calls completed each week.

A system of this nature provides an objective means for determining maintenance effectiveness. In the past, many maintenance supervisors have frequently used a "feel for what was best" attitude. Unfortunately, this method of evaluation has become too subjective and does not always provide a definitive means for measuring performance.

A more detailed evaluation of facility management is presented in chapter 20, including specific maintenance areas and sample checklists and tables for recommended maintenance procedures.

Table 14.1a   National Maintenance Management Benchmarks

Staff time allotment for common tasks
Four major facility types
% of total annual cleaning hours spent by staff on average

Task	K-12 school	College/university	Hospital	Industrial plant/whse.
Floor care (including damp and dust mopping, scrubbing, buffing, recoating, etc.)	25.4%	18.8%	23.1%	21.2%
Vacuuming	24.8%	19.2%	13.6%	15.9%
Restroom care	16.6%	20.7%	15.6%	18.0%
Trash collection	10.6%	15.1%	13.8%	22.8%
Dusting (nonfloor)	6.9%	7.5%	11.8%	7.5%
Carpet cleaning (other than vacuuming)	6.8%	7.7%	8.6%	4.5%
Other misc. tasks	8.9%	10.0%	13.5%	10.1%
Totals	100%	100%	100%	100%

Note: This information is derived from the 1995 *Cleaning & Maintenance Management* in-house survey. Results were based on 1,267 respondents who were randomly selected subscribers to *Cleaning & Maintenance Management.*

Table 14.1b   National Maintenance Management Benchmarks

Estimated annual cost per square foot

Facility type	Estimated annual cleaning cost per square foot*
Private office buildings	$1.32
Schools (K-12)	$1.98
Colleges/universities	$0.91
Hotels/motels/resorts	$3.04
Industrial plants/warehouses	$1.66
Hospitals	$2.64
Government facilities (not education or health care)	$2.39
Nursing homes	$4.40
Misc. other facilities (combined)	$1.16
National in-house average (all facilities)	$1.68

*Data from in-house, facility-wide managers only. Calculated by dividing respondent's average total annual cleaning budget by average facility interior square feet.

Note: This information is derived from the 1995 *Cleaning & Maintenance Management* in-house survey. Results were based on 1,267 respondents who were randomly selected subscribers to *Cleaning & Maintenance Management.*

Table 14.1c   National Maintenance Management Benchmarks

	Wages		
	Hourly rate/shift supervisor	Hourly wages rate/average cleaning worker	Hourly rate/starting cleaning worker
Government facilities	$13.45	$9.89	$7.89
Schools (K-12)	$11.65	$9.16	$7.55
Industrial plants/whs.	$12.06	$9.18	$7.13
Colleges/universities	$11.17	$8.40	$7.12
Private office bldgs.	$10.84	$7.82	$6.55
Hospitals	$10.05	$7.51	$6.23
Nursing homes	$ 9.02	$7.01	$5.83
Hotels/motels/resorts	$ 7.81	$6.57	$5.66
Misc. other	$ 9.62	$7.40	$6.16
1995 National Average	$10.75	$8.22	$6.79
1994 National Average	$10.37	$7.97	$6.55

PREVENTIVE MAINTENANCE

Once the maintenance program is operating efficiently, emphasize organizing and implementing a preventive maintenance program. The amount of funds invested in mechanical, electrical, and exercise equipment certainly justifies the costs of maintaining the equipment so it is safe and operational. In the health fitness business the cost of waiting until a system malfunctions is not worth the outcome.

The goal of any preventive maintenance program is to ensure the continuous operation of facility systems (HVAC, boilers, pool heaters, fire alarm, security systems, etc.) and equipment (cardiovascular, strength, computers, etc.). An organized preventive maintenance program facilitates continued operation either through completion of work that keeps equipment operating or through the identification of substandard performance, faulty parts, or equipment failure.

You can categorize each preventive maintenance action according to how it reduces or avoids costs to the facility operation. These categories are described here.

Table 14.1d   National Maintenance Management Benchmarks

Three major facility types*	Annual cleaning expenditures				
	Chemicals	Paper products	Powered cleaning equipment	Nonpowered cleaning equipment	Employee training
Schools (K-12) 831,307 sq. ft.	$36,313	$17,700	$11,545	$8,071	$3,323
Colleges/universities 1,722,729 sq. ft.	$36,351	$30,927	$12,029	$9,133	$4,696
Hospitals 462,635 sq. ft.	$35,129	$42,195	$12,571	$7,826	$12,765
Avg. all respondents 810,689 sq. ft.	$30,120	$28,233	$10,303	$7,510	$6,992

*Figures in italics are average facility size.

From "1995 In-House Survey" by publisher's staff, *Cleaning & Maintenance Management Magazine*, National Trade Publications. Reprinted by permission.

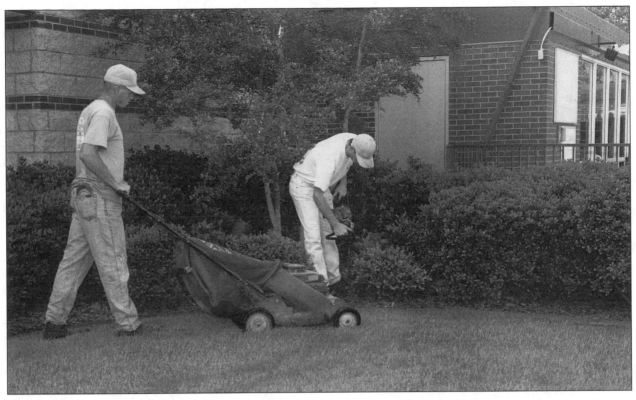

© Tom Wallace

Preventive maintenance tasks are performed whenever the financial impact of failure to perform the activity exceeds the cost of its performance. For example, the cost of maintaining an air-conditioning system often outweighs the cost of periodically replacing condensers or complete systems.

Maintain Operations

The most obvious justification for preventive maintenance is to maintain facility operations. The continued operation of a facility directly relates to the preventive maintenance tasks performed to ensure equipment reliability. However, some systems have a higher priority to keep functioning than others. For example, failure of a club's water heater could disable operations, whereas failure of a pool or spa water heater may not completely impede usage but might result in disgruntled member feedback.

Lengthen Service Life

Many preventive maintenance procedures are designed to ensure that a piece of equipment will not fail prematurely. Most equipment is designed for a specific service life. The duration of operation depends on timely servicing throughout the equipment's use.

Identify Worn Out Equipment

Because exercise equipment does not always perform like new, you should implement a system of monitoring its gradual deterioration. Schedule specific preventive maintenance tasks to detect any subtle changes and to alert maintenance personnel to major changes in equipment performance. Regular preventive maintenance will reduce overall costs if you catch mechanical problems early enough to detect signs of premature equipment failure.

Prevent Loss

Certain installed systems exist to protect the members and personnel within the facility. For example, a malfunctioning fire alarm system has no effect on the facility operation until there is a fire. Preventive maintenance performed on this equipment is justified because it prevents losses involving the protected member and facility.

Personal Safety

Regularly maintain any system or piece of equipment within a club installed to prevent bodily injury or possible death to members. Protective systems such as exit signs, fire alarms, and emergency lighting are required by local building codes or city standards. The costs of preventive maintenance for these systems are unavoidable.

Facility Protection

Some systems are installed to protect physical property. Sprinkler systems and burglar alarms reduce risk of property loss and reduce insurance premiums. For these reasons, perform maintenance even if the insurance policy doesn't require proof of maintenance for these systems.

Federal and State Compliance

Numerous aspects of a facility must comply with local, state, and federal standards. For example,

swimming pool water must meet local health department regulations. Steam room boilers must meet emission control standards to satisfy insurance companies. Paint or possible explosive materials cannot be stored next to electrical panels to comply with *Occupational Safety and Health Administration (OSHA)* requirements. In each case, the existing equipment must be maintained to perform at the levels required. Failure to comply with these organizations will result in discipline that could range from verbal warnings to closing a facility.

Preparing to initiate a preventive maintenance program begins with identifying those areas that have the greatest impact on the facility if not maintained. Examine and classify each system and piece of equipment as to its level of importance in facility operations. Those items that you consider critical to safe and continued operation of the facility receive high priority.

A primary source for identifying preventive maintenance tasks are procedures recommended by the manufacturers. Companies that mass produce cardiovascular or strength equipment include a user's manual specifying recommended service frequency and procedures. Any warranties provided with such equipment usually depend on completion of recommended preventive maintenance. Table 14.2 provides a preventive maintenance schedule for a StairMaster Crossrobics machine.

Table 14.2	Preventive Maintenance Schedule for the StairMaster Crossrobics 1650 LE			
Part	**Recommended action**	**Frequency**	**Cleaner**	**Lubricant**
Plastic side cover (exterior only)	Clean	Daily	Soap and water or diluted cleaner	N/A
Seat	Clean	Daily	Same as above	N/A
Console	Clean	Daily	Water	N/A
Weight stack belt and connectors	Inspect	Weekly or every 70 hours	N/A	N/A
Pedal arm return springs	Inspect, clean, and relube	Weekly or every 70 hours	Degreaser	Oil-dampened rag
Alternator and drive belts	Check tension and inspect for wear	Weekly or every 70 hours	N/A	N/A
Pedal arm chains and drive chain	Clean and lubricate	Weekly or every 70 hours	Degreaser	30W motor oil
	Remove, clean, and lubricate	Every 3 months or 900 hours	Degreaser	30W motor oil
Guide rods	Clean and lubricate	Weekly or every 70 hours	Window cleaner	Silicone spray
Drive shaft and hub assembly	Grease	Every 3 months or 900 hours	N/A	Heavy multipurpose grease
Bottom stop spring	Wipe clean and grease	Every 3 months or 900 hours	N/A	Heavy multipurpose grease

Note: Use of a silicone spray on parts not so specified will result in diminished performance and a shorter life span for that part.
N/A = Not applicable.

Once you determine the need for preventive maintenance for a system or piece of equipment, establish the procedures to provide that preventive maintenance task. Develop a form called the *preventive maintenance order (PMO)*, which acts as more than just a how-to guide. Properly prepared, the form describes the physical actions of performing the maintenance. The PMO is a planning document and a safety document. It provides assistance in ordering parts, and you can use it as an inspection and feedback tool. Although PMO forms have never been standardized and many variations probably exist in every health fitness setting, basic components of the form should include equipment data information, location, tools and materials required, safety procedures, maintenance procedures, and work completion data.

Each time preventive maintenance is to be performed on a system or piece of equipment, staff should prepare a PMO and forward it to the person administering the job. Once the work is completed, return the PMO to either the club operator or the maintenance supervisor. Pay close attention to any comments the worker makes that might initiate further investigation. File the completed order and establish a date for the next PMO for that piece of equipment. Record the date either manually or in a computer database file for the next scheduled preventive maintenance. Figure 14.11 shows a fully completed preventive maintenance order.

Preventive Maintenance Order		
Equipment name *Concept II Rower*	Model no. *None*	Manufacturer *Concept II, Inc.*
Frequency: daily weekly monthly quarterly annual		
Location *cardio room*	Other location information *Unit next to window*	
Tools required	*wrench* *screwdriver* *pliers*	
Materials required	*1 - lubricant tube* *1 - non-abrasive scouring pad*	*1 set - footstraps*
Safety procedures	*watch tension on chain after cleaning*	
Maintenance procedures	*Clean monrail with non-abrasive scouring pad—(daily)* *Clean and lubricate chain—(weekly)* *Check cord tension—(weekly)* *Check chain for stiff links—(monthly)* *Check tightness of all nuts and bolts—(monthly)*	
Date completed	Completed by	Time to complete
Remarks		

Figure 14.11 **Preventive maintenance order form.**

Periodically evaluate the preventive maintenance program to determine its effectiveness. Measure the effectiveness by the performance of the facility and equipment maintained and by the cost of the program. Address the following questions:

- Is the program running efficiently, or is preventive maintenance being forgotten or ignored?

- Has the number of maintenance request orders been reduced on those items receiving preventive maintenance?

- Have parts and equipment supply costs been reduced?

- Have there been fewer calls for outside repair workers?

- Have any equipment failures been the result of inadequate preventive maintenance?

IN CLOSING

The life cycle of a health fitness facility completely depends on properly implemented maintenance and housekeeping systems. Proper maintenance for a facility means keeping the facility and its components in good condition, ready to serve their intended purpose. To accomplish this goal, facility managers must first have a clear understanding of the scope of required maintenance for their setting. They must initiate a strategic management plan that incorporates a four-step process, including needs assessment, program planning, program implementation, and program evaluation. Emphasize the workforce and requirements needed to achieve the housekeeping, general maintenance, and repair tasks requiring daily attention. Hiring in-house personnel, contract labor, or a combination of both are the primary methods being used in today's fitness settings. Finally, implement a comprehensive preventive maintenance program to preclude the failure of expensive mechanical equipment, installed systems, or exercise equipment.

KEY TERMS

Benchmarking

Contract labor

Contract maintenance

Heating, ventilation and air-conditioning (HVAC)

Iterative process

Needs assessment

Occupational Safety and Health Administration (OSHA)

Preventive maintenance

Preventive maintenance order (PMO)

Purchase order system

Strategic plan

RECOMMENDED READINGS

Feldman, E. 1991. *How to save time and money in facilities maintenance management*. Latham, NY: Cleaning Management Institute.

Hoke, J.R. 1975. *Designer's guide to OSHA*. New York: McGraw-Hill.

International Health, Racquet and Sportsclub Association. 1994. *Profiles of Success*. Boston: IHRSA

Magee, G. 1988. *Facility maintenance management*. Kingston, MA: Means.

Patton, R.W., J.M. Corry, L.R. Gettman, and J.S. Graf. 1986. *Implementing health fitness programs*. Champaign, IL: Human Kinetics.

Patton, R.W., W.C. Grantham, R.F. Gerson, and L.R. Gettman. 1989. *Developing and managing health fitness facilities*. Champaign, IL: Human Kinetics.

Publishers Survey. 1995. 1995 in-house survey. *Cleaning and Maintenance Management* 32(12): 2-8.

Rice, R. 1995. Housekeeping benchmarks. *Cleaning and Maintenance Management* 32(3): 62-65.

Tatum, R. 1995. How technology is reshaping facility management. *Building Operating Management* 42(1): 24-30.

Williams, T. 1994. How top managers evaluate their facilities. *Cleaning Maintenance Management* 31(9): 40-42.

CHAPTER 15

Financial Management

A prerequisite for becoming an owner or manager of a health fitness facility is understanding the principles of financial management. Making the many financial decisions required to effectively manage the day-to-day operation of the business and to develop sound plans for its future requires reliable and pertinent information on the financial performance of the organization. This means having answers to such questions as the following:

- Is the business generating cash flow sufficient to maintain a profitable level of operations?

- Are operating costs adequately controlled?

- Is the nonprofit status (if applicable) of the organization being properly maintained?

- Is the collection rate on accounts receivable sufficient to maintain satisfactory cash flow?

- Are accounts payable effectively controlled?

The more detailed the information on how the business operates, the easier it is to provide reliable answers to these critical questions. As you'll learn from this chapter, basic financial statements (balance sheet and income statement), which accountants or bookkeepers produce, provide much needed information. You can derive other types of information from budgetary planning, tax considerations, and expense-management techniques. Despite the source of the information, the key is knowing what information you need for a particular purpose, where to find it, and how to use it. This chapter discusses some techniques for accomplishing these goals.

Whether operating in a commercial, corporate, community, or clinical setting, understanding financial management is essential. Health fitness managers must be familiar with standard financial principles and procedures to compete in today's marketplace. Traditionally in the fitness industry, management and university preparatory programs have placed more emphasis on the operational aspects (personnel management, facility maintenance, and programming) than on financial management. Unfortunately, this management style has contributed to the downfall of some established health fitness organizations.

The importance of competent financial management—making payroll, paying the bills, paying the bank, and having enough left as profit—is vital to the success and even survival of many health fitness entities. The most common reason cited for the high failure rate experienced by new health fitness ventures is a lack of financial expertise (Moscove 1981). Similarly, the importance of financial administration in nonprofit organizations (YMCAs, city-owned community and recreational centers) and government tax issues are all critical components for success in any fitness business.

Fortunately, the views and attitudes toward financial information have changed drastically over the years. In the past, financial matters were kept confidential for management's use only. However, today's owners and operators have discovered the importance of sharing financial figures and empowering employees to positively influence the performance of the business. The belief is that the more employees know about what it takes to be successful, the more they can direct their actions toward attaining that goal. This style of management allows employees to perform as business people and helps positively affect the bottom line.

This chapter introduces fundamental concepts and techniques of financial management, many of which are considered necessary components for establishing an organized financial plan. This chapter discusses the accounting process, financial statements, budgeting, income management, expense management, cash flow emphasis, and tax considerations.

We use an assortment of accounting terms throughout this discussion. To assist the readers in familiarizing themselves with these terms, a list of definitions is presented here.

Accounting Terminology

Accounting—The recording, classifying, summarizing, and interpreting of financial data.

Accounts payable—You or your company owe money to another individual or company.

Accounts receivable—An individual or company owes you money.

Assets—Properties of value owned by a business firm or by an individual.

Balance sheet—A financial statement that reveals the assets, liabilities, and owner's equity in a firm as of a specific date.

Budget—A financial plan indicating expected income and anticipated expenses for a specific time, which can be used as a means of exercising financial control.

Capital—Money, goods, land, or equipment used to produce other goods or services.

Equity—The money value of a property or of an interest in a property in excess of claims or liens against it.

Fixed assets—The land, plant, equipment, and other physical productive assets of a firm that are expected to have a useful life in excess of one year.

Fixed costs—Costs that must be incurred regardless of the level of production undertaken.

Gross profit—The profit earned on sales after deducting the cost of the goods sold but before deducting other business expenses.

Income statement—A financial statement revealing the summary of the income or loss resulting from the business transactions for the preceding period.

Ledger—Individual account books that keep a running balance of the status of each account.

Liability—Debt owed by an individual to others and the equity of creditors in business firms.

Net income—The earnings of a company after allowing for all legitimate business expenses, including taxes.

Operating expenses—Expenses incurred because of the production operations of the business firm.

Profit—Excess of sales income after deducting all related expenses.

Variable costs—Costs whose total magnitude varies directly with the level of production.

ACCOUNTING PROCESS

Before entering into a health fitness business, establish a system for tracking and recording all financial transactions. For those businesses already operational, evaluate and update this system regularly. This process is called the accounting system, and its main purpose is to provide pertinent financial information to aid in decision making. A difficult problem that every club comptroller or accountant has is being able to take all the financial data and present it in a fashion that external parties (bankers, state and federal government agencies such as the IRS, and potential investors) and internal parties (management and department heads) can understand.

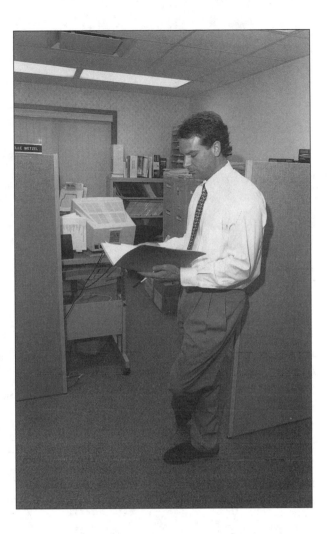

Develop a financial accounting system so that it is flexible to meet the needs of the various parties, while communicating the information in an understandable format.

The procedures for establishing an accounting system correspond with many aspects of the information phase of the I-formation management model. Perform an initial needs assessment and financial plan before you implement an accounting system. You can obtain pertinent information by conducting a comparison evaluation of similar health fitness settings, while investigating national recommendations and financial standards for the health fitness industry.

Fortunately, you do not have to develop and implement all accounting systems from a start-up phase. Depending on the setting, many accounting systems are already in place and managers are trained

to follow the preestablished accounting format. For example, hospital-based wellness centers often use the internal hospital accounting system for maintaining financial records. Corporate fitness centers have traditionally used the same accounting system as the company they are servicing. Many YMCAs and other community centers have local and regional accounting offices where facility financial information is downloaded daily into a central data processing unit. Commercial fitness centers that are franchised or have multiple site locations also follow a preexisting accounting format for all entities.

The primary group responsible for establishing their own accounting system are new, independently owned or leased, commercial health fitness centers. Fortunately, owners and managers of these organizations do not have to reinvent the wheel when adopting a financial program. Many health fitness businesses today have computerized data processing systems to aid in accumulating, processing, and analyzing financial data. Software companies have entered into the fitness industry by offering a variety of accounting programs that you can adapt to fit any setting. We provide more discussion of these software programs in chapter 19.

Establishing an Accounting System

Developing an accounting system begins with hiring a competent accountant or bookkeeper. Because people must operate a system, it is important that employees are adequately trained and able to perform efficiently with the in-house accounting system. The best planned system on paper is not effective in practice unless employ-

ees are capable of performing their assigned duties and responsibilities.

The next step is to ensure that an information system is in place for tracking daily financial transactions. Whether this system is manual or computerized, it must be reliable, flexible, user-friendly, and have systems for checks and balances to process all the financial data accumulated for an organization's financial statements. It is important to realize that each company's information system should be designed to satisfy its own decision-making needs. There are general accounting functions that all information systems must possess to satisfy the financial process. These include the following:

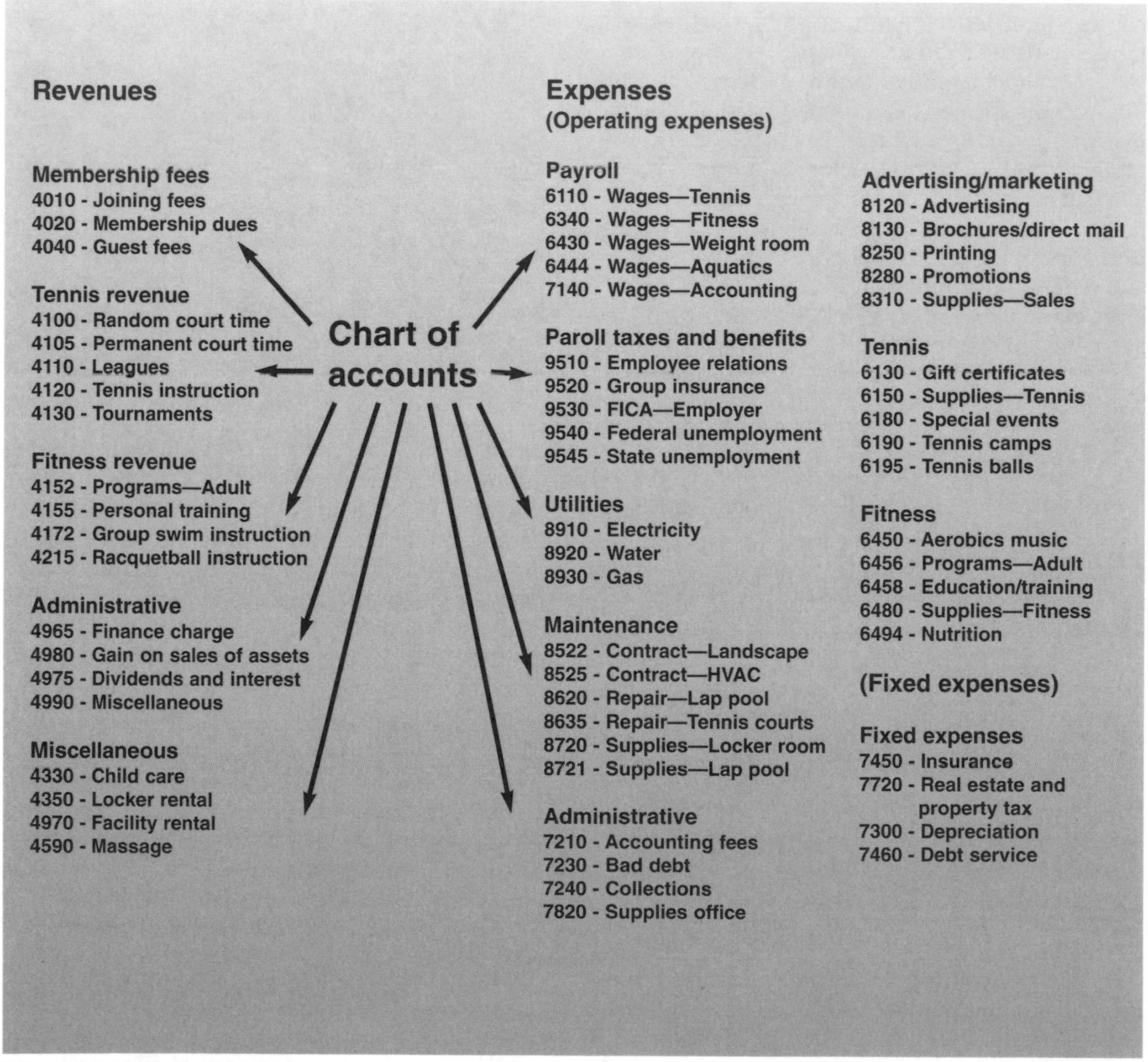

Revenues

Membership fees
4010 - Joining fees
4020 - Membership dues
4040 - Guest fees

Tennis revenue
4100 - Random court time
4105 - Permanent court time
4110 - Leagues
4120 - Tennis instruction
4130 - Tournaments

Fitness revenue
4152 - Programs—Adult
4155 - Personal training
4172 - Group swim instruction
4215 - Racquetball instruction

Administrative
4965 - Finance charge
4980 - Gain on sales of assets
4975 - Dividends and interest
4990 - Miscellaneous

Miscellaneous
4330 - Child care
4350 - Locker rental
4970 - Facility rental
4590 - Massage

Chart of accounts

Expenses
(Operating expenses)

Payroll
6110 - Wages—Tennis
6340 - Wages—Fitness
6430 - Wages—Weight room
6444 - Wages—Aquatics
7140 - Wages—Accounting

Paroll taxes and benefits
9510 - Employee relations
9520 - Group insurance
9530 - FICA—Employer
9540 - Federal unemployment
9545 - State unemployment

Utilities
8910 - Electricity
8920 - Water
8930 - Gas

Maintenance
8522 - Contract—Landscape
8525 - Contract—HVAC
8620 - Repair—Lap pool
8635 - Repair—Tennis courts
8720 - Supplies—Locker room
8721 - Supplies—Lap pool

Administrative
7210 - Accounting fees
7230 - Bad debt
7240 - Collections
7820 - Supplies office

Advertising/marketing
8120 - Advertising
8130 - Brochures/direct mail
8250 - Printing
8280 - Promotions
8310 - Supplies—Sales

Tennis
6130 - Gift certificates
6150 - Supplies—Tennis
6180 - Special events
6190 - Tennis camps
6195 - Tennis balls

Fitness
6450 - Aerobics music
6456 - Programs—Adult
6458 - Education/training
6480 - Supplies—Fitness
6494 - Nutrition

(Fixed expenses)

Fixed expenses
7450 - Insurance
7720 - Real estate and
        property tax
7300 - Depreciation
7460 - Debt service

Figure 15.1 Chart of accounts.

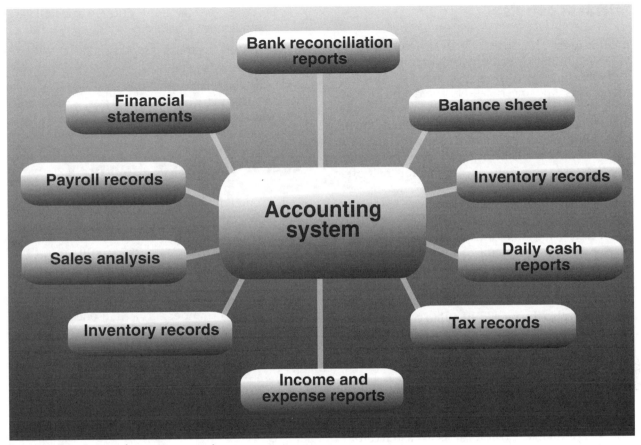

Figure 15.2 Accounting system reports.

- Accounts payable
- Payroll
- Accounts receivable
- Inventory control
- General ledger
- Financial statements
- Sales analysis
- Invoicing accounts

Also included with these functions is a chart of accounts, which is a classification list of the names and numbers of each account in the system. Generally, the accounts are organized around service or profit centers (fitness, racquet sports, pro shop, restaurant, massage) or in some cases cost centers (day care, operations). This list allows you to itemize all financial transactions under specific departments or categories and to analyze them individually. Such a system allows management to allocate the necessary revenue and expense items to one department and determine the status of its contribution to the profit or loss of the business.

Although standard reporting systems have been developed for the health fitness industry, having the flexibility to customize and adjust the chart of accounts as the business grows is essential. Figure 15.1 provides a sample chart of accounts list for a commercial fitness center.

In addition, an accounting system must provide accurate records for fulfilling legal requirements, such as filing income taxes; safeguarding assets, for example, evaluating profit and loss from monthly income statements; and planning and controlling daily operations, including marketing and promotional planning (DeThomas 1991). To obtain these records, establish various forms and reports to register relevant data about a company's financial activities. Examples of these forms include purchase orders, petty cash receipts, member applications, employee time cards, and inventory records. Maintaining these records allows you to generate reports to assist management in its decision-making process, provides federal and state tax information, and compiles payroll and inventory records. Figure 15.2 highlights reports that you can generate from a well-planned accounting system.

Internal Controls

Include internal controls within an accounting system design that contribute to operating efficiency and effectiveness. A sound internal control system safeguards a business's assets against misuse and theft. For example, misuse of office equipment could include unlimited use of a copier machine, uncontrolled long distance phone calls, and postage meter use. Without established procedures you can incur needless expenses. Internal control for theft often begins with the separation of duties; one employee acts as a check on the work of the other. For example, if a service desk attendant attempts to embezzle guest fees, a system of double checks should be in place to make it difficult to manipulate the cash records to cover up theft.

Because cash (coins, currency, and checking and savings accounts) is the most liquid of a company's assets, it is also the most difficult to control. Consequently, put a variety of systems in place to safeguard against the possibility of theft. These systems include the following:

1. Establish a business checking account.

   - Deposit all cash transactions daily.

   - Compare deposit receipts to cash receipt.

   - Attempt to have all cash transactions made by check.

   - Develop an internal system for paying all bills.

   - Consider having two check signers for payables.

2. Perform monthly bank reconciliation.

   - Compare monthly bank statements to facility account records.

   - Reconcile any differences between bank and business accounts.

   - If an adjustment must be made, have someone other than the employee who records the cash transactions make it.

3. Evaluate petty cash.

   - Establish a petty cash fund to pay for minor expenses (i.e., postage stamps, delivery charges, vending machine reimbursement).

   - Determine a maximum amount that may be used for cash disbursements.

   - Develop a petty cash voucher to use for all transactions.

   - When cash is given out, always replace it with a petty cash slip.

   - Reconcile transactions regularly, with remaining cash and vouchers equaling beginning balance.

   - Once petty cash becomes low, write a check to petty cash for the original amount.

Cash Versus Accrual Accounting

Determine whether you will use cash or accrual accounting when recording revenues and expenses. *Cash accounting* involves recording business transactions only when the accounting entity receives or pays cash (Caro 1986). In a cash-based system, record revenue when it is received, regardless of when goods are sold or services rendered. When you sell merchandise or render services in one month and collect cash the following month, cash-based accounting recognizes the revenue only when you receive cash. Similarly, accounting for expenses means that when you make a cash payment, you record the amount as an expense. For example, if a utility bill is incurred in June but not paid until July, the expense is not recorded until the month in which it is paid.

Accrual accounting records transactions in the accounting periods during which they occur, rather than when cash is received or paid. Record revenues when you earn them, whether or not you have received cash. Record expenses when they occur as opposed to when you pay them. Therefore, as in the utility bill example, record the bill in June rather than in July.

There are advantages and disadvantages to both systems. Although a cash-based system is simple and straightforward to implement, it is difficult to determine an accurate net worth because unpaid revenue and expenses are not reflected. Also, organizations that offer prepaid annual memberships will appear financially solvent when cash is received, but if funds are not properly managed the remaining 11 months of the year, a cash shortage could occur. For example, if a member of a health fitness facility prepays a year's membership for $900, the cash-based system recognizes all $900 in the month in which the cash is received. In the accrual system, $75 ($900 divided by 12 months) is recognized each month as member revenue.

Although it is not uncommon for a club to adopt a mix of the cash and accrual methods, the preferred system for commercial health fitness settings is accrual-based accounting because it provides management with a more accurate understanding of an organization's operations (Howland 1995). There are three reasons why accrual-based accounting is preferred among club operators:

1. Better cash management, because all prepaid memberships received are recorded as 1/12 of the dues for each month of the year.

2. As a management tool, accrual accounting provides a more realistic picture of the financial status of the business by including all unpaid expenses and unpaid revenues that are due.

3. You can report a club's net worth with accrual accounting, which a cash-based system cannot do. This is especially important if a club is attempting to obtain a loan or solicit investors.

A well-organized accounting system entails a number of functions, all designed to record, track, protect, and analyze the financial transactions of a business. A series of checks and balances should always be in place to account for every transaction that goes in and out of the organization. In addition, the process by which you accumulate financial information to prepare financial statements is another integral aspect of the accounting system. When discussing the various elements that an accounting system provides, Burstiner (1979) listed eight areas of importance:

- Interpret past performance.
- Measure present progress.
- Anticipate and plan for the future.
- Control daily operations.
- Uncover significant trends.
- Compare results with similar businesses and within the particular industry.
- Make decisions.
- Comply with government regulations.

FINANCIAL STATEMENTS

The purpose of financial statements is to provide a financial summary of the current status of the fitness organization. Generally, an in-house or outside accountant prepares financial statements and completes them in a timely and accurate fashion. Preparing financial statements depends on an organized bookkeeping system that tracks every transaction

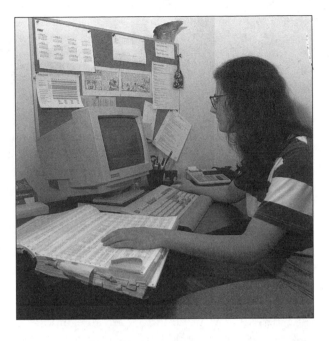

from its inception until it becomes part of the financial statement. Comparing industry trends, budget analysis, internal controls, and short- and long-term planning are all internal uses of these statements. External uses include financial information for refinancing, renovating, or expanding a facility or debt within the organization.

> *Financial statements depict the strengths and weaknesses of the business and the gains or losses arising from various transactions.*

A *balance sheet* and an *income statement* are the two major reports accountants prepare to communicate the current financial position to management. The following discussion provides the concepts and procedures involved in preparing the balance sheet and the income statement.

Balance Sheet

If an individual decided to start her own fitness facility, she would generally require a cash investment. With this money, she could purchase fitness equipment, operating inventory, office equipment, land, and a building to start the club. In buying these items, the individual may run short of cash. As a result, she might go to a bank and arrange to borrow money. Upon receipt of the loan, she can then buy the additional items needed to finish the new facility.

This simplified example illustrates what an organization's balance sheet includes. The three major financial terms included in a balance sheet are *assets*, *liabilities*, and *owner's equity*. We can best express these financial items by the following equation:

Assets = liabilities + owner's equity

Assets are anything a business owns that has monetary value. In the previous example, the cash invested, land, exercise equipment, office equipment, inventory, and building are all examples of assets. Assets are divided into two main categories: current assets and fixed assets. An accountant assumes current assets—cash, accounts receivable, inventory, and prepaid expenses—to be either cash or converted into cash within one year. Fixed assets—land, the building, office furniture, and fitness equipment—are the more long-lived resources owned by the business. With the exception of land, these assets are valued by an accountant at book value minus depreciation.

Liabilities are amounts owed to creditors. Like assets, liabilities are divided into two categories: current liabilities and long-term liabilities. Current liabilities consist of notes payable, accounts payable, and accruals (such as wages or taxes payable) that are due within one year. Long-term liabilities are obligations to be paid beyond a one-year period. A common example in the health fitness industry of a long-term liability involves repaying a loan note for new outdoor tennis courts.

Owner's equity (or net worth) represents the owner's claims on the assets of the business. This is a residual claim because owners receive only what remains after all claims, including taxes, have been paid. It is important to understand that the amount of owner's equity is not the market value of the business. As is the case with any investment, what the business is worth on the open market (the amount a buyer is willing to pay for the business) is determined by placing a value on the future cash flow it is expected to produce. Owner's equity as shown on the balance sheet reflects the book value, not the market value of the business.

The purpose of the balance sheet is to give management pertinent information about the financial condition of the business on a specific date.

To best analyze a club's financial condition, an owner or manager must have information about its assets and the sources of these assets, the liabilities, and the owner's equity. A balance sheet reflects a snapshot of an organization's financial status on a given date. Consequently, changes in balance sheet accounts between two statement dates provide important information about a club's financial health. Understanding the nature and implication of changes in financial statement accounts can help provide answers to questions such as the following:

- How much did the funds in accounts receivable and inventory increase or decrease, relative to the change in member sales for the period?
- Has the amount of debt financing increased to unsatisfactory levels since the last statement date?
- Are accounts payable rising to a level of concern?
- Has the club maintained a satisfactory level of cash flow from operations?

Figure 15.3 represents a sample balance sheet for a health fitness business.

Income Statement

The income statement or, as it is often called, the statement of profit and loss, reflects the financial results of the business operations over a specific time (month, quarter, or year). It is a summarized statement of the transactions that produced revenue for the period and the operating expenses and taxes the business incurred in generating this revenue.

The two major financial categories included on an income statement are revenues and expenses. Revenues, which can be defined as increases in a company's assets, are earned through selling products or providing a service to someone (DeThomas 1991). In the health fitness industry, revenues are

XYZ Company
Balance sheet
December 31, 2001

Assets
Current assets

Cash		185,236	
Inventory		85,693	
Total current assets			270,929

Fixed assets

Equipment	1,256,756		
Furniture and fixtures	356,458		
	1,613,214		
Less: accumulated depreciation	563,254	1,049,960	
Land		650,000	
Total fixed assets			1,699,960

Other assets

Loan fees	56,000		
Security deposits	7,500		
Total other assets		63,500	
Total assets			
			2,034,389

Liabilities and stockholder's equity
Current liabilities

Accounts payable		75,896	
Current portion of long-term debt		2,584	
Payroll taxes		6,589	
Total current liabilities			85,069

Long-term debt

Note payable—bank		953,450	
Less: current portion		2,584	
Total long-term debt			950,866

Stockholder's equity

Capital stock		1,000	
Additional paid-in-capital		25,000	
Current period profit (loss)		254,875	
Retained earnings		717,579	
Total stockholder's equity			998,454
Total liabilities and stockholder's equity			2,034,389

Figure 15.3   Balance sheet.

generated primarily through membership sales, racquet sport programs, fitness programs, profit centers, or miscellaneous income (guest fees, locker rentals, towel fees). To clearly understand the concept of revenue, note the following two points:

• Although you may think the value produced by the sale of a new club membership is cash received, an accountant measures the membership by either a cash sale or a credit sale. To an accountant, a credit sale means something of value: a claim on the new member for the amount of the membership sale. This claim appears as an asset and is classified as accounts receivable. Accounts receivable have a definite value to the club, but they are not cash and may never become cash.

• In preparing an income statement, an accountant recognizes a credit sale as revenue in the period in which the credit sale was made. This means that the revenue figures on the income statement for a given period include all credit sales made during that period, even though cash from those transactions may not be received until later. This means that there could be a significant difference between the membership sales revenue shown on the income statement and the actual amount of cash received during that time.

Comprehending these concepts is essential to properly interpreting an income statement and becoming familiar with cash flow practices.

Expenses represent the costs incurred for generating revenue and operating a fitness facility.

Typically, in the health fitness industry expenses are broken down into operating expenses and fixed expenses. Operating expenses are the costs associated with the normal operation of a club, such as payroll and benefits, administration, utilities, maintenance and repairs, advertising, marketing, and program and profit center costs. Fixed expenses are costs that remain constant over a designated time. Examples of fixed expenses include rent and lease payments, interest and financing charges, real estate and personal property taxes, and depreciation. The expenses recognized in a given period are matched with revenues for that time to determine the amount of profit or loss (net income or net loss).

> *As with revenue, measure expense value when the expense occurred, not when the cash flowed out of the club. Expenses that appear on an income statement for a certain period may actually represent cash paid in from a previous period, the current period, or possibly a future period.*

Financial Statement Analysis

Interpreting an income statement and applying the information obtained to the operation of a club is a primary on-going responsibility of every manager. Experienced owners and managers take the time each month for reviewing all revenue and expense categories to evaluate the overall business performance. Make monthly comparisons between the income statement and the projected (budgeted) income statement. Also, analyze all departments, and share the information you obtain with each department head. Either the manager or department head should investigate any significant variations between the actual and projected figures to determine the cause of the variations. A sample income statement is shown in figure 15.4.

Financial Statement Ratios

Another method of interpreting financial statements is to compare financial ratios and percentages with industry standards. Outsiders often use these measurements to determine the overall liquidity of a

business, its debt, profitability, and coverages (Caro 1986). Lenders, investors, and club operators also use this information when comparing one fitness facility with another to establish a market value for a facility. Then they can compare these ratios with industry data averages available through such organizations as IHRSA, Dunn & Bradstreet, and Robert Morris Associates.

As an example of key financial ratios for various commercial fitness settings, IHRSA has developed industry averages for determining financial performance. These key ratios not only provide benchmarks for operators to use for club comparisons but also offer insights into how the fitness industry's top performing facilities achieve success.

In IHRSA's 1996 *Profiles of Success*, eight ratios were identified as benchmarks for determining operational trends and financial standards for commercial health, racquet, and sport clubs. These ratios are as follows:

- *Revenue per square foot*—the value of membership to a facility's real estate worth (total revenue/square footage).

- *Square feet per member*—a measure of whether a facility is meeting its market potential and space allocation (total square footage/numbers of members).

- *Payroll as a percent of revenue*—a measure of staff productivity (total payroll/total revenue).

- *Membership attrition*—a measurement (percentage) of the number of members who terminate their memberships annually compared with the total number of members (number of members lost during the year or month/number of members at start of the year or month x 100).

- *Operating margin*—a measure of financial operating performance (net income before fixed expenses).

- *Net profit*—a measure of total financial performance of the business (profit after fixed expenses but before taxes).

- *Sales to assets*—a measure of performance and potential return on assets (total revenue/total assets).

- *Revenue per member growth*—(percentage) a product of many factors, including membership growth, pricing, and discounting; can be a guide in determining goals for nondues income growth (total revenue/total members).

Table 15.1, *a* and *b*, provides benchmark financial ratios for various commercial club settings.

XYZ Company
Income statement
For the period ended December 32, 2001

Acct no.	Description	Current period 2001	%	2000	%	Year to date 2001	%	2001	%
	Revenue								
4010	Joining fees	145968	4.5	131371	4.5	145968	4.5	131371	4.5
4020	Membership dues	2415984	74.7	2174386	74.7	2415984	74.7	2174386	74.7
	Total membership fees	2561952	79.2	2305757	79.2	2561952	79.2	2305757	79.2
4100	Random court time	68745	2.1	61871	2.1	68745	2.1	61871	2.1
4110	Leagues	125698	0.0	113128	3.9	125698	0.0	113128	3.9
4120	Tennis instruction	254994	7.9	229495	7.9	254994	7.9	229495	7.9
	Total tennis revenue	449437	13.9	404494	13.9	449437	13.9	404494	13.9
4155	Personal training	128952	4.0	116057	4.0	128952	4.0	116057	4.0
4172	Group swim instruction	8523	0.3	7671	0.3	8523	0.3	7671	0.3
	Total fitness revenue	137475	4.2	123728	4.2	137475	4.2	123728	4.2
4965	Dividends and interest	85694	2.6	77125	2.6	85694	2.6	77125	2.6
4990	Miscellaneous	547	0.0	492	0.0	547	0.0	492	0.0
	Total administrative	86241	2.7	77617	2.7	86241	2.7	77617	2.7
	Total revenue	3235105	100.0	2911596	100.0	3235105	100.0	2911596	100.0
	Expenses								
6110	Wages—tennis	350558	10.8	315502	10.8	350558	10.8	315502	10.8
6340	Wages—fitness	330563	10.2	297507	10.2	330563	10.2	297507	10.2
7140	Wages—accounting	75894	2.3	68305	2.3	75894	2.3	68305	2.3
	Total payroll	757015	23.4	681314	23.4	757015	23.4	681314	23.4
9520	Group insurance	295282	9.1	248269	8.5	275854	8.5	248269	8.5
9530	FICA—employer	57912	1.8	52121	1.8	57912	1.8	52121	1.8
9540	Federal unemployment	46935	1.5	42242	1.5	46935	1.5	42242	1.5
9545	State unemployment	39845	1.2	53345	1.8	39845	1.2	53345	1.8
	Total payroll and benefits	439974	13.6	395977	13.6	439974	13.6	395977	13.6
8910	Electricity	134191	4.1	120772	4.1	134191	4.1	120772	4.1
8920	Water	21781	0.7	19603	0.7	21781	0.7	19603	0.7
8930	Gas	25194	0.8	22675	0.8	25194	0.8	22675	0.8
	Total utilities	181166	5.6	163050	5.6	181166	5.6	163050	5.6
8522	Contract landscape	41142	1.3	37028	1.3	41142	1.3	37028	1.3
8620	Repair pool	32568	1.0	29311	1.0	32568	1.0	29311	1.0
8720	Supplies locker room	75105	2.3	67595	2.3	75105	2.3	67595	2.3
	Total maintenance	148815	4.6	133934	4.6	148815	4.6	133934	4.6
7210	Accounting fees	50000	1.5	45000	1.5	50000	1.5	45000	1.5
7230	Bad debt expense	115000	3.6	103500	3.6	115000	3.6	103500	3.6
7820	Office supplies	35577	1.1	32019	1.1	35577	1.1	32019	1.1
	Total administrative	200577	6.2	180519	6.2	200577	6.2	180519	6.2
8120	Advertising	42897	1.3	38607	1.3	42897	1.3	38607	1.3
8250	Printing	25478	0.8	22930	0.8	25478	0.8	22930	0.8
8280	Promotions	31913	1.0	28722	1.0	31913	1.0	28722	1.0
	Total advertising	100288	3.1	90259	3.1	100288	3.1	90259	3.1
6150	Supplies tennis	31568	1.0	28411	1.0	31568	1.0	28411	1.0
6180	Special events tennis	24569	0.8	22112	0.8	24569	0.8	22112	0.8
6195	Tennis balls	27976	0.9	25178	0.9	27976	0.9	25178	0.9
	Total tennis	84113	2.6	75701	2.6	84113	2.6	75701	2.6
6450	Aerobics music	10464	0.3	9418	0.3	10464	0.3	9418	0.3
6480	Supplies Fitness	27336	0.8	24602	0.8	27336	0.8	24602	0.8
6494	Nutrition	4256	0.1	3830	0.1	4256	0.1	3830	0.1
	Total fitness	42056	1.3	37850	1.3	42056	1.3	37850	1.3
	Total operating expense	1954004	60.4	1758604	60.4	1954004	60.4	1758604	60.4
7450	Insurance	737603	22.8	663843	22.8	737603	22.8	663843	22.8
7300	Depreciation	213517	6.6	192165	6.6	213517	6.6	192165	6.6
7460	Debt service	152050	4.7	136845	4.7	152050	4.7	136845	4.7
	Total fixed expenses	1103170	34.1	992853	34.1	1103170	34.1	992853	34.1
	Total expenses	3057174	94.5	2751457	94.5	3057174	94.5	2751457	94.5
	Net income	177931	5.5	160139	5.5	177931	5.5	160139	5.5

Figure 15.4 Income statement.

Table 15.1a Financial Benchmarks for Commercial Settings

Benchmarks by club type

	All clubs[1] 1994	1995	Fitness only[2] 1994	1995	Multipurpose[3] 1994	1995	Tennis only[4] 1994	1995	Multioperations[5] 1994	1995
Total revenue (thousands $)	1,406	1,506	885	978	1,552	1,665	987	1,036	1,623	1,761
Operating expenses	71%	69%	71%	70%	71%	69%	78%	79%	69%	66%
Operating margin	29%	31%	29%	30%	29%	31%	22%	21%	31%	34%
Fixed expenses	22%	22%	24%	23%	22%	22%	17%	17%	24%	25%
Net income before taxes	7.1%	8.4%	5.5%	7.3%	7.3%	8.8%	3.9%	4.8%	6.3%	8.5%

[1] Based on data from 320 respondents.
[2] Based on data from 62 respondents.
[3] Based on data from 164 respondents.
[4] Based on data from 22 respondents.
[5] Based on data from 87 respondents.

Table 15.1b Financial Benchmarks for Commercial Settings

Key ratios

	All clubs[1] 1994	1995	Fitness only[2] 1994	1995	Multipurpose[3] 1994	1995	Tennis only[4] 1994	1995	Multioperations[5] 1994	1995
% revenue growth (1994-1995)		7.1%		10.5%		7.3%		5.0%		8.5%
% payroll	39%	39%	42%	41%	39%	39%	39%	38%	38%	38%
% attrition	35%	35%	44%	38%	34%	34%	34%	34%	37%	36%
% net membership growth	6.6%	5.7%	11%	9.8%	4.9%	5.9%	10.4%	7.7%	5.0%	4.9%
Revenue/member ($)	686	678	575	581	708	703	821	765	647	670
Sq. ft./member	21	21	19	16	21	21	24	21	18	17
Revenue/sq. ft. ($)	41	43	49	52	39	42	60	63	44	48
Current ratio (assets/liabilities)	.98	1.12			.91	1.06			1.04	1.25
Sales/assets	.97	1.06			.90	.98			1.06	1.22

[1] Based on data from 320 respondents.
[2] Based on data from 62 respondents.
[3] Based on data from 164 respondents.
[4] Based on data from 22 respondents.
[5] Based on data from 87 respondents.

Data for tables 15.1a and 15.1b adapted, by permission, from IHRSA, 1996, *Profiles of success* (Boston: IHRSA), 10.

In summary, financial statements are the principal means for obtaining information about a fitness organization's monetary activities. The balance sheet reflects a club's financial condition on a specific date by disclosing its assets and the two sources of the assets: the liabilities and the owner's equity. The income statement shows operating results by comparing the revenues earned against the expenses incurred. Analysis of a club's income statement indicates the success or failure of that organization to increase its assets through earning a net income. The income statement and balance sheet are linked together because the net income computed is added to the owners' equity section of the balance sheet.

BUDGET PLANNING

Adequate financial planning is essential in the success of any health fitness organization. Conversely, the lack of financial planning is the reason for failure of many health fitness businesses. Projecting future financial results—budgeting—is a helpful planning and controlling tool (Moscove 1981). A *budget* provides a road map for an organization to follow.

> *Without the means to make financial projections, an organization proceeds on a blind course with the consequences of always reacting too late to financial matters.*

A budget is simply a plan for the future expressed in monetary terms. The objective of this plan is to provide a planning and control system to guide an organization for the next month, quarter, or year. We emphasize the word *control*, which allows the business to compare actions with intentions. It is unreasonable to expect a monthly budget to be 100 percent accurate over a planning period of 6 to 12 months. Rather, the intent of the budget is to lay out a plan and provide guidelines for controlling the operations of the club according to the plan.

A preliminary budget establishes how management implements its financial plan for an upcoming year. According to the I-formation management model, the implementation phase determines whether an organization maintains its current state of operations or expands into other areas. Budget preparation allows management the opportunity to diagnose deficiencies and identify areas of potential growth.

Although there are a variety of budgets businesses may choose to develop, health fitness organizations have traditionally prepared four types:

- Sales budget
- Income and operating expense budget
- Capital expenditure budget
- Cash budget

Sales Budget

The sales budget is a projection of the revenue categories directly affecting the overall business. In a profit setting, this primarily consists of initiation fees, as well as the estimated number of new and continuing members, multiplied by the price of the membership to obtain annual membership dues. You should also include the projected number of members who drop their memberships and any adjustment to monthly dues in this budget. In a nonprofit setting, in which membership dues may be priced low, projections for such categories as activity programming, child care, guest fees, and court fees may collectively represent the highest revenue percentage. Use monthly projections for these categories with associated fees to establish a sales budget. Table 15.2 represents a sample sales budget for a commercial setting.

Operating Budget

> *The goal of an income and operating expense budget is to summarize the financial projections of all phases of the business and allow management to weigh each individual budget against the overall profit plan for the year.*

A budgeted income and operating expense statement is built from previous budgets and may resemble the organization's financial statement. Each income and expense category is broken down into

Table 15.2   Sample Sales Budget

XYZ Athletic Club annual membership projections

| FYE 1996 dues projected | $191,890 |
| FYE 1996 # members | 2,675 |

	Jan	Feb	Mar	Apr	May	June
# of new members	55	45	45	45	40	35
# of members lost	30	35	40	35	30	35
Net members gained	25	10	5	10	10	0
Total # of members	2,700	2,710	2,715	2,725	2,735	2,735
Attrition rate percent	13.33	15.50	17.68	15.41	13.16	15.36
Joining fees	$22,000	$18,000	$18,000	$18,000	$16,000	$14,000
Monthly dues	$1,725	$690	$345	$690	$690	$0
Dues increase						
Commissions	$6,225	$5,025	$5,025	$5,025	$4,425	$3,825
Total dues	$193,615	$194,305	$194,650	$195,340	$196,030	$196,030
Average monthly dues						

line items that represent the various ways of receiving revenue and spending business funds. Listed here are the line items that most income and operating expense budgets include.

Revenue Line Items

- Membership revenue
- Guest fees
- Racquet sports
- Fitness programs
- Profit centers
- Miscellaneous revenue
- Expense line items
- Payroll
- Administration
- Maintenance
- Utilities
- Advertising and marketing
- Program expenses
- Profit center expenses
- Miscellaneous expenses

Depending on the size and scope of the operation, you will need involvement from supervisors or other department heads regarding revenue and expense categories if you are to perform the budgeting process accurately. Table 15.3 provides a sample of an income and operating expense budget.

Capital Expenditure Budget

The capital expenditure budget determines the future cost projections for the building and equipment. In preparing this budget, consider assets that are becoming worn out, obsolete, or inefficient as well as proposed expansion or renovation projects of the facility. The magnitude of such projects will vary annually depending on the long-term goals of the organization. Consequently, it is customary to plan a capital expenditure budget over several years and to continuously register ideas of areas needing upgrading or replacing.

According to IHRSA's 1996 *Profiles of Success*, most health fitness settings spend four to six percent of their total annual revenue on capital improvements. By reviewing capital needs you can set aside a designated amount of funds each year to reinvest into the organization. A regular investment of this nature reflects management's commitment not only to maintain but also to regularly improve the overall appearance of the facility. A sample capital expenditure budget is provided in table 15.4.

XYZ Athletic Club annual membership projections

July	Aug	Sept	Oct	Nov	Dec	Annual total
40	40	40	30	30	45	490
30	35	35	30	30	30	395
10	5	5	0	0	15	95
2,745	2,750	2,755	2,755	2,755	2,770	
13.11	15.27	15.25	13.07	13.07	13.00	
$16,000	$16,000	$16,000	$12,000	$12,000	$18,000	$196,000
$690	$345	$345	$0	$0	$1,035	$6,555
						$0
$4,425	$4,425	$4,425	$3,225	$3,225	$5,025	$54,300
$196,720	$197,065	$197,410	$197,410	$197,410	$198,445	$2,354,430
						$196,203

Cash Budget

> *Cash flow is the lifeblood of any business, and the cash budget is the most effective tool for planning and controlling cash flows.*

A cash budget is a period-by-period estimate of the amount and timing of the cash flows produced by planned operations (DeThomas 1991). The usual planning period is a year, but you may break it down into quarters, months, or weeks. Cash budgets project the estimated inflows (receipts) and outflows (disbursements) of normal operations. Cash inflows include cash sales, collection of accounts receivable, sale of fixed assets, and income earned on investments. Cash outflows consist of accounts payable, tax payments, payments for cash expenses, and any fees associated with financing, investment, or dividend activities. A summary at the end of the budget reflects the expected cash balance at the end of the period compared with the amount established as the minimum balance. The difference is the cash shortage or surplus for that period.

The importance of the cash budget cannot be overemphasized. Unexpected cash shortages may result in staff layoffs, borrowing funds under crisis conditions, poor credit ratings, and dipping into financial reserves. A cash budget forces an owner or manager to identify, evaluate, and monitor financial variables that are essential to the success of the business. A sample cash budget is provided in table 15.5.

BUDGET PREPARATION

The process used to prepare a budget varies from setting to setting. Although the size, scope, and organizational structure of the business determine the types of budgets to use, there are basic steps that you can apply to implement the budgeting procedure. The components of these steps are as follows:

Step 1 Call to Action

- In a timely fashion, announce the budget process to all department heads.
- Set direction by announcing financial goals and assumptions based on management's profit plan.
- Provide a user-friendly format by distributing specific line items to each department head.
- Provide a workable timetable to follow to have all budgets completed by year end.

Table 15.3   Sample Operating Budget

XYZ Athletic Club
Annual operating budget projections

Acct.#	Period:	Jan. 1, 2000 thru Dec 31, 2000	
Acct.#		**Account Description**	**Proj. # of members**
			260 members
		Revenue	
4010		Joining fees	$ 0
4020		Membership dues	$125,000
4040		Guest fees	$5,000
4400		Programs	$360
4420		Health/fitness instruction	$10,000
4500		Massage	$10,000
4520		Snack bar	$2,400
4580		Locker rental	$1,800
4590		Pro shop	$0
4900		Miscellaneous revenue	$1,000
		Total revenue	**$155,560**
5140		(Massage commission)	($13,500)
		Net revenue	**$142,060**
		Expenses	
6440		Wages—aerobics	$6,500
7110		Wages—management	$21,000
7160		Wages—front desk	$24,000
		Total payroll	**$51,500**
9510		Employee relations	$50
9520		Group insurance	$1,525
9530		FICA—employer	$3,940
9540		Federal unemployment	$412
9545		State unemployment	$824
		Payroll taxes and benefits	**$6,751**
9210		Electricity	$21,000
		Utilities	**$21,000**
8515		Contract services—temporary	$0
8520		Contract services—interior	$3,000
8539		Contract services—other	$0
8630		Repair—fitness equipment	$100
8690		Repair—other	$0
8740		Supplies—locker room	$300
8755		Supplies—massage	$100
8760		Supplies—laundry	$150
8775		Supplies—cleaning	$200
8790		Supplies—other	$100
8870		Pest control	$100
8885		Towels	$200
		Maintenance	**$4,250**

Table 15.3 (continued)		
7230	Bad Debt	$ 1,200
7240	Collection fee/service chg.	$1,250
7260	Contributions	$0
7270	Courses and conferences	$500
7330	Dues and subscriptions	$250
7360	Education	$0
7390	Employment advertising	$100
7400	Equipment rental and leases	$0
7625	Office equipment maintenance	$100
7640	Permits	$0
7650	Postage	$100
7670	Printing	$100
7860	Professional fees	$0
7730	Repair—office equipment	$150
7779	Repair—other	$0
7820	Supplies—computer	$100
7830	Supplies—office	$300
7880	Supplies—other	$0
7910	Telephone	$2,200
7940	Travel and entertainment	$0
7980	Uniforms	$500
4775	Cable	$450
	Administration	**$6,850**
8120	Advertising	$2,000
8130	Brochures and direct mail	$700
8210	Membership referrals	$0
8220	Membership relations	$25
8280	Special promotions	$25
	Advertising and marketing	**$2,750**
6480	Supplies—fitness	$100
6450	Music/Ascap/BMI	$300
	Fitness	**$400**
9040	Food items	$1,300
9400	Pro shop items	$0
	Food/pro shop	**$1,300**
7590	Miscellaneous	$300
	Miscellaneous	**$300**
	Total operating expenses	**$95,101**
7450	Insurance	$1,500
	Total fixed expenses	**$1,500**
	Total expenses	**$96,601**
	Net income	**$45,459**

Table 15.4   Sample Capital Expenditure Budget

XYZ Athletic Club
Capital expenditures
Year 2000

Items to purchase	Projected date	Amount
Smith machine	1/15/00	$2,229
Computer hardware	2/21/00	$3,000
Resurface outdoor pool	3/30/00	$19,000
New ball machine	4/25/00	$1,200
Security cameras	5/14/00	$4,500
Upgrade HVAC unit	6/09/00	$2,400
Two treadmills	7/20/00	$12,000
Resurface parking lot	8/01/00	$16,700
Relamp indoor tennis courts	9/15/00	$6,500
Audio—CV room	10/10/00	$2,500
Pool vacuum	11/28/00	$2,450
Grill—restaurant	12/15/00	$1,800
Total capital expenditures		**$74,279**

Note: Total capital expenditures equal 6 percent of projected annual revenues.

- Only as a guideline, distribute previous year's results.

Step 2 Draft Presentations

- Stress not basing new year's figures on previous year's numbers.
- Emphasize zero-based budgeting techniques, in which each line item amount is justified through worksheets and key assumptions.
- Review historical financial data, including previous financial statements and prior year budgets.
- Prepare break-even analysis for all programs.
- Present first draft to designated supervisor and defend budget figures.
- Management creates separate capital budget.

Step 3 Completed Budget

- Have final budget completed and, if applicable, entered into computer system by established deadline date.
- Provide a copy of each department budget to respective supervisor.
- Communicate to department heads that they are each accountable for managing their own budget. If applicable, tie compensation to performance.

Step 4 Budget Analysis

- Compare budget to actual figures monthly or quarterly with department heads.
- If analysis indicates a significant change, management may choose to make necessary modifications with existing budget.
- If a department exceeds its expense budget by a preapproved percentage, consider obtaining management approval for subsequent purchases.

Most managers study the variance between the actual financial data and the projected budget. If revenues surpass projections then the variance is favorable. The same is true if expenses are less than projected. However, unfavorable variances occur when either of these conditions are reversed and projections are negatively skewed from actual figures. Management's role is to determine the categories that have exceeded estimated levels and make timely adjustments to control spending or boost revenue generation. Conversely, monitoring the budget may reveal positive changes, such as the expense savings from a program or the increased revenues generated from an organized promotional campaign.

> *The budgeting process is only as successful as the emphasis you place on its importance. Employees must have a vested interest in the budget preparation for it to be an effective operational tool.*

Management should take the time to teach supervisors the proper techniques of budgeting. This could involve sitting down with each supervisor and discussing the club's philosophy toward the budgeting process. For example, are *zero-based budgeting* principles used, in which you must justify every category before inserting a projection figure, or is historical data with a percentage adjustment the preferred method? Also, if you do not conduct periodic review sessions in which you hold supervisors accountable for their department actions, the budget will soon lose its effectiveness. It is important to maintain account-

ability; otherwise a lack of confidence gradually deteriorates the budget purpose.

INCOME MANAGEMENT

Since 1990, total revenues generated by commercial fitness facilities has increased approximately eight percent per year. In addition, the average commercial club produces more than $1.5 million in annual revenue. The cause of this consistent growth rate has been attributed to three factors: (1) increasing new member growth, (2) lowering member attrition, and (3) increasing the average revenue derived per member. Today's managers have discovered that focusing on new member sales is only a portion of the success equation. They must place additional emphasis on retaining existing members, becoming as efficient as possible with space use, and implementing creative programming. Figure 15.5 illustrates the total revenue growth for both fitness-only and multipurpose clubs since 1988.

Membership

Membership joining or initiation fees and monthly dues continue to drive the revenue base that supports commercial, community, corporate, and clinical settings. Without a strong membership base many health fitness facilities cannot provide the necessary revenue to offset operating costs. According to industry surveys, 82 percent of the total revenues generated by multipurpose commercial fitness centers today comes from initiation fees and monthly dues (IHRSA 1996). The remaining 18 percent of nondues revenues resulted from racquet

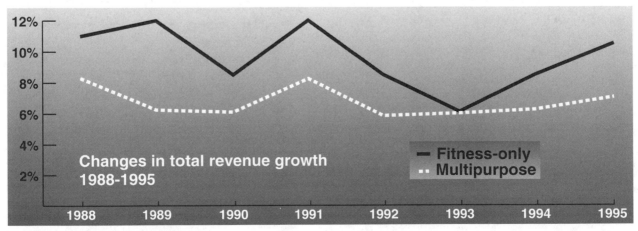

Figure 15.5   Total revenue growth.

Copyright 1995 by National Trade Publications, Inc. Reprinted, with permissioin, from Cleaning & Maintenance Management, 13 Century Hill Dr., Latham, NY 12110.

Table 15.5   Sample Cash Budget

	Period				
	January	February	March	April	May
Cash inflows					
Membership fees	70,000	70,000	65,000	65,000	65,000
Racquet sports	13,400	13,400	12,000	12,000	12,000
Fitness programs	9,600	9,600	9,600	9,600	9,600
Profit centers	7,000	7,000	7,000	7,000	7,000
Total inflows	100,000	100,000	93,600	93,600	93,600
Cash outflows					
Payroll/taxes	37,000	37,000	37,000	37,000	37,000
Utilities	8,000	8,000	8,000	8,000	8,000
Administration	6,500	6,500	6,500	6,500	6,500
Maintenance	4,600	4,600	4,600	4,600	4,600
Advertising	3,500	3,500	3,500	3,500	3,500
Program expenses	1,300	1,300	1,300	1,300	1,300
Profit centers	2,600	2,600	2,600	2,600	2,600
Total operating	63,500	63,500	63,500	63,500	63,500
Insurance	2,200	2,200	2,200	2,200	2,200
RE and PP taxes	2,300	2,300	2,300	2,300	2,300
Rent and lease	8,300	8,300	8,300	8,300	8,300
Total fixed	12,800	12,800	12,800	12,800	12,800
Total outflows	76,300	76,300	76,300	76,300	76,300
Net cash flow	23,700	23,700	17,300	17,300	17,300
Beginning cash	10,000	10,000	10,000	10,000	10,000
Total cash	33,700	33,700	27,300	27,300	27,300
Minimum balance	15,000	15,000	15,000	15,000	15,000
Excess cash	18,700	18,700	12,300	12,300	12,300

sport programs (31 percent), fitness programs (6 percent), profit centers (7 percent), and other miscellaneous revenue (2 percent).

Although membership fees have traditionally been the backbone of industry revenues, today's fitness managers are focusing on nondues revenue as the key for future profits. Lower attrition rates are a significant benefit associated with clubs offering a wide array of nondues-related profit centers. Clubs most successful in nondues revenue reported an average attrition rate of 25 percent versus the industry average of 35 percent. Improved retention rates positively affect net revenue while eliminating some marketing expense associated with replacing lost members.

Industry analysts believe that health fitness facilities that continue to rely on member dues for 80 percent or more of their revenues may soon find themselves at a competitive disadvantage with profit-driven clubs.

Organizations with additional sources of revenue have less need to raise membership fees and may choose to even lower the price of dues. As the

			Period			
June	July	August	September	October	November	December
60,000	60,000	60,000	62,500	62,500	65,000	65,000
10,000	10,000	10,000	12,000	12,000	13,400	13,400
12,000	12,000	12,000	9,600	9,600	9,600	9,600
7,000	7,000	7,000	7,000	7,000	7,000	7,000
89,000	89,000	89,000	91,100	91,100	95,000	95,000
37,000	37,000	37,000	37,000	37,000	37,000	37,000
8,000	8,000	8,000	8,000	8,000	8,000	8,000
6,500	6,500	6,500	6,500	6,500	6,500	6,500
4,600	4,600	4,600	4,600	4,600	4,600	4,600
3,500	3,500	3,500	3,500	3,500	3,500	3,500
1,300	1,300	1,300	1,300	1,300	1,300	1,300
2,600	2,600	2,600	2,600	2,600	2,600	2,600
63,500	63,500	63,500	63,500	63,500	63,500	63,500
2,200	2,200	2,200	2,200	2,200	2,200	2,200
2,300	2,300	2,300	2,300	2,300	2,300	2,300
8,300	8,300	8,300	8,300	8,300	8,300	8,300
12,800	12,800	12,800	12,800	12,800	12,800	12,800
76,300	76,300	76,300	76,300	76,300	76,300	76,300
12,700	12,700	12,700	14,800	14,800	18,700	18,700
10,000	10,000	10,000	10,000	10,000	10,000	10,000
22,700	22,700	22,700	24,800	24,800	28,700	28,700
15,000	15,000	15,000	15,000	15,000	15,000	15,000
7,700	7,700	7,700	9,800	9,800	13,700	13,700

health fitness industry continues to expand into all markets, the ability to be flexible with membership rates provides a strong competitive edge over other dues-driven facilities. In addition, club managers have found that they can expand their target market by implementing programs and adding profit centers that attract new members from outside the regular membership. For example, some clubs have found that by renovating a racquetball or tennis court into a youth fitness center, they can attract the family market thus expanding their revenue base.

Another popular source of income for those organizations providing a corporate membership plan is capitation pricing. Within the health fitness industry, capitation refers to the practice of pricing a corporate membership as though only 20 to 40 percent of a company's workforce will use a club's facilities, while officially extending use to all employees. For example, if a company has an employee base of 100 executives, the club would offer access to all employees, but charge for only 20 to 40 employees. Because formulas for determining the percentage of the workforce to charge for varies from organization to organization, there is no industry standard that has been established to fit every situation. Fitness analysts believe that the potential increase in revenue generated by a one-year or multiyear contract is worth estimating the number of employees who will actually use their memberships.

Fitness Programs

Fitness programming today is positioned to be one of the best avenues for incrasing overall revenues. The introduction of programs such as personal training, aquatics, youth programs, physical therapy, and spa services have caused annual fitness revenues to increase 20 to 30 percent since 1994. The addition of specialty classes for boxing, yoga, karate, and ballet provide opportunities for fitness directors to add variety to their schedules while inserting additional funds to their bottom line. Figure 15.6 lists the breakdown of fitness revenue in 1995.

Racquet Sports

Although racquet sport programs rank behind fitness programming in recent growth, the annual revenue generated from racquet sports has been greater (4 percent) than all fitness activities combined. The racquet sport category primarily represents tennis, racquetball, and squash income generated through court fees, private and group instruction, leagues, clinics, tournaments, and special events.

Profit Centers

Additional profit centers, such as food and beverage, pro shops, child care, and other services, now account for approximately 7 percent of total revenues. Although these services have been considered a member amenity first and a profit center second, annual revenues are expected to increase to 10 to 12 percent of total revenues by the year 2000.

Corporate Clients

Because companies underwrite much of the income derived from operating a corporate program, they have placed little emphasis on selling memberships as a primary source of income. Traditionally, corporate fitness centers have been viewed as providers of exercise programs and facilities for a specific group of executives. However, today's corporate executives have a more comprehensive vision for their physical and mental well-being. They now emphasize such topics as ergonomics and wellness benefits. The result is a wide array of services and products designed to meet the needs of the corporate client.

Ergonomics has become a topic companies are increasingly interested in because a growing number of employees spend more time at their desks. Consequently, companies are contracting programs relating to stress and back problems to outside agencies and underwriting them. In addition, companies want more than just fitness options available to executives, thus the increased interest in wellness services. Health-risk appraisals, blood and cholesterol screening, on-site exercise programs, and corporate retreats are all services verifying that preventive medicine is now accepted as a legitimate component of health care.

Hospital and Wellness

According to the Association of Hospital Health and Fitness (AHHF), in Evanston, Illinois, the number of hospital-based fitness centers has doubled from 175 in 1990 to approximately 350 in 1997. Revenues derived from hospital-based wellness centers continue to come from physician

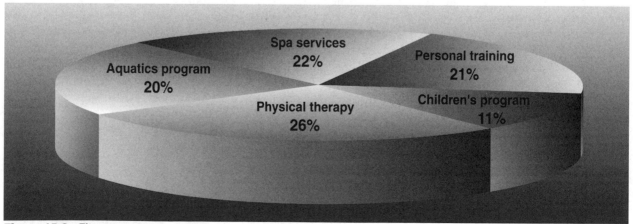

Figure 15.6   Fitness revenue in 1995.

referrals of patients, third-party reimbursement, programming for special populations, and health promotion services. In addition to providing the facilities and services of a commercial fitness center, hospital-based wellness programs offer cardiac rehabilitation, postrehabilitative therapy, and physical therapy services, as well as dietary counseling and classes for special populations.

Hospital-based wellness programs have the lowest attrition rate in the health fitness industry, averaging between 20 and 30 percent a year. The reason for this low rate is based on being affiliated with the positive image of a professional and trustworthy hospital. Consequently, revenues are expected to increase into the year 2000, since a study by the American Heart Association (1995) found that approximately 7 million people in the United States have coronary artery disease, 11 million suffer from diabetes, 13 million are overweight, and 58 million have hypertension. Industry analysts believe individuals in these categories will choose a hospital-based wellness program over a facility with no medical affiliation.

Once you have identified the income sources for a particular setting, organizing an internal system for receiving funds for services rendered is the next component of the accounting process. Identifying, tracking, and monitoring accounts receivable is a standard accounting practice used in all businesses.

ACCOUNTS RECEIVABLE

Accounts receivable is an amount that is owed a business, usually by one of its customers or members, as a result of the ordinary extension of credit (Caro 1986). Receivables are generated primarily from funds for membership fees and dues, programming and service fees, and miscellaneous profit center charges over a designated time. Being able to control the funds invested in accounts receivable is an important component of income management. In addition, the system you create for tracking accounts receivable plays a major role in establishing an organization's credit policy. A credit policy involves decisions on how to collect, manage, and control receivables.

Accounts Receivable Management

The health fitness industry is no different than most small businesses in which a percentage of its funds are regularly tied up in receivables created from credit sales or membership dues. A continuing problem for organizations that obtain revenue from membership and initiation fees is collecting these funds. Typically, you would mail bills before a member's anniversary date (i.e., monthly, quarterly, biannually, or annually). Cash flow problems occur when the time that passes between sending the bills and receiving payments is extensive. Until the point of collection, an unpaid account represents a drain on an organization's financial resources. To achieve effective management of accounts receivable, it is necessary to incorporate the three following tools.

Sales Analysis

It is effective to produce a regular sales analysis that breaks down the total sales figures into components so you can evaluate the performance for each. By tracing sales revenue to the individual category, management can identify trouble spots and take action before trouble arises. Table 15.6 provides a sample sales analysis that categorizes membership types and the amount billed for each payment cycle.

Aged Trial Balance

It is important to stay apprised of the length of time individual accounts have been outstanding. You can accomplish this by generating an *aged trial balance*, which lists the total of all outstanding balances falling into established past due categories. Generally, the past due categories are from 1 to 30 days, 31 to 60 days, and 61 to 90 days. From this report a manager can determine which accounts are past due and which accounts exceed established credit limits. A sample aged trial balance is shown in table 15.7.

Credit Policy

Establish and enforce a sound collection policy and effective procedures for dealing with delinquent accounts. Create a policy that provides a balance between generating the pressure needed to obtain payment from delinquent accounts and not jeopardizing future business by offending members. Unfortunately, there are no industry standards or rules that guarantee an acceptable approach to collections. However, there are some guidelines health fitness organizations follow that have provided a nucleus for an effective collection policy.

1. Base your collection policy on clear, effective communication between the organization and the member.

Table 15.6   Sample Sales Analysis

Member type	Member status summary					
	Active	Susp.	Term	Del.	Total	Last month
20-Ind. annual	173	1	1	0	173	170
21-Family annual	362	0	0	0	364	362
22-Ind. midday ann.	8	0	0	0	8	7
23-Fam. mid. ann.	5	0	0	0	5	5
24-Sr. ind. annual	12	0	0	0	12	10
25-Sr. fam. ann.	20	0	0	0	20	20
26-Cor. ind. ann. TE	53	0	0	0	53	54
28-Yng. adult ann.	1	0	0	0	1	1
29-Cor. fam. ann.	11	0	0	0	11	12
30-Ind. semiann.	8	0	0	0	8	8
31-Fam. semiann.	4	0	0	--	4	4
40-Individual	719	10	0	1	730	715
41-Family	964	6	0	0	970	950
60-Midday ind.	60	1	0	0	61	52
61-Midday fam.	15	1	0	0	16	15
70-Corp. individual	39	0	0	0	39	40
71-Corp. family	40	0	0	0	40	39
75-Individual TE	30	0	0	0	30	29
76-Family TE	48	0	0	0	48	48
80-Nonresident	13	0	0	0	13	13
81-Nonres. family	20	0	0	0	20	20
90-Senior individual	41	0	0	0	41	42
91-Senior family	51	1	0	0	52	52
93-Leave medical	4	8	0	0	12	4
94-Leave other	4	15	0	0	19	4
95-Drop	6	1	32	267	306	6
96-Employee ind.	107	0	0	0	107	103
97-Employee fam.	26	0	0	0	26	26
98-Corporate	28	0	0	0	28	28
99-Nonpay	34	0	0	0	34	33
Subtotal	2906	44	33	268	3251	2872
02-Family member	3353	10	92	28	3483	3403
Totals	6259	54	125	296	6749	6288.86
Average dues						

	Member status summary			
Change	Joined this month	Estimated dues	Last month dues	Change
3	3	110	0	110
0	4	0	0	0
1	1	0	0	0
0	0	0	0	0
2	0	43	31	12
0	0	89	89	0
−1	0	29	29	0
0	0	0	0	0
−1	0	0	0	0
0	0	0	0	0
0	0	0	0	0
4	21	45511.97	45256.97	255
14	18	83946.30	82698.30	1248
8	5	2100	1820	280
0	0	750	750	0
−1	1	2420	2485	−65
1	1	3469.20	3377.20	92
0	0	1881	1816	65
0	1	3601	3606	−5
0	0	499	499	0
0	0	801	801	0
−1	0	1962	2014	−52
−1	0	3321	3394	−73
0	0	0	0	0
0	0	0	0	0
0	0	0	0	0
4	4	0	0	0
0	0	275	275	0
0	0	20	20	0
1	2	0	0	0
34	62	150828.47	148961.47	1867
−50	68	2168	2118	50
−15	130	152996.47	151079.47	1917
		24.46	24.09	0.37

Table 15.7	Sample Aged Trial Balance								
Member #	Name	Phone no.	Last payment	Current	30 days	60 days	90 days	Net due
6317	JohnDoe	555-3433	2/09/96	2.39	2.36	2.34	236.31	243.40
3227	Jane Doe	555-6590	11/08/96	17.76	87.81	54.53	521.12	681.22
5946	Austin Jones	555-7117	12/01/96	13.84	0.04	0	3.96	17.84
9658	Martin Smith	555-0053	4/02/96	10.54	10.54	0	1053.64	1074.72
6211	Becky Wilson	555-2365	6/06/96	105.17	104.15	672.65	106.21	988.18
8076	Jim Jacobs	555-6347	1/06/96	102.38	101.38	100.39	293.54	597.69
9776	Mary Walter	555-9521	4/27/96	87.81	54.53	521.12	17.76	681.22
1205	George Perkins	555-7782	5/22/96	751.17	0.03	0	3.45	754.65
3499	Samuel Johnson	555-7811	1/19/96	190.51	97.33	102.12	331.17	721.13
5674	Daniel Patrick	555-3603	5/08/96	65.89	65.03	79.88	79.91	231.71
Final total				1347.46	523.20	1533.03	2647.07	5991.76

2. Establish specific procedures to follow for delinquent accounts that reach 30, 60, and 90 days.

3. Secure a collection agency to handle problem accounts that management cannot rectify.

4. Internally control a member with a delinquent account from using the facility.

Electronic Funds Transfer

As a means to improve the collection of accounts receivable, an *electronic funds transfer (EFT)* method of billing can make payments as easy as possible for members while expediting the collection of funds for the business. This alternative method of billing is the system predominately used in the health fitness industry today for collecting receivables.

EFT debits a checking, savings, or credit card account for the payment of monthly fees. Members authorize a predetermined membership fee deduction or other incidental charges that are automatically withdrawn from their account or credit card company on an established date. You can deposit collected funds in a club's account in five days or within a 24-hour period if necessary.

Some Advantages of Electronic Billing

• The cost of paper billing (e.g., monthly statements and coupon books) represents 12 percent of the total billing cost, whereas EFT billing ranges between 4 and 7 percent.

• Payments are automatically deposited into a facility's account within a matter of days, thus securing a predictable cash flow.

• Easier process for members to pay monthly fees, consequently increasing member adherence.

• Reduced administration and collection fees.

Some Disadvantages of Electronic Billing

• Members' negative perception of having fees deducted from their account each month.

• The time involved with correcting clerical errors.

• Proper communication of member terminations so drafts can be stopped on time.

There are four recommended EFT services available to club managers:

1. *EFT provider.* A manager contracts with an EFT provider who keys in all member data from hardcopy membership forms sent by the business. The service provider updates all member files, performs the billing service, and credits the organization's account. Although this is considered a labor-saving method for personnel, it is generally the most expensive form of EFT service.

2. *Software-supported EFT.* An organization is responsible for keying in all member information and bank account or credit card numbers. This information is then downloaded to the EFT provider via modem. The EFT provider debits the members' accounts, minus the provider's service fee, and credits the account. Software-supported EFT is the most widely used service in the health fitness industry.

3. *A bank as an EFT provider.* All services that an EFT provides a bank can also perform. Although

this method is the most inexpensive, it does not provide some customized reports or other customer service options available through an EFT provider.

4. *Do it yourself.* Depending on the size of operation, some club operators, through an internal computer system, have taken on the role of an EFT provider. The amount of internal administration and communication with various banks makes this option difficult to administer and more costly than hiring an EFT provider.

EXPENSE MANAGEMENT

Understanding the *expense management* side of operating a health fitness business is an important component of financial management. Traditionally, managers have focused on income issues such as advertising, marketing, and new member sales as a means to increase overall profits. The health fitness industry has always been a market-driven business, emphasizing the revenue side more than controlling spending. However, over the years, managers have realized that cutting costs is more tangible and predictable than estimating member sales. Rick Caro, president of Management Vision Inc., a fitness consulting company based in New York City, estimates that unnecessary expenditures for soap, utilities, towels, payroll, and so on cost the average commercial multirecreational facility an extra $100,000 a year. Unnecessary expenditures result from not providing such things as proper accounting controls and security, regular bidding and negotiating with vendors, questioning every expense as though it were coming out of your own pocket, performing internal maintenance, and eliminating costs when necessary.

Controlling expenses starts with categorizing all costs associated with operating the business. Then divide each expense into subheadings that represent standard industry expense categories. As an example of these categories, table 15.8 provides an expense model of a commercial fitness setting. As previously mentioned in this chapter, expense categories are separated into operating expenses (varied costs according to the number of memberships) and fixed expenses (those incurred whether or not an individual uses a fitness facility). They are not dependent on the volume of the business.

According to the 1996 IHRSA *Profiles of Success*, the total expenses for an average commercial setting are 70 percent operating and 22 percent fixed. The most common expense categories to regularly monitor are payroll, renting or leasing, administration, and utilities; combined, these expenses represent

Table 15.8 Expense Model for a Commercial (Multipurpose) Health Fitness Facility

Expense categories	Average (%)
Operating expenses (% of total revenue)	1995
Payroll	39.0%
Administration	9.4%
Maintenance and repairs	5.5%
Energy and utilities	6.6%
Membership sales and marketing expenses	3.0%
Program expenses	1.6%
Profit center expenses	3.0%
Other operating expenses	1.9%
Total operating expenses	70.0%
Operating margin	30.0%
Fixed expenses (% of total revenue)	
Interest and financing	4.1%
Rent and leasing	8.7%
Real estate and personal property taxes	2.2%
Depreciation	6.6%
Other fixed costs	0.8%
Total fixed expenses	22.4%
Net income before taxes	8.1%

Reprinted, by permission, from IHRSA, 1996, *Profiles of success* (Boston: IHRSA).

the majority of expenses. An acceptable net income (profit) before taxes is approximately 9 percent. Profit margins (operating expenses expressed as a percentage of total revenue) measure management's ability to control operating expense spending. If management can hold the growth of operating expenses to a rate lower than the growth of total revenue, then net profits will increase. As reflected in table 15.8, the average operating margin for commercial fitness centers in 1995 was 30 percent.

Depreciation

A term often seen listed on financial statements but seldom totally understood is *depreciation* (the process of allocating the cost of an asset to the periods benefited).

> *Because the health fitness industry has its share of deterioration and repairs to equipment and the facility, depreciation needs to be listed as a* real *expense. In other words, reflect depreciation in an income statement in the regular expense category.*

Neglecting to list depreciation as an actual cash expense (although technically it is a noncash expense) could prevent allocating the proper amount of funds to cover the annual wear and tear of building and property. Health fitness centers today should expect to spend funds similar in amount to that year's depreciation total for repairs and replacement costs.

> *To fully comprehend depreciation, understand that the total cost of a new piece of exercise equipment or a building represents an asset, which has present and future value to the business.*

A depreciable expense is the allocation of the cost of these long-term assets over their estimated useful life as an expense (Moscove 1981). If a fitness center purchases a new treadmill for $5,000, this machine is an asset because it represents potential business value to the organization. As members use the machine, recognize an expense each accounting period for the service value received from this asset. Before you can determine depreciation you need two important estimations:

1. An estimate of the asset's useful life. The expected useful life represents how long the business plans to receive service benefits. For example, the useful life for most fitness equipment has been estimated at five to seven years. The Internal Revenue Service has its own depreciation tax guidelines of recommended useful life for different categories of building and equipment assets.

2. An estimate of the asset's expected salvage value. The salvage value is the amount that the business can reasonably expect to receive from selling the asset at the end of its useful life. In the open market, fully depreciated fitness equipment yields from 10 to 40 percent of original purchase prices.

Although we recommend that you have an accountant's assistance in preparing these estimates, management's knowledge must also help determine these values. Remember that depreciation rules change from year to year; however, the rule that was in effect when you purchased an asset is the rule that you use to determine the write-off period.

Another aspect of expense management is becoming familiar with all costs associated with operating the business. Knowing each vendor, what is being supplied, and the respective charge for each item are prerequisites for good expense control. Review and scrutinize each invoice as though you were paying it from a personal account. Take steps to ensure consistency and predictability from one month to the next. Question monthly variances, determine reasons for each variance, and take actions to minimize excessive variances.

Health fitness professionals must understand the effect expense management can have on business profitability.

> *Managing expenses provides a more tangible method of controlling costs than trying to generate additional revenue.*

For example, if you could reduce a credit card discount by three percent and projected sales for the year was $1 million, you would immediately notice a savings of $30,000. However, nobody can predict the financial outcome of the next marketing campaign or how many new members will join a facility the next month.

Learning to control the expenses of a health fitness facility should be the goal of every manager or owner. To date, there is not a comprehensive method for completely controlling the expenses of any business. However, there are industry standards and management procedures that provide a gauge for expense management.

Twelve Tools of Expense Management

A financial profile comparing the most profitable commercial health fitness centers with less successful operations indicates that the most successful clubs control expenses better than others. Although the successful clubs' operating expenses increase more than those of an average club, their revenues increase much faster, whereas other clubs' expenses outgrow their revenue (Gangemi 1996).

> *By being creative and embracing change, managers can positively affect their organization's bottom line. Closely evaluating and identifying cost-saving opportunities while implementing ways to control costs are factors for ensuring higher net income for the future.*

Checklist to Assist in Expense Management

1. **Accounting controls and security**
   - Use purchase orders that include an estimated cost for the purchase and management approval.
   - Control access to cash by limiting access and including a drop safe, three-part receipt forms, and control sheet verifications.
   - Provide physical plant security by including alarm systems, entry gates, and security cameras.
   - Provide computer security by including password protection, limited access, and room security.
   - Install management controls by preparing procedure manuals, providing a manager on duty at all times, and obtaining management's approval on large purchases.

2. **Value analysis**
   - Have a cost-benefit mentality. Weigh results versus costs; consider the return on investment and what the payback includes.
   - Ask key questions. Why are we purchasing this? Is this the best value for the money? What did we purchase that we didn't need?

   - Review the method of funding, for example, leasing versus buying, paying cash versus borrowing from the bank.

3. **Bidding**
   - Bid everything—signs, insurance, office supplies, garbage removal, carpeting, construction.
   - Obtain at least three comparison bids.
   - Buy in bulk.
   - Do comparison shopping every three to six months for selected goods and services.

4. **Negotiating**
   - Vendors expect negotiations.
   - What you can negotiate—total price, payment terms, delivery date, service (guarantee, contract), guarantees, options or extra features, and training.

5. **Doing it yourself**
   - Use internal resources.
   - Use in-house maintenance team for carpentry, basic HVAC, electrical and plumbing, carpet cleaning, and court floors.

(continued)

- Communication needs—printing, photography, and desktop publishing (newsletters, in-house flyers, forms).

6. Eliminating

- Jobs (not functions)—investigate using full-time employees for part-time work, avoid double overlapping jobs, and regularly analyze staff schedules.
- Mass media advertising (shift to other marketing vehicles).
- Office supplies and unused services.
- Unnecessary cost centers.

7. Buying used

- Items that you could purchase used include restaurant equipment, computers, and maintenance equipment.
- Consider the following when purchasing used equipment: name brands, appraisals, and guarantees.
- Locate used equipment by attending auctions and reading trade periodicals and local newspapers.

8. Contracting out

- Reasons for contracting out include lack of expertise, internal tasks that are unprofitable, and outside resources that could improve business performance.
- Examples of areas to contract out include restaurant, pro shop, lawn care, and HVAC service.
- Advantages include predictable return, re-claim use of staff, less risk, greater knowledge of a particular service.

9. Trading or bartering

- Determine value of the trade by comparing a full (initiation fees and dues) membership fee with a company's normal charge for the service.
- Examples of trades include photography, printing, supplies, advertising and promotion, and architectural and legal services.

10. Substituting

- Lower wattage light bulbs.
- Generic replacement parts.
- Accountant's review statement instead of a full audit.
- Private labels versus name labels.

11. Donating

- Offer a free (limited) membership to charitable organizations requesting donations.
- Offer free fitness evaluations or an invitation to a club party.
- Avoid giving cash.

12. Using space more efficiently

- Convert cost centers into profit centers; contract out restaurant after internal failure of running; or convert offices to a pro shop.
- Convert underused space to a usable (i.e., revenue-generating) function; convert a lounge to a sales office or storage space to a massage room.

Reprinted, with permission, from Rick Caro, Management Vision, Inc. (1995).

TAX CONSIDERATIONS

To understand the full nature of financial management, it is important to understand the tax environment within which a health fitness center owner or manager must operate. Taxes impact the financial planning and decision-making process of every business. It is essential for management to understand the tax system and its connection with financial planning and tax planning to successfully function in the business world today.

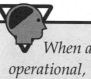
When a health fitness facility becomes operational, it is automatically subject to being taxed under the three levels of government: federal, state, and local.

Because the tax laws are complex and the revisions by congress are frequent, we recommend assistance from either an accountant or the Internal Revenue Service (IRS) to complete tax forms and maintain record keeping. The ever-present possibility of an IRS audit is incentive enough to keep good accounting records and receipts of all bills.

Federal Taxes

The legal form of ownership (as delineated in chapter 3) has a major impact on the way tax regulations—especially income tax regulations—apply to a business. The federal income tax assessment for sole proprietorships, partnerships, corporations, and S-corporations are listed here.

Sole Proprietorship

- The profits from a sole proprietorship are taxed as personal income to the owner.
- Legally, the owner and the business activity are inseparable and are taxed as though the owner is an employee.
- A sole proprietor is expected to estimate income tax each year and pay estimated quarterly taxes.

Partnership

- As with the sole proprietorship, tax liability is only assessed for the earned incomes of the individual partners and not against the business.
- Each partner files a separate form, noting his or her distributive shares of the profits.
- A report of the business must be submitted to the IRS each year. This is only an information report; no tax payment accompanies its submission.
- As with the sole proprietorship, each partner also files an estimated tax.

Corporation

- Tax reporting becomes more elaborate and complicated with this form of ownership.
- As an employee of the corporation, you report annual income and company dividends to the IRS.
- As a separate entity, the corporation must also file a return to the IRS.
- Make estimated tax payments to an authorized bank depository or to a regional Federal Reserve Bank.

S-Corporation

- The IRS code allows some incorporated businesses to be taxed as a sole proprietorship or partnership.
- The main requirements to qualify for S-corporation treatment are as follows:
  1. The company must not have more than 35 stockholders, and the company may have only one class of stock.
  2. The company must be a domestic corporation and must not be affiliated with any group eligible to file consolidated tax returns.
  3. The corporation may not derive over 20 percent of its gross receipts from royalties, rents, dividends, interest, annuities, and gains on sales of securities.

State and Local Taxes

The rates for state and local taxes on health fitness facilities vary from state to state. Common among these taxes are the state tax on gross income; real estate taxes; sales on retail goods, food, and services; and membership fees, which some states consider an amusement or entertainment tax. Currently, 22 states tax membership dues as an amusement or entertainment tax. The charges for these taxes range between 3 and 8 percent, depending on the state.

An additional local tax assessed against every for-profit health fitness center is a *property tax* or, in some states, both property and personal property taxes. City tax assessors calculate property taxes three ways:

1. *Cost approach.* The value of the property is the selling price of the land, plus the cost to construct the building, minus depreciation caused by facility wear and tear. States that tax personal property also include the value of the equipment, furniture, and fixtures.

2. *Income approach.* The value of the club property is the value of its earning potential. In this approach you could use a club's gross income or, if the facility was being rented, the property's rental value.

3. *Market or comparable sales approach.* The value of the club is predicated on the selling price of other land and similar businesses in the area. This approach is not used as often as the two previously mentioned, because most city assessors do not have realistic information on club sales.

Every owner or manager of a for-profit health fitness center should monitor property tax assessments closely. On the average, three percent of a club's gross revenues are paid annually for property taxes. For example, consider the average commercial club that grosses $1.5 million in revenues. From this amount, $45,000 would be paid in property taxes. Appealing property taxes is a right afforded any owner or manager of a business. You can obtain assistance for questioning or appealing property taxes by contacting a CPA or by inquiring with a representative from your local city assessors office.

> *In the fitness business appealing a property tax is one of the few ways to cut costs without affecting member service, staff morale, or facility upkeep.*

Note to reader—the previous section on tax considerations was a brief review of some tax codes as they relate to the health fitness industry. You can obtain further information on these codes from a CPA or through the Internal Revenue Service.

IN CLOSING

This chapter has described the major issues of financial management that every owner or manager must confront when operating a health fitness program: the accounting process, financial statements, budget planning, income management, expense management, and tax considerations. Although these topics represent some principles of financial management, they are in no way totally inclusive of the financial process. Employ additional resources (e.g., workshops, seminars, educational classes) and assistance (accountants and bookkeepers) to develop the financial skills necessary to operate a health fitness business.

KEY TERMS

Accounts receivable

Accrual accounting

Aged trial balance

Assets

Balance sheet

Budget

Cash accounting

Depreciation

Electronic funds transfer (EFT)

Expense management

Income statement

Liabilities

Owner's equity

Property tax

Zero-based budgeting

RECOMMENDED READINGS

American Heart Association. 1995. Exercise standards: A statement for healthcare professionals from the American Heart Association. *Circulation* 91: 580-615.

Burstiner, I. 1979. *The small business handbook: A comprehensive guide to starting and running your own business.* Englewood Cliffs, NJ: Prentice Hall.

Caro, R. 1986. *Financial management.* Boston: International Health, Racquet and Sportsclub Association.

DeThomas, A., ed. 1991. *Financial management techniques for small business.* Grants Pass, OR: PSI Research/Oasis Press.

Droms, W. 1990. *Finance and accounting for nonfinancial managers.* Reading, MA: Addison-Wesley.

Gangemi, R. 1996. Pumping up your profits. *Club Business International* 17(8): 26-27, 34-39.

Howland, W. 1995. Know your numbers. *Club Business International* 16(7): 22, 49.

International Health, Racquet and Sportsclub Association. 1995. *Profiles of success.* Boston: IHRSA.

———. 1996. *Profiles of success.* Boston: IHRSA.

Keeny, B. 1994. By the numbers. *Club Business International* 15(10): 26-30, 42-43.

Kochanek, R., and D. Hillman. 1990. *Financial accounting.* Orlando, FL: Harcourt Brace Jovanovich.

Moscove, S. 1981. *Accounting fundamentals for non-accountants.* Reston, VA: Reston.

Patton, R.W., W.C. Grantham, R.F. Gerson, and L.R. Gettman. 1989. *Developing and managing health/fitness facilities.* Champaign, IL: Human Kinetics.

Pinches, G. 1990. *Essentials of financial management.* New York: Harper Collins.

CHAPTER 16

Payroll and Compensation

As operators of health fitness programs rush to embrace innovative ways to improve management practices, most organizations overlook a critical component of successful change: how they pay their employees. Even though the health fitness industry has undergone major changes over the last decade, organizations are still compensating most employees the same ways they did 25 years ago. Standard merit pay raises, length of service, and organizational rank are still the norm today. However, today's creative managers are attempting to modify existing pay systems to fit their changing environments. For some organizations this could include such things as *performance-based pay*, retirement benefits, or bonus plans. Whatever the situation, the challenge with pay systems is to keep them flexible and focused on the premise for which they were founded.

In this chapter we explore the basics of a compensation program and how to develop one to fit your program. Further discussion centers on the various elements of compensation, surveys and job pricing, job evaluation, and pay-for-performance issues. Finally, we discuss the most commonly used pay practices in the health fitness industry today.

The health fitness business is a customer service driven industry. Adhering to the needs and expectations of members and guests requires a skilled and knowledgeable staff. The human talent of a club's personnel is the most important resource an organization has in today's competitive market, and managers should consider it an asset. Successful health fitness managers realize that no matter how state of the art the facility, sophisticated the equipment, or extensive the services, businesses cannot survive without highly motivated employees.

To attract and retain the caliber of individuals needed to work in the health fitness field, you need a well-designed and properly implemented compensation plan. Organize the plan to show the value of each employee and reward their contributions to the organization. All too often employees feel a lack of recognition for the work they perform. For this reason, it is the responsibility of every owner or manager to ensure that the compensation package developed for personnel is fair and equitable for both the employee and the employer.

> *Whether managers can substantiate or perceive employees' feelings of under-appreciation, they can negatively impact overall employee morale if left unattended.*

COMPENSATION AND MANAGEMENT

Compensation is considered a vital component of management. Specifically, it contributes to the success of any health fitness operation and provides the mechanism to compensate employees for their productivity. You should view compensation as a part of management, so the management style must be reflected visibly in the method of compensation. Does the compensation plan consist of salaries and hourly wages only, or are there performance-based incentives, benefits, or a bonus plan included? Addressing these issues reflects management's commitment to employees.

Five Compensation Suggestions

A well-developed compensation program can impact the success of a health fitness organization in a number of ways: it can set you apart from the competition, assist in recruiting candidates for employment, help retain existing personnel, and contribute significantly to employee morale. To ensure a compensation plan that contributes to the operation's success and is supported by employees, consider these five suggestions:

1. *Make certain that pay is competitive with similar positions in the health fitness field.* With the increasing number of health fitness facilities and the decreasing number of hourly wage employees, more attention has been directed to the competitiveness of pay. Industry surveys are now available listing national salaries and wage scales, so you can compare similar positions in the health fitness field. Managers should monitor comparable facilities within their community to maintain a competitive pay scale. As the health fitness industry has matured, the price paid for labor has increased along with the demand for additional services and facilities.

2. *Recognize that employees are income-producing assets.* View each employee of a health fitness organization as a major contributor to the overall success of the organization. Because the terms health and fitness are not considered tangible products, it is the responsibility of every employee to assist in creating the overall value or image associated with belonging to a facility. For this reason, managers of all settings must recognize that compensation has to do with acquiring and using a club's most important asset—human talent.

3. *Balance payroll costs with employee productivity.* Unfortunately, traditional accounting practices have impeded the way most managers view personnel. On a balance statement employees are considered liabilities, and on an income statement they are treated as an expense. Rarely do you hear managers talk about the income-producing potential of employees; instead, emphasis centers on wage cost containment. With this view, there is inevitably an overemphasis on cutting payroll and little emphasis on increasing the output per payroll dollar.

> *Today's managers must recognize the fragile balance needed between payroll costs and the individuals who produce the income for the business.*

4. *Manage payroll costs, not just pay-rate levels.* The single largest expense in the health fitness industry is payroll. Currently, salaries and wages, benefits, and payroll taxes represent 35 percent of a commercial fitness center's total expenses. For this reason, you should manage payroll costs like any other expense, even though payroll costs are not like other expenses. For example, if a successful member-retention program is the result of trained and enthusiastic employees, management should seriously consider the negative impact of reducing payroll, or eliminating training and development programs. In this scenario, if management reduces payroll costs, then the overall business will suffer. Payroll management involves weighing the impact of each dollar of payroll cost against the business's financial results.

5. *Consider payroll costs as an investment in the future.* An accountant views every dollar of payroll as an expense. Although this is considered sound accounting, a good manager takes into account other factors when determining appropriate compensation. These factors include weighing the direct payroll costs against the overall performance of the business. If, for example, a club compensates employees by paying a straight wage, this is considered a direct expense: pay for time worked, regardless of the output of the work performed. However, if another club decides to incorporate a profit sharing plan as an incentive for employees to receive higher pay while contributing to the increased profits of the business, this is considered an investment opportunity for the business as well as the employee. Although both options are recognized compensation plans, one is considered an expense and the other is an investment.

> *Controlling compensation means optimizing the margin between output and payroll costs.*

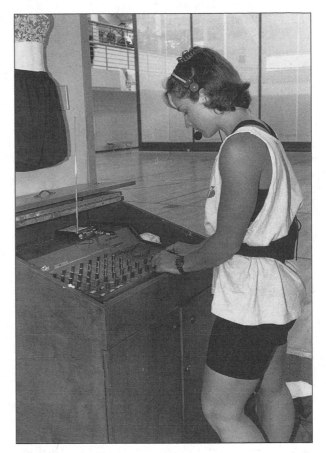

© Tom Wallace

Compensation Policies

Once management has developed its views and strategies on compensation, establish policies that reflect the values of the organization. Identify and answer compensation policy issues to ensure all personnel are treated fairly and consistently during their employment. Basic policy issues that you should address include the following:

- What should be the pay for jobs compared with similar positions in the health fitness field?
- What is the policy with respect to pay for performance?
- Is there a standard policy for performance review pay adjustments?
- Will the organization provide health and retirement plans? If so, what will the employee contribute?
- What will be the compensation policy differences for full-time, part-time, and independent contractors?

- As a form of compensation, are employees able to use the facilities without charge? If so, when are acceptable times of usage?

- Which positions will be designated salaried, hourly wage, commissioned, or payment per class?

Although in every setting there are additional compensation issues that you must address, these seven items represent the major policy issues for most health fitness organizations. The compensation policies that evolve from answering these questions should meet certain requirements. First, they should be specific enough to act as a screen. When an employee makes a proposal regarding some action, you can screen it against the policy statements. Policies must be the basis by which supervisors or department heads make specific decisions and judgments about compensation matters. Finally, policies must be specific and comprehensive enough so they become an important communication tool.

Accountability to Employees

Part of being a health fitness manager is providing accountability when necessary. This should include accountability to employees. Answering compensation-related questions by saying, "I'm sorry, but that's our policy," might have worked in the industrial age of the 1950s but not in the knowledge age as we enter the 21st century.

> *Employees today are a vital and influential force in the workplace. Their actions affect everything that goes on in the business, whether it is positive or negative. With this in mind, management should recognize the importance of maintaining proper accountability to employees.*

Because pay is such a personal matter, managers have the obligation to justify, report, or explain any issue relating to compensation. Being accountable means having the authority to act and the responsibility to exercise that authority if needed. If, for example, an employee brings up a policy that is deemed unfair among other personnel, management has the responsibility to investigate and act on the issue in a timely manner.

Being accountable to employees is not meant to restrict or dilute the manager's position. The final decision maker in any compensation issue is always the manager. However, being accountable only enforces that the organization wants to show fairness and a commitment to its employees.

BASICS OF A COMPENSATION PROGRAM

Essentially, every health fitness setting is unique, different not only in terms of the type, size, location, and services offered but also in more subtle ways. For example, some health fitness settings have different management styles: they perform tasks differently and make decisions in various ways. As a result, each setting should tailor its compensation programs and practices to fit the organization's specific situations.

Successful compensation plans are simple in design, yet adaptive to an organization's management philosophy. The procedures for providing employee pay should be easily understood and implemented by the payroll administrator and be flexible enough to facilitate the employees' needs. New employees should be able to register easily into the plan, and existing employees should be able to receive appropriate remuneration depending on management's requirements. For example, health fitness managers will often cross train employees to work in two or more divisions of an organization. The pay associated with working in separate divisions may differ; consequently, the compensation program must be flexible enough to identify the areas worked and provide the appropriate pay. This is just one example of the importance for having a payroll system that is adaptive to the needs of the organization.

Grouping Employees

Before establishing a compensation plan, make a list of every employee position. This list assists in determining how to group each employee in various divisions. A sample employee position list for a commercial health fitness setting is provided in table 16.1.

Table 16.1   Employee Positions—Commercial Health Fitness Setting

#	Staff positions	#	Staff positions
1	Ownership group	29	Child care supervisor
2	General manager	30	Child care attendant
3	Administrative assistant	31	Martial arts instructor
4	Accounting/business office manager	32	Gymnastics director
5	Accounts payable services	33	Gymnastics instructor
6	Member accounts services	34	Operations manager
7	Accounts receivable coordinator	35	Housekeeping supervisor
8	Data entry clerk	36	Locker room attendant
9	Human resources director	37	Maintenance assistant
10	Service desk manager	38	Building engineer
11	Service desk attendant	39	Assistant building engineer
12	Athletic director	40	Pool maintenance
13	Fitness director	41	Food and beverage manager
14	Fitness/weight training instructor	42	Snack bar attendant
15	Personal trainers	43	Pro shop staff
16	Aerobics director	44	Marketing director
17	Aerobics instructor	45	Marketing assistant
18	Junior aerobics instructor	46	Massage therapists
19	Aerobics training coordinator	47	Membership representative
20	Junior programming director	48	Member relations
21	Sports camp counselor	49	Court sports director
22	Aquatics director	50	Squash and raquetball pro
23	Head lifeguard	51	Head tennis pro
24	Lifeguard	52	Tennis pro
25	Swim instructor	53	Tennis desk attendant
26	Water aerobics coordinator	54	Basketball coordinator
27	Water aerobics instructor	55	Basketball monitor
28	Children's programming director	56	Manager on duty

Grouping employees into an organizational structure that is easy to administer and classifies employees based on management's goals is the next step. Various job categories may require different pay programs and practices.

For management purposes, group jobs so that work tasks and responsibilities are appropriate for each category, and the training and recruiting methods required to fill the jobs are similar. This process is part of the information phase of the I-formation management model in which you determine employment needs. Once you complete this, you can develop many personnel practices, such as recruiting, training, employee communication, and payroll, to meet the requirements of the job.

In the health fitness industry there are at least five groups of employees to consider: upper management and supervisors, full-time staff (salaried), full-time staff (hourly wage), part-time staff (hourly wage), and outside contractors.

Within each category there are subgroups that include employees from various divisions of the organization. For example, upper management includes the general manager, the sales and marketing director, fitness director, aerobics director, and tennis director. Employee subgroups vary depending on the type and size of an organization. Table 16.2 represents a sample employee list for the fitness industry.

Developing a Compensation Program

A recommended approach for developing compensation programs follows. This is the traditional approach commonly used for problem solving in many businesses.

Table 16.2	Sample Employee List—Fitness Setting		
Upper management	**Full-time staff (salaried)**	**Full-time staff (hourly wages)**	**Part-time staff (hourly wages)**
Ownership group	Maintenance manager	Aerobics instructors	Aerobics instructors
General manager	Front desk manager	Aquatics instructors	Aquatics instructors
Sales/marketing director	Food and beverage manager	Personal trainer	Personal trainer
Sales representatives	Sales representative	Fitness center personnel	Fitness center personnel
Fitness director	Controller/business office manager	Tennis instructor	Tennis instructor
Aerobics director	Manager on duty	Racquetball instructor	Racquetball instructor
Tennis director	Assistant general manager	Service desk attendant	Service desk attendant
		Bookkeeper	Bookkeeper
		Office staff	Office staff
		Maintenance/cleaning	Maintenance/cleaning
		Child care staff	Child care staff
		Food and beverage staff	Food and beverage staff
		Pro shop staff	Pro shop staff

Reprinted, by permission, from IHRSA, 1995, *1995 industry data survey* (Boston: IHRSA).

Recommended Process for Developing Compensation Programs

1. Perform a needs analysis. Identify the questions, problems, or opportunities by focusing on the following:

   - Discussions with department heads or supervisors.

   - Discussions with employees.

   - Reported issues, member or staff related.

   - Personnel audits.

2. Develop objectives.

   - Set specific goals.

   - Consider impact on all phases of the operation.

   - Consider schedule format.

   - Determine if there is staff available to meet these goals.

3. Construct the program.

   - Align the program to fit the way business is managed.

   - Make the program flexible to change.

   - Keep the program simple.

   - Have a way of measuring results.

   - Don't make compensation a bad word.

4. Test the program layout.

   - Consider the legal, tax, and accounting ramifications.

   - Play devil's advocate, consider "what if" possibilities.

   - Determine if it will stand the test of time.

   - Compare the program against alternative answers.

5. Implement the program.

6. Evaluate the program's effectiveness.

7. Review.

▼ *All three components (information, implementation, and innovation) of the I-formation management model are incorporated in developing a compensation plan.*

Identify Compensation Needs

Developing a compensation program begins with identifying needs. An organization might be in a start-up phase when it must install an initial pay program. Others may need a change in their compensation system due to problems with an existing system or new opportunities. Despite the reason, identifying the needs is the most crucial aspect of compensation.

Although there are many ways to identify needs, it is critical to have a reliable process that you can use regularly to obtain the information you need.

In accordance with the I-formation management model, identifying compensation needs involves regular monitoring and observation, feedback from reliable sources, and obtaining information on current trends in the health fitness industry.

Some methods that organizations should use to determine specific compensation needs include the following:

- Observing the compensation experiences and problem areas that employees encounter in their work.
- Using opinion or focus polls with managers and employees.
- Performing personnel audits in which you question all aspects of personnel management, not just compensation.
- Using statistical analysis and personnel data to determine needs. Obtain benchmark surveys from industry organizations (IHRSA, Fitness Management). Consider using an information bank that has downloaded job titles, responsibilities, and salary levels from similar settings into a computer file to determine compensation rates.

Develop Goals and Objectives

Accomplishing these goals starts with setting specific objectives. Because much of personnel management is based on knowledge obtained from experiences, it is sometimes difficult to set specific objectives. Often objectives such as "improve employee morale," "provide greater internal consistency," or "create a better quality of work environment" are used to quantify the desired objectives of an organization. Unfortunately, these nonspecific objectives are meaningless and can confuse rather than clarify a specific intent.

The goals of a compensation program are to meet the needs of the organization, resolve problems, and meet the reasonable aspirations of employees and owners.

Set specific, quantifiable goals such as "reduce the employee cost of health care by 25 percent" or "delegate pay decisions to department heads or supervisors." Once you have identified goals, set up appropriate systems to evaluate cost and value.

Construct the Program

Based on the needs assessment data and the stated goals and objectives, the next step is to construct the compensation program. Having a formal compensation system in which everything is spelled out for every possible situation is highly unlikely. However, we recommend establishing predetermined standards in writing that serve to guide individual pay decisions. Such elements of a compensation program should contribute to better decision making, more consistency, and greater fairness.

A compensation program should never mean that the program itself makes the decisions and that the

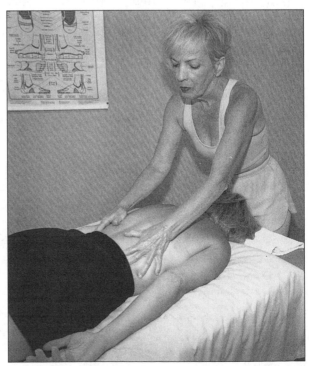

© Tom Wallace

Table 16.3a   Compensation for Fitness Upper Management—Commercial Facilities

| | Upper-management taxable earnings | | |
	Average	Top 25% (earn >)	Bottom 25% (earn <)
Ownership group	$72,750	$120,000	$37,709
General manager	$48,000	$65,000	$37,466
Sales director	$33,751	$44,625	$27,000
Sales representative	$25,000	$38,000	$21,000
Fitness director	$29,500	$35,000	$22,100
Aerobics director	$17,000	$23,000	$8,125
Tennis director	$41,400	$52,500	$31,750

program becomes mechanical. Neither the program nor its procedures can be the decision-making process.

We mention here suggested standards to follow when developing a compensation program:

1. Align compensation programs to fit the way you manage the business. As with any business, health fitness organizations are unique. Management styles, operating systems, and personnel issues vary from setting to setting. A properly tailored compensation program reflects each of these factors and is developed with these values in mind.

2. Make the program flexible to change. A compensation program should adapt to a rapidly changing world. Develop the program so you don't have to reinvent the wheel if you make a change. Whether you incorporate wage scales, cost-of-living increases, pay for performance, or commission-based pay, each of these is subject to change at any time.

3. Keep the program simple. Consider all the supervisors and other managers who are to support and administer the plan. It should make their job easier, not more difficult.

4. Have a way of measuring results. There is no way of incorporating pay to performance if you can't manage performance. Use measures dependent on your organization's goals. Possible measurements may include financial performance, productivity of a division, economic value, quality control, and customer service ranking.

5. Don't make compensation a bad word. Empower employees to understand the compensation process. If pay is to truly motivate employees to perform, then bring it into the open to be understood. This doesn't mean sharing privileged pay information on employees. However, it does mean communicating and updating employees on the process.

Also consider two cornerstones of compensation management, surveying and *job pricing*. The data obtained from these processes are readily accessible, provide specific pay comparisons, and list current salary levels. Only through these methods can pay be sufficient to ensure competitiveness for the organization and fairness to its employees.

Obtaining compensation information is the basis for determining competitive pay and is vital for

Table 16.3b   Compensation for Fitness Upper Management—Commercial Facilities

| | Upper-management compensation by club type (total taxable earnings) | | | |
	All clubs	Multipurpose	Fitness-only	Multioperations
Ownership group	$72,750	$76,750	$65,477	$117,250
General manager	$48,000	$54,500	$36,500	$64,000
Sales director	$33,751	$34,000	$33,000	$38,500
Sales representative	$25,000	$31,680	$23,500	$33,250
Fitness director	$29,500	$30,000	$27,000	$31,350
Aerobics director	$17,000	$18,315	$8,250	$20,500
Tennis director	$41,400	$37,500	N/A	$42,000

Table 16.3c Compensation for Fitness Upper Management—Commercial Facilities

	Upper-management compensation by club size (total taxable earnings)		
	Small < 25 K sq. ft.	Medium 25-50 K sq. ft.	Large >50 K sq. ft.
Ownership group	$117,500	$53,500	$109,500
General manager	$38,500	$47,500	$64,000
Sales director	$29,050	$34,800	$34,500
Sales representative	$18,500	$28,340	$33,750
Fitness director	$26,750	$28,000	$33,000
Aerobics director	$8,600	$18,650	$17,680
Tennis director	$19,250	$33,000	$42,000

dealing with issues relating to fair pay. In response to the need for more and better compensation information, the health fitness industry has invested a great deal of time and effort in developing survey information to improve compensation management. As a result, a variety of information is now available for managers of all settings to review and compare before establishing a quality compensation program.

When compared with more established businesses, the health fitness industry is still in its infancy regarding salary data. Professional journals and industry organizations have primarily been responsible for the salary surveys published today. The data obtained from these surveys can assist managers in establishing comparative benchmarks when recruiting and conducting performance evaluations (refer to chapter 11 for further information on this subject). Keep in mind that pay variations exist between similar positions, depending on the region, type, and size of facility and whether the organization is considered a low revenue performer (25 percent < earnings) or a top performer (25 per-

cent > earnings). Table 16.3, a through d, illustrates these compensation differences between commercial health fitness facilities in 1994.

A word of caution when using published salary information; it is essential that the data obtained from any survey be closely scrutinized before adjusting or setting wages and salaries. Managers need to know the size of the survey, how was it conducted, when, and by whom. Determine the sample size of the organizations participating in the survey. The goal is to find reputable and reliable surveys used by most health fitness managers.

Perhaps the most common method for establishing wages and salaries is to perform job pricing. This system starts by identifying all compensated positions, followed by a brief written description of each position (usually one paragraph). Next, prepare an organizational flow chart, which illustrates position hierarchy and establishes a career path for employees to follow. Once you have completed this information, start pricing the jobs based on management's experience and salary information

Table 16.3d Compensation for Fitness Upper Management—Commercial Facilities

	Upper-management compensation by region (total taxable earnings)			
	Northeast	North Central	South Central	West
Ownership group	$76,750	$115,000	$48,368	$109,500
General manager	$52,250	$40,000	$46,509	$54,000
Sales/marketing director	$33,750	$49,500	$33,751	$31,450
Sales representative	$25,750	$21,350	$29,500	$32,090
Fitness director	$27,696	$30,000	$26,000	$30,000
Aerobics director	$17,000	$12,980	$18,800	$14,318
Tennis director	$29,600	$40,000	$42,000	$50,000

Data for tables 16.3 a-d adapted, by permission, from IHRSA and the University of Massachusetts Amherst Sport Management Department, 1995, *1995 industry data survey: Sales & marketing, membership retention, payroll & compensation* (Boston: IHRSA), 15. Copyright 1995 by IHRSA.

obtained from similar settings. Frequent methods supervisors use to obtain compensation information include personal visits to other clubs, questionnaires, and telephone interviews with other managers.

Test the Program

After designing a compensation program, testing the program is the next step. A major component of testing is reviewing and questioning the legal and tax implications of the program. This process often requires working with an attorney and accountant to make sure the organization is in compliance with the Fair Labor Standards Act.

During this time, you need input from all levels of employees. Take a "what if" approach, questioning each aspect of the plan and deciding on any changes before implementing the program.

Implement the Program

As a component of the I-formation management model, implementation means putting the program into operation and establishing the various procedures and reviews necessary to any new program. The ongoing application of the program illustrates if it is achieving the original goals established by management and employees. Of course, this phase never ends because implementation is dynamic—expect regular changes and modifications. Finally, the nature of administrative and operational work involved in implementation will change, and the staffing required to perform the work must similarly change to meet modified requirements.

Review and Revise the Program

The continuous review of a compensation program will undoubtedly necessitate revisions or major changes. Causes for these revisions may be a change in operations, payroll regulations, financial status, or in management. Managers will want to stay abreast of economic conditions affecting inflation. Monitor factors such as cost of living changes and consumer price index fluctuations quarterly. Annually review the state of the health fitness industry. Are pay rates for all positions staying constant or oscillating? Are the number of employees needed to operate various sizes of facilities staying the same or is a downsizing trend occurring? Is there still a high demand and supply need for health fitness professionals? Is the overall growth of the industry continuing to reflect a posi-

tive change, or has growth slowed? Consider all these factors when reviewing and revising compensation programs.

Making changes to an established compensation program is never easy, especially if the program has been successful and is understood by management and employees. However, waiting too long to make revisions may cause larger problems over time.

> *Remaining innovative includes updating technology, staying in compliance with changing payroll laws, and being adaptive to the ever-changing needs of the organization.*

Thus, it is necessary to realize regular revisions and act on them.

You can adapt this process for developing compensation programs to fit any health fitness setting. Although you can use this process as a basic management tool, the real challenge is to make the program reflect the personality of the business. Because the cultures of fitness centers are so unique and dynamic, clearly understanding the club's profile, including short- and long-term goals and objectives, is essential.

FORMS OF COMPENSATION

Employees in the health fitness industry receive their pay in various ways. Each form of compensation reflects an organization's philosophy, managerial style, and commitment to its employees. Some elements of compensation for employees in the health fitness field include *wages* or salaries, overtime pay, commissions, bonus or profit sharing payments, pay for time not worked, *benefits*, nonfinancial rewards, and compensatory time off.

The compensation elements mentioned in this section have the most practical value in compensation management. Managers of health fitness facilities should identify the specific elements of compensation that best fit their organization. Once identified, determine a value or cost for each item. Although this is sometimes difficult to do, it is the only way to fully understand and manage a compensation program.

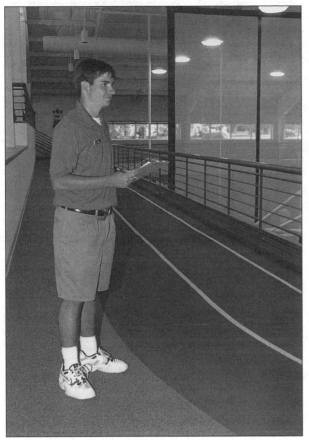

© Tom Wallace

worked in excess of 40 during a week. You cannot combine or average work weeks beyond a one-week period, and you cannot give compensatory time off (details follow) outside of a work week in lieu of overtime.

Most health fitness organizations pay either time-and-a-half or double-time for work on holidays or scheduled vacations. For those employees who occasionally work overtime, the additional pay they receive increases their overall rate of pay. For example, a service desk attendant, making $5.00 an hour, who works 7 hours of overtime per week for only 10 weeks a year increases his rate of pay by 5 percent. However, if the same desk attendant worked one hour of overtime each workday (assuming a 40-hour work week) for a year, his rate of pay would increase by 19 percent.

The economics of overtime pay are important business considerations.

Regularly monitor employee overtime and instigate a procedure for obtaining overtime approval from supervisors.

Without these safeguards in place, an annual payroll budget may erode quickly.

Wages and Salaries

The term wages usually applies to payment for employee services rendered on an hourly or daily basis. Depending on the setting, this form of payment is generally paid to such positions as service desk attendants, maintenance personnel, weight-room trainers, and child care attendants. *Salaries* refer to compensation paid weekly, semimonthly, or monthly and describes the earnings usually paid to the ownership and management group and to fitness, tennis, sales, and aerobics directors. Each form of compensation represents a fixed cost to the business and a basis for administering other forms of compensation.

Overtime Pay

Service desk attendants, weight-floor personnel, day care workers, and most other nonsupervisory employees who are nonexempt are eligible for overtime. By law, these employees must be paid time-and-a-half their regular base pay for each hour

Commissions

Commission-based pay has become a popular method for compensating specialty employees in the health fitness industry. Sales personnel, massage therapists, personal trainers, tennis pros, and aquatics personnel are some employees who might receive remuneration from commissions. A straight commission plan pays employees a percentage of what they obtained in total sales. The rate of commission pay depends on industry standards and the estimated volume of sales generated. For example, a massage therapist could start at a commission rate of 60 percent (to the therapist) and 40 percent (to the club). As the volume of massage sales increases, management could increase the commission to 70/30 to reward the massage therapist for her increased client base, allowing the therapist to earn more money and the club to receive additional revenue through increased sales.

> *The biggest advantage of the commission approach is that it provides the highest level of motivation for employees to sell the greatest volume of their services.*

Although commission-based pay can motivate employees, commission-only plans may cause employees who depend entirely on sales for a weekly paycheck to sell more aggressively, sometimes generating unfavorable member reaction. Under this plan, an organization might find it more difficult to get commission-based personnel to perform other necessary duties.

Another plan gaining wide acceptance is the salary plus commission combination. Management provides a basic salary to cover living expenses, and the employee earns a smaller percentage of sales as a commission. This combination guarantees employees funds for paying current expenses and provides an extra incentive to sell their services.

Bonuses and Profit Sharing

Bonuses or profit sharing plans involve periodic lump-sum payments. The payments may be in the form of an annual or quarterly payment for meeting predetermined financial goals or a monthly bonus to sales personnel for reaching a preestablished new member goal. Bonuses may also provide an incentive for such achievements as cost savings. For example, the bonus structure for the employees of the Little Rock Athletic Club is based entirely on quarterly net profits. Employees have learned that they can positively impact their quarterly bonuses if they are constantly watchful of all expenses associated with their division.

For an employer, all such payments represent a variable cost. More important, many health fitness organizations believe that some type of bonus plan contributes significantly to improving overall operations and member services by providing financial motivation to the employee. An example of a club-sponsored bonus program is explained here.

Ojai Valley Racquet Club Employee Profit Sharing and Point System

The plan

Each quarter, on April 1, July 1, October 1, and January 1, our accounting department will compute the net profit (after all expenses) during the prior three months. We will designate 20 percent of that profit number for employee distribution as a cash bonus, no sooner than 30 days but no more than 45 days from the end of each quarter.

For the first three quarters of one's employment, we will pay 50 percent of this profit sharing bonus to employees directly and hold back the other 50 percent to offset possible quarterly losses until computing the final annual profit at year end. At this time we will pay the remainder of the 50 percent antiloss fund (net) to the eligible employees in addition to normal quarterly bonuses, if any.

Who is eligible?

All hourly employees and some salaried personnel.

What determines the bonus?

1. Your quarterly minireview results.
2. Overall productivity with respect to others in your department.
3. The number of hours of work per week.
4. Attitude toward each other.
5. Length of employment.
6. To what degree your department meets its expense budget.

What's the purpose of the profit sharing plan?

The purpose of the plan is to send each eligible employee an important message. The message is specifically spelled out in the amount of the employee's check (with respect to others in each department) and in the substance of your quarterly minireview.

1. A check for a large percentage means you are meeting or exceeding your job requirements.
2. A check for a smaller percentage means that you are a valuable person but could use improvement in some areas.

3. A check for a small percentage means that your performance is not always what it should be.

4. No bonus means you should consider seeking employment elsewhere.

The overall objective of the plan is to help create a higher level of team effort and to tangibly reward those employees who are doing the best job for the club in their department.

What is the criteria for the best job?

1. Meeting expense budgets rates high for the department as a whole and exceeding expense budget goals will result in a larger share of the total profit allocated to each department.

2. Meeting the needs of the members with regard to the function and purpose of each department.

3. Supporting company policies, rules, and regulations and offering constructive criticism, in writing, to your supervisor when policies need changing.

Point system

The profit sharing plan is based on a point system. We have found that without the point system, the profit sharing becomes an entitlement rather than an incentive.

In the point system, each employee may receive both positive and negative points. Positive points include attending a club event, performing a special act for a member, suggesting an idea to improve the club, and any other positive acts to benefit themselves and the club. Negative points include tardiness, complaints, failure to attend a mandatory staff meeting, and any other acts that fail to meet the daily requirements of an employee.

We give each item a certain number of points, which are logged in each employee's workbook. We then total the points each quarter. Any negative net is used as a percentage, which is multiplied by the profit sharing amount. For example, if an employee has -50 points, then he or she only receives 50 percent of his or her profit sharing amount. Positive net is carried into the next quarter and eventually to the end of the year.

At the end of the year, the employee may exchange these positive points for vacation days or additional bonuses.

Performance-Based Pay

The logic behind performance-based compensation is that improved performance should result in greater employee productivity, which in turn should result in improved business results. If this logic is correct, there is a financial return for improvement in employee performance. Managers must remember that pay increases for improved performance are considered investment spending. There are few investment opportunities in a business or fitness setting that yield a higher return for such a low risk. However, until recently, this form of compensation was rarely discussed by health fitness managers. Over the years, owners and managers have realized that by rewarding individual performance, the company and the employee both benefit. Performance pay creates a system of self-management. Employees not only perform their own tasks but also become watchful of the whole club's operations. Over time, they understand that their productivity is linked to their success and income, and to the company's success and income as well.

> *A popular trend in the health fitness industry today is finding innovative ways to reward employees who contribute significantly to the overall success of the business. The approach most commonly used is a performance-based pay system.*

The disadvantages associated with pay-for-performance compensation centers on accountability. The measurements used for identifying performance improvement as it relates to increased business productivity are not precise and are rarely easy to assess from one day to the next. Supervisors must establish tangible goals that they can measure at least monthly. Possible goals could include increase in monthly fitness revenue by 3 percent, decrease in monthly fitness expenses by 2 percent, or increase in the annual participation rate for fitness programs by 5 percent. Once management determines goals, they must decide how each employee contributes to achieving these goals.

Another problem associated with pay-for-performance compensation results in the merit approach to productivity. Personal traits may be deemed as meriting a pay increase, however, they may have no impact on work effectiveness.

> *Define performance clearly in all forms of compensation so you can view actual work performance as a means to provide greater work output.*

> *In some cases, employer-sponsored benefits provide coverage at a level the employee could not obtain as an individual.*

Administering a performance pay plan involves establishing a performance rating system that identifies the methods of evaluation and how you will conduct the rating system. Once you complete the rating plan, determine how to link compensation to performance. Will you make compensation through salary increases, bonus payments, or a higher commission percentage? Will you reduce poor performers' pay if they do not achieve goals? After you have formalized this information, it is essential to communicate the plan to the employees making sure they understand the process.

Pay for Time Not Worked

Pay for time not worked includes vacation time, holidays, sick-leave days, and special time off for such things as jury duty and military service. There is also pay for time not worked during working hours, such as scheduled rest breaks. Sick-leave days represent a form of self-insured sickness pay, providing employees with continued income in the event of a short-term illness. Vacation and holiday payments allow for a paid rest from work. For the employee, providing payment for these nonworked periods allows them more time for families, recreation, and sometimes more importantly a needed break from the customer service business.

Benefits

Employee benefits provide protection against economic risks, including death, disability, and illness. Many of these are insured benefits, with the employer paying some or all of the insurance premium. For additional information on employee insurance refer to chapter 18.

Offering benefits to employees as a group provides needed protection at a lower cost than would be available individually.

Providing benefits can assist in meeting the needs of the organization. For example, starting a 401(k) plan can help employees begin to save for the future. Awarding a designated number of paid vacation days for each year worked can also show employees that management wants to reward them for their years of service. In today's market, providing a sound benefit package is considered a necessity to attract and retain employees.

Each form of compensation can represent a significant portion of the overall remuneration of an employee. You can express only the financial elements of compensation in dollar terms; therefore, when you pay employees, all they see is the paycheck amount. They give little thought to the added benefits the employer pays for. Consequently, benefits are often viewed as *soft* costs to employees. Employers should calculate a tangible *hard* dollar cost for such items as taxes (FICA, unemployment, workers' compensation, disability), health and life insurance, holiday and vacation pay, sick leave, retirement plans, bonuses, training and education, employee uniforms, and the price of club membership. Only through this approach can employees see the total value of wages and benefits. Figure 16.1 provides a sample employee benefit work sheet, which any organization can adapt to reflect an individual's complete compensation and benefit package.

In this model, an additional 32 percent was added to the employees' base pay as a result of the benefit package. Understandably, most managers would view this figure as excessively high. However, a consideration when creating a similar model for employees is turnover. Often people do not stay long enough to earn all vacation pay, sick pay, or holiday pay. Others decide against taking health or life insurance. Consequently, depending upon turnover rates, a correction factor should be included to adequately represent payroll taxes and benefits.

Little Rock Athletic Club
Employee compensation and benefits worksheet
(Assistant Athletic Director—full-time)

	Hourly rate $10.00	Annual hours 2080	Base annual earnings $20,800	% of base
Taxes	**BAE**	**Factor**	**Total**	
Federal unemployment	$20,800	0.008	$166	0.80%
State unemployment	$20,800	0.016	$333	1.60%
FICA (social security)	$20,800	0.0765	$1,591	7.65%
Worker's comp insurance	$20,800	0.024	$499	2.40%
		Total	**$2,590**	**12.45%**
Medical insurance	**Monthly**	**Annual**	**50% Pd. by LRAC**	
Health Advantage HMO				
Employee	N/A	N/A	N/A	
Health Source HMO				
Employee	$128.00	$1,536.00	$768.00	
	Total	**$768.00**		**3.69%**
Dental insurance				
$14.64/staff/mo. @ 12 mo. = $175.68				
$7.32 pd. by LRAC/mo. @ 12 mo. = $87.84		$87.84		0.42%
Paid holidays*				
Salaried				
(daily rate × 7)		$560.00		2.69%
Hourly employees				
(hourly rate × 2.5)				
(hourly rate × 1.5 × # of holidays)		$0.00		0.00%
Paid vacation*				
Salaried				
(hourly rate × 13 days)		$1,040.00		5.00%
Hourly employees (20⁺ hrs./wk.)				
(hourly rate × average hrs./wk. × 7-20 days)		$0.00		0.00%
Paid breaks*				
(hourly rate × 86.6)		$0.00		0.00%
Paid sick leave*				
(hourly rate × hrs. taken) up to 32		$320.00		1.54%
Employee staff shirts				
($8.00/shirt @ 4 shirts/staff/yr.)		$32.00		0.15%
Training and educational courses*				
($12,000/yr. for qualified staff)		$1,000.00		4.81%
	Total benefits	**$3,807.84**		**18.31%**
	(less benefits			
	included in	$2,920.00	salaried	14.04%
	base earnings)	$0.00	hourly	0.00%
	Net benefits		**$887.84**	**4.27%**
	Bonus plan		**$3,200.00**	**15.38%**
Total compensation and benefits pd. by LRAC			**$27,477.44**	**132.10%**

*Represents cost for nonproductive time.

Figure 16.1   Employee compensation and benefits worksheet.

> *Although wages and salaries continue to represent the key elements of compensation, we can no longer look on employee benefits as a minimal cost to the organization.*

A work sheet similar to figure 16.1 can assist employees in understanding that if the organization incurs an increase in health care cost, employees might have to share some of the additional cost.

Nonfinancial Rewards

Although money is the driving force for most employees to work, there are some instances in which nonfinancial elements of remuneration are important and should be an integral part of a compensation program. In the health fitness industry, working in a fitness environment is a perceived value to the employee. This value can relate to the social merits of helping people become physically fit or improving their self-image.

The job itself can be another area of great worth to the employee. Those entering the fitness field consider the opportunity to have a job that combines physical and social skills an added benefit. Having the opportunity to regularly use the club's facilities for personal workouts can be an additional value. Thus the work itself not only determines direct pay but also has a psychological value.

Other forms of nonfinancial pay elements include club discounts, continuing education assistance, and in-house contests. It is the responsibility of an owner or manager to identify each of these areas for their organization and include them in their personnel manual as an added benefit (refer to chapter 11 for additional information on this subject).

PAY PRACTICES IN THE HEALTH FITNESS INDUSTRY

As reflected in table 16.4, compensation for employees in the health fitness industry is generally reflected as either an hourly wage or salary-based pay (full- and part-time). A third category that also should be included is *outside contractors*. There are

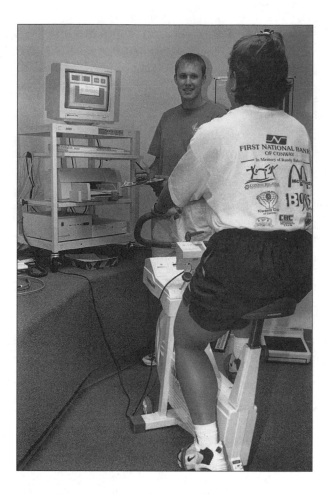

specialty variations within each group depending on the setting, but you can group most employees under these categories for the purpose of managing payroll.

Salaried Compensation

Salaried jobs are those in which the individual's input and decision-making judgments significantly impact the success of the business. As an example, salaried positions in the commercial health fitness industry include the ownership group, general manager, sales and membership director and representatives, fitness director, aerobics director, tennis director, aquatics director, and others. Depending on the size of organization, the salaried group can represent anywhere from 5 to 10 percent of the total number of employees. The average compensation can range from 15 to 20 percent of total revenues.

Organizations pay this group in three ways: salary, bonus or profit sharing, and benefits. Managers usually compensate sales and membership personnel through either a base salary, commission structure, or a combination thereof. Performance pay plans have also become popular with management by achieving preestablished goals set at the start of a fiscal year.

Hourly Wage Compensation

In the health fitness industry, hourly wage employees serve in a number of positions. They can be front-line employees serving members, perform operational duties, or be in administration assisting in the internal aspects of the business. Included in this group are service desk personnel, weightroom instructors, child care staff, restaurant and pro shop employees, operations and housekeeping personnel, and clerical staff. Some of these positions require experience, certification, or education, whereas others require a short training period.

Although hourly wage positions have historically been the lowest paid, managers today are seeing the importance of fair compensation for those individuals providing face-to-face service to members. Currently, average pay for hourly wage employees ranges from minimum wage to $20 an hour, depending on the position.

Hourly wage jobs pay a single rate or have step raises. In these jobs, the work is often learned quickly or in a predetermined time. Job duties can be set and the work standards achieved within a few months.

In these circumstances, when all employees must perform and produce the same, you should pay them at the same rate. It is only fair to have equal pay for equal work. Consider a wage progression scale for each position of this nature. Table 16.5 provides a sample wage scale for evening housekeeping personnel.

Outside Contractor Compensation

When developing and planning compensation matters, much discussion centers on full- and part-time employees. However, a large percentage of workers in the health fitness field are neither full- nor part-time employees. Many are subcontracted (e.g., aerobics instructors, activity instructors, massage therapists, personal trainers). Some are hired for a specific time or task, and others are companies hired to provide a specific service (e.g., landscaping, HVAC, legal, computers, sales, and marketing). This form of compensation has been increasing annually in the health fitness industry and will continue to do so because of the advantages it provides.

Subcontractors are generally paid per hour, per class session, or on commission. Usually, these individuals are not covered by group benefit or retirement plans. Liability insurance is generally the responsibility of the contracting firm, which reduces employee risk. Placement of personnel also becomes the responsibility of the contractor instead of the contracting company.

A disadvantage of using an outside contractor is the lack of internal loyalty associated with being a part- or full-time employee. Contractors leave the premises once they have completed their class, client session, or task. Consequently, it becomes difficult to establish communication lines and to develop a sense of camaraderie or cohesiveness among coworkers. Because compensation amounts for outside contractors should be compatible with those who are full time, resentment could result if an employee were passed over for a position now being held by an outside contractor. Also, continually adhering to the IRS statutes based on what constitutes an employee-employer relationship is a difficult task for managers and supervisors. If the IRS ever audits a club that is not adhering to these statutes, they can assess back tax penalties.

Pay for outside vendors is based on a preestablished contract agreement for services rendered. This agreement has conditions that specify the terms of payment (monthly, quarterly, or annually).

> *Contracting with outside vendors has become popular because of the lower costs, better caliber of employee, no governmental paperwork involved, and no severance or union problems for the contracting business.*

A summary of the pay practices for the commercial health fitness industry is provided in table 16.4. On an average, most salaries and wages are expected to increase annually between 3 to 7 percent. Some positions, however, are expected to stay the same or even decrease, depending on an organization's profitability and regularly adjusted pay scales. A word of caution to managers of health fitness centers who are experiencing continued revenue growth—do not fall into the practice of developing a make-and-spend mentality. Reduced operating margins, combined with creating new positions and continual pay increases, can cause payroll expenses to slowly erode a club's economic growth.

Table 16.4   Pay Practices in the Health Fitness Industry

Employee category	Pay ranges	Projected—year 2000	Additional pay options	Optional benefits
Upper management—salaried				
Ownership group	$38,000-$120,000	$40,000-$125,000	Profit sharing/bonus, based on revenue growth	Health, dental, life ins. (prem. 100%); 401(k)
General manager	$30,000-$65,000	$33,500-$73,000	Profit sharing/bonus, based on revenue growth	Health, dental, life ins. (prem. 100%); 401(k)
Tennis director	$30,000-$53,000	$32,000-$56,500	Plus commission, bonus or profit sharing	Health, dental, life ins.; 401(k) (matching)
Sales/marketing director	$25,000-$45,000	$29,500-$49,000	Plus commission, bonus or profit sharing	Health, dental, life ins.; 401(k) (matching)
Fitness director	$22,000-$35,000	$28,000-$44,500	Profit sharing/bonus + based on programs	Health, dental, life ins.; 401(k) (matching)
Aerobics director	$8,000-$23,000	$8,000-$23,000	Profit sharing/bonus + commission on # of participants/class	Health, dental, life ins.; 401(k) (matching)
Full-time staff—salaried				
Operations manager	$20,000-$32,000	$24,500-$39,000	Bonus, tied to expense savings	Health, dental, life ins.; 401(k)
Service desk manager	$18,000-$24,000	$20,500-$27,500	Bonus/profit sharing based on revenue growth	Health, dental, life ins.; 401(k)
Food and beverage manager	$18,000-$30,000	$26,500-$44,000	Bonus/profit sharing— division net profits	Health, dental, life ins.; 401(k)
Sales representative	$20,000-$38,000	$25,000-$40,000	Plus commission, bonus/ profit sharing	Health, dental, life ins.; 401(k)
Controller/business office manager	$25,000-$33,000	$27,000-$35,000	Bonus/profit sharing	Health, dental, life ins.; 401(k)
Manager on duty/ assistant general manager	$21,000-$34,000	$25,500-$41,500	Bonus/profit sharing based on revenue growth	Health, dental, life ins.; 401(k)
Full-time staff—hourly wages				
Aerobics instructor	$12.00-$25.00/ class	$13.00-$27.00/ class	Bonus, # of participants/ class	Insurance, 401(k), emp. discounts, service awards
Aquatics instructor	$9.00-$15.00/ class	$11.00-$18.00/ class	Plus commission/bonus; # of participants/lesson	Insurance, 401(k), emp. discounts, service awards
Personal trainer	$15.00-$30.00/ session	$18.00-$40.00/ session	Plus commission/bonus	Insurance, 401(k), emp. discounts, service awards
Fitness center personnel	$7.00-$10.00	$8.00-$11.50	Bonus/profit sharing	Insurance, 401(k), emp. discounts, service awards
Tennis instructor	$15.00-$30.00/ lesson	$16.50-$33.00/ lesson	Plus commission, bonus or profit sharing	Insurance, 401(k), emp. discounts, service awards
Racquetball instructor	$8.00-$18.00/ lesson	$10.00-$20.00/ lesson	Plus commission, bonus or profit sharing	Insurance, 401(k), emp. discounts, service awards

Table 16.4 (continued)

Employee category	Pay ranges	Projected—year 2000	Additional pay options	Optional benefits
Full-time staff—hourly wages (continued)				
Service desk attendant	$6.00-$8.00	$7.00-$9.50	Bonus/profit sharing	Insurance, 401(k), emp. discounts, service awards
Bookkeeper	$8.50-$12.00	$9.75-$14.00	Bonus/profit sharing	Insurance, 401(k), emp. discounts, service awards
Office staff	$6.50-$10.00	$7.50-$11.50	Bonus/profit sharing	Insurance, 401(k), emp. discounts, service awards
Maintenance/ housekeeping	$6.50-$9.00	$7.50-$11.00	Bonus/profit sharing	Insurance, 401(k),emp. discounts, service awards
Child care staff	$5.15-$6.50	$5.75-$7.50	Bonus/profit sharing, based on total revenue	Insurance, 401(k), emp. discounts, service awards
Food and beverage staff	$5.15-$7.50	$5.75-$8.50	Bonus/profit sharing, based on division growth	Insurance, 401(k), emp. discounts, service awards
Pro shop staff	$5.50-$7.00	$5.75-$8.00	Bonus/profit sharing, based on division growth	Insurance, 401(k), emp. discounts, service awards
Summer camp staff	$5.50-$7.50	$6.25-$8.50	Bonus/profit sharing, based on camp revenues	Insurance, 401(k), emp. discounts service awards
Part-time staff—hourly wages				
Aerobics instructor	$12.00-$20.00/ class	$13.00-$23.00/ class		Emp. discounts, service awards, emp. asst. prog.
Aquatics instructor	$7.50-$15.00/ class	$8.50-$17.25/ class		Emp. discounts, service awards, emp. asst. prog.
Personal trainer	$15.00-$30.00/ session	$18.00-$40.00/ session	Bonus or profit sharing based on hours worked, revenue potential, and length of employment	Emp. discounts, service awards, emp. asst. prog.
Fitness center personnel	$6.00-$8.00	$7.00-$9.00		Emp. discounts, service awards, emp. asst. prog.
Tennis instructor	$14.00-$25.00/ lesson	$14.00-$25.00/ lesson		Emp. discounts, service awards, emp. asst. prog.
Racquetball instructor	$8.00-$18.00/ lesson	$10.00-$20.00/ lesson		Emp. discounts, service awards, emp. asst. prog.
Service desk attendant	$5.25-$6.50	$6.00-$7.50		Emp. discounts, service awards, emp. asst. prog.
Bookkeeper	$7.00-$10.00	$8.00-$11.50		Emp. discounts, service awards,emp. asst. prog.
Office staff	$6.00-$8.00	$7.00-$9.25		Emp. discounts, service awards, emp. asst. prog.
Maintenance/ housekeeping	$5.50-$7.50	$6.25-$8.50		Emp. discounts, service awards, emp. asst. prog.
Child care staff	$5.00-$6.00	$5.75-$7.00		Emp. discounts, service awards, emp. asst. prog.
Food and beverage staff	$5.00-$7.00	$5.75-$8.00		Emp. discounts, service awards, emp. asst. prog.
Pro shop staff	$5.00-$6.25	$5.75-$7.25		Emp. discounts, service awards, emp. asst. prog.
Summer camp staff	$5.00-$6.00	$5.75-$7.00		Emp. discounts, service awards, emp. asst. prog.

Table 16.5 Sample of a Wage Scale

ABC Athletic Club
Wage scale —evening housekeeping

Note: The following wage scale was established to provide supervisors with starting pay rates, incremental performance review pay changes, and wage caps for each respective position in their division. This scale is based on average to good performance ranking for employee's performance review. You can adjust the recommended pay rate accordingly if an employee exhibits either poor or excellent work habits. In some cases, starting pay rates are negotiable depending on an individual's education, past experience, and level of certification.

Remember, ABC management must preapprove all starting wages and performance review rate changes before you hire an individual or perform an employee's performance review.

Scale #1 Part-time/full time

Length of service	Hourly pay
Starting wage	$5.15/hr.
30 days	$5.50/hr.
90 days	$6.00/hr.
1 year review	$6.25/hr.
2 year review	$6.50/hr.
3 year review	$6.75/hr.
4 year review	$7.00/hr.—maximum wage cap for position

While providing regular wage and salary adjustments, many club operators will also continue to improve on additional pay options and benefits. Managers will implement more creative pay for performance bonuses and commission structures to retain and continually motivate employees. In addition, organizations will continue to increase their spending by using outside contractors.

IN CLOSING

In summary, offer employee compensation for value created, not for years of service, time spent on a project, rank, or position. The intent of a sound compensation program is to improve productivity for the business, while communicating to the employees that their work is noticed and appreciated by the employer.

KEY TERMS

Benefits

Commission-based pay

Job pricing

Outside contractors

Performance-based pay

Salaries

Wages

RECOMMENDED READINGS

De Pree, M. 1989. *Leadership is an art*. New York: Bantam Doubleday Dell.

Flannery, T., D. Hofrichter, and P. Platten. 1996. *People performance and pay*. New York: Free Press.

Fraser, J. 1995. Tis better to give and receive. *Inc.* 17(2): 84.

Lancaster, P. 1994. Incentive pay isn't good for your company. *Inc.* 16(9): 23.

Lasser, J. 1983. *How to run a small business*. New York: McGraw-Hill.

Rausch, E. 1979. *Financial management for small business*. New York: American Management Association.

Sibson, R. 1990. *Compensation*. New York: American Management Association.

Stewart, G. 1991. The quest for value. *Harper Business* 32(8): 5.

CHAPTER 17

Legal Issues

Modern American society is frequently described as being more litigious (quick to file a lawsuit) now than at any previous period in history. Regardless of whether this observation is true, it is clear that a prudent manager should be aware of a wide range of issues that give rise to legal rights, obligations, and liabilities. The purpose of this chapter is not to provide specific legal answers to issues related to managing and operating a health fitness facility. Rather, the objective is to identify the major areas that are most likely to generate legal questions and provide basic concepts and definitions that allow the health fitness manager to identify, evaluate, and define levels of risk and determine when to obtain formal legal advice from competent counsel.

WORKING WITH LAWYERS AND LAW FIRMS

A health fitness manager must be able to determine when a circumstance requires outside legal advice. It is a common perception by many in the health fitness industry that using lawyers and law firms is expensive and they should avoid it if at all possible. The reality of the situation is that this decision, like many other management decisions, requires a balance of risks and resources. It may be true that to have an attorney review every contract is more expensive than an organization's budget will allow. On the other hand, is the cost-saving measure of operating without competent legal advice worth it, if the risks involved in multiyear leases, large insurance contracts, employee labor decisions, and long-term vendor contracts have the potential to destroy the economic viability of your organization? This chapter looks at the steps to take to select a lawyer, different ways to pay for legal services, and areas of potential legal risk for a health fitness organization.

How to Select a Lawyer

The first step in working effectively with a lawyer is to select one who understands the special needs of a health fitness organization.

The best way to locate an attorney with a special type of experience is to obtain recommendations from other professionals within the industry, business associates, vendors, friends, family, or the local bar association.

If it does not appear that a lawyer with experience in the health fitness industry is available in your immediate market, ask about lawyers with experience in service or retail industries that have similar legal concerns about employees, contracts, vendors, equipment, insurance, and premises liability.

Once you've identified a prospective lawyer, schedule a meeting to interview the lawyer or representatives of the law firm. Before the meeting, review over the telephone the purpose of your visit and what you wish to discuss. If you are interviewing several attorneys or firms, say so. This should not offend the attorney, and in fact, indicates the seriousness of your search. Ask in advance whether there is any fee for the initial meeting. There is not usually a fee for an introductory meeting, but by asking, you avoid confusion and illustrate that you understand the attorney's time is valuable.

The attorney is likely to ask whether your health fitness organization has been represented by another attorney or law firm in the past and the status of the relationship. In some cases a release may be needed from a previous attorney and a formal request made for prior files, documents, or information related to your organization.

Be prepared to briefly describe your most immediate needs and your potential needs. Time is money when working with attorneys. You and your attorney will be more satisfied with the results if you have your information well organized, copies of needed documents available, lists of questions prepared, and initial expectations thought through. Ask questions about staffing, scheduling, fees, and process. Be sure that you understand the respective roles and responsibilities of the lawyer, management, staff, and other professionals (i.e., accountants, consultants, and bankers) in addressing the legal issues in question. Do not hesitate to ask for references and a description of the lawyer's experience with the type of legal issues in question. You might also consider checking with the state or local bar association to determine whether grievance or malpractice violations are on record for the attorney or the law firm.

Once you have completed the initial meeting, assess whether you believe that the demeanor of the lawyer is a good fit with you and your organization. It is important that you believe the lawyer understands you and your organization's needs and will respond in a manner that will meet these needs.

Once you select a lawyer, have a written agreement prepared that specifies fees, rates, costs, and all other major factors related to the legal representation.

Developing a Legal Services Plan

Once you have selected a lawyer, it is important to develop a legal services plan that outlines the areas of legal representation your organization needs. The plan you develop is much like the marketing plan discussed in chapter 5. The plan identifies the legal needs, outlines the action steps required, stipulates anticipated results, and identifies the necessary resources to accomplish the objectives.

A typical plan, whether it is to initiate or defend litigation or for transactional business such as contracts and licenses, should be in writing and should be the common product of the lawyer and the client. It should include the following elements:

1. Definition of the problem

2. Gathering of facts

3. Initial identifications of the legal issues involved

4. Statement of client goals and expectations

5. Prescription of steps necessary to succeed

6. Listing of uncertainties, unknowns, and possible alternatives

7. Definition of the scope of the work

8. Determination of required resources

9. Forecast of schedules

10. Definition of client's duties

11. Definition of lawyer's duties

12. Determination of the range of dollar values and the importance of what is at stake

13. Evaluation of the risks

14. Determination of the billing method to use

15. Procedure for modifying the plan, providing for contingencies, unknowns, factors beyond control, changed conditions, and the need for possible revision in the case; transaction planning to meet changing conditions

For example, a summary plan for evaluating the membership contracts of a health fitness organization might include some of the following elements:

Summary Legal Service Plan for ABC Fitness Club

1. Definition of the problem. Review all contracts to determine whether they comply with local, state, and federal laws and regulations.

2. Gathering the facts. The health fitness organization will provide current copies of all contracts and any pertinent forms, documents, and materials. The attorney will review the applicable laws and regulations.

3. Initial identification of legal issues involved. Legal issues include contract law issues, consumer protection issues, and consumer credit issues.

4. Statement of client goals and expectations. All contracts, forms, materials, and documents will be in compliance with applicable state and federal laws and regulations.

5. Prescription of steps needed to proceed. After the initial review, the attorney will provide a summary of any major areas of noncompliance. If major changes are required, the attorney will provide a listing of the types of changes and an estimate of the cost to bring the current contracts into compliance.

6. Listing of uncertainties and possible alternatives. If major rewriting of contracts is required, a review of the costs will be made to see if the client prefers to have in-house staff do the initial re-drafting to reduce cost.

7. Definition of scope of work. The initial step is a review for compliance. Additional steps may include partial or total revision or re-drafting of contracts.

8. Determination of required resources. The initial review will be done by an associate attorney under supervision of a partner to minimize costs. Re-drafting may require partner involvement.

9. Forecast of schedule. The attorney will provide an estimate of the time necessary to complete the initial review and the proposed revisions, if any.

10. Definition of client duties. The client is to provide copies of all pertinent contracts, documents, and forms. The client will also provide copies of the pertinent state laws that regulate health fitness facilities in each of the markets where the client has facilities.

(continued)

11. Definition of lawyer duties. The lawyer will provide an initial review at a pre-determined fee. The lawyer will review with the client the status of each area potentially needing changes and discuss alternatives and possible liabilities. The lawyer will provide an estimate of the time/fees required to complete any recommended revisions.

12. Determination of dollar values. The lawyer will complete the initial review based on rate charges of $125.00 per hour, but total charges will not exceed $2,500 unless authorized by the client. The lawyer will provide a specific estimate for making revisions after the initial review and before undertaking any additional legal work. It is also agreed that the total cost of reviewing and revising the existing con-tracts, forms, and materials will not exceed $10,000.

13. Evaluation of risks. The attorney will provide an analysis of the potential risks associated with not modifying the existing contracts.

14. Billing method. See #12. Bills will be submitted at the conclusion of the initial review and from that point forward on a monthly basis.

15. Modifications. The attorney and club general manager will meet after the initial review to discuss options for revising existing contracts, review associated risks, and discuss the costs and timing for making any recommended changes. All additional work after the initial review will be subject to the approval of the club general manager.

The legal needs plan is a method to allow clients to receive the most cost- and results-effective service from a lawyer or law firm. It requires active participation by the client throughout the process and should be reviewed and updated regularly.

Methods of Paying for Legal Services

Attorney fees can be a significant element of an operational budget. In a typical commercial health fitness setting, total professional fees for legal and accounting run approximately two to four percent of all expenses. For many health fitness organizations this translates to $20,000 to $40,000 in professional fees per year. Although many health fitness managers do not have prior experience in dealing with attorneys, it is important to understand that there are alternative methods of obtaining and paying for legal services (see figure 17.1). The following section describes several common alternatives available and provides a summary of the situations in which they are most likely appropriate.

Fixed or Flat Fee

A *fixed* or *flat fee* is a single price for the completion of a single legal project or a series of similar legal projects. For example, an attorney may quote a flat

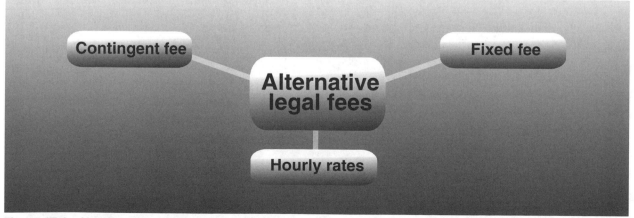

Figure 17.1 Alternative legal service payments.

fee to revise an existing set of membership contracts and make recommendations for improvements. Flat fees are also common for creating the standard legal documents you need to establish a company, such as the Articles of Incorporation and Bylaws, and stock certificates. Flat fees are most effective for routine services in which both parties have experience estimating the level of work required and can accurately foresee and define the legal services needed. These types of fees are also effective for volume work of a repetitive nature, such as routine collection work for membership contract defaults. Flat fee arrangements allow the health fitness organization to know in advance the amount to budget for legal services (see table 17.1).

Contingent Fee

The *contingent fee* is a legal fee based on the percentage of money that is recovered in a lawsuit, or in defense cases, the percentage of money not having to be paid if liability is not proven. Contingent fees are not allowed in criminal matters. Contingent fees are most common in personal injury lawsuits where the fee is a percentage of the dollar recovery.

Although not as common, you can also use contingent fees for legal representation in business-related lawsuits. Consider the following example. A large, well-established health fitness organization obtains a copy of proprietary programming materials developed by a contract labor fitness professional and uses the materials without compensating the developer. The contract labor professional may not have the financial resources to hire an attorney on an hourly basis, but may consider seeking an attorney to represent him on a contingency basis for a percentage of the potential damage recovery. The greater the potential for a substantial recovery, the more likely the lawyer will consider a contingency fee representation.

Contingent fee agreements are most effective when a potential client cannot otherwise afford to pursue or defend the legal matter and when significant dollar damages are involved. Contingency fee arrangements can be effective because there is considerable incentive for the lawyer to work efficiently and effectively to minimize her out of pocket expenses and to pursue the best result possible for the client (see table 17.2).

Hourly Rates

In the past quarter century, hourly billing for legal services has become the most popular method (for lawyers) of paying for legal representation. It requires the lawyer to keep detailed and accurate records of time spent on behalf of the client by lawyers, legal assistants, and other staff members. To some extent, *hourly rates* are market driven and should represent differences in expertise, number of years in practice, and the fees of comparable attorneys providing similar services. Many lawyers or firms have different rates for each lawyer in the firm and for different types of services they provide. If requested, the lawyer or firm should be willing to provide a schedule of standard fees and hourly rates. Hourly rates are most effective when you can use no other fair alternative method. It is also the way to obtain legal representation if an attorney is not willing or interested in sharing the risks or rewards associated with the outcome (see table 17.3).

Table 17.1 Advantages/Disadvantages of a Flat Fee Arrangement

Advantages

Forces agreement between lawyer and client about the specific services that are required.

Client knows exactly what the cost of services will be.

Client can compare the costs to other lawyers.

Allows the service to be measured in terms of the value of the specific result.

Disadvantages

Does not take into consideration unexpected circumstances or the possible need for extra work.

Encourages the use of standard forms versus customized approach.

Does not encourage flexibility between the attorney and the client.

Should not be used when there are foreseeable uncertainties.

Table 17.2   Advantages/Disadvantages of Contingent Fee Arrangement

Advantages

Client does not pay unless favorable result is achieved.

Clients who are otherwise unable to pay can obtain legal representation.

Payment depends on results, not on time expended in obtaining results.

Terms of representation can be clearly defined in fee agreement.

Disadvantages

Not all legal representation is based on dollar damages.

Many corporate attorneys will not accept contingent fee work.

Payment based on a percentage is likely to exceed the amount charged for a flat fee or hourly fee.

Attorney may have incentive to seek the least difficult result to minimize work or expenses.

In summary, it is important for the health fitness manager to be comfortable with the process of seeking legal advice. In most cases, the risk of operating without appropriate legal representation is far greater than the cost of obtaining timely advice. Health fitness managers should be willing to openly review their needs with an experienced attorney and expect the attorney to assist them in developing a legal services plan that includes the following: evaluating the merits of their claim or nature of their risks, estimating the cost of the legal services, and clearly describing the process through which the attorney will obtain the results. Finally, the legal services plan, including the method for calculating fees, should be in writing and reviewed frequently. The frequency of review should be appropriate to the type of legal work the lawyer provides. In some cases an annual review will be adequate, whereas in other circumstances a monthly review may be required to monitor and manage the legal services and fees.

Table 17.3   Advantages/Disadvantages of Hourly Rate Fees

Advantages

The system is simple and can easily be calculated: hours spent working for client $\times$ rate = fee.

The client can select lawyers with appropriate expertise and rate for specific projects.

Billing records are easy to review and represent the actual time spent on behalf of the client.

Subjective judgments in billing are not required.

The lawyer does not participate financially in the results obtained.

Provides a method of paying fees when the scope of representation is unpredictable.

Disadvantages

The client does not know at the outset what the total charges will be.

All risks related to the outcome are borne by the client.

The fee charged may have little relationship to the value of the benefits received.

The fee does not recognize or reward extraordinary, priority, or emergency services.

The method of payment does not encourage innovation and efficiency.

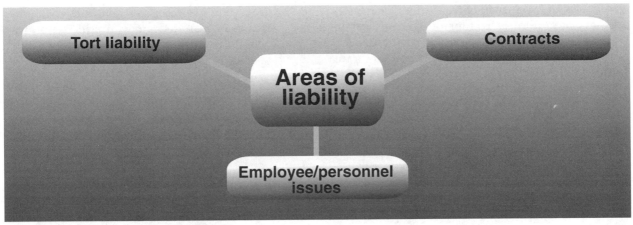

Figure 17.2 Potential areas of legal liability.

AREAS OF POTENTIAL LEGAL RISKS

Let's review some common areas of legal risks for health fitness organizations. Although it is tempting to provide simple answers and recommendations that will minimize legal liabilities for health fitness organizations, it is not practical or appropriate to do so. Legal liabilities and risks are based on the myriad of issues surrounding each circumstance. The purpose of this discussion of legal issues is to raise the awareness and sensitivity of health fitness managers to possible areas of risk that they should address to maintain effective management control over potential liabilities (see figure 17.2).

Contracts

In today's world, each of us is surrounded by *contracts*. Individually, we enter into contracts to buy or lease a home, purchase or rent automobiles, use credit cards, purchase goods and services, acquire insurance, and become employers or employees. As a manager in a health fitness setting, many of the same types of contracts come into play. In most cases, the principles of contract law are the same for personal and business contracts. Frequently the only difference is that the numbers and liabilities are larger for business contracts. Some of the most common contracts found in a health fitness setting include membership contracts, vendor contracts, employment contracts, warranties, independent contractor agreements, leases, and joint venture agreements.

Essentials of a Contract

A contract is a legally enforceable promise between two or more people or between two or more legal entities. Individuals, corporations, and partnerships are all recognized legal entities that can enter into contracts and be legally bound by the terms of a contract. Individuals can also act in the capacity of

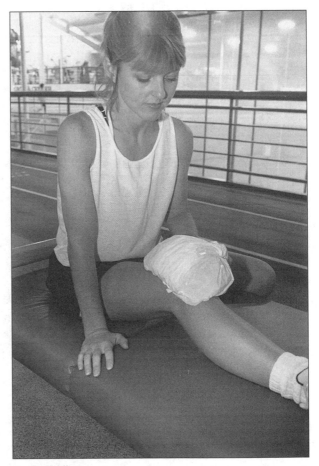

© Tom Wallace

an officer, employee, or agent of another legal entity and have the authority to enter into contracts on the entity's behalf. As a rule, parents or legal guardians must authorize any agreement with a minor for the contract to be binding.

Not all promises are legally enforceable contracts. Social agreements, illegal agreements, vague and unspecified agreements, and agreements entered into under duress or incapacity are examples of circumstances in which an agreement may be in the form of a contract, but will not be enforceable in a court of law.

> *With a few exceptions, a contract does not need to be in writing to be valid. However, it is difficult to prove the specific terms of an oral contract.*

There are five basic criteria that must be met for a valid contract to exist:

1. A valid *offer* to enter into a contract that includes the terms of the contract
2. A valid *acceptance* of the offer under the terms of the contract
3. An exchange of *consideration* from each party that may include money, products, services, actions, or promises to pay, act, or not act in a specific manner
4. A *legal purpose* that does not require an illegal act or violate public policy
5. Genuine *assent* between both parties that is not forced by duress, misrepresentation, fraud, or involve incapacity

Although most contracts do not need to be in writing to be legally enforceable, there are six categories of contracts that must be in writing and signed by the party being sued to be enforceable.

1. Contracts that by their terms cannot be performed within one year
2. Contracts for the sale of an interest in real estate
3. Contracts for the sale of personal property worth $500 or more
4. Contracts promising to answer for the debt of someone else
5. Contracts of executors and administrators of estates
6. Contracts made in consideration of marriage

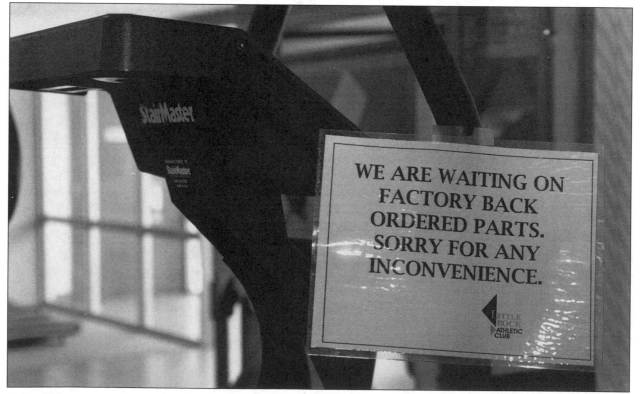

© Tom Wallace

In a health fitness setting, the most likely category requiring a written contract is multiyear agreements with members, vendors, employees, landlords, or joint venture partners.

Membership Agreements

All relationships between a health fitness organization and members are based on the existence of a contract. This is true whether a written signed agreement exists or members are merely paying a daily entry fee each time they visit the facility. It is also true if an employer is providing the facility at no additional cost to an employee, but as part of an employee benefit package. The only cases in which a membership contract relationship does not exist would be a free public facility or where the person is visiting as a nonpaying guest.

Because of the wide range of health fitness settings, it is difficult to generalize about membership contract requirements. Some states have passed specific laws requiring fitness clubs to include certain contract terms related to duration of the contract, canceling a contract, getting refunds of deposits, using automatic billing to checking ac-

Recent court decisions have stated that to be effective, a waiver and release must state a clear and unambiguous intent of the member to release the health fitness organization from liability.

counts and credit cards, and transferability of the contract. Because these laws are enacted at the state level, it is important for each health fitness manager to obtain copies of their state's laws and regulations related to spas, fitness centers, and health clubs.

In general, it is to the mutual benefit of the health fitness organization and the member to have a clearly worded, complete written agreement that identifies the respective obligations of the health fitness organization and the member. Vague contracts rarely work to the benefit of either party and frequently cause unnecessary confusion and conflict. Examples of issues that a membership contract should address include the following:

Basic Contract Terms

- Names and addresses of the parties.
- Duration of the contract with clearly stated starting and ending dates.
- Signatures and dates of signatures.
- Location of the facilities; specific facility access issues such as time of day, days of the week; facility use limitations (i.e., tennis only, cardiovascular areas only, aerobics and classes only).
- Membership fees and terms of payment.
- Rights, penalties, and fees associated with cancellation or transferability.
- Renewal options.
- Direct billing terms for checking accounts or credit cards.

Promises by the Health Fitness Organization

- Maintain a safe, clean environment.
- Provide prompt maintenance and repair.
- Maintain properly trained and supervised staff.

Promises by the Member

- Pay amounts due in a timely manner.
- Abide by all rules and regulations.
- Operate equipment safely and cautiously.
- Notify health fitness management immediately about any observed unsafe condition or practice.
- Notify the health fitness management of any personal health or fitness conditions that impact the member's ability to participate in health or fitness activities, programs, or use of equipment.

Waivers and Releases

The membership contract should include a separate waiver and release of liability that expressly waives the member's right to make a claim against the health fitness organization for any injury, damage, or loss caused to the person or property of the member while on the premises or while participating in activities sponsored by the health fitness organization. The waiver should be clearly worded and as explicit as possible to be effective.

If the intent of the waiver and release is to have members release the health fitness organization from all claims, including those based on negligence of employees (as described in the next section of this chapter), the waiver must specifically include "negligence" as part of the waiver language. Review specific release and waiver language carefully in light of the state laws and case rulings. An example of waiver and release language is as follows:

Use of our facilities is at your own risk. Participating in health fitness activities and programs and using health fitness facilities and equipment are inherently dangerous. By entering into this contract, the member waives all claims and releases the [health fitness organization] from all liability for any injuries or damages to person or property resulting from using the [health fitness organization]'s facilities or participating in the [health fitness organization]'s sponsored activities or negligence of [health fitness organization]'s employees.

Vendor Contracts

Health fitness organizations develop vendor relationships with a variety of service and product suppliers. The contracts between the health fitness organization and vendors are frequently written using standard forms the vendor provides. Although these contracts appear to be fixed by the terms of the standard forms, it is important for the health fitness manager to consider all contract terms negotiable. Of course, a vendor has the right to refuse to sell you services or products if changes to the contract are not to the vendor's liking. However, the manager has a responsibility to review the terms of each contract and determine the organization's rights and liabilities under the agreement. Critical terms in vendor agreements include the health fitness organization's right to terminate the agreement without cause, return unused goods without charge, maintain a nonexclusive relationship that allows the organization to use other products or services, and be indemnified by the vendor for any loss or damage caused by the vendor's services or products.

In some cases, the health fitness organization may select a vendor to subcontract operation of one or more membership or operational services. Examples of operations areas frequently contracted out to vendors include pro shop, food and beverage, vending machines, specialty health services (i.e., massage therapy, health and beauty services, sports medicine services), facility maintenance (night janitorial services), and towel laundry service. In each circumstance, establish written contracts that outline the relationship of the parties. Because of the critical nature of these services, seriously consider having an attorney review these contracts.

Employment Contracts

The employer-employee relationship is based on contract law. Whenever one individual agrees to work for another individual or legal entity in exchange for wages and other benefits, an employment contract is in place. The rights and obligations of the employer and employee are governed by a combination of general contract law, and state and federal regulations and statutes. In many states, unless a written employment contract is signed, employment is considered to be *at will*. Employment at will means that, absent a discriminatory motive, an employer may terminate an employee at will and without cause. Likewise, the employee is not required to give notice or reasons for quitting and may do so at any time without liability.

If health fitness organizations do not use employment contracts to specify the characteristics and expectations of specific jobs, how are job expectations communicated? The most effective method of defining the employer-employee relationship is to use employee manuals and handbooks. As a prerequisite of employment, many organizations require that all new employees sign a document stipulating that they have read or been provided a copy of the organization's employee handbook or manual. Although the manual commonly provides specific information on policies related to employee benefits, vacation, safety, drug use, smoking, performance reviews, dress codes, on the job behavior, termination, and discipline, in employment at will states the manual or handbook is not considered part of an employment contract. Because of the importance of these issues in determining employer liability, the last section of this chapter reviews areas that an employee handbook or manual should include.

In certain circumstances, health fitness organizations may consider using an employment contract that includes a noncompete agreement to protect the organization from an employee leaving the company and taking proprietary knowledge to a competitor. Although each state is different in this area of law, most states are restrictive in allowing an

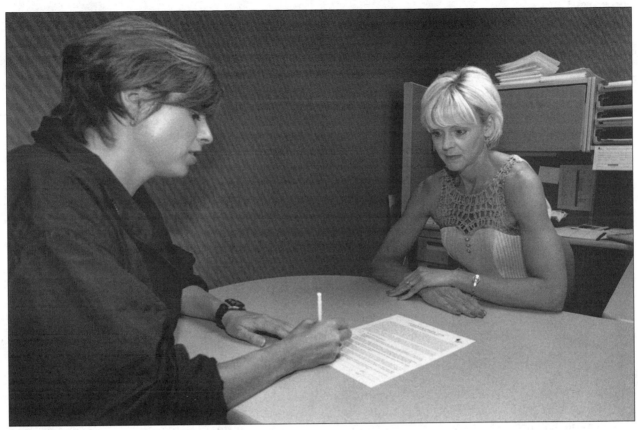

© Tom Wallace

employer to limit the opportunity of an individual to seek gainful employment. Noncompete agreements must be narrow in their geographic definition and reasonable in the length of time during which competition is prohibited. These agreements are generally limited to key officers of a company, developers of specific proprietary products or services, or individuals with access to extremely sensitive information that would damage the company if shared with a competitor.

Independent Contractors

An *independent contractor* is, by definition, not an employee of the health fitness organization. As the title describes, the individual is independent from the organization and provides specific services on a contract basis. As we've discussed throughout the book, the health fitness industry creates many opportunities for independent contractors (aerobics instructors, dance instructors, tennis and sport instructors, independent coaches and trainers, specialty therapists, nutrition specialists, and a range of specialty consultants) to provide services. Why is the distinction of independent contractors important? The most important issues relate to paying taxes, employee benefits, and liability.

> *If an individual is classified as an independent contractor, the health fitness organization is not required to pay FICA (Federal Insurance Contributions Act or Social Security), FUTA (Federal Unemployment Tax Act), or state unemployment taxes.*

In addition, an independent contractor does not receive health care benefits, retirement benefits, vacation pay, sick-leave pay, or any other employee benefits. The health fitness organization is not held liable for injuries or torts (see next section of the chapter) an independent contractor causes.

With all these benefits, why not designate all workers in a company as independent contractors and save money and reduce risk? The answer is the Internal Revenue Service (IRS). To ensure that employers are paying appropriate unemployment and social security taxes, the IRS has increased scrutiny of the designation of workers as independent contractors.

> *Improperly designating an individual as an independent contractor subjects the health fitness employer to potential back taxes, interests, and penalties.*

Although the status of independent contractor is defined by tax rulings rather than a specific checklist, the following list provides some general measures used to determine a worker's status. An independent contractor

- is not on the regular payroll,
- does not receive employee benefits,
- does not work exclusively for one employer,
- provides own tools and equipment,
- schedules own work, and
- works independently from direct supervision.

Torts and Civil Liability

The law of torts concerns itself with private wrongs or injuries (other than a breach of contract) for which a court awards damages. A tort is committed when a person fails to observe a *duty of care* or responsibility not to infringe on another's rights, by either intentionally or carelessly causing harm or injury. The harm could be physical, emotional, or to property. In a health fitness setting, examples of possible torts include injuries to members or guests due to unsafe facilities, injury from faulty or defective equipment, failure to properly supervise, and unsafe practices of members or guests. There are so many circumstances that give rise to tort liabilities that it is only possible to define torts in general terms. The determination of whether a tort has been committed requires that a court review the circumstances of each case and render a decision. The definitions of torts are established by the process of case-by-case decisions that collectively are known as *case law*. Judges and juries in civil disputes generally use the prior decisions of other courts, termed *precedent*, as authority for setting standards of care and determining liability in current cases.

> *The law of torts exists to let wrongfully injured people collect damages from those who have injured them.*

Tort law does not punish wrongdoers (that is the primary objective of criminal law) but compensates people for legal wrongs they suffer at the hands of others. The ultimate goal of tort law is to put the wronged party back into a position as close as possible to the position he or she was in before becoming the victim of a tort.

Civil Versus Criminal Liability

A common area of confusion is the difference between *civil and criminal liability*. It is possible that the same activity may give rise to both criminal and civil liabilities. For example, if an angry member strikes another member during an argument and causes physical injury, the injured party may bring a civil lawsuit (tort of battery) to recover medical costs and file a separate criminal complaint asking that charges of assault be brought by the district attorney. The difference between a *tort* (civil law) and a crime (criminal law) is that in a tort, one *individual* is suing another to recover money damages. In a crime, the *state*, acting through a prosecutor, is suing an individual to punish an act or failure to act. Civil and criminal cases are for the most part handled by different judges, in separate courts, and under separate rules. In civil cases, the remedy for a violation of the law is payment of money damages. In criminal cases, the remedy may be incarceration (jail or prison) or a fine. In the case of a criminal fine, the money goes to the state (although restitution to an injured party may be included as part of punishment), not to the injured party. In a civil matter, the money goes to the injured party, and not to the state.

Duty of Care

Before we can examine the potential liabilities associated with torts, it is first important to review the legal concept of a duty of care.

> *A tort will not arise unless there are two elements present: the existence of a legal duty and a breach of that duty. Even if there is an injury, if no legal duty is breached, no tort is committed.*

Consider the following example: A guest walking by the pool sees another guest fall into the pool, thrash around in the water violently, and call out for help. The guest also calls for help, but makes no attempt to jump into the pool and assist the person in the water. If the person drowns, is the guest who witnessed the incident liable for not attempting a rescue? Under tort law, the clear answer is no. There is no legal duty of care that requires an innocent bystander to take action in an emergency. Therefore, without a legal duty of care, the witness is not legally obligated to take any action and not liable for any injury to another person. However, if the situation is changed to a lifeguard or club manager observing the incident, the result is different. Both the lifeguard and the club manager have a legal obligation to provide a safe environment and to appropriately respond to dangerous incidents or conditions. Because a legal duty of care exists, if either fails to properly perform his or her duty, each may be liable for injuries sustained by the guest. In addition, because they are employees, they may create a liability for the health fitness owner as well.

There are many relationships that give rise to a legal duty of care. The following list provides examples of relationships that create a duty of care and may come into play in a health fitness setting.

- Employer to employee
- Employer to guest or member
- Employee to guest or member
- Independent contractor to guest or member
- Vendor to guest or member
- Parent to child
- Child care attendant to child
- Teacher, coach, trainer to student
- Landlord to tenant
- Property owner to individuals with access to the property
- Manufacturers to consumer
- Retailer to consumer

In each relationship there exists a legal duty of care that varies based on the circumstances involved. Specific cases in state and federal civil court set the level of care.

Categories of Torts

In a health fitness setting, the most likely areas of tort liability will be issues of negligence. Negligence occurs when a duty of care is unintentionally breached causing injury or damages. The two other general categories of torts include intentional torts and strict liability.

Negligence Torts

Negligence torts occur when a duty of care is breached unintentionally, causing harm. For example, if a club fails to place a warning sign on or remove a known, damaged piece of equipment, and a member, unaware of the damage, is subsequently injured trying to use the equipment, the club has committed an unintentional tort of negligence. The club may not have intended to injure the member, but by inaction when a duty to act existed, the club committed a tort and may be liable for the injury.

> *In the area of negligence, if an employee causes an injury while acting within the scope of his or her employment, the employer is generally held liable. The defense to negligence liability for an employer is to prove that the employee was acting outside of the scope of his or her job when causing the injury or damage.*

Many courts will examine the issue of contributory negligence when considering the cause of injury or damages. In these circumstances, the court will consider the actions of the injured party, employee, and other individuals when determining the extent to which each party is liable for damages. From the standpoint of employer liability for *employee negligence*, issues involved in determining contributory negligence include evaluating

1. the adequacy of training and supervision;
2. the existence of established guidelines and procedures;
3. the hiring of appropriately experienced personnel; and
4. proof of adequate instructions, notices, warnings, and other necessary information directed toward minimizing injury risk.

The duty of care related to negligence torts may be affected if the injured party has affirmatively accepted an assumption of risk. Individuals may shift the risk related to potential injury from one party to another by proving that a specific activity or type of activity is inherently risky and that the injured individual, after being made aware of the known risks, personally accepted the risk of injury. The legal test of whether an assumption of risk has occurred requires that notice was provided about either a known risk or that the risks assumed could have been reasonably anticipated. Included in consideration of proper notification of potential risks are posted notices, warnings, instructions, and documents such as informed consent forms. (See chapter 13 for a further discussion of informed consent forms.)

> *Minors (children under the age of 18) are not legally allowed to assume additional risks without the specific knowledge and approval of a parent or guardian.*

Intentional Torts

Intentional torts, as the name implies, arise out of an intentional or willful breach of duty. If a club member violently and intentionally strikes another member during an argument, the violent member has committed the intentional tort of battery. The legal remedy is to force the violent member to pay for any damage caused and possibly impose punitive damages to deter the activity from being repeated. Other intentional torts include slander (false and defamatory verbal statements), libel (false and defamatory written statements), fraud (intentionally misleading someone to cause a financial loss), false imprisonment (wrongful detention), trespass (unlawful use or injury of property), and conversion (unlawful taking and keeping of property).

Strict Liability Torts

Strict liability torts arise when someone suffers an injury, not from a specific negligent act, but from an inherently dangerous activity or, under certain circumstances, from the manufacturing of an unsafe product. For example, a health fitness organization decides to commercially produce a new weight-loss dietary supplement that has been successful for select individuals in one of its special weight-loss programs. If the product is later determined to cause health problems for certain users, the organization as a manufacturer is likely to be held to strict liability for injuries. It is not necessary for a consumer injured by a defective product to prove that the manufacturer was negligent or intentionally created a risk of injury. The consumer merely needs to prove that the defective product was the cause of the injury and was produced by the manufacturer.

Legal Status of Guests, Members, and Program Participants

Health fitness members and guests are legally classified as business invitees. Generally, business invitees are individuals invited or allowed to enter a facility for a purpose that is beneficial to the facility owner, lessor, or tenant. For example, making a facility available to individuals who pay dues or fees to use the facility classifies the members as business invitees.

A business invitee is owed a high duty of care when on the premises. To meet the duty of care, the owner or occupier

1. must warn of any known defects on the premises,

2. is responsible for any unknown defects that could reasonably be discovered, and

3. must make the premises safe and free from such defects or dangers.

Although the standard of care may not be as high for other guests on premises, such as an uninvited guest, trespasser, vendor, salesperson, or delivery person, injuries to these individuals due to failure to meet these standards will also create a level of liability for the health fitness facility.

When considering this duty, it becomes apparent that frequent facility and equipment inspections are necessary to meet the legal standards of care required. Inspection procedures, written reports of unsafe conditions, and records of maintenance and repair (see chapter 14) are extremely important in proving the organization's efforts to meet the legal standards of care.

Facility Dangers

Litigation, particularly in relation to suits involving claims of negligence related to facility upkeep, is often complex and frequently depends on matters of proof. Consequently, logging detailed, written records that track facility repair and maintenance (see chapter 14) is important to minimize potential legal risks associated with litigation following participant injury or death. Such records can support other testimony and assist in the successful defense of suits against the organization.

Some of these documents are significantly more important than others. Acknowledgment of proper use of facility and equipment; health risk appraisals; informed consent forms; and proper documentation of employment rules and regulations related to equipment use, training, and supervision are areas most likely to be involved in legal claims against the health fitness organization. Regardless of the efforts of the organization, certain areas of the facility create inherent risks. Wet floors, complex and heavy equipment, and variable conditions inside and outside a facility create an environment that can easily cause an unexpected injury to a member or guest.

Floor Surfaces, Preparations, and Coverings

Make every effort to provide proper floor surfaces throughout a health fitness facility to avoid what is commonly called slip-and-fall situations. Slippery, oily, overwaxed, wet, dusty, or damaged floors can cause serious falls or collisions and related injuries. Liability can attach from injuries and falls, particularly when the injured party can establish knowledge of the dangerous condition or that improper maintenance or repair created an implied knowledge of the danger. Upon discovering a dangerous situation, the club should immediately either

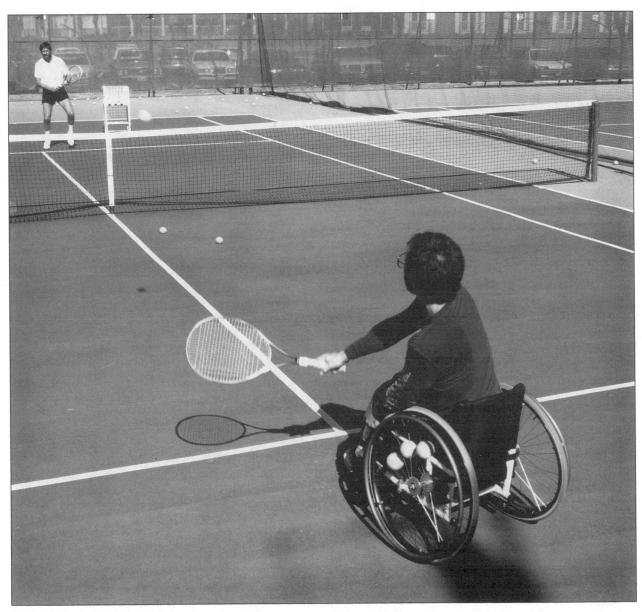

Courtesy of the Cooper Fitness Center

correct the condition, inform participants of the temporary hazard with signs or by posting a staff member at the location, or limit access to the location until correcting the problem.

Inside Facilities and Special Equipment

Some program activities require special services and precautions. For example, certain flexibility and muscular toning exercises require floor mats of a particular minimum thickness or resilience to avoid friction burns of the skin or possible trauma to soft tissue and bone. Failure to provide such mats, or insisting on exercise without mats, can result in liability for injuries.

We can cite many other examples of risk in relation to program facilities, including those associated with locker rooms, shower areas, steam rooms, saunas, hot tubs, and swimming pools. Inappropriate and harmful conditions in these areas increase risk of lacerations related to sharp objects that protrude into participant pathways or access ways. Physiologically stressful levels of heat, humidity, and air pollutants coupled with poor air circulation represent additional conditions that the facility must address. Serious communicable diseases may be transmitted, particularly in hot tubs, and the risk of this occurrence increases when the design, structural material, or maintenance are inappropriate or when a lack of personal hygiene prevails. Also, allowing extended heat exposure or alcohol consumption in hot tub facilities, without concurrently providing proper supervision, can result in drowning accidents.

In general, your facilities must be properly designed, equipped, and maintained in all program areas if you are to control liability. Regularly check all areas and keep them free of defects and nuisances to minimize the chances of participant injury, illness, or death.

Outside Facilities and Property

Circumstances such as accumulation of ice, snow, dirt, or water can result in dangerous conditions outside a facility. Individuals have a responsibility to exercise caution in conditions that are obviously dangerous, such as ice on an outside parking lot or sidewalk. However, potential liability exists for the facility owner or operator if the dangerous condition is caused by improper maintenance or is concealed by a hidden defect, such as a weak surface in a parking lot or sidewalk that gives way and causes an injury. If outdoor jogging trails, par courses, and sport facilities are part of the activities the facility promotes, injuries related to improper repair and maintenance, pedestrian and vehicular traffic, unavailability of lighting, inadequate water, and personal security may create situations of liability.

Equipment Use

The equipment used in a health fitness facility is integrally related to the facility. Litigation in cases related to equipment injuries is frequently based on allegations of improper instruction in equipment use or inadequate supervision by the staff. Less frequently, alleged liability may be based on design or manufacturing defects in the equipment or on improper or negligent installation of the equipment.

It is extremely important that members and staff are aware of and follow manufacturer instructions for installation and use of equipment and products. Although primarily aimed at promoting the desired exercise and conditioning outcome, the club can also use these instructions to limit allegations of liability. Such instructions must be comprehensive and readily communicable to the participants. To ensure consistent and accurate communication by program personnel, they should be written, posted, and made known to users before initial participation. The language must be clear, concise, and easily understood, and the information content must be comprehensive. This is no simple task. At a minimum, the presentation should include

1. a full and complete description of the mechanical function of the equipment,

2. a complete step-by-step procedure indicating proper use,

3. adequate warnings of reasonably foreseeable and known risks associated with use, and

4. adequate warnings about the risks related to improper use.

Initially review these instructions with all participants, generally as part of a new member orientation. At the conclusion of the orientation, it is a good practice to have new members sign an acknowledgment that you have provided proper instructions and warnings. Even if you have provided proper instructions, facilities are under an obligation to provide adequate supervision. In the event that equipment misuse or a potentially dangerous activity is noticed, it is important that facility staff stop the activity, provide appropriate correction, and in serious cases prepare a written record of the incident.

Equipment Design or Manufacturing Defects

Many issues surround liability relative to program equipment. Liability can be predicated on one or more possible grounds encompassing one or more potential defendants. Typically, the equipment used in a facility is not designed, manufactured, or built by program personnel. Consequently, any injury alleged to be due to design, manufacture, or assembly defects will be primarily directed against the equipment engineers, manufacturers, designers, or installers.

Primary liability for injuries due to defects lies with the equipment manufacturers and their associates. Commonly, the related actions are lumped together under the heading of products liability. Although legal responsibilities in products liability cases primarily lies with entities outside the program, liability can also attach to the health fitness facility under one or more of the following theories:

1. Failure to inspect equipment for possible defects

2. Failure to select appropriate equipment for the anticipated use

3. Failure to disclose inherent dangers in the manufactured equipment

4. Provision of equipment in an unreasonably dangerous condition

Even though liability for equipment defects in design or manufacture are primarily directed against equipment producers, wholesalers, retailers, and providers, the program and its personnel are likely defendants due to the mentioned legal responsibilities involving the equipment, which are separate from those of manufacturers. For example, a duty clearly exists with the exercise staff to inspect the equipment on receipt, to test it for defects, and to properly assemble and install it. Failure in these duties can create independent liabilities beyond those of the manufacturer or designer.

In cases for which wholesalers and retailers are found liable to injured participants as a result of defects that are independent of design or manufacturer responsibilities, liability can also attach to the program and its personnel as a result of agency principles flowing from the manufacturer or designer to the provider. Thus, program personnel along with equipment providers can incur costly defense and related expenses as a consequence of participant injury due to faulty equipment. Although liability insurance can limit litigation costs in such cases, take all reasonable precaution to limit the deleterious effects arising from product-liability claims.

Personnel Liabilities

Although liability related to facility and equipment are important, also pay close attention to labor and employment liabilities.

Establishing and Following Written Standards

The most prominent groups to publish written standards that impact the operation of health fitness activities include the American Medical Association, the American Heart Association, the American College of Sports Medicine, and the American Physical Therapy Association. The guidelines developed and published by these and other organizations are influential in defining the standards of care for professionals and other staff in a health fitness setting. Where appropriate, incorporate these standards into the written policies of the organization, including employee manuals, job descriptions, and training procedures.

Employee Negligence

Health fitness organizations are generally liable for the negligent activities of their authorized employees. Liability can be from specific actions or, in some cases, from a failure to act if there existed a responsibility to do so. Examples of areas of risk include the failure by staff to

• properly monitor activities within the facility;

• adequately and competently instruct participants about the safe performance of exercise activities or the proper use of exercise equipment;

• properly and competently evaluate the participants' capacity to participate in certain exercise or sport activities;

• properly supervise participants' exercise during program sessions or advise individuals regarding any restrictions or modifications they should follow during unsupervised periods; and

• maintain a safe exercise environment, including proper lighting, safety features, equipment maintenance, and health standards.

In those settings where exercise prescriptions are developed, additional risk is involved related to administering exercise testing and properly designating exercise activities. In cases where the claim of negligence is made against an individual employee and the organization, a judge or jury will determine respective liability, depending on case law within each state.

Employee Handbook Versus Personnel Policy Manual

To decide whether to have an *employee handbook*, a *personnel policy manual*, or both, it is first necessary to distinguish between them. Handbooks and manuals differ in the intended audience, in scope, and in the degree of detail. Employee handbooks are addressed to employees. They generally are shorter and simpler than personnel policy manuals, communicating in clear, direct terms only the more important policies that govern employment. For example, equal employment opportunity, vacation, sick leave, holidays, and discipline.

Personnel policy manuals, by comparison, are addressed to managers and personnel professionals who must administer the employer's policies. The manuals not only describe the policies, but also designate administration procedures. Personnel policy manuals, therefore, are more comprehensive in scope, address a larger number of policies, and address each in greater detail. Each department maintains personnel policy manuals for access by all employees, but they usually do not distribute them to each employee.

Table 17.4　Checklist of Policies to Include in Employee Manual

[ ] Introduction to the manual

[ ] Equal employment opportunity

[ ] Employment at will

[ ] Orientation/probationary period

[ ] Hours of work, overtime, and payday

[ ] Vacation

[ ] Holidays

[ ] Sick leave

[ ] Other leaves of absence, including disability and family and medical leave

[ ] Internal complaint review procedure

[ ] Termination, discipline, and rules of conduct

[ ] Employee classifications

[ ] Performance and pay review

[ ] Personnel records

[ ] Dress and grooming standards

[ ] Smoking

[ ] Recruitment and selection, employment of relatives, rehires

[ ] Safety program

[ ] Security, confidential information

[ ] AIDS and airborne pathogens in the workplace

[ ] Employee benefits

[ ] Nonfraternization

[ ] Conflicts of interest

[ ] Proof of right to work

[ ] Medical examinations

[ ] Inspections for prohibited materials or substances, including concealed weapons

[ ] Drug-free workplace

[ ] Harassment

[ ] Employee assistance program

Whether to have one or both depends on the organization's needs. Large health fitness organizations traditionally have both an employee handbook and a personnel policy manual. Many small facilities have neither. We recommend an employee handbook for most health fitness organizations. It tells employees what they may expect of their employer and what the health fitness organization expects of them. In the absence of any written guidelines, an employer is more likely to encounter problems arising from ignorance of its policies, inconsistent application, and confusion about what is expected. An employee handbook can help avoid some of these problems.

Developing a personnel policy manual is a detailed and extensive process. Large organizations consider policy manuals necessary to maintain consistency and to ensure compliance. For all employers, personnel policy manuals are a two-edged sword. To the extent that the manual defines standards and procedures for discipline, performance evaluations, and payment of wages and to the extent that these policies and procedures are followed, they can help avoid legal problems. However, if the personnel policy manual is overly complex, not properly distributed, or not enforced, different legal issues and liabilities may arise.

For example, each time a health fitness organization gives one employee a special privilege, the organization may be creating exceptions to published rules and creating an obligation to accord all employees the same privilege or risk charges of discriminatory treatment. The health fitness organization can find its good intentions used against it by a disgruntled employee alleging that the organization failed to follow its policies.

In short, each health fitness organization must achieve a balance between adequate standards and guidance for fair and consistent treatment, and creating unnecessary legal problems. Table 17.4 shows the most critical areas that an employee handbook or policy manual should address.

Termination, Discipline, and Rules of Conduct

The health fitness organization should develop an employee handbook including guidelines defining inappropriate conduct that may result in disciplinary action. It also should list the circumstances under which the company will consider an employee to have voluntarily terminated employment and notify the employee of the potential results of a termination or temporary layoff.

The grounds given in the handbook that justify involuntary termination include poor performance, general misconduct, and engaging in any specific misconduct listed. In addition to listing specific types of misconduct that may result in discipline, the handbook should contain provisions that describe what might constitute unacceptable job performance, including below average work quality, failure to follow established rules or regulations, high levels of absenteeism, or repeated tardiness.

The handbook may also include a nonbinding disciplinary procedure or mediation process in which the employee would receive an opportunity to correct perceived deficiencies in conduct or performance. The handbook may outline the provisions for an exit interview that a manager might ask employees to attend before leaving the organization.

Providing Warnings and Notice

A warning regarding poor performance should address four issues: (1) the nature of the unacceptable performance, (2) steps required to correct the unacceptable performance, (3) specific time the employee has to correct the unacceptable performance, and (4) the consequences of failure to correct the unacceptable performance. If initially delivered orally, create a written memo that includes the date, the name of the employee, the subject discussed, a summary of the discussion, and specific issues identified here. Give a copy of the memo to the employee and place one in the employee's personnel file. The employee's signature on the memo is advisable but not required. These types of memos should state the issues and discussions in objective terms and should not editorialize or make personal comments outside the scope of the warning.

Americans With Disabilities Act of 1990 (ADA)

The *Americans with Disabilities Act of 1990 (ADA)* potentially limits a health fitness organization's right to discipline or terminate an employee for performance problems or misconduct attributable to a disability. Therefore, whenever considering termination or discipline, health fitness organizations should determine whether an employee has an underlying mental or physical disability that might explain the employee's problems. However, the organization should conduct an investigation only if it reasonably believes that an underlying mental or physical problem may be causing the performance problems or misconduct.

When an employee's excessive absenteeism or tardiness is related to a disability, the health fitness organization may be required to make reasonable accommodations in the form of leave or modified work schedule. Although reasonable accommodation is a term defined by courts, many courts have held that if regular attendance is an essential job component, an organization is not required to accommodate a disabled employee's high rate of unpredictable absences if it would result in an undue hardship. Organizations facing these issues would be well served to consult with legal counsel before disciplining a possibly disabled employee for absenteeism or tardiness.

Drug-Free Workplace Act of 1988

The *Drug-Free Workplace Act of 1988* requires that certain federal contractors and recipients of federal grants certify to the federal contracting or granting agency that the organization will provide a drug-free workplace. Texas has also enacted a drug-free workplace provision in the Texas Workers' Compensation Act. This provision requires health fitness organizations that maintain workers'

compensation insurance to adopt a policy to eliminate drug abuse in the workplace. Failing to establish and maintain drug-free policies may eliminate a health fitness organization's opportunity to serve as a contractor providing services such as fitness testing, training, and other wellness programs to city, county, state, public school, federal, and other governmental organizations in the community.

Policy Against Harassment

Harassment in the workforce based on sex, race, color, religion, national origin, age, or disability is prohibited under both state and federal law. To discourage such behavior and to protect against potential legal liability, all health fitness organizations are encouraged to include a policy in their employee handbook (1) stating clearly that the organization is committed to providing a work environment free from any type of harassment, (2) describing the types of behavior that may constitute impermissible harassment, and (3) encouraging all employees to report any incident to an appropriate manager.

Table 17.5 Checklist of Legal Liability Issues

[ ] Do professional staff have appropriate credentials?

[ ] Are all staff CPR certified?

[ ] Are adequate staff available in the exercise and activity areas?

[ ] Do all new members go through a thorough orientation program?

[ ] Are safety notices clearly posted on or near all equipment?

[ ] Are all public areas regularly inspected for unsafe conditions?

[ ] Is all equipment inspected regularly?

[ ] Is a standard procedure in place to respond to discovery or notification of an unsafe piece of equipment or dangerous condition?

[ ] Are safety inspection records documented and kept current?

[ ] Has equipment layout been evaluated to determine safety issues related to location and arrangement?

[ ] Are internal and external lighting adequate to enhance safety?

[ ] Is a standard health fitness screening protocol used to screen for unsafe medical conditions?

[ ] Does the facility have a written emergency plan that is available for review?

[ ] Does the facility have adequate first aid supplies that are checked and refreshed regularly?

[ ] Are all areas of the facility free from physical hazards?

[ ] Are all activity areas free from environmental hazards?

[ ] Does the organization have written personnel policies that are available to all employees?

[ ] Has the organization provided training for all staff in the areas of discrimination and harassment?

[ ] Does management have clear procedures for responding to and documenting violations of personnel policy?

[ ] Do all staff participate in safety training and review sessions for emergency procedures?

[ ] Is a formal policy in place for making statements on behalf of the organization?

We encourage that the policy include the organization's commitment to review and investigate all complaints as thoroughly and confidentially as possible and a statement that no retaliation will be permitted against employees who file a complaint. The handbook should identify the potential discipline or termination process for any employee determined to have engaged in harassment and include a policy that covers harassment by nonemployees, such as members or vendors. Health fitness organizations should be aware that they may be liable for harassment conducted by nonemployees if the organizations knew or should have known of the offensive conduct and failed to take appropriate corrective action.

> *Because of the inherently sensitive and volatile nature of issues and incidents related to harassment, we encourage each health fitness organization to designate and provide appropriate training for at least one manager who will investigate and resolve complaints of harassment.*

IN CLOSING

There are many major areas likely to generate legal questions related to rights and liabilities in a health fitness setting. Within each area, it is the responsibility of the health fitness manager to identify, evaluate, and define levels of risk and determine when to obtain formal legal advice from competent counsel. The health fitness manager should review the checklist in table 17.5 in an ongoing effort to keep on top of areas of potential legal liability. Although the checklist is not intended to be comprehensive, it provides a framework for identifying major areas of risk.

One of the most important decisions a health fitness manager must make is determining when a circumstance requires outside legal advice. Although using a lawyer may appear expensive, the cost-saving measure of operating without competent legal advice may be a short-lived gain when you consider the potential liabilities of contract obligations, tort liabilities, and employment law issues. Poor decisions in areas that create legal liabilities have the potential to destroy the economic viability of your organization.

KEY TERMS

Americans With Disabilities Act of 1990 (ADA)

At will case law

Civil and criminal liability

Contingent fee

Contracts

Drug-Free Workplace Act of 1988

Duty of care

Employee handbook

Employee negligence

Fixed or flat fee

Harassment

Hourly rates

Independent contractor

Intentional torts

Negligence torts

Personnel policy manual

Precedent

Strict liability torts

Tort

RECOMMENDED READINGS

Herbert, D.L., and W.G. Herbert, eds. 1993. *Aspects of preventive and rehabilitative exercise programs.* 3d ed. Canton, OH: Professional Reports.

———. 1987-1997. *Exercise standards and malpractice reporter.* Canton, OH: Professional Reports.

———. 1989-1997. *Sports medicine standards and malpractice reporter.* Canton, OH: Professional Reports.

Maslanka, M.P. 1996. *Texas employer's guide to employee policy handbooks.* Nashville: Smith.

CHAPTER 18

Insurance Considerations

Insurance exists because the world is filled with uncertainty. Every day each of us experiences some uncertainty due to the unpredictability of weather, political events, activities of a coworker, and even actions of our family and friends. Some uncertainties can lead to financial loss. Wind damage to a local health fitness center, new laws eliminating certain tax benefits, injury on the job caused by a coworker's negligence, and payment to a member who fell and injured himself due to housekeeping carelessness all result in financial loss.

Although there are many types of uncertainty with various effects, this chapter identifies the risks involved with operating a health fitness business. We provide information on the reasons and benefits for purchasing property and casualty insurance, how to choose an insurance carrier, and how to implement a well-designed risk-management program.

As discussed from the legal perspective in chapter 17, operating a health fitness facility presents an inherent condition of risk for members, guests, and

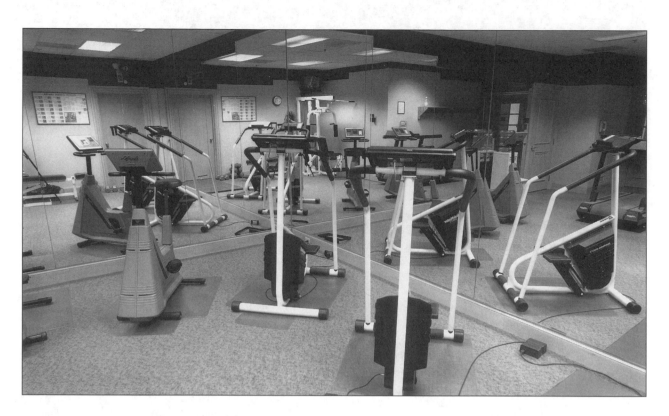

personnel. An environment with cardiovascular machines, resistive weight-training equipment, locker rooms with wet areas (i.e., showers, saunas, whirlpools, and steam rooms), and a pool all possess the possibility for accidents. Combine these facilities with a membership comprised of men and women of every age range, fitness level, and health status, and the risk potential is significant.

Most personal injury losses incurred by health fitness operators have resulted primarily from not repairing or replacing faulty or outdated equipment, providing inadequate supervision in activity areas, and adopting poor maintenance standards within a facility. However, history has also shown that insurance claims brought against health fitness owners have no boundaries and can occur at any time. Even the most successful, well-managed clubs cannot guard against accidents and physical hazards. For this reason, having the right insurance to cover such incidents is essential.

This chapter provides an overview of insurance as it relates to the health fitness industry. We discuss aspects of *risk management*, facility insurance, and employee insurance. We will cover information on choosing an insurance carrier and the recommended guidelines to follow when purchasing insurance. Readers should be aware that numerous articles and texts have been written about insurance. It is beyond the scope of this chapter to provide a comprehensive overview of insurance.

For this reason, we encourage you to engage in additional reading to further your knowledge in this area.

UNCERTAINTIES OF THE HEALTH FITNESS BUSINESS

Insurance exists primarily for the uncertainties of managing any business. Each day conditions exist that provide concern due to the unpredictability of weather, building and mechanical conditions, activities of members, and even actions of coworkers. Some risks may lead to financial loss. Fire damage due to a faulty steam room boiler, a member who slips and falls in a shower and fractures a shoulder, or an injury caused by maintenance negligence can all result in financial loss for the organization.

Although there are many uncertainties with various effects, this chapter focuses only on those that cause financial loss. A financial loss is an unexpected decrease in value arising from an event. Financial losses result when property is destroyed, damaged, or stolen; when money or other financial assets must be paid to injured individual(s) due to legal liability of the business; and when income is lost or medical expenses are incurred due to death or disability (Smith, Trieschmann, and Wiening 1988).

A financial loss generally occurs when an entity is susceptible to loss or the possibility of loss. It is the probability (not certainty) of a financial loss that creates insecurity and the need for insurance.

HEALTH FITNESS FACILITY RISKS

During the evening of January 1, 1981, a fire ignited by a gas dryer nearly burned down the Cooper Activity Center in Dallas, Texas. By the time the blaze was under control, most of the facility had sustained substantial fire and smoke damage. Although the fire was considered an accident, the Activity Center was criticized for failing to install a sprinkler system and to have appropriate fire walls. Because the fire occurred in the middle of the night there were no members present; however, a housekeeping crew was completing their work and some workers experienced smoke inhalation. This incident illustrates the four major types of *loss exposures* (property loss, net income, liability, and personnel losses) that identify and categorize potential loss.

Property Losses

Property loss exposures exist because property exists. Families and businesses own property, depend on it as a source of income or services, and rely on its value. For all practical purposes, property is any item with value. It can decline in value or become worthless if it is lost, damaged, or destroyed.

A health fitness facility's property consists primarily of the building(s), fitness and office equipment, furniture and fixtures, money, inventory, boilers, and machinery. General causes of property loss include fire, smoke, explosions, windstorms, hail, vandalism, and vehicle damage of a company car. Many property insurance policies cover these events. However, property loss resulting from maintenance causes such as normal wear and tear, rust, water seepage, and termites are not covered. These hazards are considered preventable through proper care and maintenance. In the Activity Center fire, damage to the building and its contents was reported in millions of dollars. Although much of the fitness and office equipment had been used for some time, replacement value reflected new equipment and furniture cost. Unfortunately, incidents of this nature find many owners underinsured due to replacement cost values and a lack of diligence in

updating insurance policies to reflect increased contents purchased annually.

> *We highly recommend that health fitness managers regularly evaluate (at least annually) their insurance policy and update current replacement cost values for all contents.*

Net Income Losses

Property damage can also reflect net income losses. As discussed in chapter 15, net income is the generated income (or revenue) minus expenses during a designated time. For any business to stay operational and profitable it must generate an excess of income over expenses. A net income loss consists of either a reduction in income or an increase in expenses as a result of an event.

Often the net income losses to a business greatly exceed the property loss that caused it. Although the Activity Center had insurance to cover business interruption, revenues decreased because the organization was unable to collect membership dues, the restaurant and pro shop were closed, and other nondues-related programs (massage, activity programs) were discontinued. Some lost revenue was permanent, a result of some members joining another club while the new building was being constructed. In addition, the Activity Center incurred increased expenses from the costs associated with an accelerated rebuilding process.

Liability Losses

A *liability loss exposure* occurs when an individual or business may be sued by another individual or firm for alleged wrongdoing. The most serious form of a liability loss is bodily injury, which can lead to medical expenses, lost income, rehabilitation expenses, and possibly damages for pain and suffering. Property damage losses can result in direct damage to or loss of use of another person's property. Other kinds of personal injury, such as damage to another person's reputation, can lead to liability losses. Finally, many liability claims lead to defense costs, including legal fees, investigation expenses, and other expenses to defend a claim.

In the Activity Center fire, the liability losses included payments for medical and rehabilitation costs for those employees who suffered smoke inhalation. In some incidents, once these direct costs are paid, a liable party must pay additional damages for pain and suffering to the individuals involved. Although the fire was contained within the Center's property, a more severe fire might have caused adjacent property damage, which could have resulted in a greater loss of property expenses.

Personnel Losses

Personnel or human losses result from events such as death, disability, and unemployment. Although injury to members of the public is a liability loss, injury to coworkers is considered a personnel loss. A coworker's loss could result in a loss of income, especially if there was a death to the primary revenue producer. Many businesses fear the loss of an employee due to death, disability, or resignation, especially if that person cannot be readily replaced.

In the Activity Center incident, no deaths occurred; however, there was partial disability paid to one employee for lung damage and unemployment to another for smoke inhalation. Understanding the possible risks and uncertainties involved in operating a health fitness facility is important in determining the type and amount of insurance to obtain.

> *Realizing that a fitness center has a higher degree of uncertainty and risk than most other businesses, club operators should regularly evaluate their annual loss records and learn where accidents and losses are occurring.*

A summary of where clubs are experiencing accidents and suffering losses, their frequency, and the dollars associated with the losses is provided in table 18.1.

Table 18.1   General Loss Liability for Fitness Facilities*

Slips and falls	# of claims 262 (31%)	Incurred cost $2.4 million (48%)	Largest claim $211,434	Average $9,220
Wet floor area				
Shower/locker room	44	$504,350	$211,434	$11,463
Pool, hot tub, sauna, etc.	34	$203,400	$60,790	$5,982
Walking surfaces				
Steps/stairs	38	$338,600	$80,790	$8,911
Sidewalk/parking lot	26	$326,300	$143,280	$12,550
Floor surface (general)	47	$150,000	$31,676	$3,191
Equipment				
Treadmill	29	$250,200	$48,029	$8,628
Other	3	$10,833	N/A	N/A
Recreational sports				
Basketball	18	$217,264	$62,256	$12,094
Tennis	12	$104,000	$34,148	$8,667
Racquetball	7	$248,742	$94,136	$35,535
Volleyball	4	$61,900	$31,382	$15,475

Struck by	# of claims 72 (8%)	Incurred cost $735,100 (14%)	Largest claim $151,828	Average $10,210
Equipment use	26	$427,400	$151,828	$16,429
Weightlifting	36	$307,700	$148,866	$8,547

*This chart depicts the loss analysis of liability claims occurring in U.S. fitness facilities from January 1991 to February 1995, the latest period for which statistics are available.

Reprinted, by permission, from National Fitness Clubs Insurance Program, 1996, *General loss liability for fitness facilities: A study reported by Royal Insurance* (Charlotte, NC: Royal Insurance), 47.

BENEFITS OF INSURANCE

Insurance provides a variety of benefits for both individuals and businesses.

> *One obvious benefit of insurance is that it provides payment for losses, which helps people and businesses recover from misfortune.*

To understand the importance of paying for a loss, consider what happens to people or businesses who have no insurance. Families burned out of their homes or apartments find themselves on the street, without money, clothes, or a place to stay. A health fitness business that suddenly goes bankrupt creates an unemployment status without an immediate source of income for the employees and owners of that facility. Members who have prepaid their membership dues are also affected because they have paid for a service that is not available.

The primary benefit of insurance is providing financial compensation for covered losses. The fear of a fire destroying a health fitness center or the death of the family breadwinner is almost completely eliminated through the transfer of loss to an insurance company. This factor alone greatly reduces anxiety and stress for individuals and business owners.

A second benefit of insurance is that insurance companies contribute to the control of loss by adopting strict risk-management standards for facility operations. In the health fitness industry, insurance investigators and engineers assist club operators in identifying and evaluating loss exposures and recommend ways to minimize the frequency and severity of potential losses. Insurance companies also have the benefit of sharing years of knowledge and experience with managers to assist them in maintaining a safer, more efficient operation.

CHOOSING AN INSURANCE CARRIER

Before purchasing insurance for a health fitness business, find either a risk manager, *broker*, or agent to help determine the most appropriate insurance carrier for your facility. Without a broker's assis-

tance the manager is left to negotiate in a maze of competitive insurance companies on such items as the specific insurance coverage needed, the associated premium costs, the company ratings and solvency situation, and history of claims payments.

> *An insurance broker's objective is to convince insurance carriers to accept the potential loss exposures of a business in exchange for the lowest premium payment, while still ensuring proper coverage to the business if an exposure should ever become a loss.*

It is the broker's job to sell insurance companies on the positive aspects of underwriting a particular business. The broker accomplishes this task by doing the following:

- Establishing criteria for selecting an insurance carrier.

- Analyzing an organization's potential loss exposures and identifying which insurance contracts can best cover them.

- Making oral or written presentations to selected companies regarding the organization's exposures and insurance requirements.

- Playing an active role in negotiating insurance coverage. In most cases the broker is the primary salesperson for an account and must be the spokesperson for the business.

- Negotiating the final terms of the various insurance contracts the organization purchases and the corresponding premium rates.

In addition to performing these roles, a broker working for a health fitness business should be familiar with the fitness industry and the club insurance marketplace. Agents who have previously served other health fitness organizations have a specific understanding of the loss exposure in a fitness facility and can better advise clients on a course of action.

Traditionally, an insurance broker receives a commission from the insurance companies from which the coverage is placed. These commissions are computed as a percentage of the premiums collected. These are generally 10 to 15 percent but can vary

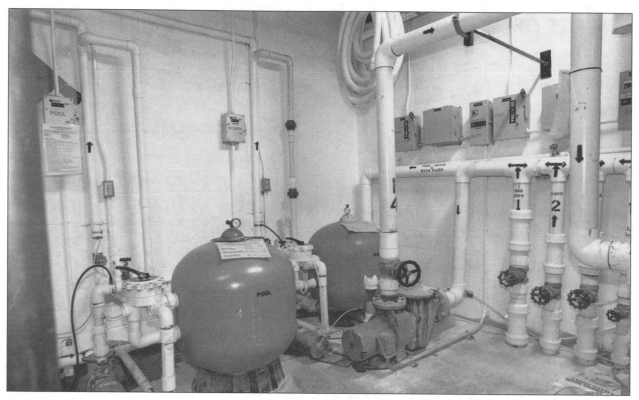

© Tom Wallace

from one insurer to the next and by the amount of insurance written. Some brokers are compensated with a flat fee from the client based on the value of the services provided.

With the increasing emphasis on range of risk management services, some health fitness operators are opting for this form of payment. Providing insurance is only one phase of a total risk management plan; other areas include risk retention programs, providing safety services, and administering claims. These activities are of considerable value to an operator but are not directly related to the volume of premiums generated. Therefore, an increasing number of brokers consider fees a more appropriate compensation system than commissions.

Determining Your Facility's Insurance Needs

Determining the insurance needs for a health fitness facility is complex and time consuming. The first step involves identifying and analyzing the potential loss exposures within the facility. This step includes conducting research, preparing an evaluation, and analyzing and reporting the data.

It is the broker's responsibility to identify the facility exposures, then weigh the potential financial loss to the organization. However, managers are often asked to assist brokers by providing pertinent specifications on equipment and specified facilities. Brokers evaluate the amount and type of equipment used in the mechanical room, the number of wet areas within the club, the use of an air-inflated pool bubble during the winter months, weight-room specifications and equipment, floor surfacing, types of lockers used, and aerobics studio layout with average number of participants per class. Each of these areas is susceptible to accidents and potential losses.

In addition to identifying the potential loss exposure areas, it is helpful to compile lists of all programs, facilities, and special equipment. These lists will ensure that proper coverage is given to the areas mentioned and guard against possible gaps in the policy. Such services as massage, blood cholesterol screening, child care, and tanning beds are generally not covered by a standard insurance policy unless you request it.

Once these specifications have been completed, a broker can informally test the evaluation of an organization's insurance needs by asking other brokers or agents to review the specific recommendations. This step confirms that nothing has been overlooked and that the specifications are consistent with any recent developments in the insurance industry. It also ensures that each insurance carrier receives a preapproved list of specifications, which can easily be adapted into a bid proposal.

Purchasing Insurance

Once you have established insurance needs, purchasing insurance is the next step. Spend some time diagnosing coverage needs, obtaining and analyzing insurance bids, and ensuring that the coverage decided on provides the necessary security to operate the business.

> *Once you have established insurance needs, purchasing insurance is the next step.*

Entering into a new insurance contract or renewing an existing one consists of five steps coordinated by a broker or risk manager.

1. The broker assists the manager in determining coverage needs and develops specifications.

2. The broker makes presentations to insurance carriers and obtains at least three bids for coverage.

3. The broker develops coverage proposals and submits them to the manager in a timely fashion.

4. If the policy is a renewal, the broker submits a list of all claims against the business for the previous year.

5. The manager selects a proposal and enters into an insurance policy contract. The broker provides a list of what the insurance policy specifically excludes for the manager's reference.

This sequence ensures that all parties involved (insurance carriers, broker, and client) possess enough information to reach an agreement on insurance coverage, policy awarding, and price. The cyclical aspect of the insurance industry dictates the importance of allowing adequate time for brokers and managers to review policies before deciding on a company. As with the stock market, insurance carriers experience buyers' and sellers' markets.

> *A* buyers' market *pressures carriers to provide businesses with more coverage for less money, whereas a* sellers' market *provides less coverage for more money.*

For this reason, brokers must have enough time to shop around for the right climate and company to fit their client's needs. This process should begin at least five months before the expiration date of an existing policy. The activities that take place during each of these months are shown in figure 18.1.

Selecting Proposals

About two months before the deadline date for insurance coverage, the broker should begin receiving proposals from carriers interested in providing the desired coverage. Most often, the broker asks insurance companies to submit bids by a predetermined time. After receiving each insurer's offer and

Months before renewal	Activity
5	Determine insurance needs, develop specifications
4	Make presentations to insurer intermediaries
3	Develop and present coverage proposals
2	Select proposals
1	Finalize insurance contract

Figure 18.1   Insurance plan time line.

making sure each proposal is complete and conforms to the specifications of the organization, the broker can either decide which proposals to accept or reject, or the manager may make the decision.

During this phase, the broker also has the responsibility for obtaining insurance carrier ratings. The five major rating agencies are A.M. Best, Standard & Poor's Corporation (S&P), Moody's Investors Service, Duff and Phelps Credit Rating Company (D&P), and Weiss Ratings. These ratings are the primary means for determining the financial viability of an insurance company. The mission of these companies is to provide ratings based on a carrier's financial strength (on a numerical scale), including such factors as quality and diversification of assets, liquidity, leverage, and profitability. In addition, service performance is also rated (on an alphabetical scale), by product and geographic diversification, parent company affiliation, adequacy of reserves, and management philosophy and experience. An ideal insurance carrier rating would be A+15, with the A+ indicating solid financial strength and the 15 reflecting excellent service. With insurer insolvency and professional liability lawsuits against agents increasing, the reliability of insurer ratings has never been more critical.

The following list provides some warning signs that an insurer's financial condition is deteriorating. By monitoring these indicators and other data, and taking the appropriate precautions, brokers can assist managers in reducing their exposure to insolvency risk. However, the ultimate responsibility still rests with the owner or manager.

Warning signs when investigating potential insurance companies include:

1. Unusual growth in premiums written, relative to surplus

2. Premiums that are too good to be true

3. Excessive delays in settling small claims

4. Many complaints filed against the company with the state insurance department

5. An unusually high rate of management turnover

6. Downward trend in ratings over a two- to five-year period

7. Below-average ratings in the most recent year by two or more top rating agencies

Entering Into Insurance Contracts

Once you have selected the coverages for purchase, it is customary for the broker to notify all companies involved in the bidding process to confirm those carriers who were selected and to notify those who were rejected. Depending on the size of the organization and the amount of coverage needed, it is rare for one carrier to underwrite all the insurance needs of a club.

It is common for a health fitness center to enter into multiple contracts with various agencies to meet all insurance needs. For example, you could contract one company to underwrite only the building and contents insurance while another provides coverage for the general liability insurance.

Because no two insurance policies are alike, study each policy before signing any contract to determine the areas specifically covered by the policy and, more importantly, to identify the areas not covered by the policy. Because it generally takes between two and three months for an organization to receive its policy once purchased, it's a good idea to request a sample policy to study when you make a bid. The key in reading a policy is to study all the exclusions and understand what is not covered.

Once you have signed all insurance contracts, have your broker prepare a written summary of all insurance policies. This summary should include pertinent information on coverage, limits, deductibles, major exclusions, premiums, and effective as well as expiration dates. Update the summary annually so you can keep all information current and easy to access in case of accident.

Although entering into a contract represents the final stage of the annual insurance process, take time during the year to include changes or additions to the summary for the following year. Only in this way can operators stay ahead of an ever-changing insurance market while providing the necessary coverage for a growing and dynamic business.

PROPERTY AND CASUALTY INSURANCE

Purchasing adequate and affordable insurance can be a frustrating task for health fitness professionals. Determining the type of insurance to purchase for the best possible price is the goal of every organization. Minimal coverage for any business should consist of at least two types of insurance: property coverage and general liability coverage. Most professionals in the health fitness industry, however, prefer a facility insurance package consisting of a variety of coverages. These package policies are called *property and casualty insurance.* Components of the property and casualty are illustrated in figure 18.2. Additional insurance coverage is recommended for worker's compensatioin, automobile, and umbrella liability.

- Package policy
- Building (commercial property)
- Contents (commercial property)
- General liability
- Business interruption
- Crime (by outsiders or employee dishonesty)
- Boiler and machinery
- Automobile (liability, comprehensive, and collision)
- Umbrella liability

Commercial Property Insurance

Commercial property insurance covers accidental losses resulting from damage to property of the insured. In a health fitness setting, the insured is usually the owner or manager of the business. When the insured experiences a loss, such as fire damage to a facility, the insured deals directly with the insurance company in the settlement process.

Property insurance is necessary for many business operations. Insurance requirements are commonly imposed by financial institutions when money is loaned or property mortgaged. Not only is insurance required, but the lending agency frequently insists on being named in the policy as a payee in the event of a loss. This practice assures the financial institution that restitution will be made in case of an accident or a catastrophic event. Without insurance of this nature, it is doubtful that large shopping malls, office buildings, or health fitness centers would be built.

The two primary areas covered by commercial property insurance are the building, and business and equipment contents.

Buildings

A commercial property policy covers the buildings or structures the owner lists and describes in the specifications the broker provides. Additional building property also includes the following:

1. Completed additions to covered buildings

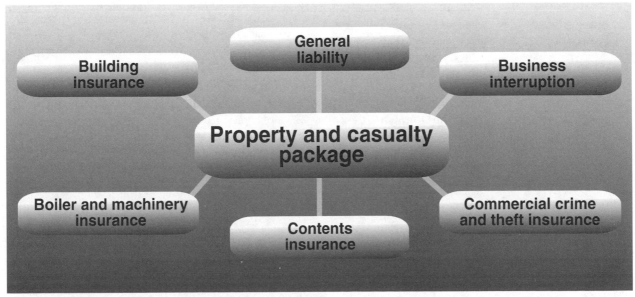

Figure 18.2   Basic property and casualty insurance package.

2. Permanently installed fixtures, machinery, and equipment

3. Outdoor fixtures

4. Personal property owned by the organization and used to maintain or service the facility, for example, fire extinguishers, outdoor pool furniture, floor coverings, and washers and dryers

Basic property insurance limits any coverage on outdoor signs, outdoor trees, shrubs and plants, outdoor fences, and radio and television antennas or cable lines. These items may specifically be insured, but do not consider their value in determining the amount of insurance on a building.

Understanding the property included in the building definition of a policy is essential to determining a proper amount of insurance and charge of premiums.

Contents

Most insurance agents refer to business personal property as *contents*. Contents applies to personal property contained within designated buildings. Examples of personal property covered by most insurance policies are the following:

1. Furniture and fixtures.

2. Machinery and equipment.

3. Supplies and inventory items.

4. In addition to building coverage described in the policy, protection extends to property in the open or in vehicles within 100 feet of the described premises.

Contents insurance protects the owner against loss or damage to the personal property of others while such property is in the custody of the insured. In a health fitness facility this would include loaned or leased equipment, which is not owned by the business but would be covered in the case of a loss. Personal property is covered only while it is (1) in the insured's care, custody, or control; and (2) in or on the building or grounds described in the policy or within 100 feet of the described premises. This property is not covered while being transported from the premises.

General Liability

Liability insurance is necessary to cover the risk of incurring legal liability and possibly paying monetary damages.

> *Liability insurance guarantees financial protection to an owner who might be required to pay damages resulting from negligent conduct that causes personal injury, death, or property damage.*

Liability for negligence may result not only from the actions of the owner but also from the conduct of the employees. Liability insurance is often referred to as third-party insurance, because the insurance company protects the owner against suit by a third party.

In the health fitness industry, acts of negligence resulting in liability occur in a variety of activities. A four-year study (January 1991 to February 1995) by the National Fitness Clubs Insurance Program and reported by the Royal Insurance (Charlotte, NC) agency (1996) discovered that slips and falls accounted for 31 percent of total claims filed against clubs and 48 percent of the claims cost. Royal Insurance officials recommend the following guidelines to assist club owners and managers in evaluating existing conditions and to implement appropriate loss control measures:

- *Swimming pools.* Provide a well-drained, slip-resistant apron, preferably one that is at least four feet wide.

- *Hot tub, sauna, whirlpool, and Jacuzzi.* Install handrails where steps are used to enter equipment and slip-resistant materials on steps. Provide slip-resistant mats or coatings where floor surfaces are always wet. Post wet floor signs whenever appropriate.

- *Showers and locker rooms.* Floor surfaces, showers, and entrances to showers should have slip-resistant floors, be coated with slip-resistant material, or be covered with mats. Install handrails in shower stalls.

- *Floor surfaces (general).* Regularly inspect all floor surfaces (at least monthly) and maintain records of inspection. Repair or replace torn carpet immediately. Clean up spills (e.g., water, soda, coffee) promptly. Post "wet floor" signs whenever appropriate.

- *Sidewalks and parking lots.* Regularly inspect for potholes or cracks. Make repairs and clean up

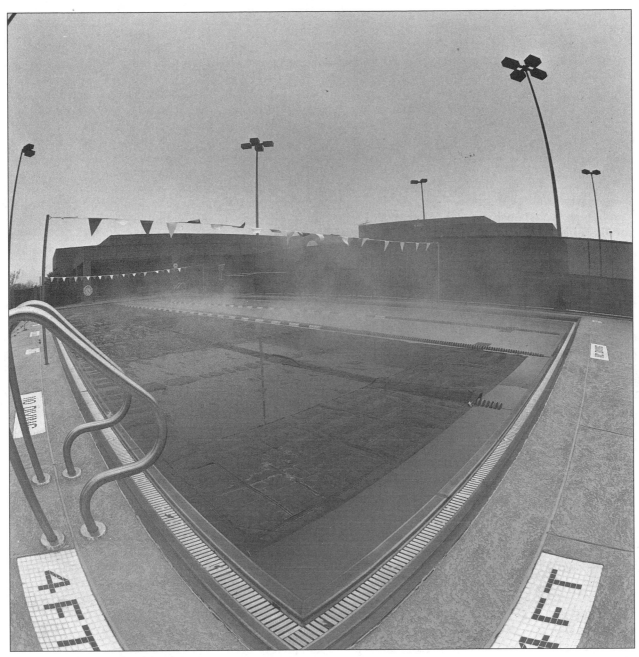

Courtesy of Dallas Texins Association

debris promptly. Arrange for prompt snow and ice removal.

- *Cardiovascular equipment.* Give all members instruction on proper usage, such as how to work the machines' controls, prevent the equipment from suddenly stopping, and how to slow down and step off the machines.

- *Selectorized equipment.* Maintain all equipment in accordance with manufacturer's recommendations. Inspect daily for loose pins and fasteners, frayed cables, and stability. Mark equip-

ment that needs repair with an "out of order" sign or remove it from the fitness floor until fixed. In addition, maintain enough space between stations so users can easily get on and off machines.

A liability insurance policy generally provides for investigating and negotiating private settlements. In addition, the policy covers the defense of lawsuits brought against the owner and the payment of judgments up to the limit of the policy.

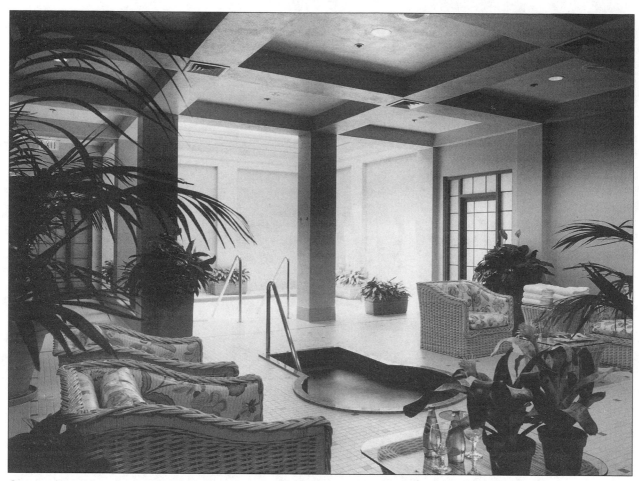

Courtesy of Four Seasons Resort and Clubs at Las Colinas, Irving, Texas

Independent Contractor Liability

Another form of liability insurance that both health fitness operators and independent contractors (i.e., aerobics instructors, racquet sport instructors, and personal trainers) should be aware of is *owner's and contractor's protective coverage.* Currently, health fitness insurance policies do not cover independent contractors while working on the premises of a club. Consequently, club managers now require self-employed individuals to obtain owner's and contractor's protective coverage.

A fundamental rule regarding liability is that responsibility lies with the person who commits the act and causes the damage or injury. If a personal trainer injures a client, the trainer is responsible for the client's injuries or damages. However, under the term *vicarious liability,* in some cases, the liability will be placed with someone other than the person committing the act. Vicarious liability gives the client an additional party to proceed against, presumably someone more able to pay any damages awarded by the court.

Generally, a health fitness center's liability insur-ance covers the employer's liability for negligent acts by employees. However, an independent contractor must be distinguished from an employee. An independent contractor is hired to perform specific tasks, and management should exercise little or no control over their method of performance.

> *Only the independent contractor is responsible for his or her actions.*

Unfortunately, some operators, either knowingly or unknowingly, assume a supervisory role over their independent contractors. This practice establishes an employee-employer relationship and may be viewed adversely by the courts. In addition, if the club operator provides equipment or supplies, the courts are likely to interpret an employee-employer union rather than independent contractor. Under this scenario, club owners can be held responsible for the actions of their independent contractors. Consequently, it is wise to add these individuals to the club's insurance policy as an additional insured.

If an employee is classified as an independent contractor, require her to show proof of liability insurance. In addition, she should include the club as a Name Insured *on the policy. This means the contractor's insurance carrier will have to fight any related claim, and it will not affect an organization's premium even if it is named as part of the claim.*

Typically, the club's insurance agent requests copies of independent contractor's insurance certificates before underwriting their liability insurance. Because the liability exposures associated with being an independent contractor vary from the standard commercial liability policy, insurance companies have established different policies for specific groups. For example, companies specializing in the health fitness insurance market have prepared a separate personal trainer insurance program. Figure 18.3 provides a sample personal trainer insurance application.

Event Liability Coverage

It is the responsibility of managers of health fitness settings to contact their insurance agent anytime there is a major addition to, or renovation of the facility, or if the club is planning a special event that may not be covered under the existing policy.

If a business offers off-site trips, it should ask the coordinating outside party to provide the necessary insurance. This applies to ski tours, white water rafting companies, and even the charter bus company that transports members to an event. Generally, such companies do not have to pay anything extra to name the club on their insurance coverage for an outing or event. However, if the outside party chooses not to provide insurance coverage, it is the responsibility of the club to obtain an insurance rider on the club's liability policy to cover the event.

Business Interruption

Most insurance policies offer *business interruption* or loss of earnings coverage for disasters that tempo-

rarily affect the daily operations of a health fitness facility. This can be significant if, for example, an organization is damaged by a fire and must wait 9 to 12 months to finish construction documents, obtain permits, solicit bids, and rebuild. The damage is not just the cost of renovation. It also involves the cost of expenses that are ongoing, even when the club is not operational (i.e., debt service, real estate taxes, insurance, and the demand portion of utilities). In some situations, key employees will need to be retained during the reconstruction phase. A temporary trailer or rented office and furniture may be required.

Business interruption insurance reimburses the club for lost revenues sustained by the loss. This is important coverage because initiation fees and membership dues cannot be collected when a club is inoperable. Also members may decide to join another club and consequently cause additional loss of income during the reconstruction phase. Fortunately, for this type of insurance coverage business income is determined by net profit or loss that would have been earned if the loss had not occurred and normal operating expenses, including payroll, that continue during renovation.

The amount of profit and loss that would have been earned if the loss had not occurred is estimated from past and prospective performance of the business. Consequently, estimated membership revenues are determined from normal operating conditions rather than actual occurrences during the restoration period. In addition to business interruption insurance, many managers choose to pay for extra expense coverage during the renovation phase. Extra expenses are those costs over and above those that may have been incurred for the normal operation of the club. The two types of extra expenses that may occur as the result of a loss are the following:

- *Extra expenses that reduce the loss.* These expenses can include advertising fees to announce a fire sale or expediting costs to speed reconstruction. If the amount spent is smaller than the revenue derived from the expenditure, the overall amount of the loss is reduced.

- *Extra expenses to remain in operation.* Some extra expenses exceed any revenue they may produce but are necessary because the business must continue to operate. For example, an organization can incur expenses for the cost of renting a temporary building until construction is complete. Payment for overtime work and the cost for bringing in temporary employees are other examples of this kind of extra expense.

Professional Liability Insurance
for Personal Trainers and Aerobics Instructors

Markel Insurance Company offers the coverage you need...
Our policy covers professional liability and personal injury. Coverage applies to each occurrence and there is no deductible. This policy is designed for professional fitness trainers, aerobic instructors, and dance instructors who are considered sub-contractors with health clubs, community centers, and corporate facilities, and who do not own or lease any premises for this purpose.

Only $145 for $500,000 coverage... no policy fees, no dues, and no taxes (CA add 3.35% to premium). Markel Insurance Company is A-rated ("Excellent").
Note: All trainers and instructors must be certified by a nationally recognized board. We will not cover the following: any premises you own or lease, martial arts, sports medicine, gymnastics, trampoline, tanning devices, body wrapping, massage therapy, physical therapy, and any medical or chiropractic treatment. (These activities may be covered under other Markel programs. Call for information.) To enroll, simply complete and return this application along with your check made payable to Markel Insurance Company. **Send to:**   **Markel Insurance Company**
Health & Fitness Division
4600 Cox Road
Glen Allen, VA 23060

★ ★

Liability Application for Professional Fitness Instructors

Markel Insurance Company • 4600 Cox Road • Glen Allen, VA 23060 • (800) 431-1270 • Fax (804) 273-6144

Application for: ❑ Aerobics instructor   ❑ Personal trainer   ❑ Both   ❑ Other _____

Your name: _____

Your business name (if applicable): _____

Are you: ❑ Individual   ❑ Corporation   ❑ Prtnership

Mailing address: _____

City/state/zip: _____

Business phone: (_____)_____ Home phone (_____)_____

At which facility do you work?   Name of facility: _____
              Street: _____
              City/state/zip: _____

Does the facility require a certificate of insurance?   ❑ Yes   ❑ No

Have you ever had a liability claim brought against you?   ❑ Yes   ❑ No (If yes, attach a letter explaining all details.)

I am certified by: ❑ NHCA   ❑ ACE   ❑ AFAA   ❑ NFPT   ❑ ACSM   ❑ Other _____
(*Note:* You must have a current certification in order to qualify.)

Current insurance carrier (if applicable): _____

In addition to professional fitness instruction, please explain any other services you provide (i.e., diet counseling, martial arts, supplements or product sales) _____

_____

Liability limit desired: ❑ $500,000 (premium $145)   *Note:* Premium is fully earned.

Coverage shall not be bound until the company approves the applicant's completed application and premium payment is received. The company's receipt of premium does not bind coverage until the completed application is also approved. In the event the company does not approve your application, your premium payment will be refunded.

FRAUD WARNING: Any person who knowingly and with intent to defraud any insurance company or other person files an application for insurance containing any false information or conceals for the purpose of misleading, information concerning any fact material thereto, commits a fraudulent insurance act which is a crime.

Signed: _____ Date: _____/_____/_____

Figure 18.3   Personal trainer insurance application.
Reprinted, by permission, from Markel Insurance Company.

When applying for business interruption insurance, a manager is asked to estimate the annual operational income and expense figures on the application form. Realizing that the premium charged for this insurance is predicated on the figures provided, club operators have been known to low-ball their estimates to obtain a lower quote. The rationale behind this thinking is that the chance of having a catastrophic event is so remote, why pay a high premium every year. Essentially, the choice is to gamble with this coverage. This thinking leads to a feeling of false security and, consequently, we do not recommend it.

Crime

Commercial crime insurance covers two types of crime: those committed by employees of the organization and those committed by outsiders. Not all types of crime losses are considered insurable (e.g., theft by a partner of property belonging to the club), and some losses are covered under other insurance forms (e.g., vandalism or malicious mischief coverage in the commercial property forms).

In a health fitness setting, a commercial crime policy covers direct loss of money and securities. Money includes currency, coins, and bank notes in use, which have a face value. Securities mean negotiable and nonnegotiable items, and contracts representing either money or property. For example, securities can include charge tickets issued for programs, products, or services rendered; tokens; gift certificates; credit card debt; or a stamp used for monetary value. Securities do not include money.

There are 10 causes of loss that most widely used crime coverage policies can cover (see figure 18.4).

Of these 10 causes of loss, employee dishonesty is having the greatest impact, not only in the health fitness industry but in other businesses as well. Claims associated with criminal acts by an employee or in collusion with others are increasing annually. Employee dishonesty insurance provides coverage when there is intent by an employee to cause the employer a loss and to obtain a financial benefit for the employee or someone else. Although employee dishonesty usually involves taking cash, it can also involve taking property, such as equipment, or allowing unauthorized discounts on merchandise.

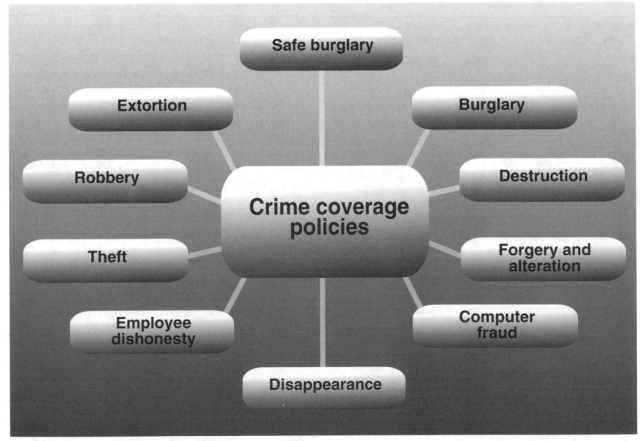

Figure 18.4 Causes of loss covered under crime insurance.

Boiler and Machinery

Steam boilers, used primarily for steam rooms and other types of machinery (air conditioners, electrical equipment, and refrigeration systems), contain tremendous amounts of potential energy. In the rare event that a steam boiler explodes or a piece of machinery undergoes a sudden breakdown, several types of loss may result. The facility owner or manager may incur the following losses:

1. Damage to the boiler or machinery
2. Damage to other property belonging to the owner
3. Loss of income resulting from either or both of the previously listed items
4. Legal liability for damage to property of others in the owner's care, such as member and guest property
5. Legal liability for bodily injury to members and guests

As a result of these potential losses, boiler and machinery insurance is necessary because commercial property policies exclude explosion of steam boilers and breakdowns of machinery.

A key element of boiler and machinery insurance is the inspection service and loss control recommendations that insurance companies provide in connection with obtaining this insurance. In many states, inspection by an authorized insurance company representative satisfies state requirements for the periodic inspection of boilers and certain types of machinery.

For a claim to occur under boiler and machinery insurance, there must be an accident to a piece of machinery covered under the policy. An accident has occurred, for example, when a boiler suddenly explodes during its operation, resulting in damage that necessitates its repair or replacement. However, this type of insurance does not cover accidents due to wear and tear, deterioration, corrosion, valve leakage, the breakdown of data processing equipment, or structure breakdowns. These exceptions reinforce the idea that covered accidents are to include only sudden and accidental incidents as opposed to losses that happen over the life of a mechanical device, such as its components wearing out over time.

Commercial Automobile Insurance

A significant liability exposure facing all businesses today comes from operating automobiles. In the United States, automobile accidents produce the greatest number of liability claims and account for most of the liability awards higher than $1 million. Even businesses not owning an auto can be held liable for the operation of an auto by others. For example, an employee could take the day's cash deposit to the bank and have an accident on the way. If the employee is at fault, the business can be held responsible because the employee was acting on behalf of the business.

Commercial automobile insurance policies assume the risk of financial loss arising from liability for bodily injury or property damage to third parties caused by automobile accidents. The liability exposure exists if the organization has to defend itself against suits alleging negligent ownership, maintenance, or use of autos. Liability can arise from using rented or borrowed autos or even from the operation of employees' autos on behalf of the business.

When applying for business auto insurance, a representative of the organization must identify and list those employees who are to be insured. In addition, the business is to indicate its legal form of organization (corporation, partnership, franchise, etc.) and determine the autos to be covered, how much coverage for each auto, limits of liability, and deductibles. This information is all provided on a declaration form, which becomes part of the automobile insurance policy.

In addition to liability and physical damage coverage there are several other coverages available that you can add to a standard commercial auto policy. We recommend that a club representative meet with the broker to discuss all the vehicle-related situations that may exist with the daily operation of the club. This will ensure that you obtain proper coverage at the best rate.

Umbrella Liability

Health fitness organizations are exposed daily to legal liability because of the physical hazards (exercise equipment, wet areas, and mechanical equipment) associated with operating a facility. Although managers can obtain liability policies covering these exposures, the policies are subject to limits of insurance that ordinarily do not exceed $500,000 to $1 million. These policies, which provide the first layer of coverage, are referred to as primary policies.

Financial awards to injured persons, in severe cases, may exceed the limits of primary liability policies. For example, a catastrophic loss suffered by an organization could easily result in a court award exceeding $1 million. If the business was only insured under its comprehensive general liability policy with a cap of $1 million, it would be liable for any amount over $1 million. Although many operators are not likely to experience such a large liability loss, the possibility exists for virtually any business.

You can insure exposures to large liability losses with an additional policy known as umbrella liability. An umbrella liability policy provides excess coverage for several areas of insurance, such as commercial general liability, auto liability, and employer liability. In addition, umbrella liability policies usually provide broader coverage than most underlying policies, thus providing primary coverage for certain occurrences that would not be covered by an existing policy.

An umbrella liability policy is used primarily as excess insurance that is broader than ordinary liability policies.

Because umbrella insurance is not subject to rate regulations as are other types of insurance, underwriters have considerable freedom in setting prices. Umbrella coverage rates for health fitness centers generally depend on loss history, the existing coverages and limits, and competition with other insurance companies. As a rule, umbrella insurance is rated at a percentage of the premium for the underlying insurance, subject to a minimum premium per $1 million of coverage.

Health fitness consultants Rick Caro and Joseph Acciavatti have developed a checklist of recommendations for operators when purchasing or renewing annual property and casualty insurance policies. Establish a timetable to complete this list and to use the full services of your broker or agent.

EMPLOYEE INSURANCE

Deciding what types of insurance to offer as a benefit for employees can be a difficult task. With the cost of group health insurance increasing 350 percent from 1980 to 1990, and with the average cost of health care alone rising 21 percent in 1991, many managers are questioning how they can minimize their insurance costs while maximizing their benefits to employees (Hildreth 1991). Numerous insurance companies now provide an assortment of coverages designed to protect employees from accidents, illness, disability, and to provide families with compensation in case of early death. However, each plan has annual premiums that are either shared by the employer and employee or simply offered to the employee at a group rate.

Unfortunately, with the spiraling cost of health care comes higher annual premiums, which have caused employers to seriously consider what benefits, if any, they can provide.

Despite the fact that fitness professionals generally lead a healthier than average lifestyle, some insurance companies categorize them with professional athletes and other high-risk groups, consequently demanding even higher premiums.

The two types of insurance most often considered for employees are group health insurance and life insurance. Often each plan includes optional coverage such as disability, dental, and cancer insurance, which can be provided for an extra cost. Currently, you can purchase insurance to obtain coverage for virtually any type of medical expense. It is beyond the scope of this chapter to explain each optional coverage; however, we provide a summary review for health and life insurance. Figure 18.5 lists the types of insurance available for employees.

Workers' Compensation

Most work-related accidents, diseases, and disabilities are subject to state *workers' compensation* statutes, which require employers to provide compensation for covered injuries without regard to fault. The scope of coverage varies in each state with respect to

Checklist for Buying or Renewing Insurance Policies

Check when completed.

Step 1 ❏

Have your agent prepare a written summary of all your insurance policies giving key information (i.e., coverages, limits, deductibles, major exclusions, premiums, dates). *Note:* This must be updated annually.

Step 2 ❏

Ask your agent for a listing of all claims and losses for the prior three completed policy years plus the current year. This should be broken down by type of insurance, with full details for each claim of loss, including whether the claim has been paid or is still pending.

Sometimes, there are questionable claims brought against a club. Make sure the amount of reserves created by the insurance company is reasonable while the claim is going through what might be a multiyear process until it is finally settled.

Key point is to track open and pending claims. Check the amount reserved by individual claim. Make sure it's realistic based on the facts of the claim. You're entitled to this information

The listing should be updated every six months. Your agent should go over this listing with you in person.

Step 3 ❏

Check on the amount of insurance you are presently carrying on the building if you own it. Is the amount sufficient, based on today's costs to rebuild the structure? Then do the same for the contents and equipment. What will be the costs to replace these items at today's market prices? If you lease the building, make sure you are covering any improvements and betterments you have made. Classify them properly between building versus contents.
Make sure you are not insuring the depreciated book value but rather today's replacement cost, including the need to meet today's building codes, Americans With Disabilities Act, and other requirements imposed by various laws.

Step 4

Review the total limits of liability insurance you now have for general liability and automobile liability. This would include the primary policy and any umbrella liability policy.

If you don't have an umbrella liability policy, ask for a quotation. Ask for one at various limits ($1,000,000, $2,000,000, and increments up to at least $5,000,000). If you currently carry an umbrella liability policy, ask for a quotation for a higher limit.

Step 5 ❏

Consider preemployment procedures: This would include physicals for new employees, and checking driving records and references. *Note:* Check the laws in your state to determine any possible limitations.

Step 6 ❏

Implement a loss control and safety program. Your insurance company should do this as part of their services at no charge. It's included in the premium you pay.

Many insurance companies have created written loss control guides. Ask your agent to see if your insurance company has published one; then involve your staff in using it as an ongoing educational training tool.

Preventing claims is vital. Managing claims after they happen is critical in keeping the costs down. *Loss control and safety are the most important steps you can take in gaining control over your insurance costs.*

Step 7 ❏

Extensions and exclusions. The following is a partial list of extensions and exclusions usually associated with fitness club policies. Check each one against your current insurance policy:

- Glass (interior and exterior, any limitations)
- Locker room liability for property of members and guests
- Summer camps
- Child care facilities
- Sexual harassment
- Professional liability
- Computer software and hardware

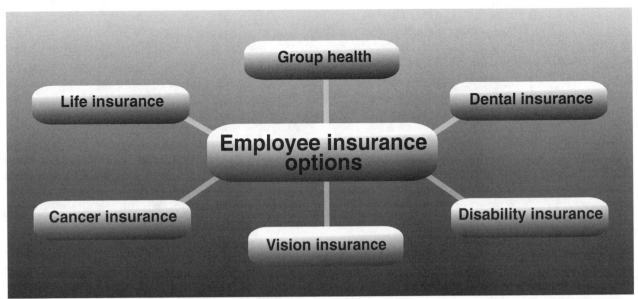

Figure 18.5 Employee insurance options.

benefits payable in the case of early death, total disability, and partial disability due to specific injuries. For an injury to be covered by workers' compensation, it must have the following conditions:

1. Cause an impairment
2. Be the result of an accident or an occupational disease
3. Be work related

The benefits paid in the event of a valid workers' compensation claim include medical expenses, disability income or death benefits to replace lost wages, and rehabilitation services to assist the employee in getting back to work.

Today some form of compulsory workers' compensation is in force in practically every country in the world. Although the federal government and every state have enacted workers' compensation laws in the United States, recent changes in some state statutes no longer require workers' compensation to be mandatory. Instead, these states have made workers' compensation elective; that is, the employer may elect to be governed by the provisions of the act. An employer electing not to be governed cannot use as a defense employee's negligence as a contributing factor, or that the accident was due to the actions of a coworker, or that the accident was a normal risk of the business.

Group Health Insurance

Of the various types of insurance available to employees, a group health plan is the most preferred by employees. Health insurance provides protection to employees and their families for financial losses resulting from sickness and accidental injury. One major difference between various kinds of medical insurance policies is the specific type of medical costs covered.

We can divide health insurance into three categories—medical expense insurance, dental insurance, and *disability insurance.*

Health Insurance Providers

Health insurance has traditionally been provided by private insurance companies and by service associations such as Blue Cross and Blue Shield. With this variation in providers comes different ways in which services are reimbursed to an employee or employer. For example, in a basic policy commonly offered by Blue Cross and Blue Shield, medical services, including hospitalization, are generally free to the user up to a certain limit (for instance, 15 days in the hospital), and the physician or hospital agrees to accept a certain fee schedule. Additional benefits are paid for services such as laboratory tests, X-rays, and operating room usage, as well as drugs.

Alternatively, a comprehensive major medical policy may cover all prescribed medical expenditures, in and out of the hospital. Such policies, issued by either Blue Cross and Blue Shield or by a commercial insurance company, typically require the patient pay an initial deductible fee and a percentage of any amount above the deductible, which is called the coinsurance rate.

Other policies have internal limits, which pay, for example, up to $20 per office visit or $150 per hospital day. Benefits of this type are called indemnity benefits. A more popular alternative to an indemnity benefit is a copayment; the employee pays a set amount (for example, $5 per office visit), and the insurance company pays the remaining fee.

All these insurance plans cover the services of any physician who bills on a fee-for-service basis. A different type of plan is known as a *health maintenance organization (HMO)*. Basically, HMOs combine health care delivery and health care financing. For a monthly fee, an HMO provides all the necessary medical services that a business requires. Under most HMOs, employees must designate a physician as a primary physician and have all medical treatment performed by that physician.

In recent years, private health insurance companies have established *preferred provider organization (PPO)* plans. These plans were designed to help control health care costs and compete with service associations and HMOs. PPO plans have two basic characteristics. First, a private insurance company enters into contracts with selected physicians and hospitals to provide medical services according to a reduced fee schedule. These physicians and hospitals become the preferred providers under the plan. Second, the insurance company provides incentives to employees to use the plan when medical care is needed. A major difference between a PPO and an HMO is that reimbursement for medical services will still occur even if a physician is not on its preferred list.

C.O.B.R.A. Compliance

Any health fitness organization providing group health insurance to its employees should be aware of and comply with the *Consolidated Omnibus Budget Reconciliation Act (C.O.B.R.A.)* of 1985. This law was enacted to protect employees against loss of health insurance due to job termination, death of a spouse, divorce or legal separation from a spouse, or spouse becoming eligible for medicare. Initially, the law was written to provide coverage under the organization's plan for a specified period (initially 60 days). However, in 1989 the law was revised to provide for continuation of coverage of either 18, 29, or 36 months, depending on the qualifying event. For example, if an employee either voluntarily or involuntarily terminates her employment, 18 months of health insurance coverage would be given. If on the other hand, an employee quits his job due to a divorce or a legal separation, the employee's health insurance benefits would be extended for 36 months.

C.O.B.R.A. continuation coverage is typically paid 100 percent by the employee or employee's family. It is an option offered that the employee may choose to accept or decline.

It is the responsibility of a health fitness organization to not only be familiar with the provisions under C.O.B.R.A. law, but also appoint an administrator who oversees the continuation coverage for qualified employees. Failure to provide this coverage can result in a variety of penalties by either the IRS, Department of Labor, Department of Health and Human Services, or civil lawsuits.

Policy Coverage Guidelines

Before purchasing a group health insurance plan we recommend that you discuss the following items with either a broker or insurance agent to ensure that the plan satisfies the needs of both the employee and employer:

1. Identify exactly what services the policy covers.

2. Identify the items excluded from the policy and the corresponding limitations.

3. Obtain information on the optional coverage available.

4. Identify the various deductibles for each coverage.

5. Determine the coinsurance provisions, what percentages the employee pays, and what the employer pays.

6. Is there a stop loss provision, and if so how much is it?

7. How are preexisting conditions handled?

8. What type of premium payment options are available?

9. Obtain the definition of disability.

10. What claims procedures are used?

Life Insurance

Another type of insurance usually made available to employees is life insurance. Probably the most severe cause of financial loss to a family is the premature death of a family member, especially the primary wage earner. Life insurance reduces the financial consequences of premature death by providing funds to replace lost income and to pay expenses associated with outstanding financial

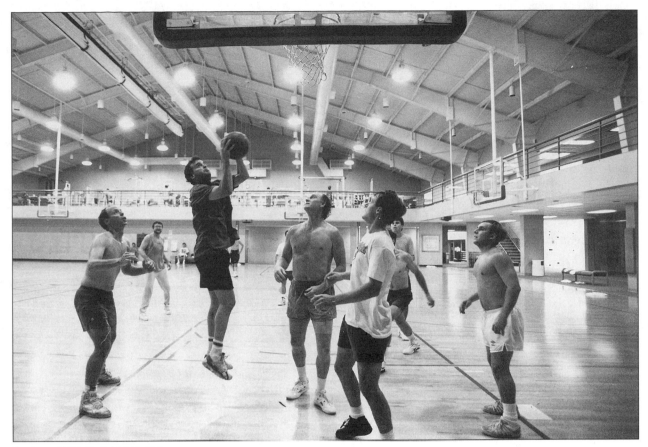

Courtesy of Little Rock Athletic Club

obligations, such as a mortgage, family members to support, and children to educate.

Today there are two traditional types of life insurance policies: whole life insurance and term insurance. Other policies written by life insurance companies are combinations of these basic types.

Whole life insurance provides lifetime protection (the whole of life) and is considered permanent insurance. Whole life policies accrue a cash value that may be borrowed against after a policy has been in effect for a specified number of years. Whole life insurance is recommended when lifetime protection is needed and when a savings element (cash value) is desired.

Term insurance provides coverage for a specified time, such as five or ten years and, therefore, is not permanent insurance. Term life insurance has no cash value. Term insurance is appropriate when the maximum amount of life insurance protection is needed at the lowest cost.

Some life insurance plans are sold directly to the employee, whereas other plans cover an entire group of employees. Such group policies are usually term insurance arranged through an employer.

As with health insurance, life insurance policies encompass a number of provisions that are important to understand before entering into a contract, items such as ownership clauses, incontestable clauses, suicide clauses, grace period, and reinstatement clause. These are just some areas in which a broker or agent should assist a manager or employee in fully comprehending the provisions.

IN CLOSING

We cannot stress enough the importance of obtaining appropriate insurance for operating a health fitness business. We recommend that operators of new health fitness facilities hire a broker who can assist in obtaining a commercial property package that complements the setting. Facilities that are already operational should have a manager who regularly reviews and evaluates the current policies and follows the suggested guidelines outlined in this chapter.

KEY TERMS

Broker

Business interruption

Buyers' market

Consolidated Omnibus Budget Reconciliation Act (C.O.B.R.A.)

Contents

Disability insurance

Health maintenance organization (HMO)

Loss exposure

Name insured

Owner's and contractor's protective coverage

Preferred provider organization (PPO)

Property and casualty insurance

Risk management

Sellers' market

Vicarious liability

Workers' compensation

RECOMMENDED READINGS

Caro, R. 1990. Club insurance: "10 truths" you need to know. *Club Business International* 11(12): 23-25, 45-49.

Head, G., and S. Horn. 1985. *Essentials of the risk management process*. Vol. I and II. Malvern, PA: Insurance Institute of America.

Hildreth, S. 1991. Employee health insurance—Minimizing costs/maximizing benefits. *Club Business International* 12(11): 41.

———. 1994. Inside insurance—Our experts explain all you need to know. *Club Business International* 15(9): 14, 47-48.

Kensicli, P., R. Smith, T. Marshall, S. Waranch, and D. Close. 1986. *Principles of insurance production*. Vol. I and II. Malvern, PA: Insurance Institute of America.

National Fitness Clubs Insurance Programs. 1996. *General loss liability for fitness facilities: A study reported by Royal Insurance*. Charlotte, NC: Royal Insurance

Rudd, A. 1995. Insurer solvency. *The Risk Report* 17(12): 1-8.

Smith, B., J. Trieschmann, and E. Wiening. 1988. *Property and liability insurance principles*. Malvern, PA: Insurance Institute of America.

Webb, B., S. Horn, and A. Flitner. 1990. *Commercial insurance*. Malvern, PA: Insurance Institute of America.

CHAPTER 19

Computer Applications

In a short period computers have infiltrated almost every aspect of health fitness operations, from member check-in to the monthly billing process that keeps the revenue stream alive. In this chapter we briefly review the history of computer use in our industry, discuss current trends and opportunities for informed managers and organizations, and look at the endless possibilities computers offer for the future. We present basic needs assessment information to assist the health fitness manager in determining individual computer needs and offer an overview of applications available to the industry. We consider computer purchases and assist in the tedious and confusing task of differentiating the intricacies of hardware and software purchase options. Finally we take a ride on the *information superhighway* to discuss possible implications and opportunities the *Internet* offers for organizational and professional growth.

    Without question, computers and the technology that drives them are developing at a pace few other industries have experienced.

> *Technology that was state-of-the-art five years ago is now antiquated as the power of the computer chip doubles approximately every 18 months (Gates 1995).*

It took huge mainframe computers, 10 to 15 years ago, to solve what are now considered simple calculations. Currently computers that are smaller than some textbooks and completely portable can handle such problems in seconds. The amazing and intimidating fact to many is that this explosive development is still in its infancy. In a relatively short time, the use of computers will infiltrate every aspect of our daily activities, making us more efficient and keeping us better informed. The dawning of a new millennium is occurring, not only on the calendar, but also in the development of an information age orchestrated via computer technology.

COMPUTER EVOLUTION

The development of the personal computer, a powerful computing device small enough to fit on a desk or in a lap and affordable for the average individual, introduced new blueprints for the way we accomplish tasks and conduct business. Software that has made the operation of personal computers user-friendly brought computers to the mainstream business environment as recently as the 1980s. Fifty million personal computers are now sold each year worldwide (Gates 1995). As more individuals have access to personal computers, information and re-

sources that once took several days or possibly weeks to obtain will be available in seconds. The continuing development of hardware and software will result in faster, easier to use, more powerful systems that will be indispensable in daily business and personal life. The evolution process is just beginning. In the near future, we will use computers for needs not yet realized. The health fitness industry must embrace this wealth of possibility to fully capitalize on opportunities this technology offers.

COMPUTERS IN THE HEALTH FITNESS SETTING

Using computers in the health fitness industry to conduct many daily tasks previously handled manually began in the late 1970s and early 1980s. Repetitive assignments, such as member billing of monthly dues, were the first tasks to be computerized using general business software applications modified to fit the task. The use of word processors to handle clerical tasks quickly followed. Software applications specific to the industry began to appear on a larger scale in the mid-1980s. These applications were designed to assist in club management functions, such as improved member billing, member database management, front desk check-in, and specialty programming areas, such as fitness testing and exercise prescription. Many companies first to arrive on the scene still operate today, but the products they offer differ dramatically from that of 5 or 10 years ago.

It is without question these developments will continue. In this chapter we provide some specific information regarding applications currently available and some insight to the possible direction this development may take (see figure 19.1).

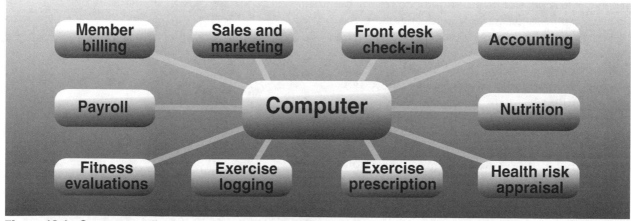

Figure 19.1   Computer applications in a health fitness setting.

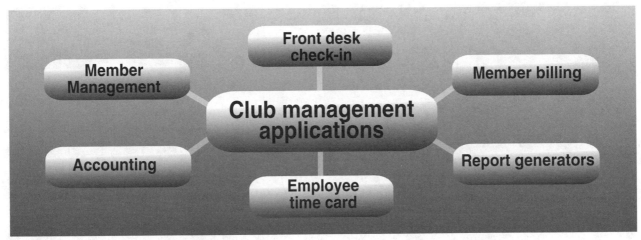

Figure 19.2   Club management software.

> *Software applications today are faster, easier to use, and integrated with other applications vital to an efficient operation.*

> *When developing your organization's computer systems it is important to determine your software needs before purchasing any computer hardware.*

HEALTH FITNESS SOFTWARE APPLICATIONS

A myriad of computer programs are available on the market to assist health fitness managers in efficiently and professionally delivering health fitness services. Each program vendor emphasizes one or more features that distinguish its program from its competitor's.

> *As a potential buyer, keep firmly in mind your goals for computerization and locate the vendors with the programs that best fit your needs.*

The following is a brief, descriptive listing of the types of software applications on the market, their basic functions, and relevant issues or features to consider when researching applications and vendors.

Club Management

Club management software refers to software applications that assist and enhance the business functions of the club. Typically, these applications center on accounting-based responsibilities and tasks. These programs ensure that the business of running a health fitness organization is handled as efficiently and effectively as possible (see figure 19.2).

Member Management

All club management programs must have a member database component providing a foundation for the various applications. As mentioned previously, you can store all member demographic, medical history, and payment history in this component. The ability to search records and print reports on various pieces of data stored in this component often assists the health fitness manager in operating the club. Carefully review the information that you can capture by this component. Ask the vendor the questions on the next page regarding the member database:

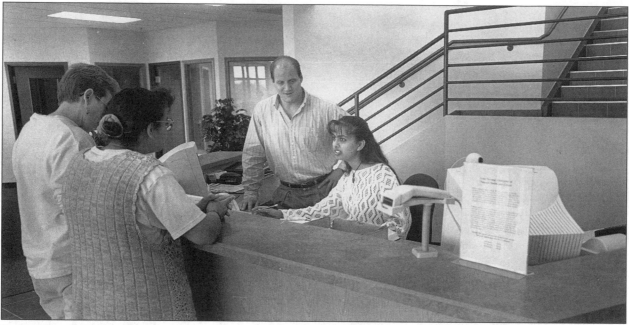

© Mary Langenfeld

- Are there user-defined fields that allow you to gather information you specifically require that this system does not currently capture?

- Can you generate reports from these user-defined fields?

- Can you generate address labels from this system?

- Can you merge various fields of captured data with a word processing application to speed the generation of letters, delinquent notices, or direct mail?

Front Desk Check-In

Member check-in at the service or front desk is a crucial function of the club. An efficient check-in process that controls access to the facility offers the member a positive, professional first impression. An unorganized, laborious check-in process that slows members' entry to the club or allows entry of members currently in arrears presents a less than optimal first impression, sure to cost the club memberships and revenue. The front desk check-in component of club management software ensures the first scenario is the one your members consistently experience. Front desk check-in software offers efficiency to the service desk. This component offers features such as the following:

- Instantaneous member recognition to speed the access of a member in good standing to the club

- Recognition of members who currently have suspended or terminated membership privileges

- Member message services to alert the service desk staff of a member entering the club who has a message waiting

- Member tracking systems that allow staff to access check-in records and run daily traffic reports to set appropriate staffing levels or know the exact time a particular member entered the club

Front desk check-in software technology is rapidly advancing. Using identification cards with bar codes or magnetic strips for scanning is giving way to using video imaging, in which a photographic likeness of the member is displayed on the screen when he or she checks in.

Touch screen and voice recognition technology, as well as fingerprint and handprint scanners, which totally eliminate the need and expense of member identification cards, represent technology currently being refined.

New technology, if it is affordable, will continue to be available on the market to meet the needs and demands of the health fitness industry.

Member Billing

The numerous methods in our industry for billing members complicates the installation of a member billing system. Electronic funds transfer (EFT, see chapter 15), credit card draft, coupon books, sliding scales depending on usage, off-peak charges, multiple membership types and rates, incidental charges, split billing, corporate billing, billing that occurs at different intervals (biweekly, monthly, quarterly, annually), and more are prevalent in clubs across the country. A member billing application that fits the current and future needs and membership configuration enhances the efficiency, productivity, and professionalism of the club's accounting department.

A regular and predictable revenue stream should be the primary goal of member billing software. Whether this billing is handled by EFT or traditional methods of billing and collection, a software program that carefully monitors the type of membership and the payment status of that membership, generates listings of those currently delinquent, and produces that regular and predictable income stream is a valuable asset to the club.

Accounting

Accounting functions, such as general ledger, accounts payable, and accounts receivable, are often offered in conjunction with member billing software. These programs allow the in-house accountant or controller to conduct the essential accounting functions to keep the business operating efficiently. Often the existence of such programs reduces the staffing requirements to handle these behind the scenes, yet vital, functions. Primary considerations regarding accounting software include the ability of these packages to integrate with the member billing component and their ease of use and modification to the facility's currently accepted accounting practices.

Point of Sale

Point of sale (POS) software is important for the club operating one or more profit centers. The ability to charge members' accounts for incidental purchases made in the pro shop, food and beverage outlet, or spa enhances the profitability of these outlets. Many club management software packages offer point of sale application components. Point of sale applications typically offer features in addition to member signing privileges, such as inventory control and tracking, integration with member billing systems, and the ability to take alternative forms of payment, such as credit cards, gift certificates, checks, or cash. Point of sale systems are connected to cash drawers that offer security and staff accountability for outlets that handle cash. Reporting capabilities of point of sale systems are often elaborate. Reports indicating daily, weekly, and monthly sales totals; inventory on hand or back ordered; items on order; sales totals by staff member; and so on offer the creative health fitness or profit center manager multiple opportunities to optimize the profitability of the outlet. Point of sale systems streamline the laborious tasks associated with managing profit centers and offer the health fitness manager an excellent means to closely monitor the profitability of these outlets.

Employee Time Card

Another challenge for the health fitness industry is the many payment methods for employees. Full-time salaried staff and part-time hourly staff are often the minority in an industry that creatively uses contract labor, internships, and bartering. Often the compensation structures for these employees differ dramatically (see chapter 16). Using an employee time clock system provides the organization with a basis from which to optimize payroll procedures. Employee time card systems provide a clock by which employees can register their attendance. These systems then automatically calculate gross earnings based on hours worked and compensation structure, eliminating the arduous task of calculating earnings manually. Many employee time card systems offer flexibility that is essential in the health fitness environment. Situations in which an employee is paid different wages for different jobs is common in our industry. These systems are designed to efficiently handle this and many other scenarios and provide accurate, detailed payroll information for the paymaster. Reviewing current compensation packages and structures and an application's ability to handle these configurations should be the focus of the research and review process for this software application.

A word of caution regarding the use of these systems. Wage and hour laws differ from state to state. Many applications generate only gross totals that must undergo taxation, social security withholding, and any optional pretax deduction programs. Although you can program some employee time card systems to handle this taxation and deduction, it is necessary to regularly monitor changes in wage and hour laws that may necessitate updates in payroll software.

Report Generators

The ability to generate reports from the data the different components of the club management software package collect and store is an often underestimated benefit of computerization. Although most software vendors offer many reporting options, the ability to generate reports you desire is a tremendous benefit. Including a user-friendly ad hoc report generator and the documentation detailing its operation can be tremendously valuable to the creative and curious health fitness manager. Information stored in computer systems should be available in the format desired. Discuss reporting capabilities in detail with any vendors whose product you are seriously considering.

Wellness Applications

Wellness applications allow the fitness professional to automate the calculation of certain fitness parameters, track exercise participation, analyze nutritional intake, and enhance wellness programming. These software programs, often operated by the fitness or wellness personnel rather than the business office staff, provide health fitness staff the opportunity to present results of various wellness criterion in a professional and educational format. Figure 19.3 shows the wellness programs commonly used in the industry.

Fitness Evaluation and Exercise Prescription

Fitness evaluation and exercise prescription software allow the fitness professional to input figures from various fitness exercise testing protocols. They can produce test results comparing the individual to industry-accepted norm tables and produce an exercise prescription based on the results of the fitness evaluation. Fitness evaluation software typically handles fitness-related parameters, such as functional capacity, body composition, muscular strength, muscular endurance, flexibility, and some programs can track pulmonary values and blood chemistry results. As mentioned, when you enter the results of selected testing protocols, values are calculated instantaneously and compared on the printout with a selected norm table for the individual's gender and age group.

Although most fitness evaluation software programs are similar in the parameters measured or tracked, they differ dramatically in the output generated, the norm tables used, and the testing protocols available.

When considering fitness evaluation software for your testing program, look closely at the educational quality, the ability to define the text, and the professional quality of the printout.

Evaluate the selection of the norm tables used. Do the norms fit your demographic profile or are you

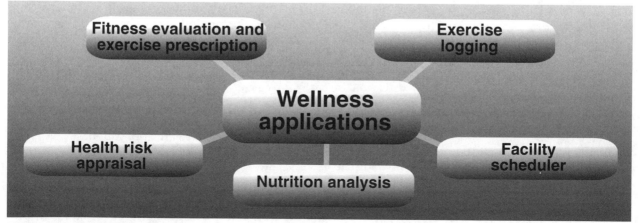

Figure 19.3 Wellness applications.

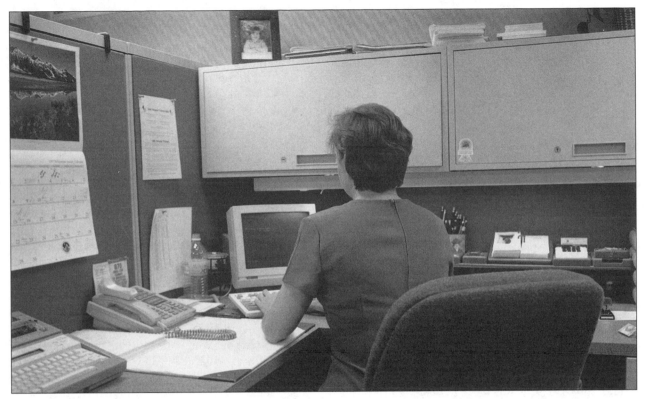

© Tom Wallace

comparing 40 to 50 year olds to norm tables developed testing college students? Ask the vendor if the ability to select or change the norm table is available, what the scientific basis is for the norm tables, and if user-defined norm tables are available. Finally, look closely at the available testing protocols. If your fitness testing program uses a testing protocol not available on the software package, you face a decision to redefine your testing program or continue the search for software. Typically, most software vendors have built in the standard laboratory treadmill and cycle tests as well as field tests, such as step tests, 1.5-mile runs, or 12-minute walk-run tests. Be sure that you can input all the parameters currently measured. Check for protocols for all parameters, functional capacity, body composition, muscular strength, and so on. Question the vendor for detailed information regarding how results are calculated and the possibility of including any modified protocol you may be using in the testing program.

Exercise prescription software uses the results generated in the functional capacity testing conducted previously, weighs information entered in the individual's medical history, and generates an exercise prescription based on industry standards for the activities the individual plans to participate in. The exercise scientist should carefully review these exercise prescriptions before presenting them to the client. Exercise prescriptions are used almost exclusively for aerobic activities. Generating an exercise prescription for strength training involves too many uncontrollable variables such as technique, weight variances based on biomechanics of the different lines of equipment, and the different pieces of equipment available in fitness centers.

Exercise Logging

Exercise logging software allows members to input their daily activity, the amount of activity completed, and the approximate intensity. In return they get information such as caloric expenditure, pace per mile, and aerobic points earned.

To be effective, most exercise logging programs must be incorporated into an activity program or contest that provides members incentive to continue entering their activity. Exercise logging software programs are designed to continually provide members with positive feedback.

Members can use some exercise logging software programs interactively with the assistance of a personal trainer, exercise professional, or computer coach. The member enters what activity was done; the specific parameters appropriate for that activity such as miles, distance, sets, time elapsed, workload; and the personal trainer or coach reviews the activity and provides suggestions to improve the quality of the workout to achieve predetermined goals. Several of these interactive or coaching software programs are now available for home PC use through retail vendors and magazine advertisements.

Health Risk Appraisal

Health risk appraisals (HRA) are software programs that analyze risk of morbidity and mortality based on the responses to a series of pencil and paper questions regarding personal health and safety habits. Health risk appraisals, although they may assess physiologic parameters, do not inherently require a physical assessment. Consequently, HRAs are excellent tools to positively motivate large groups of people to adopt healthier lifestyle habits.

Health risk appraisals require the client or member to complete a detailed questionnaire on topics such as personal medical history; family medical history; personal health habits such as exercise frequency and intensity, cigarette smoking, and seat belt use; as well as life circumstances such as the miles one must drive daily and the type of car driven. The software program then determines the individual's risk of death from certain disease processes or incident scenarios. It then compares this risk to the Centers for Disease Control and Prevention (CDC) norm tables for the top 10 or 12 reasons persons of that age and gender die. The software program generates a comparative analysis of the individual's chronological age, or their age in number of years, versus their health risk age, or their age when all their health and lifestyle habits are accounted for. Some programs take this information a step further and provide the client with an achievable age if all controllable negative health habits, such as cigarette smoking or poor seat belt use, were positively modified. These programs, when implemented properly, allow an individual to see the long-term risk of certain health and safety habits and provide information for positive lifestyle change.

Nutrition Analysis

Nutritional analysis, much like fitness assessments, evaluate the nutritional habits and intake of the client. Typically the client will keep daily food intake records

and systematically use these records to indicate the foods eaten and the amount consumed on a weekly basis. This information is then combined with information about the person's eating habits, such as time of day food is consumed, the circumstances around the consumption of food, and habits, such using salt or sugar, to provide a nutritional analysis for the client. This analysis can indicate an estimate of the current intake as it relates to calories consumed, fat intake, and vitamin or mineral intake. With a clear picture of current eating habits, a program or menu plan can be assembled, typically using ADA guidelines to place the member on a path to improve the nutritional value of the foods consumed.

Many other nutritional programs exist that provide an analysis of a particular recipe or meal menu. The ingredients of the recipe or menu are entered into the computer, the number of servings are indicated, and the software prepares a nutritional analysis of that dish or menu. These programs are particularly helpful when determining the nutritional value of a meal or a favorite dish and what, if any, minor modifications in the recipe can improve its nutritional value. Usually these programs are used individually to assist in the education process of the member. Free-standing terminals in the wellness area allow members to access these nutrition databases and enter their daily intake or favorite menus on their own time. Although a baseline nutrition evaluation is appropriate during the initial health assessment, free-standing terminal access often proves more successful as the members can attain their personal nutrition information when they are ready.

Facility Schedulers

Scheduling systems can serve as reservations systems for tennis courts, racquetball courts, or a massage room. They can maintain control of space rental commitments and keep on a waiting list a record of interested clients not able to book space. These systems assist in managing all aspects of facility and space rental. Look for flexibility and user-defined space and time guidelines when researching these applications.

With the proliferation of multi-purpose facilities offering a variety of programming options, a facility scheduling system saves time, prevents mistakes, and efficiently controls several outlets in the facility.

Custom Programming

After exhaustively reviewing the software applications on the market, your facility may desire to customize an existing program or write a program in its entirety. Be prepared to expend a great deal of time, effort, and money in this process. Custom programming is not generally profitable for existing software vendors unless the enhancement you suggest increases the value of the product they are selling. If the enhancement you desire improves the product they offer, many times the vendor can recoup the cost of programming. If the enhancement you desire is specific for your facility and not widely needed, the programmer would be required to maintain and update two versions of the same software. If several customers desire custom applications, multiple versions of the software must be maintained, a costly and time-consuming process for the vendor. Consequently, the vendor may not be motivated to incorporate your customization unless it has wide appeal.

Writing a custom computer program from scratch is a time-consuming exercise, not only for the programmer, but also for the individual driving the design of the package. Although the programmer may spend hundreds of hours writing code, an individual intimately familiar with the desired goals and outcomes for the software must commit many hours to determining specifications and processes.

One should never initiate this assignment without first doing a great deal of research. Current and future needs must be heavily weighed and planned for. Select a programmer carefully, and assure the protection and exclusivity of the finished product. This procedure can either produce the ultimate software program for your needs or be a nightmare of expense and wasted time.

Available Vendor Resources

Software vendors are plentiful in the health fitness industry. They are common exhibitors at national fitness and wellness conferences. Their advertisements are readily found in trade magazines and journals, and many are listed in the annual product and services guides. When a particular vendor or software package is of interest, cautiously investigate the company, its length of time in business, the make up and turnover of its staff, and its commitment to service of its customers. Problems and bugs will undoubtedly arise in the daily use of software applications. The commitment level of the vendor to provide service and keep programs functional is vital to a smooth operation. Be sure to call the company's references and ask detailed questions about such issues as its installation and training process, the time the system is not functioning when a bug or error occurs, and the availability of

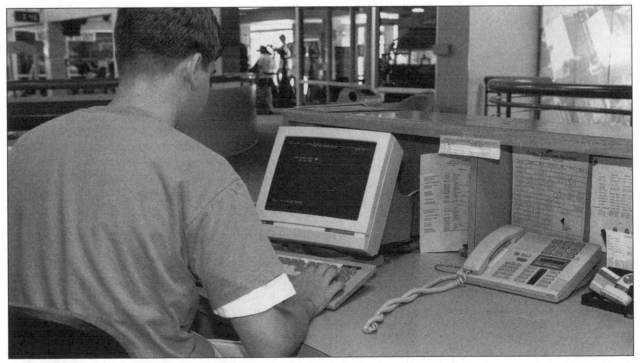

© Tom Wallace

on-line help, if needed. Inquire about the impact the program has made on profitability, member retention, and employee morale. Fierce competition for your business puts the buyer in the driver's seat. Take time to research and negotiate the best deal possible.

COMPUTER NEEDS ASSESSMENT

Using computer technology offers advantages in both efficiency and accuracy for the health fitness operation. Most fitness and wellness centers are computerized in some way. Some may use computers to handle clerical and accounting functions only, whereas others have implemented fully integrated programs in every area of the facility.

> *The fitness manager who keeps abreast of developments in computer technology and aggressively implements applications to meet the needs of the operation undoubtedly provides a valuable service to the organization.*

However, interpreting promotional literature detailing the capabilities of this rapidly developing technology is often difficult. Understanding key features of new *software* and *hardware* developments and determining if these often highly priced features fit your current and future business needs are the primary goals in conducting a computer needs assessment (see figure 19.4).

Health Fitness Applications

Several types of software programs or applications are necessary to efficiently manage and operate a successful health fitness operation. We review here some primary applications and their functions. Careful review and selection of the program best suited to your facility is important for long-term success. Following are the primary types of health fitness software and tools to assist you in determining the best program for your needs.

• *Member database management.* These databases should not only store important demographic and medical history information but also be able to be mined for purposeful means, such as member retention programs or direct mail campaigns. See table 19.1 for issues to consider when reviewing membership database components.

• *Business and financial applications.* Maintaining a single software program that tracks current member database information as well as billing and payment records can save the organization time and money. Most club management software available today builds the programs around this task. See table 19.2 for issues to consider when reviewing accounting software applications.

• *Wellness applications.* These applications can enhance current programming or provide a foundation for developing new member retention programs. Wellness applications include such software programs as fitness evaluation, health risk appraisal, nutrition evaluation, and exercise logging. These programs provide a professional touch to services offered by activity departments. Although wellness software is not required to operate a professional fitness evaluation program, it assists the professional staff in delivering a quality product. See table 19.3 for issues to consider when selecting the most appropriate wellness programs for your setting.

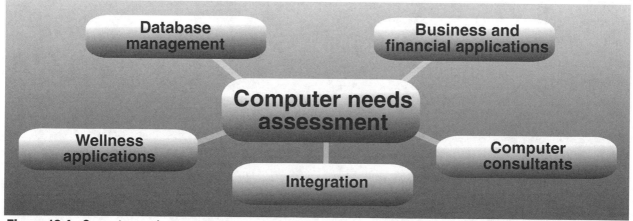

Figure 19.4 Computer needs assessment.

Table 19.1   Member Database Needs Assessment

Rank the objectives listed here from 1 to 5 (with 1 being low and 5 being high) in relation to their importance to your needs and the capability of the software to accomplish those needs.

Objective	Your needs	Capability
• User-defined fields for data or comments		
• Ability to handle current ID system		
• Complete, yet concise for efficiency		
• Ability to capture all vital information		
• Ability to capture vital marketing information		
• Ability to track guests and prospects		
• Ability to report on programming information		
• Ability to scan current ID cards		
• Video imaging capabilities		
• Security of member information		
• Integration with other programs in use		
• Tracking inactive accounts		
• Member's guest tracking and referrals		
• Generation of membership statistics		
•		
•		
•		
•		
•		

Notes:

Table 19.2 Member Billing and General Accounting Needs Assessment

Rank the objectives listed here from 1 to 5 (with 1 being low and 5 being high) in relation to their importance to your needs and the capability of the software to accomplish those needs.

Objective	Your needs	Capability
• Accommodate current billing method		
• Accommodate multiple billing methods		
• General ledger capability		
• Accounts receivable tracking		
• Accounts payable tracking		
• Ability to generate required reports		
• Ability to integrate with member database		
• Ability to assist with staff payroll		
• Notify at check-in if account is in arrears		
• Credit tracking and account history		
• Point of sale systems		
• Security features		
• Inventory control		
• Cash drawer support		
•		
•		
•		
•		
•		

Notes:

Table 19.3   Wellness Applications Needs Assessment

Rank the objectives listed here from 1 to 5 (with 1 being low and 5 being high) in relation to their importance to your needs and the capability of the software to accomplish those needs.

Objective	Your needs	Capability
• Fitness testing and exercise prescription		
• Nutrition evaluation and meal planning		
• Exercise logging		
• Facility/activity scheduler		
• Health risk appraisal		
• Ability to handle current testing protocol		
• Norm tables match current population		
• Ability to modify educational information		
• Ability to modify norm tables		
• Fit with current programming		
• Ease of administration		
• Security of member information		
• Multiple test improvement tracking		
• Member usage tracking		
•		
•		
•		
•		
•		

Notes:

Integrating Applications

Facilities with an existing software system that is vital to the operation must consider integrating new applications into their existing computer environment. For example, assume the health fitness center is part of a large resort or hospital facility whose existing software applications handle member or patient database management and billing functions. The addition of a new software program to handle point of sale for the pro shop must be able to link to this existing database and billing system or you will duplicate efforts to process charges. Each time the effort is duplicated, the possibility for error and the labor expense required to offer the service increases. Perhaps the staff member forgets on a busy day that this particular invoice must be reentered into a separate system for billing, resulting in a charge never collected.

Integration is also important if you consider purchasing modules from different vendors. For example, during the research phase of purchase, a particular club management system from vendor A seems to provide the best fit for the current operating processes for the organization. However, you are also in the market for a wellness software program to assist the programming staff

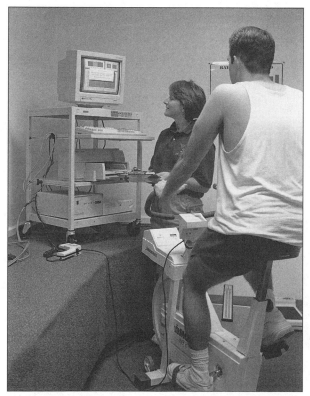

© Tom Wallace

with fitness testing. The program you find most advantageous for your organization is available through vendor B. Discussions between these vendors is crucial. The membership database component of each software system must be able to communicate with the other so that if an address change is made in the club management software, duplicate entry is not required for the wellness software.

Software vendors should be able to arrange real time or delayed download interface to share information and prevent duplicate entry. Writing a link to integrate two programs may be an additional up-front charge, but the cost is well worth the time and effort saved in the long run. Openly discuss with the vendors any existing or additional applications you have or are considering to ensure integration is achievable before making a purchase decision.

Using Computer Consultants

If the thought of sorting through the maze of application software, hardware components, and local area networks is overwhelming, consider hiring a computer consultant. A competent consultant can accomplish the task of research in an efficient time, ensure you purchase products that fit your needs, and oversee proper installation and training.

In most cases, the hardware or software vendors provide their expert to assist in implementing their product. This individual works with health fitness managers to ensure their product is considered valuable. The issue to remember is that this expert is a member of the sales team of that vendor. Although they may have extensive computer knowledge and be able to assist in one of the many roadblocks that hinder computerization, they are not obligated to assist and may not offer assistance that is in the best overall interest of the organization.

Using an independent computer consultant, hired by the organization, will ensure the initial goals of the organization remain in focus.

Additionally, following the installation and training phase, the consultant remains a member of your team to continue training; handle bugs in the hardware, software, or network; and assist in the laborious process of establishing the member database.

Using a computer consultant may seem like an unnecessary expense at the outset; however, when you break the implementation of facilitywide computerization into tasks, the effort required to successfully achieve this goal can be exhausting. You can hire the computer consultant to accomplish a limited number of specific tasks or to take the project from inception to completion. Some tasks a computer consultant can assist with are listed here. Without question, using a computer consultant in the large-scale computerization of a facility is money well spent.

Computer Consultant Tasks

- Research available software applications, and prepare an overview of this research for review.

- Coordinate with software vendors and prepare bids.

- Prepare hardware bids for review.

- Work with vendors to ensure integration of applications.

- Select the most effective hardware configuration to fit current and future needs of the club, including local area network configuration, printer locations, point of sale cash drawers, and so on.

- Prepare an overall proposal for hardware and software installation, coordinate with vendors regarding installation dates, and so on.

- Coordinate efforts to install a local area network, including running necessary cables and making dedicated phone lines available.

- Oversee installation and configuration of software to ensure efficiency.

- Work with software vendor to download or key in existing member demographic and billing information.

- Coordinate and oversee training of staff.

- Continue on a contractual arrangement to assist with troubleshooting.

PURCHASE CONSIDERATIONS

Consider several important issues when purchasing computer hardware and software.

Understanding computer technology and terminology should be a prerequisite to investing money in computerization. Issues to keep in mind when researching available software and hardware include the following:

- Evaluate and document your current and future computer needs and desires. Clearly understanding your computerization goals is necessary to purchase only what you need, not every expensive bell and whistle on the market. Review the needs assessment section of this chapter to carefully define your computerization goals.

- Locate and purchase your software first; then purchase the necessary hardware that meets the configuration demands of the software.

- If possible, purchase the software and hardware from the same vendor. By doing so, the same vendor handles the support of both the software and the hardware, preventing the frustrating situation in which one vendor blames the problem on the other and claims no responsibility.

- Look for software and hardware that will grow with your organization. Hardware expandability and a regular schedule of software upgrades allow the organization to grow and change as technology improves.

- Know the environment in which your software will exist. Before researching hardware or software, establish if you will use a DOS, Macintosh, or Windows environment.

- Ask for a demo disk of the software of interest. The vendor should provide you with an interactive demonstration disk with a limited member database or life expectancy so that you may experiment with the software in your own environment and on your own time. Many vendors may charge a fee for the demo disk, which is refundable with purchase of the software.

- Ask questions. No question should be considered silly. Do not risk purchasing a system that is not optimal for your program for fear of asking a question. Be sure you understand all aspects of purchase, installation, training, and support.

- Be sure your vendor specializes in computer hardware or software. Is the vendor committed to providing hardware or software to the health fitness industry?

- How long has the vendor been in business? Longevity is a sign of a solid product with an excellent support system. Typically, the longer a vendor has been in business, the fewer bugs remain in the system, as many of these errors have been documented and eliminated. What happens if the company goes out of business? Does the vendor have a plan if this unfortunate incident occurs?

- How many current users does the vendor support? How many other club operators have selected this product as the best available on the market?

- Look at the lifetime cost of computerization, not initial cost. When comparing products and vendors, consider the long-term cost of initial hardware and software purchase, support agreements, extended warranty packages, training expenses, and potential customization.

- Remember, you get what you pay for.

Hardware Options

Hardware options seem never ending. Pentium, PowerPC, speed in Mhz (megahertz), upgradability, expansion bus, memory (Mb—megabyte) capacity, 1.44 Mb, 3 1/2-inch floppy drive, super VGA color card, tape drive backup system, CD-ROM drive speed, standard 14-inch VGA color monitor, mouse, internal modem, multimedia, high-quality color ink-jet printer, laser jet printer—how do you choose? Discuss the selection of specific hardware to meet your needs in detail with a computer consultant or someone familiar with the latest in computer hardware technology. Although a detailed explanation of these components is beyond the scope of this text, it is important that anyone considering a large-scale computer purchase understand the contribution each of these parts make to the computer as a whole. Several books and periodicals are available on the newsstand or through a local bookstore that explain in simple terms the function of each component. Consider the following suggestions when shopping for computer hardware.

- *Buy the most powerful technology you can on your predetermined budget.* As mentioned previously, hardware is developing rapidly. Look for the latest technology you can afford.

- *Be sure the hardware configuration matches or exceeds the software specifications.* Each software application comes with minimum and optimum hardware requirements.

- *The more memory, the better.* As soon as you assume you will never be able to fill the available hard disk space, it is gone. Software applications continue to grow in size and complexity. Purchase the most memory your predetermined budget allows.

- *The faster, the better.* Purchase the fastest processor and the largest amount of RAM (random access memory) your predetermined budget will allow. Although the slower systems may run your application adequately, software developments may tax a slower system.

- *Shop all available vendors.* The software vendor you select may be able to acquire more hardware for the money through volume purchase direct from the manufacturer or from a used computer dealer. In addition to your selected software vendor, shop for hardware through computer stores, computer superstores, advertisements in computer magazines for purchase directly from the manufacturer, or from a used computer dealer.

Lease Versus Purchase

The lease versus purchase debate has raged for computer hardware just as it has for cars. Leasing and purchasing both have inherent advantages and disadvantages. Consider the advantages presented in table 19.4.

Single- Versus Multiuser

Single-user versus *multiuser* refers to the number of computers that can access a single database or software application. Most home computers operate as single-user systems. This means that one user has access through communications using a keyboard or mouse to the software applications and data stored by that computer. In business environments it is often necessary to have several individuals access a single database or software application. Multiusers most frequently use a network to accomplish this task. A *local area network*, or *LAN*, is the method of choice when all computers needing access to a single database are housed in one physical location. LANs typically use cables pulled from the server to each computer communicating on the network. This allows persons in the accounting office to access the billing records of a particular member in the member database while the membership office is adding a new member or updating the address of a member who has recently moved in that same

Table 19.4 Advantages of Lease Versus Purchase	
Lease advantages	**Purchase advantages**
1. With the rapid development of computer hardware, leasing allows easy replacement of outdated hardware with little or no additional capital expense.	1. Ownership eliminates monthly payments.
2. Lower initial financial commitment.	2. Lower lifetime cost.
3. Maintenance agreement ensures hardware is properly functioning for the duration of the lease.	3. Maintenance and support agreement with purchase ensures proper functioning for period of warranty.
4. Expense can be operationalized.	4. Expense can be capitalized.
5.	5.
6.	6.
Notes:	

database. The use of the network allows the club to maintain a single database of member records instead of maintaining one database in the accounting office and another in the membership office.

In contrast, a *wide area network,* or *WAN*, allows computers that are spread over a large distance to communicate via telephone lines or satellites. A club chain with multiple locations might need a WAN to offer club privileges for each member to any of their multiple locations or to monitor sales figures at the corporate office.

Networks offer the club efficiency and accuracy, but an experienced network administrator must maintain them. To implement a network, specific network software and hardware requirements must be met. Hire an experienced network administrator to oversee the installation of the cabling, computer hardware, and software necessary for operation. The club can then retain this network administrator to oversee the maintenance and error-free operation of the network. See the previous section on computer consultants for more information.

Installation and Training

The installation process must be well thought out and scheduled appropriately. Often cables must be run throughout the club to link multiple terminals. Schedule cabling outside the operating hours of the club to avoid displacing or inconveniencing a member. Installation of the hardware and software should also occur at a time that will not interrupt daily operation. Establish a temporary training area during installation to provide the staff with a private location in which uninterrupted initial exposure and training can take place.

> *Installation and training are important aspects of the success of computerization. The staff must receive a positive first impression of computerization and the benefits it will provide.*

Software training can either be exciting or frustrating. Depending on the computer skills and interest of the staff member, the training process can be engaging or disconcerting. Be sure to provide all staff members who will interact with the new system as a part of their daily responsibilities with uninterrupted training and practice time. Provide a supportive environment in which to learn and experiment. Arrange a flexible schedule to avoid overstimulation and burnout. Begin preparing staff members who are not computer literate well before the vendor training representative arrives. A positive training experience will result in a staff excited about the system and a membership that receives positive feedback and support from staff regarding the effort to computerize.

Maintenance, Support, and Warranties

The quality and comprehensiveness of software support programs should be a major focus during the hardware and software purchase process. Problems and bugs will occur. The ability of the vendor to restore full function of the system quickly is essential. Questions to pose to vendors and issues to carefully consider regarding maintenance and support include the following:

• *What is the warranty for hardware?* Typical manufacturer hardware warranties cover parts and labor for one year. Extended warranties of three to five years are commonly offered for an additional fee. In-house or in-home warranty packages are also available, covering the cost of a technician to come on site to investigate and repair hardware failures.

• *Is there an additional fee for support on top of software purchase?* Often support and software upgrades are included in the initial purchase for one year. Thereafter, an annual support fee is typical. Inquire about the structure of the support agreement. Is it included in the initial price or additional? What is the annual fee? What does this fee entitle the user to? This is often a potential negotiating point during the purchase process. Estimate the lifetime cost of the software when comparing available packages.

• *What are the hours of the vendor support services?* Does the vendor provide 24-hour support or is it limited to 9:00 A.M. to 5:00 P.M. eastern time? Ensure the hours of the support team meet the needs of your club. If the system fails at 5:00 P.M. on the West Coast and the support office closed at 5:00 P.M. eastern time, the operator is left with a computer failure during prime time. Is 24-hour support offered via a paging system? Call the support line before purchasing the software to measure response times.

• *How often are software upgrades provided?* Customarily program upgrades are provided to clients with a current support agreement. These upgrades typically fix errors that have been found and provide new functions to enhance the value of the software. Inquire as to the frequency of previous upgrades and the anticipated upgrade schedule. As technology develops, new graphics and speed capabilities should be incorporated into the product.

• *Is modem support provided?* Does the vendor load fixes and upgrades via modem and test those files once loaded, ensuring proper functioning while eliminating involvement and anxiety on the part of the staff member, or is a diskette sent that the user must load and test?

• *Is there an 800 number for support?* When a problem or question exists with the software and you make a call to the vendor, can you use an 800 number or does the club pay for the cost of the call?

• *What are the qualifications of the support personnel?* Are the support technicians programmers or health fitness professionals? If a bug exists in the system, the support of a programmer to find and fix the problem is essential. If a question arises regarding the use of a particular fitness testing protocol, will the programmer field this question or is there a qualified exercise professional who can assist? How long have the support staff been with the company? Is there a high rate of turnover?

Cost

The cost of computerization is significant and for that reason alone should not be considered lightly. Hardware costs per system have remained relatively constant during the past 10 years; however, money spent today purchases more computing power than thought possible 10 years ago. With the continuing pace of development, money spent today is likely to be for a hardware system that is out of date in the next three to five years. See the lease versus purchase section of this chapter to optimize the dollars spent on the purchase of computer hardware.

Software continues to develop at the same rapid pace. However, purchasing a maintenance agreement with the software vendor ensures a continuous stream of upgrades and improvements that should keep pace with the development of computer technology. Software vendors often offer different pricing structures to meet the needs of a diverse market. Although some vendors offer a flat rate for a comprehensive program, others offer cafeteria-style plans that allow you to select the components you need and can afford. Other vendors offer a database option that bases the price of the software on the number of expected records in the member database. This system allows the personal trainer to purchase the same software system a large club may purchase. The personal trainer, however, pays significantly less for a maximal database of perhaps 50, whereas the large club may set their database at 5,000. This system allows the club to purchase an initial database size they can currently afford and upgrade to a larger database as needed.

Shopping for software and hardware is somewhat like shopping for a car. The models and styles are numerous, with the possible upgrades and options virtually limitless. The frugal computer buyer can make large improvements on manual systems for less than $5,000, and the buyer looking for the best system possible can spend more than $100,000.

> *Clearly define the goals of computerization and purchase the system that best fits your needs and budget.*

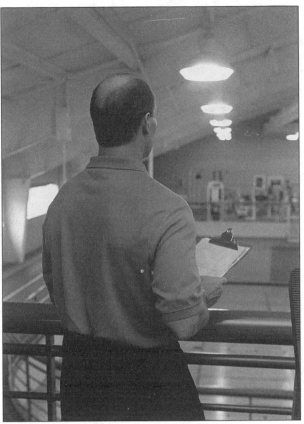

© Tom Wallace

Security

Confidentiality is a growing concern in the realm of computers. As computers around the world gather and hold every imaginable bit of information about us, concern mounts regarding the confidentiality and access to that information. The club member has similar concerns regarding the information he or she has provided to the club. Carefully control personal financial information, including credit statements, credit card numbers, checking account numbers, and member account numbers, to prevent unauthorized use. Also, closely guard health history information. A condition such as hypertension could inhibit an individual's chances for promotion if that information was provided to another member, a coworker, or supervisor.

Most confidentiality issues involving computers fall into two areas. The first is the accuracy of the information provided. In the age of e-mail and the Internet, where anonymity is high, confirming the accuracy of the information or the identity of the individual is often difficult, if not impossible. The second area is accessibility. This area is of greater concern for most than accuracy. Are private e-mail messages really private if others can access them? When ordering an item over the Internet, how many others will be able to access your credit card number as you offer it as a method of payment? These issues and many others are now topics of hot debate and continuous development. New software applications are available on the market daily to increase the confidentiality of information by scrambling code, increasing the levels of password security, and destroying information as it is used. As in the past, it will be a race to keep the methods of security one step ahead of those who try to gain unauthorized access.

To improve the security of your computer system, adhere to the following suggestions:

- Fully implement any security systems available in software purchased.

- Select a unique and random password that cannot be easily guessed.

- Change your password often.

- Do not share your personal password with anyone for any reason.

- Do not use the same password for multiple uses. Select a unique password for each computer system, ATM card, telephone card, and so on.

- Fully implement the management security measures available with all club management software, ensuring that confidential information is not available to nonmanagement personnel.

- Never assume confidentiality.

INTERNET

The Internet as a dynamic, rapidly changing environment is difficult to define. Started as a communication network in the late 1960s by the U.S. government to assist during wartime, the Internet was developed primarily in the university setting. The goal of the defense department was to increase the stability and reliability of what was then called the ARPAnet, after the Advanced Research Projects Agency, the agency overseeing this development. This network grew as computers and operating systems became more standardized, allowing the transfer of electronic mail and files. Little commercial intent was given to the ARPAnet during that time.

The Internet now represents the fastest growing and most dynamic commercial medium of the day. Companies are going on-line to offer information about their products or services to literally millions of people, worldwide, for less than it costs to run an ad in the local yellow pages. The Internet is changing how we market and advertise our products and how we research and locate products for personal consumption. On today's Internet, a small business can produce information on its products and services that is comparable in quality, quantity, and market penetration to a Fortune 500 organization. Health fitness managers must embrace this technology and mobilize it for their benefit or face the consequences of being left behind.

Resources

The Internet offers a world of information for the individual with the patience and willingness to attain it. Information regarding everything from airline flight availability and cost to camping sites in the national forests is available. You can access the contents of many of the finest libraries in the world from the Internet without ever leaving your home or office. The industrious health fitness manager can easily access bulletin boards with information about every type of programming activity imaginable. You can post questions regarding health club operation, allowing health club managers from around the world to assist you through their experiences and efforts. You can access and print in seconds the latest popular magazine articles about a particular activity or journal articles of interest, eliminating the waste of valuable hours researching a topic. The resources available on the Internet are mind-boggling. Once a user goes on-line, the time spent learning to navigate the Internet for topics of interest is minimal. You will recoup the time you spend many times over.

Electronic Mail

Electronic mail is the most popular aspect of communicating on-line. Electronic mail, or *e-mail*, is a basic feature of the Internet, and it is easy to use. The ability to communicate with anyone, anywhere in the world for the cost of a local telephone call and with amazing speed makes e-mail popular. Because it is instantaneous, e-mail dramatically increases the ability to send and receive multiple short communications during the workday, increasing productivity. You can copy e-mail to all members of a specified work group with the click of the mouse, eliminating the need to make hard copies or send multiple fax messages. You can organize and save e-mail in specified files, allowing easy access of past messages, both sent and received. You can establish an e-mail mailing list of your club members, allowing instantaneous sending of direct mail or marketing information regarding a particular program you are offering. Imagine communicating with your membership and your prospect list simply by typing a message and sending it with the click of a mouse to everyone on an established mailing list. The options and opportunities are immeasurable for the organization that uses electronic mail to its advantage.

IN CLOSING

The future of computerization lies in establishing and using networks. The ability to use your computer to access limitless information, communicate instantaneously anywhere in the world, and research boundless products and services is all tied to the use of worldwide networks.

The information superhighway is in its infancy. Using this analogy, the Internet as we know it can be likened to the dirt road system in the early days of the automobile. The continuing development of the

Internet depends on the construction of an infrastructure of satellites, high-capacity or bandwidth cables, and high-speed modems that will allow digital information to travel farther and faster. The merging of efforts between cable companies and telephone companies will lead this effort while the development of more powerful computer processors continues.

Although most users of the Internet are in the United States, the future will bring large numbers of users from all over the world, enhancing communication by eliminating distance in miles. Tomorrow's powerful computers will be connected to an infrastructure that will bring information, entertainment, and services into your home or office from anywhere in the world, 24 hours a day. The development of technology will allow us to carry pocket-sized computers, much more powerful than today's top machines, to help us manage every aspect of our daily personal and professional lives. The implications of this development are far reaching.

> *Keeping pace with technological growth and development through education and experience should be a goal of every health fitness organization.*

KEY TERMS

E-mail

Hardware

Information superhighway

Internet

Local area network (LAN)

Multiuser

Single-user

Software

Wide area network (WAN)

RECOMMENDED READINGS

Anderson, T. 1994. Integrated club management software. *Fitness Management* (November): 24-28.

Dvorak, J.C., ed. 1995. *PC magazine 1996 computer buyer's guide*. Emeryville, CA: Ziff-David.

Gates, B. 1995. *The road ahead*. New York: Viking.

Hauss, D.S. 1994. Club management systems. *Club Industry* (October): 75-79.

Hoffman, P. 1995. *Destination Internet and World Wide Web*. Dallas: Compaq Press.

Loyle, D. 1995. 10 questions to ask when shopping for an EFT service provider. *Club Industry* (December): 23-25.

McDowell, S.G. 1995. Club management software. *Club Industry* (August): 37-44.

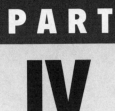

EVALUATION AND STRATEGIC PLANNING

CHAPTER 20

Evaluation

This chapter presents evaluation as an element of the I-formation management model introduced in chapter 4 and as an element in the control function held by most management theories. It defines evaluation; presents several methods of execution; and shows how managers can evaluate programs, personnel, and management techniques. The evaluation instrument developed in this chapter is a generic approach to outcome-oriented management practices and permits a snapshot view of the organization's performance, which is useful to managers in planning for the future.

Within every health fitness setting, there is a growing awareness of the need to develop meaningful standards and quality controls and to measure the extent to which a program has achieved its stated objectives. This process is commonly referred to as evaluation. Evaluation helps document the outcomes, impact, and processes involved in health and fitness services.

EVALUATION DEFINED

Evaluation is carried on within all settings of the health fitness industry—corporate, commercial, clinical, and community. It is the process of determining the extent to which an organization has achieved its stated objectives. In the health fitness field you can use evaluation to measure the efficacy of a given program offered for the first time or to gauge the overall performance of an organization to determine its value based on industry standards.

> *In an era of budget cutting, downsizing, and increased demand for accountability, it is essential that managers in all settings document the outcomes and impact of their offerings—whether by participation rates or profitability.*

Evaluation is essentially a form of practical research, and, like other forms of research, it does not seek to prove a case. Instead, the evaluator asks a series of questions and gathers evidence as systematically and objectively as possible to determine whether the program has met its goals or has achieved its appropriate standards of practice. If evaluation is performed honestly, it may yield negative rather than positive findings and ultimately result in program downsizing or elimination. Evaluating racquetball court use, for example, has recently resulted in significant reduction of available courts by retrofitting some for other functions, including retail space, free-weight studios, physical therapy services, or child care.

Another aspect of evaluation is gauging program improvement. Clearly defined goals and objectives are essential components for evaluation; consequently, you must measure them to determine program effectiveness. Elements such as program participation rates, attrition, postprogram behavior changes (e.g., weight loss, fitness improvements, stress reduction), and staff satisfaction are just some areas that you can measure to determine a program's success. Regard evaluation as part of the control function of managers.

> *Evaluation involves continual monitoring, reporting, and assessing with corrective measures or on-the-spot action taken when necessary to improve program performance.*

Goals of Evaluation

The overall goals of evaluation in the health fitness industry are as follows:

1. To determine how effective a program is in meeting predetermined goals and objectives.

2. To provide comprehensive information about the full range of the program's achievements and outcomes, as well as possible areas of weakness and inadequacy.

3. To measure the quality of a program, based on accepted standards and criteria.

4. To appraise the quality of organizational management, such as the performance of staff or the effectiveness of policies and procedures.

5. To provide feedback for improving programs once executed and recommending a direction for future reference.

6. To provide information for internal and external marketing of program achievements.

Models of Evaluation

There are many approaches for evaluation in the health fitness industry. In practical terms, the following three evaluations are designed to measure

1. the effectiveness of programs in meeting their stated goals;

2. the overall quality of programs, based on professional standards and criteria; and

3. the level of satisfaction of members regarding such factors as personnel, facilities, equipment, services, and program offerings.

Figure 20.1 depicts an evaluation model for the health fitness industry that incorporates all three outcome measurements mentioned. For this model to be effective the nine elements of evaluation listed

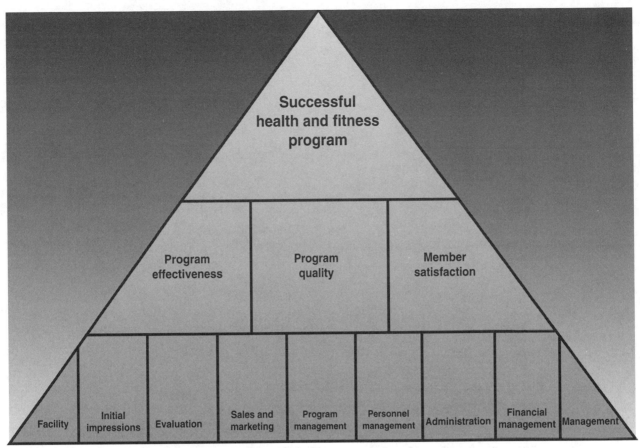

Figure 20.1   Evaluation model for the health fitness industry.

at the bottom of the pyramid in figure 20.1 must positively interact and contribute to program effectiveness, program quality, and member satisfaction.

This chapter focuses on evaluating program effectiveness and program quality. You can approach these aspects in a generic fashion that applies to many settings in the health fitness industry. However, the third aspect regarding member satisfaction would necessitate adaptation to specific settings to be applicable; therefore, we do not cover this form of measurement in this chapter.

In addition to the evaluation model illustrated in figure 20.1, the I-formation management model in chapter 4 can assist operators in the evaluation process.

> *The interrelationship of the three dimensions, information—implementation, and innovation—applies when evaluating an organization.*

By collecting pertinent information derived from such methods as surveys, focus groups, and employee committees, management can apply this data to improve program implementation and create new and innovative ways to stimulate business growth. You should perform this cycle periodically throughout the year.

Summative and Formative Evaluation Models

In the past, evaluation was primarily thought of as summative, that is, carried out at the end of a program to measure its success or failure and make recommendations for the future. An example of this form of evaluation is a fitness assessment program in which members sign up for a 16-week session with a personal trainer. They take a series of assessments (nutritional analysis, body composition, flexibility, strength, aerobic capacity, etc.) before and after the program to determine physical changes during the 16-week period. A *summative evaluation* would be conducted at the end of the program to decide if it was successful and whether changes are needed before the next program offering.

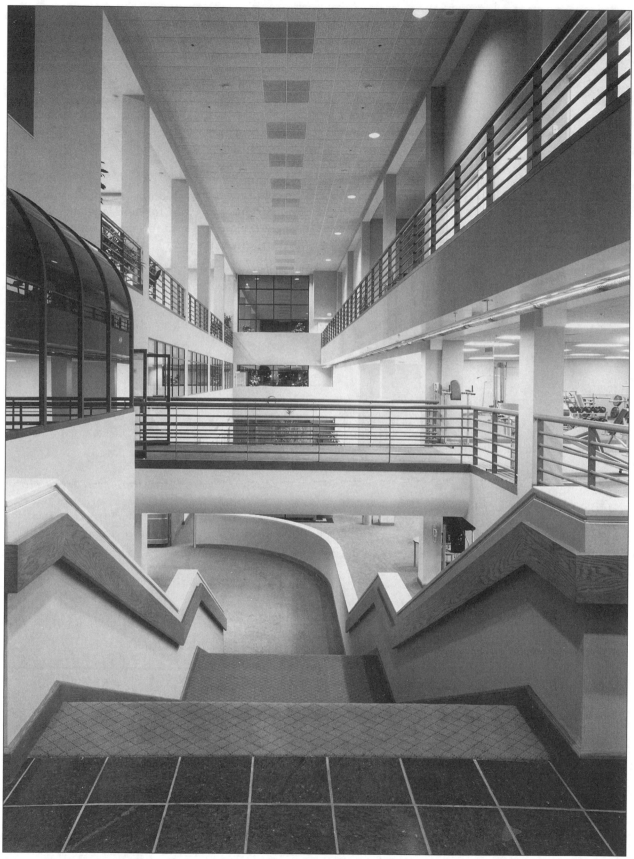

Courtesy of North Dallas Athletic Club

Today, however, much of the evaluation process is formative, with continuous monitoring of a program while it is being planned and implemented. Using the example of the fitness assessment program, the trainers routinely evaluate the program during the 16-week session and make individual adjustments to obtain the desired results. The *formative evaluation* process establishes whether goals and objectives are being met, modifying them as necessary.

Unfortunately, the approach to evaluation in most health fitness settings lacks organization; consequently, it is not used to its fullest potential.

> *As the fitness industry matures, organizations wanting to maintain their competitive edge should routinely conduct evaluations on all aspects of the business and regularly adjust the mode of operation to fit the needs of the consumer.*

Process and Preordinate Evaluation Models

Another approach to auditing programs is to use the process and preordinate models of evaluation. *Process evaluation* models delineate a set of steps and procedures to use in conducting an evaluation without identifying the judgment criteria. Preordinate models provide a process and specify the judgment criteria to use in determining the worth of a program. In other words, some evaluation models involve the application of standardized instruments, such as checklists, rating scales, or questionnaires. An example of the process model might be the locker-room attendant using a cleaning checklist to accomplish assigned work tasks, and the supervisor using the attendant's initialed responses on the checklist to evaluate his or her cleaning performance.

Other *preordinate evaluation* models begin with a process in which the program's staff determine exactly why they need to carry out an evaluation, the type of information that will be required, and the best way to gather it. An example of the preordinate model might be the aerobics coordinator meeting with all the instructors before a new aerobics program and planning the evaluation criteria and the types of information collected during the new program implementation. Member participation, interest, and feedback, as well as instructor evaluation, could be examples of preordinate evaluation.

No single approach is correct in all situations. A combination is often used in evaluating health fitness programs. Franchised commercial environments tend to have summative and process-oriented evaluations. Sole proprietorship commercial environments have formative and preordinate evaluations. Hospital-based programs strive for accreditation and have structured summative and process-oriented evaluations. Corporate and community programs look for high-level member participation and focus on formative and preordinate evaluations. An example of an evaluation that incorporates aspects of each model is presented here with guidelines on how to use the instrument for effective evaluation and long-range planning.

HEALTH FITNESS EVALUATION MODEL

You should view maintaining a competitive edge over similar facilities as a matter of survival. The quest for excellence separates the marginal operator from the successful operator. Whether a facility is small, medium, or large, striving to be the best should be the goal.

> *The pursuit of a well-managed, safe, and financially successful operation should be the driving force behind every owner, manager, supervisor, and staff member in the health fitness industry.*

You can measure the elements of quality in various ways. You can compare an existing business with the industry standard of the ideal setting. Determine a numerical rating by quantifying the operational elements of success and measuring those against an existing organization, using a predetermined scale to obtain an overall score. Another method is to perform a self-appraisal in which you compare the policies and procedures used in a business with proven management practices to determine the strengths and weaknesses of an organization.

Despite the measuring system used, the end result should be to identify those areas that meet or surpass acceptable industry standards and pinpoint areas needing further investigation and improvement.

As an example, the most widely used system for measuring quality within the health fitness industry today is called *total quality management* (TQM, see chapter 4). TQM involves observing and measuring everything that occurs within an organization (compared with an ideal setting), so you can identify weaknesses and improve operations. It also involves reviewing and revising all operational procedures and policies and examines how, and by whom, decisions are made and carried out within the organization.

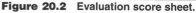

> *TQM has introduced a new measurement system with respect to teamwork, problem-solving techniques, the cost of quality, and employee-employer relationships.*

Incorporate principles of TQM if you aim to improve worker performance, productivity, customer service, and profitability.

The evaluation model for the health fitness industry illustrated in figure 20.1 lists nine categories of evaluation. In the remaining section of this chapter, we have established questions for each category to help evaluate a respective health fitness setting. The questions listed are not designed as a test to determine a specific rating or grade; rather they are meant as a guide for self-appraisal. The questions are similar to those that an outside consultant would address when evaluating an existing health fitness setting. Owners or managers should ask these questions when comparing their program with established industry standards and accepted professional criteria.

The purpose of this evaluation model is to develop an awareness of the management policies and procedures used in various health fitness settings; provide a means to measure the quality of those policies and procedures against proven methods; and point out the need to assess, improve, and change any areas deemed deficient. Use the model as a vehicle for improvement and as an indicator of where to concentrate efforts within the business.

The evaluation model covers the management practices considered most important for operating a health fitness organization. Each question is designed for a yes or no response. Answer all questions as openly and honestly as possible, while keeping in mind the current business practices. From the answers, you can draw specific conclusions regarding the adequacy of an organization's operation.

Not all questions will pertain to every health fitness setting. Questions critical to one environment may not pertain to another. For example, the questions relating to inventory will not be important for organizations that do not own or manage pro shops, restaurants, spa facilities, or salons. Adapt the evaluation model to meet the needs of your setting. A sample evaluation form is presented in figure 20.2.

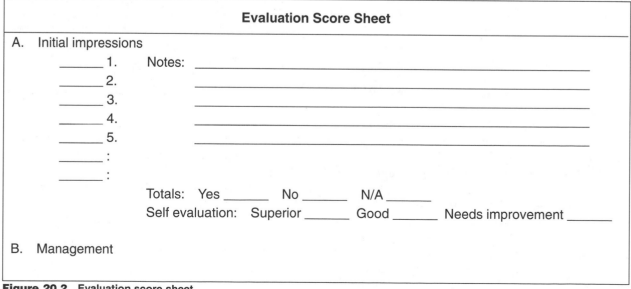

Figure 20.2   Evaluation score sheet.

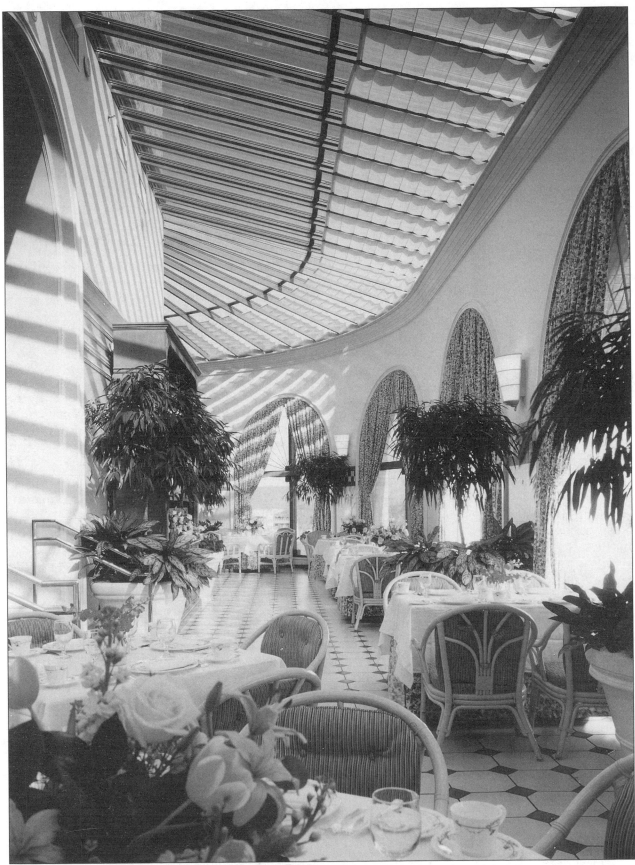

Courtesy of Four Seasons Resort and Clubs at Las Colinas, Irving, Texas

> *Because the health fitness evaluation model is a subjective self-rating tool, we recommend that a team of staff members, outside consultants, advisory board members, or a combination of these groups conduct the rating procedure. This approach should reduce any personal bias or favoritism entering into the evaluation process.*

Evaluation Questions

A number of the categories listed here will incorporate two sets of evaluation questions: one for profit organizations and another for nonprofit organizations. Depending on the type of nonprofit organization and the sources of funding, various forms of registration, reporting, and licensing are required. Although there are similarities that exist between these entities, there are also some basic differences that you should address. Several questions pertaining to profit settings can be applicable to a nonprofit environment and should be answered accordingly. However, questions that are unique to the nonprofit entities will be separated in the instrument. Separate questions pertaining to each entity are listed under denoted topic headings. Answer the questions that coincide with your organization.

Initial Impression

The following questions are a prospective customer checklist to determine if an organization meets basic fitness, social, and safety needs. Looking at an organization from the consumer's viewpoint allows management to recognize and stay focused on the key elements of a successful operation. This section summarizes areas a prospective member or guest deems important when touring a facility.

1. Does the facility provide adequate parking at all times and is the parking lot lighting sufficient for member and guest safety?

2. Are members and guests greeted in a friendly and courteous manner by service desk personnel?

3. Does the facility provide vehicles for communicating to members (e.g., bulletin boards, monthly newsletter, program guides, flyers, and posters)?

4. Is the physical environment of the facility well controlled (consider temperature, humidity, ventilation, interior and exterior lighting, space utilization, etc.)?

5. Are new members of the organization provided with an orientation and instruction in how to use equipment?

6. Does the organization provide baby-sitting or day care facilities?

7. Are there times when the facility is overcrowded (look at equipment lines, group exercise classes, locker availability, swimming lanes, etc.)?

8. Do the traffic flow patterns of the facility appear logical and smooth in transition from one area to another (consider traffic flow from the parking lot to the service desk, to locker rooms, and to activity areas)?

9. According to the guidelines established by the American College of Sports Medicine (ACSM) and the International Health, Racquet and Sportsclub Association (IHRSA), does the organization hire staff who have acceptable educational backgrounds; appropriate levels of certifications; and who provide coaching, instruction, and spotting as necessary?

10. Does the organization offer group exercise classes and activity programs geared to many fitness levels and varied in nature?

11. Does the organization provide acceptable maintenance for its resistive and cardiovascular equipment (consider the condition of upholstery, cables, belts, chains, hand grips, weight stack lettering, equipment cleanliness, etc.)?

12. Is the overall appearance of the facility clean and well maintained?

13. Is the facility conveniently located for usage at a specific time (before work, lunch, or after work)?

Management

The management section addresses questions that pertain to planning, organizing, coordinating, maintaining, and evaluating actions for the benefit of an organization. You can obtain a strategic profile from these questions that defines the direction of the program and its commitment to members. Adopting a planning strategy allows a program to establish goals and plans for the future.

For-Profit Organizations

1. Has management developed and communicated to staff a written mission statement defining the organization's purpose and structure?

2. Has management developed with staff an organizational flowchart that identifies the divisions of the enterprise and is regularly updated when organizational changes occur?

3. Does management regularly perform strategic planning sessions with staff to assess market and programming needs and to prepare short- and long-term goals and objectives?

4. Does management have a communication vehicle for obtaining feedback from members (i.e., member suggestion box, focus groups, membership committee, member surveys)?

5. Does management conduct periodic department head meetings to ensure proper communication between supervisors and employees?

6. Do management and department heads spend at least 30 percent of their time supervising and motivating employees?

7. Does management maintain a proactive status in searching for opportunities and initiating improvement projects (purchasing new equipment, renovating and remodeling, acquiring additional land, etc.) to bring about change?

8. Does management stay abreast of current industry trends by attending industry conferences, reading industry trade journals, and initiating observational tours of other facilities?

9. Does management transmit information received from outside sources (conferences, verbal contacts, committees, etc.) to professional personnel (internal memos, staff newsletters, staff meetings, etc.)?

10. Does management become actively involved with internal conflicts and resolve such matters in a timely fashion?

11. Does management have a system for initiating and approving the allocation of resources (supplies, repairs, petty cash requests, purchase orders, signing checks, etc.)?

12. Does management assume the negotiator role when working out contracts and agreements with outside organizations (janitorial contracts, HVAC contracts, insurance policies, etc.)?

Nonprofit Organizations

13. If incorporated, has a board of directors been formed to meet the requirements of incorporation?

14. Have articles of incorporation been filed as a nonprofit entity?

15. Have bylaws been established and formalized that must accompany the application for tax exemption?

16. Have officers (president, vice president, secretary, and treasurer) been nominated and elected according to the bylaws of the corporation?

17. Has management ensured that the department mission, goals, and objectives are consistent with the goals and objectives of the company?

Administration

The following questions on administration determine the policies and procedures established by an organization to accomplish its overall goals and objectives. The approach for building a quality operation is to know the strategic profile of the business, categorize the jobs to be done into tasks, and coordinate the actions to accomplish these duties. The evaluation questions mentioned here summarize the recommended administrative duties associated with a health fitness organization.

For-Profit Organizations

1. Does the organization offer a standardized health history questionnaire to all new members?

2. If a member is found to have health risk problems, does personnel recommend that medical clearance be obtained before beginning an exercise program?

3. Does the organization provide a fitness evaluation system for assessing fitness levels, identifying health and fitness goals, developing individualized exercise programs, and monitoring progress?

4. Does the organization use informed consent forms on new member applications, fitness evaluations, and guest passes?

5. Does the organization have an emergency plan that is readily accessible to all fitness center staff?

6. Does the organization provide at least one CPR-certified employee on duty at all times?

7. Does the organization provide a fully stocked first aid kit and a biohazard first responder kit that are readily accessible to staff?

8. Does the organization post telephone numbers for police, fire, and emergency assistance by all phones?

9. Has management prepared a written service desk training manual?

10. Does the service desk follow a formalized guest policy procedure?

11. Does the organization have written house rules identifying policies and procedures for members?

12. Does club management annually review its property and casualty insurance policy and obtain comparison bids?

Nonprofit Organizations

13. Has the organization established a record-keeping system for preserving documents, reports, and board meeting minutes?

14. Has the organization filed for a nonprofit bulk-rate mail permit from the post office?

15. Has the organization filed a charitable trust registration with the state?

16. Has the organization developed and submitted fund-raising proposals to obtain government grants or to solicit private foundations?

17. Does the organization initiate policy review concerning health issues, smoking policies, what is sold in the snack machines, work and family policy reviews, ergonomic reviews, and so on?

Financial Management

The financial management portion of the evaluation determines if basic accounting and record-keeping systems are in place and provide the necessary information for management to measure and report the financial status of the operation to external parties. Properly organized accounting records make it easy to develop financial information for preparing financial statements, budgets, and tax returns.

For-Profit Organizations

1. Does the organization use a formalized accounting system?

2. Does management prepare an annual operating budget?

3. Does management compare actual to budget variance figures and discuss this periodically with department heads?

4. Is a capital budget prepared annually for improvements to the organization?

5. Are monthly computerized financial reports (balance sheet and income statement) prepared for review?

6. Has management established procedures for accounts payable, such as filing invoices by due date to take advantage of discounts offered?

7. Does the organization practice good expense management by comparing current bills for utilities, supplies, and other expenses with budget figures?

8. Has management established procedures for accounts receivable, and is the current amount of bad debt tracked by management in 30-, 60-, and 90-day increments through an aged trial balance report?

9. Is a cash report prepared monthly?

10. If the club operates a pro shop, restaurant, salon, or spa facility, does it take inventory on schedule and reconcile it with accounting records?

11. Does management provide a formalized system for tracking daily cash transactions (i.e., daily deposits, monthly bank statement reconciliation, petty cash fund, point of sale registers)?

12. Is the average ratio of total payroll, payroll taxes, and employee benefits to total revenue less than 40 percent?

13. Are operating expenses 70 percent or less of total revenues?

14. Is the operating margin (net income before fixed expenses) 25 percent or higher?

15. Are fixed expenses 25 percent or less of gross revenues?

16. Is revenue per square foot $30 or greater?

17. Does management have an outside accounting firm conduct an annual audit or review of the financial status of the club?

Nonprofit Organizations

18. Has the organization filed an application with the IRS to obtain 501(c)(3) tax exemption from corporate income taxes?

19. If appropriate, has the organization filed for a state sales tax and property tax exemption?

20. Has the organization prepared an annual budget, listing projected revenues generated through fees for services, contributions, grants, and all fixed and variable expenses?

21. Is the bookkeeping and accounting system able to track various donated funds (restricted and unrestricted) and account for donated services and materials?

22. Does the organization practice program accounting by determining the individual costs associated with each program it offers?

23. Does the organization provide annual financial reports and an audited financial report performed by a certified public accountant (CPA) to fundors (in some states this is a requirement by law)?

24. Does the organization practice good internal controls regarding bookkeeping and accounting procedures (i.e., dual-signature checks, approval of expenditures, controlled handling of cash, and good fiscal responsibility by the board)?

25. As a tax exempt business, is unrelated business income (UBI) (i.e., facility rental, massage, or cosmetic services through a beauty salon, etc.) less than 10 to 15 percent of total income?

26. Has the organization developed reporting and accounting systems for filing UBI tax information, and does it maintain separate revenue information on UBI activities?

Personnel Management

Evaluating personnel issues calls for measuring such functions as personnel planning, recruitment, selection, training and development, compensation, health and safety, and cross-training of duties. The following questions should help in designing a personnel package that assists the organization in achieving its objectives while providing the means for employees to satisfy their personnel goals.

For-Profit Organizations

1. Are written job descriptions prepared for all positions, and are they updated with changes in the organization?

2. Has the organization prepared a personnel manual that it updates regularly?

3. Does the organization provide an employee benefit package (health insurance, paid vacations, bonus, profit sharing, etc.) available to qualified staff?

4. Has the organization established job qualifications for all positions relating to educational background, professional certification, personality characteristics, and experience?

5. Does the organization check and verify all prospective employee's references, conduct criminal background checks, and perform drug screening before hiring?

6. Does the organization comply with federal, state, and local laws regarding new hire regulations and personnel records?

7. Has the organization established salary and wage ranges consistent with industry standards?

8. Does the organization provide training programs based on job descriptions for all positions?

9. Does the organization cross train employees to work in other departments of the business?

10. Do employees of the organization know who to report to regarding such things as performance reviews, promotions, salary changes, vacation approval, and leaves of absence?

11. Has the organization established a formal probationary period for all new employees?

12. Does the organization provide periodic performance reviews for personnel?

13. Does the organization provide opportunities for continuing education for professional staff?

14. Is there a succession plan established to prepare designated employees for other positions when vacated?

Nonprofit Organizations

15. Has the organization registered with the state unemployment insurance program?

16. Has the organization filed employer registration with federal and state government agencies for income tax withholding?

17. Has the organization decided whether it will contribute to Social Security for employees? If so, have the necessary forms been completed for the IRS or Social Security Administration?

Programming

Health fitness programming has been shown to increase member adherence, provide a necessary social component, and assist in health education and fitness awareness. Participants are exposed to higher levels of health and fitness through individualized needs assessment, customized programming, and support services provided through counseling and regular activity classes. These questions address an organization's commitment to programming and the emphasis placed on the variety and scope of programs offered.

For-Profit Organizations

1. Does the organization offer a variety of fitness and activity programs (leagues, contests, seminars, or events)?

2. Does the organization have an annual program calendar to project timely and seasonably appropriate programs and special events?

3. Does the organization provide a variety of group exercise classes (bench, aerobics, aquatics, sports conditioning, stretch and relaxation, etc.)?

4. Does the organization offer private and group instruction to teach members a sport or an activity (tennis, swimming, racquetball, squash, etc.)?

5. Does the organization offer continuing education or health sessions for members (weight management, smoking cessation, wellness education, stress management)?

6. Does the organization offer social events to members (new member mixers, parties, potluck dinners, etc.)?

7. Does the organization support, either internally or externally, charitable and community events?

8. Does the organization provide programs to attract and retain active older adults (50 years or older)?

9. Does the organization offer children's programming (sport skills, camps, birthday parties, group activities, etc.)?

10. Does the organization provide personal training?

11. Does the organization offer spa services to members (massage, skin care, salon services, etc.)?

12. Does the organization have established methods for promoting and marketing programs to members (program guides, flyers, brochures, bulletin boards, etc.)?

13. Does the organization conduct program evaluations following each program?

14. Are periodic program surveys conducted with members to determine program interests and obtain feedback?

Non-Profit Organizations

15. To satisfy the requirements of a tax exempt 501(c)(3) organization, are most programs offered based on charitable needs; that is, do they serve the public rather than the private sector and are they of an exempt purpose?

16. Are resource audits performed on each program offered to ensure that the costs associated with the program were spent appropriately?

17. Has a program planning process been established that identifies the specific programs to be offered during a calendar year?

18. Has there been an integration of programming with other company departments (for example, a healthy back program for the safety department, a cancer screening program for the medical department, or a prenatal program for the benefits department)?

19. Has the programming been expanded to family members? Are programs flexible enough so that individuals who cannot or do not visit the facility in person can use the information?

20. Has the programming been integrated with the company's medical benefit provider? (Companies today are working hard at becoming partners with managed care companies or primary care physicians who work directly with employees and their families.)

Sales and Marketing

Sales and marketing accelerate the perception of value and services to members. Many health fitness settings offer a wide array of facilities, programs, and fitness products, but the owners and managers of these organizations recognize that success depends on providing good customer service. Ways of accomplishing this goal include advertising, promotion, publicity, sales, and public relations. Providing a sales and marketing strategy that incorporates a mix of these activities ensures management that they are communicating the mission of the organization to the public. Remember,

member satisfaction is based on the perceived value of services being offered and how well the service satisfies customer needs.

For-Profit Organizations

1. Does the organization conduct an industry analysis every three to five years to determine trends and consumer preferences?

2. Does the organization perform a market analysis every three to five years to identify or clarify the target market?

3. Does management conduct periodic comparative analysis on competitive clubs (comparing pricing, reviewing programs, and evaluating facilities and equipment changes)?

4. Do management and sales personnel prepare an annual marketing and promotional plan that includes, but is not limited to, television and radio spots, newspaper ads and articles, direct mailings, brochures, and newsletters?

5. Does management aggressively seek public relation opportunities such as speaking engagements, community service projects, adopt a school program, and so on?

6. Do management and sales personnel prepare a corresponding advertising and promotional budget annually?

7. Are membership reports prepared monthly, listing the number of new members, members who terminate, and the average adherence rate?

8. Is the annual attrition rate for the organization under 35 percent (members who annually leave the club)?

9. Does the organization use a sales and marketing reporting system that tracks the number of phone calls, walk-ins, tours, and new member sales monthly?

10. Does the organization offer a computerized check-in procedure for all members who enter the facility?

11. Does the organization use a membership tracking system that lists daily member usage (by month, time of day, activity, or by individual member)?

12. Does the organization provide a system for tracking guests?

13. Does the organization maintain member data records (computerized or manual) on each membership?

14. Are there written termination procedures for members to follow when leaving the club?

15. Are exit surveys conducted for members who terminate their memberships?

Nonprofit Organizations

16. To satisfy the requirements of a tax exempt 501(c)(3) business, does the organization follow the community benefit test by offering a membership fee structure that does not restrict community accessibility (are fees representative of community income levels)?

17. As a tax exempt business, does the organization offer wellness programs (i.e., smoking cessation, stress management, weight-management programs), reduced rates for family members, daily guest rates for guests, require no long-term financial commitments, and charge fees comparable to or less than commercial health fitness facilities within the community?

18. Has the organization planned a marketing strategy for promoting programs to senior management, middle management, employees, and their families?

Physical Facility

The operational duties, safety issues, and equipment selection are critical factors of a health fitness business. Management must select and organize personnel, materials, and contract services to provide the necessary quality and quantity of services. At the same time the facility and equipment layout must meet the needs of the members, employees, and management.

For-Profit Organizations

1. Does the facility signage (both inside and outside) comply with the ADA (Americans With Disabilities Act) and meet federal, state, and local codes (signs warning members of the potential risks involved in swimming pools, whirlpools, saunas, steam rooms, weight rooms, and other exercise areas)?

2. Are all chemicals and hazardous materials stored in a room that complies with OSHA (Occupational Safety and Health Administration) standards and regulations?

3. Does the facility meet federal, state, and local codes and regulations regarding fire safety (including a fire alarm system, fire extinguisher, and sprinkler system)?

4. Does the facility meet the following standards regarding electrical safety?

   • The facility provides grounded electrical outlets for all electrically operated equipment.

   • In areas where electrical equipment may come in contact with moisture (locker rooms, pool, bathrooms) the facility uses ground fault outlets as a safety measure to prevent electrical shock.

5. Is the exercise equipment adequately spaced (about 50 square feet per station, with adequate user circulation space), and are there member instructions and signs for all equipment?

6. Is there a system for either removing defective equipment from the floor or placing an "out of order" sign on it until repaired?

7. Does the organization provide a maintenance management program that incorporates maintenance checklists, preventive maintenance care, and daytime and evening cleaning schedules?

8. Does the pool area conform to the following standards?

   a. Water temperature ranges between 78 and 84 degrees Fahrenheit.
   b. Chlorine level maintained between 1.0 and 3.0 ppm.
   c. Level of pH maintained between 7.4 and 7.6; alkalinity range from 80 to 120 ppm.
   d. Calcium levels maintained between 200 and 300 ppm.
   e. Deck space covered with a slip-resistant material or texture.

9. Are the following temperatures maintained in the wet areas?

   a. Whirlpool 102 to 105 degrees Fahrenheit.
   b. Steam room 100 to 120 degrees Fahrenheit.
   c. Sauna 170 to 180 degrees Fahrenheit.

10. If the organization offers day lockers, can the number of available lockers accommodate 15 percent of the members in the facility at any time of the day?

11. Do most areas within the facility meet these environmental standards?

    a. Temperature 72 to 78 degrees Fahrenheit.
    b. Humidity 60 percent or less (does not include enclosed pool area).
    c. Air circulation 8 to 12 exchanges per hour.

12. Although specific lighting requirements vary from one activity area to another, does the lighting throughout the facility average between 50 and 60 foot-candles?

13. Do the number of parking spaces meet state and local codes, usually requiring one space for every 200 to 300 square feet of the facility?

14. Is the facility periodically reviewed by city officials (health department, fire marshal, OSHA) to ensure compliance of all local codes and regulations?

15. Is there adequate space to provide wellness classes (cooking classes, stress-reduction classes, etc.)?

16. Is there adequate storage space for materials, CPR mannequins, and exercise class equipment?

17. Is there adequate office space for staff to provide counseling or coaching to employees or members in a semiprivate atmosphere?

18. Does staff have access to temperature controls and are they easy to adjust?

Evaluation

Regularly evaluating an organization allows management to contemplate all aspects of the business. Integrating an evaluation philosophy emphasizes the need to continually search for improvement and implement actions to convert improvement opportunities into reality. To properly evaluate an organization there must be a good understanding of the customer and the internal operations of the business. A continuing cycle of reevaluation must exist to maintain quality standards.

For-Profit Organizations

1. Are periodic evaluations performed annually?

2. Does management involve supervisors and staff in the evaluation process?

3. Are the results of the evaluation shared with employees and customers or members?

4. Is the evaluation instrument used considered valid and reliable regarding the information that it obtains?

5. Does management take the results of the evaluation and incorporate changes to improve the operation of the business?

6. Does the evaluation process compare program outcomes and determine the programs that are the most cost effective?

7. Is the data collected from each evaluation entered into a computer-based system to help manage and interpret the findings?

8. Do strategic planning sessions involving short- and long-range goals result from periodic evaluation findings?

9. Does the evaluation identify areas in which customer expectations are not satisfied?

10. Is the evaluation tool periodically revised to accommodate new technology, trends, and to compensate for the new goals and objectives following each evaluation?

Using the Evaluation Model

As discussed in chapter 4, managers and supervisors of health fitness organizations have at least four activities they are responsible for: planning, organizing, leading, and controlling. Each activity is important and questions in this evaluation probe them all. As reflected in figure 4.14, the responsibilities mentioned are considered cornerstones of the management process and are prerequisites for anyone interpreting the results of the evaluation process.

> *The goal of the evaluation process is to provide a measurement system to determine if the organization is incorporating accepted methods of business management and operational elements of success.*

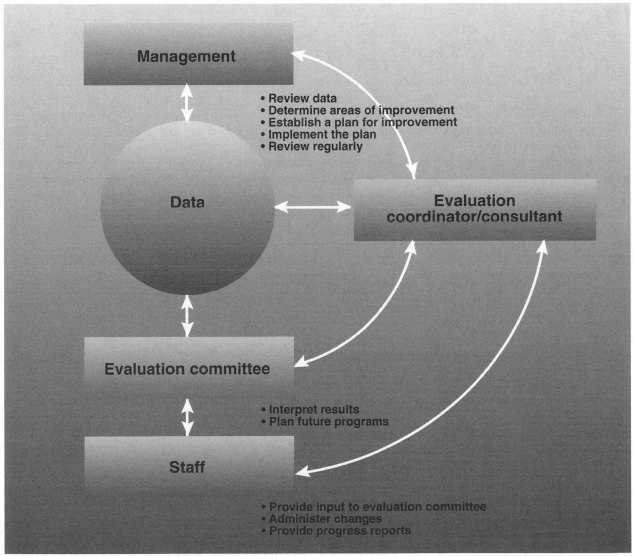

Figure 20.3 Communication network for evaluation.
Adapted, by permission, from Association for Fitness in Business, 1992, *Guidelines for employee health promotion programs* (Champaign, IL: Human Kinetics), 83.

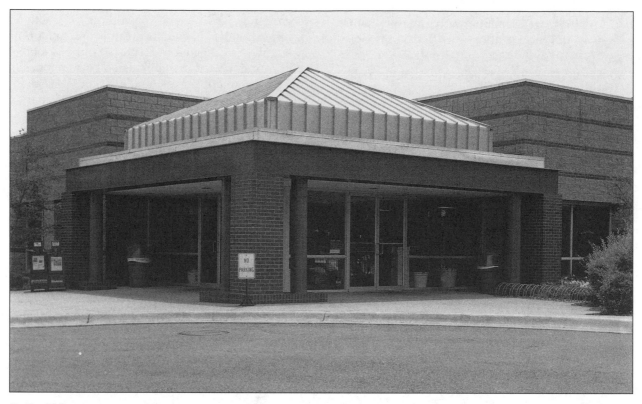

© Tom Wallace

For organizations who answer most questions positively, you are following the principles of quality management. We recommend maintaining and regularly updating these principles. Reevaluation of the organization should be ongoing.

Questions answered negatively indicate possible organizational shortcomings. Because many sections covered coincide with chapters of the text, we suggest referring to these chapters for further explanation. You can then make a decision whether to incorporate these policies or practices, depending on the setting. View the evaluation only as a tool for indicating areas that need attention and review. We wrote each question on the evaluation from the perspective of an ideal program setting, with no defined parameters or limitations. Consequently, not every principle addressed may be practical for every situation; however, it does help to appraise an organization from an industrywide perspective.

You can use the information obtained from an evaluation to report to owners, corporate CEOs, hospital administrators, or community board members as an audit of the overall program. You can measure current performance against past evaluations and can list specific suggestions for improvements as future goals. Within most health fitness settings there are various levels of communication important to the success of the business. When conducting a facility evaluation, the groups involved in the evaluation process generally include management, an evaluation committee, evaluation coordinator or consultant, and staff. Figure 20.3 illustrates how the flow of information obtained from a facility evaluation reaches the appropriate individuals.

The various roles of these groups are discussed here:

• *Management.* It is the responsibility of management to take the data obtained from the evaluation and use it to monitor established goals. Managers should look for areas considered deficient, establish a plan for improvement, implement the plan with the assistance of personnel, and regularly review the results. Having the support of management for short- and long-term planning is essential; consequently, a strong line of communication is needed between managers and other members of the evaluation group. You can obtain interaction through regular presentations and reports focusing on significant findings and recommendations for improvement.

• *Evaluation coordinator or consultant.* The role of the evaluation coordinator is to be the intermediary between management and staff. This task is often performed by an independent consultant who has no ties to the organization and can be impartial toward the findings of the evaluation. If you use an in-house employee, we recommend that both parties approve the selection. The individual chosen to manage this process will be responsible for data analysis, reviewing results, comparing data with industry benchmarks, and determining pertinent conclusions.

• *Evaluation committee.* The evaluation committee usually consists of supervisors or personnel who have a vested interest in the evaluation process. They are responsible for developing and administering the evaluation, reviewing the results with the evaluation coordinator, and providing recommendations for improvement. The committee performs these tasks through regular meetings and brainstorming sessions for solving problems associated with the evaluation process. Committee members obtain input from other staff to incorporate their ideas and to make them feel a part of the operation.

• *Staff.* Staff members assist the evaluation committee in planning and conducting the evaluation, but, more importantly, they are primarily responsible for administering the changes approved by management. We cannot overstate their involvement in the evaluation process. Providing a sense of ownership during the evaluation phase helps ensure that staff members implement planned program, facility, or operational changes positively. Staff are also responsible for providing regular feedback on these changes so the organization can make refinements as needed.

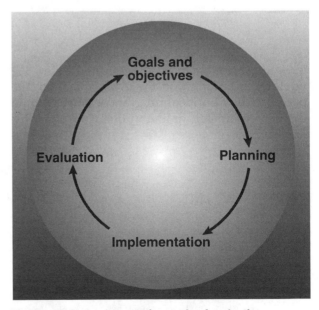

We encourage managers and supervisors to revise organizational goals and objectives to coincide with data obtained from periodic evaluations.

Strategic planning is another use for evaluation results. For example, if you were to implement programming changes, the planning process might involve defining target populations for various health fitness services, identifying specific programs to deliver, and estimating the cost for each service you provide. We offer additional information on strategic planning in chapter 21.

You can also use evaluation findings as an external marketing tool. You can incorporate promotional and advertising vehicles, such as newsletters and direct or private mailings, to communicate evaluation results to members. Reflect information pertaining to management's actions as a result of evaluation findings in prospective member packets or list them for members and guests to view.

Perform follow-up evaluations periodically throughout the year. Depending on organizational needs, we recommend that you conduct an evaluation quarterly, semiannually, or annually. If problems occur during this time, you can use specific sections of the model to identify areas needing immediate attention. Maintain a policy of long-term continual evaluation, rather than using the process for a short-term fix.

As shown in figure 20.4, we suggest an ongoing, self-renewing cycle for evaluation implementation. Use the information you obtain to define new goals and objectives, establish strategic planning, and follow up with implementing the plan. This cycle allows management to continually evaluate every aspect of the business to ensure that they are incorporating proper managerial techniques. This evaluation should not take the place of other forms of analyses that management performs. Instead, consider it a supplement to such things as financial audits and market research.

If conducted appropriately, the findings should reinforce the opinions of those using other data as

Figure 20.4 Implementation cycle of evaluation.

their primary resource for evaluating and managing the organization.

IN CLOSING

This chapter established a method for determining an organization's strengths and weaknesses compared with the ideal health fitness setting. The results of the evaluation model presented provide a snapshot of an organization's operational skills. For an evaluation model to be useful for long-term planning one must consider major trends and forces impacting our culture. Only then can we be responsive to anticipated changes or trends affecting the dynamics of the health fitness industry.

KEY TERMS

Formative evaluation

Preordinate evaluation

Process evaluation

Summative evaluation

Total quality management (TQM)

RECOMMENDED READINGS

De Pree, M. 1989. *Leadership is an art*. New York: Bantam Doubleday Dell.

Flannery, T., D. Hofrichter, and P. Platten. 1996. *People performance and pay*. New York: Free Press.

Fraser, J. 1995. Tis better to give and receive. *Inc.* 17(2): 84.

Lancaster, P. 1994. Incentive pay isn't good for your company. *Inc.* 16(9): 23.

Lasser, J. 1983. *How to run a small business*. New York: McGraw-Hill.

Rausch, E. 1979. *Financial management for small business*. New York: American Management Association.

Sibson, R. 1990. *Compensation*. New York: American Management Association.

Stewart, G. 1991. The quest for value. *Harper Business* 32(8): 5.

CHAPTER 21

Trends Affecting Strategic Planning

In an industry fraught with explosive growth, it is important to remain flexible in planning for the future. It is also important to feel the pulse of the forces acting on the industry. There are several influences acting on the health fitness industry in America, and they impact the strategic planning of the industry decision makers. The graying of our population will have a major impact on the nature of facilities and programs as they move to accommodate services for the older members. The inevitable move toward softer fitness programs and an emphasis on the mind-body connection programs will increase. The children of *baby boomers* are now challenging all aspects of the health fitness industry. The maturing of the health fitness industry will influence the structures of business, the types and credentials of staff in the programs, and the industry standards being adopted to assure consistent standards of care.

The consumers of our services are becoming more knowledgeable as they subscribe to similar literature and are exposed to the same media as the professional staff in programs. Management will be challenged to provide more qualified and better-trained staff. Advancing computer technology is constantly changing the facility and program landscape with new equipment and information systems. The health care system impacts the health fitness industry as it inevitably embraces wellness and prevention as an essential part of the delivery system. The contemporary professional needs to take these trends into account as we move into the 21st century. We must strategically plan for the future developments of our industry and enhance the quality of our lives.

Any book attempting to break new ground in a field experiencing explosive growth would be negligent if it did not address trends that will affect long-range program planning. The introductory chapter of this book provides a status report for the health fitness industry, as well as discussion regarding current trends and issues. Many subsequent chapters allude to specific trends within the scope of their chapter content.

This chapter addresses major trends in our society that will have a long-term impact on strategic planning for the health fitness industry. These trends more clearly define our current status and provide a clearer focus on the direction health fitness programs will likely take in preparing for the future. This information, along with periodic program evaluation discussed in chapter 20, should help chart an effective course for program development well into the next century.

CHANGES IN THE HEALTH FITNESS MEMBER

There is a sea change in the health fitness industry due to our country's changing *demographics*. We are growing older as a nation. The childbirth explosion shortly after World War II created a high-density population segment in our culture we call baby boomers. The baby boomers have been the focus of our national attention for the past half-century as they have grown from infants and matured to middle age. Every marketable product in our society has been directed at the baby boomer. The health fitness industry has tracked the baby boomer by giving birth to the hard-core running and bodybuilding boom in the past few decades and graduating to spa services and golf more recently. Let's take a closer look at this development.

Demographic Trends

The baby boomers began making a dramatic impact on the health fitness industry as they graduated from college and started careers. In the 1970s, the health fitness industry experienced explosive growth by focusing on the young urban professional, commonly called the yuppie. Fitness industry development at that time centered in urban areas where young, fast-paced professionals could get fitness services close to work and home. Indeed, the fitness boom was an urban phenomenon and left rural America untouched until recently. Commercial fitness centers were developed in apartment and residential areas where the yuppie market was concentrated. Corporate employee fitness programs were developed in the workplace to accommodate this new interest in fitness, presumably facilitating employee recruitment and retention as well as promoting morale and productivity. Corporate decision makers responsible for developing employee fitness and wellness programs were hopeful that these programs could stem the spiraling costs of health care. Many studies were conducted to evaluate the cost benefit and cost effectiveness of corporate wellness programs, to eventually conclude favorably regarding such investments of resources (Kaman and Patton 1994). Community programs flourished as well. YMCA organizations developed urban fitness centers located downtown where workers could get a needed fitness and recreation break from the workday. Every major metropolitan area in the country eventually sported a new YMCA located in their urban centers to accommodate the fitness needs of the young urban professional. The suburban Y facilities addressed the fitness interests as well; however, the major focus was, and remains to this day, on family programming.

In the 1980s, the leading edge of the baby boomers were approaching 40 and no longer fitting the description of a yuppie. Indeed, the boomer was approaching middle age. Broader health fitness programming was designed in all venues to accommodate both a keener consumer interest in matters such as nutrition and additional services, including child care. The long-standing projection of a shortened work week was not coming to pass. In fact, we were working longer hours and had less free time. Both adult family members were now required to work in order to support perceived needs. Time urgency was an ever-present attitude, born of the need to keep workplace and home front matters from falling through the cracks. Accordingly, the fitness industry began developing multipurpose facilities providing services, including spa, food and beverage, laundries, travel, and child care, designed to embrace the home away from home concept.

Every consumer outlet was vying for this market segment's discretionary time and money. This was the golden era for commercial fitness facility construction. Large facilities averaging 25,000 square feet were built to accommodate the multipurpose needs of the aging consumer. In extremely large urban areas, megaclubs approaching 100,000 square feet were developed, providing even broader ranges of services.

Also during the 1980s, our hospitals became interested in the fitness business. Health fitness facilities were developed to complement expanding outpatient services such as cardiac rehabilitation and physical therapy. Membership-based fitness facilities were developed to market hospital services to the increasingly affluent and influential baby boomer. As profits began declining in hospitals owing to controlled reimbursement, reduced length of stay mandated by insurance agencies, and the initiation of *managed care*, health fitness programs were viewed as a new profit center. Hospital wellness programs flourished, primarily because they were viewed as a community outreach tool for marketing a desirable segment of the prospective patient population.

In the 1990s the baby boomers began turning 50. Annual membership growth in the commercial setting continued above the 10 percent level despite significant member attrition brought about by poor compliance, occupational relocations, or disinterest. However, the baby boomer now began dominating the membership growth. Current projections indicate that from 1995 through 2010 the 55 and older age group will grow 13 percent annually, while the 18 to 34 age group will decline significantly.

In 1995, the median age of members in the multipurpose facilities was in the 35- to 44-year bracket, and the 50 and older age membership grew at an annual rate of 21 percent. Programs have begun to reflect this demographic trend. Low-impact water programs are back in full force, and clubs are starting to maximize the revenue potential of their pools. Swim classes, swim clubs, water fitness, water walking, master's swim, and water aerobics—all of which do not traumatize bones and joints—are thriving as never before. Massage and other spa services are abounding to accommodate this older market segment. Personal training is a recent phenomenon directed at the older and more affluent member

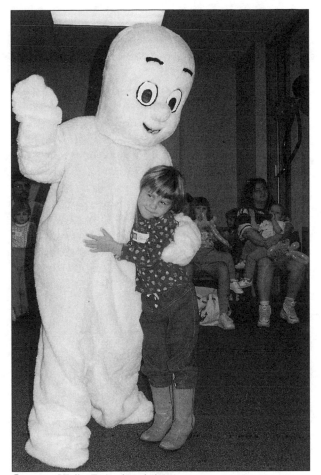

Courtesy of Dallas Texins Association

needing more personal attention with less time to spend. Because we are a market-driven business, it is highly likely that the health fitness industry will continue to respond to an aging population through creative facility, personnel, and programming development directed at less intensive exercise and broader health concerns.

Incremental Upgrades in Memberships

It is common knowledge that as the typical American grows older and more affluent he or she tends to trade up automobiles, homes, and other consumer items. The recent college graduate buys a subcompact car and rents a modest apartment. As he or she matures, resources permit upgrades to higher-priced automobiles and a nicer home. A parallel exists in the fitness industry. The average American tends to trade up when it comes to health fitness center membership. The recent college graduate starts off with a low-priced monthly membership in Spartan facilities, graduates over time to more lavish health fitness facilities, and eventually joins an expensive country club.

It is interesting to note that the average age of members in health fitness centers and those in country clubs in America are growing closer each year. Historically, the perception of a fitness member was that of a young professional, and the perception of a country club member was that of a middle-aged or older professional or retiree. There is now less than a decade difference in average age between the fitness center members and the country club members in this country. This narrowing of membership age differences obviously places both environments in competition for similar markets. Consequently, fitness centers are beginning to look and act like country clubs without expansive tennis complexes and golf courses, while country clubs are beginning to add fitness facilities and services.

> *The difference between the upscale fitness center and the country club has blurred to the extent that one might say that the golf course is all that distinguishes one from the other.*

There is evidence that some fitness centers across the country are joint venturing with public parks and country clubs to offer their fitness members preferential pricing and scheduling at selected tennis centers and golf courses. This phenomenon has had a significant impact on the finances of the for-profit fitness programs in this industry.

Historically, the dues in commercial fitness centers accounted for approximately 90 percent of total revenues, whereas the dues in country clubs accounted for only 50 percent of revenues. Fitness facilities have started adopting the country club model in program delivery by introducing value-added services to shore up the revenue generation of the club. Value-added services, such as personal training, massage and other spa services, and retail outlets in fitness centers are a direct result of this country club approach to member service. Recent evidence of the impact of these nondues revenues on the fitness industry has been positive—clubs with the highest percentage of nondues revenues are growing twice as fast in revenue and profitability as clubs with

lower percentages of nondues revenue. Also, these service-oriented clubs have had lower member attrition (31 percent versus 36 percent in 1995) than low nondues-revenue clubs.

> *It is highly likely that the increased emphasis on value-added service elements of the business will continue to impact member retention.*

Personnel play an important role in the quality and success of programs as well. Recent evidence suggests that there is a positive correlation between the employment longevity of part-time staff who make the day-to-day contact with members and the club's retention rates.

> *The longer a part-time fitness instructor stays employed, the longer a member retains his or her membership.*

Although this may seem intuitive and supports the contention that the quality of a program is no better than the people delivering the program, managers frequently fail to recognize the critical role that part-time staff play in ultimate success and profitability of programs. It is essential for health fitness organizations to establish relationships with professional preparation institutions through internships and work-study programs to get well-qualified staff. Initiating ongoing staff development programs also helps improve member retention.

The nonprofit environments are responding to the same pressures as the commercial programs regarding value-added services and quality personnel. Corporate and clinical settings are upgrading their programs, personnel, and services to respond to a competitive environment. However, specialized organizations such as bodybuilding, martial arts, dance, and other niche market facilities continue to rely predominantly on dues for revenue sources and do not provide significant value-added programs and services.

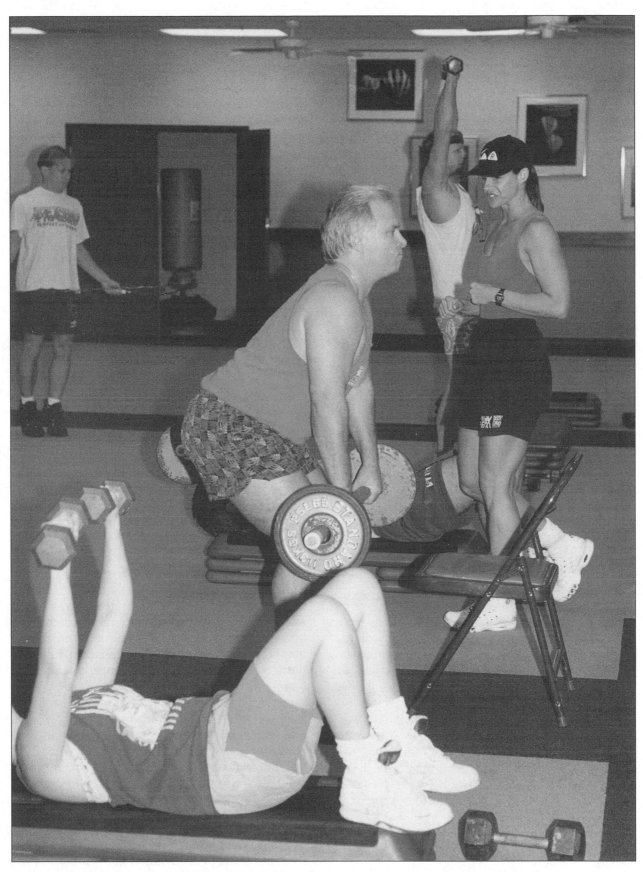

Courtesy of Dallas Texins Association

Hotels and Health Fitness

The fitness- and health-conscious baby boomers who travel as part of their business have made a significant impact on all forms of travel and entertainment. Airlines, car rentals, and other travel services are yielding to the demands of the health fitness–conscious consumer. No smoking venues are now the mode. Vendors no longer consider heart healthy food menus novel and bothersome. Hotels designed to market the business traveler are expanding to provide fitness facilities. Historically, the hotel provided only a pool to accommodate family recreation needs. Now, hotels with fully equipped exercise facilities are becoming commonplace. The upscale hotels with an affluent guest market and convention trade are frequently developing full-scale spa services to supplement their fitness facilities. Some are even attempting to become destination resorts where they provide golf, tennis, and spa services. Hotels without direct access to such services as golf and tennis frequently develop joint ventures with clubs where guests may use their golf and tennis facilities on a preferred or reduced-cost basis. Most hotel-based facilities combine a membership program comprised of local residents and nearby business professionals to complement the hotel resort clientele. In short, the traveling public is expecting no compromise to their lifestyle when away from home on business or for pleasure. This trend will probably continue for the foreseeable future.

Retirement Communities and Health Fitness

Retiring Americans will spend approximately one-third of their lives in retirement—most of these years as healthy active residents. As the life span lengthens and health care technology increases, so will the need for leisure health and fitness pursuits for the elderly. Although some individuals may be economically challenged in their later years, many will have considerable discretionary time and money. The retirement communities being developed for active seniors will need to focus on creating facilities and services beyond that of a room for checkers and card games. Professionals managing these programs will need to develop widespread facilities and services for these clients who ushered in the fitness boom in America. These aging but active individuals will not "go gently into the night." They will demand a modified extension of their lifestyle de-

veloped during the previous decades of vigorous activity. This active senior market will expect golf, tennis, dance classes, and hiking and biking trails. An entire industry surrounding the active elderly will surface in the coming years. There are several communities currently developing across the country that embrace this concept of active seniors and provide facilities and programs accommodating their lifestyles.

> *As our older citizens approach retirement, it is likely that communities developed for active seniors will spawn a whole new setting for the health fitness industry.*

Mind-Body Programs

The harried lifestyle of Americans is exacerbating stress-related diseases and disorders. Many health fitness programs have been introduced in recent years to offset or minimize the impact of our stressful lives. We presented a detailed discussion of the types of mind-body and spa programs in chapter 10. These programs are among the fastest growing in the health fitness industry and will undoubtedly keep growing as we continue to lead a time-urgent and stress-laden existence.

Baby Boomlet Programs

The babies of the baby boomers are called the *baby boomlets*. These children—school aged in the mid- to late 1990s and entering college as we approach the new century—are currently challenging the capacities of schools and their delivery systems. Unfortunately, the response of most school systems to this burgeoning segment in physical education programs is to diminish the activity requirement. In high school, for example, enrollment in daily physical education classes dropped from 42 percent in 1991 to 25 percent on 1995. Only 19 percent of high school students were physically active for 20 minutes or more in physical education classes every day of the school week This trend is pervading all levels of the public school physical education programs and is creating a huge need in the health fitness industry (U.S. Department of Health and Human Services 1996). Children and youth programs are abounding and facilities are retrofitting spaces such as racquetball and tennis courts to accommodate these new programs. Broad ranges of services are being introduced—even specialized academic programs during after-school hours until the remaining family members meet at the club. The services being offered are age specific and tend to become a glue to bind the family members to the health fitness organization. As this market segment matures, the industry must remain abreast of its changing needs.

MATURING OF THE HEALTH FITNESS INDUSTRY

Every industry experiences a slow start, followed by a rapid growth, and eventually stabilizes for a long period of maturity. This growth curve and life cycle is predictable. The fitness industry is no exception. The health fitness industry started slow, grew rapidly, and has reached a stable but mature period. The health fitness industry in this country is alive and well. It is here to stay. What started as a fad has become an integral part of the lifestyle for millions of Americans. There are more than 20 million Americans currently holding memberships in health fitness programs across the country. There is a huge number of individuals who are exercising at home. Recent data suggest there are at least the same number of home exercisers as club exercisers.

> *We have now gleaned the active individuals in the marketplace and are reaching beyond the low-hanging fruits to harvest new members from the underactive and older markets.*

The underactive and somewhat older market is the new frontier for our industry. For example, only 20 to 25 percent of the total population is getting enough regular exercise to promote their health status and prolong the quality of their life. Another 25 percent of Americans are openly resistant to the prospect of regular exercise. This leaves 50 percent of the American population from which we can successfully market our services. This underactive segment—who are on the cusp of launching a healthy and fit lifestyle, but are not members of programs and do not regularly participate in activity—will be the challenge to our continued growth in the health fitness industry. Better marketing of more appropriate services to those who are underactive and less amenable to physical exertion will influence the continued development of our industry.

Business Structures

There is a predictable change taking place in the business structures within the health fitness industry. The Mom and Pop fitness centers, initially representing most of the commercial enterprises, have increasingly been replaced by franchised or incorporated business chains. Each year the sole proprietorship or partnership is closing its doors or is being bought out by large corporate entities. For example, in 1992 there were no stand alone publicly held health fitness companies in the United States. In 1997, there were five publicly held health fitness companies and numerous others planning for expansion. However, the overall number of major corporate players in the industry is winnowing down to a precious few. These major players are not in a single market; niche markets have emerged to accommodate corporations with special interests. Club Corporation of America, still privately held, has become identified with the more upscale markets of country clubs, and urban fitness and dining facilities. Bally Total Fitness has identified itself with the mid- to lower-scale markets of large fitness centers located in diverse communities. Hospitals are merging into megagroups and large companies; some are beginning to develop management contracts with corporate fitness programs. Other corporate players will inevitably be created to achieve market dominance in yet undefined segments of the industry. While there is evidence of growth in the community settings, the bulk of the growth was seen in the commercial environment. For example, membership in all health fitness settings grew by a significant 39 percent from 1987 to 1996, but the membership in commercial centers skyrocketed by 81 percent during the same period. The growth trend for the health fitness industry is clearly focused in the commercial sector at the present time.

There is still a place, however, for the sole proprietorship in certain markets in the health fitness industry. An interesting phenomenon is taking place to foster the small business owner because of the increased burdens related to health care costs. Large health fitness programs approaching 40 percent of their expenses as payroll and experiencing spiraling

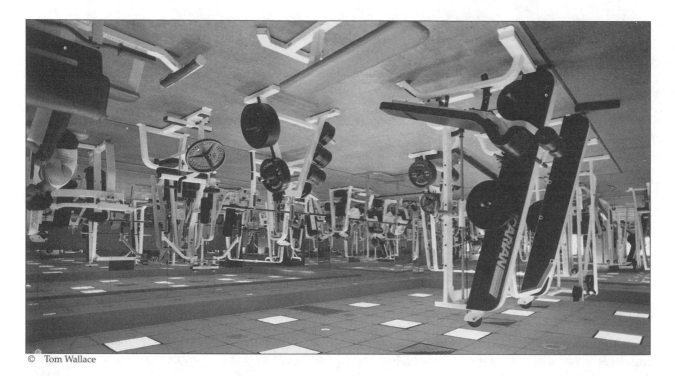

© Tom Wallace

increases in benefits associated with health care are shedding themselves of full-time employees and, thus, some of their health care expenses. Many managers turn around and hire the same individuals on a part-time contract without the burden of benefit packages. The typical scenario is that a club will downsize its staff receiving benefits to economize on payroll costs, thereby opening the door for entrepreneurial employees to contract with their employer as sole proprietors. This situation is frequently manifested in the personal training services of a club. The club's full-time employees (receiving benefits) handle the ongoing programs and services, while selected part-time contractors (not receiving benefits) provide personal training, massage, and other such services. These entrepreneurs frequently contract with multiple facilities and seek opportunities in the untapped home markets, where they can take their services directly to the consumer's residence. Inevitably, some entrepreneurs are forming partnerships and even corporations to achieve the economies of scale afforded by larger organizations.

Therefore, it would seem that the industry is growing divergently to become both larger and smaller in its business structures. The midsized business is diminishing; it will be interesting to see what the future holds for this trend. Certainly a nationalized health care program would eliminate or minimize the perceived need of employers to contract with individuals for selected services over

which they exercise minimal quality control. Other factors such as professional licensure may also impact the nature of business structures in the health fitness industry. The future relationship of health fitness professionals with health care providers, to be discussed later in this chapter, will undoubtedly influence this issue as well.

Professional Preparation

Because educational systems operate on a lag with market demand, it has taken years for needs in the health fitness industry to be translated into academic courses and programs to meet those needs. Moreover, traditionally trained physical educators and exercise physiologists whose tenure extends for decades are ill equipped to gear up for instructional programs in health fitness, especially the business aspects of operating facilities and programs. Despite this lag in curriculum and program development for health fitness professionals, there is reason for optimism. Two books by Patton et al. (1986, 1989) on the subject of health fitness have been adopted by over 50 higher education institutions. Programs are being developed to accommodate the need to train health fitness professionals. Therefore, it seems that some progress is being made to train and educate professionals in the health fitness industry. However, there are other avenues for securing trained professionals for the health fitness workplace.

> *Colleges and universities are now adapting their traditional physical education programs to accommodate professional preparation programs in the health fitness industry.*

Certification and Licensure

Certification programs now abound for health fitness professionals. In fact, many discerning professionals feel there are far too many certifications of varying types and differing expectations. It is difficult for the aspiring professional with limited resources to make good decisions regarding which certification(s) to secure. There are specialized certifications for such things as aerobics, strength training, and swimming pool operation. There are also generic certifications such as personal training and health fitness instructors. As the health fitness industry matures, it is likely that some certification will emerge as the definitive process recognized by most professionals and their employers. Clinical settings are beginning to require *licensure*. Licensure is a state-mandated requirement limiting practice to only those with defined credentials in a given professional arena. Licensure provides the quality assurance so essential in maintaining standards of care in the clinical setting. Yet, the nonclinical settings for health fitness professionals have yet to address licensure. It is likely that future developments for the profession will focus on the issue of licensure, ensuring quality control for professional practitioners.

Industry Standards

The industry is becoming mature enough at this juncture to begin setting standards regarding facilities, programs, and personnel. We have evidence of these standards in publications such as those advanced by the American College of Sports Medicine: *ACSM's Health Fitness Facility Standards and Guidelines* and *ACSM's Guidelines for Exercise Testing and Prescription*. The Association for Worksite Health Promotion, formerly called the Association for Fitness in Business, has published *Guidelines for Employee Health Promotion Programs*. Other organizations, such as the International Health,

Racquet and Sportsclub Association (IHRSA), American Association of Cardiovascular and Pulmonary Rehabilitation (AACPR), and the Young Men's Christian Association (YMCA), have internal documents that address guidelines or standards.

> *Each year there is more concern for standards of care for members, clients, and patients in this industry.*

The industry has yet to develop a document that all pertinent organizations endorse. This is sorely needed, and attempts are currently being made to accomplish some consensus among key organizations in the industry.

NATIONAL AWARENESS OF HEALTHY LIFESTYLES

There is an ever-broadening realization among the public and popular press that regular exercise is an integral, rather than a discretionary, part of a healthy and productive life. In July 1996, the Surgeon General's report (U.S. Department of Health and Human Services 1996) regarding exercise was released and will undoubtedly have a continuing impact on the need for exercise and healthy lifestyles. Yet there is much remaining for us to do.

> *Almost 60 percent of Americans engage in little or no leisure activity, and total and saturated fat intake remain high.*

We need to direct educational efforts at dispelling misinformation that can serve as a barrier to exercise and dietary change. Although the amount of time and effort invested in lifestyle change necessary to improve health is low, it may be that most Americans look at the high cost of achieving the ideal body image and feel defeated before or soon after initiating the effort.

Whether long-term compliance to modest lifestyle change can be achieved and whether modest lifestyle change will be sufficient to affect morbidity and mortality are unclear. According to the latest National Health and Nutrition Examination Survey, approximately $33 billion is spent annually in the weight-loss industry, and Americans are gaining rather than losing weight. Indeed, one-third of our adult population is considered overweight. Approximately 10 percent of U.S. adults currently exercise at levels recommended for improved cardiorespiratory fitness. Less than 25 percent of us exercise sufficiently to improve health and quality of life. Research shows that 50 percent of participants drop out of exercise programs within the first three to six months. We should view these barriers to physical activity and healthy lifestyles as the glass that is half full. Without a market to penetrate, we would have no room for growth in our industry.

The good news is that we are beginning to make a dent in these demoralizing statistics regarding exercise. Both health club membership and home-based exercise programs have been growing consistently during the past few years. The commercial setting is now able to extend its prime selling season of January into February (up 21 percent in 1995) and March (up 18 percent in 1995), and the summer membership declines that have plagued the industry have recently stalled. There is no recent published data to support definitive trends that fitness participation is no longer seasonal and sporadic; however, IHRSA's Report on the State of the Health Club Industry (1997) revealed that general interest is growing in permanent commitments to healthy lifestyles. Fifty-five percent of Americans surveyed indicated that they were more interested in fitness than they were two or three years ago. The study further revealed that Americans believe

- older people exercise just as often as younger ones (86 percent),
- people who exercise regularly will probably live longer than those who don't (85 percent),
- regular exercisers are happier (73 percent), and
- regular exercisers are more productive on the job (70 percent).

Home-based exercise programs have increased dramatically during the past five years, suggesting that we are beginning to embed exercise into our home life. The challenge ahead is to tackle the underactive populations that are amenable but have yet to initiate a personal fitness program. Remember, 20 to 25 percent are active; 20 to 25 percent will probably never be active; and 50 to 60 percent are

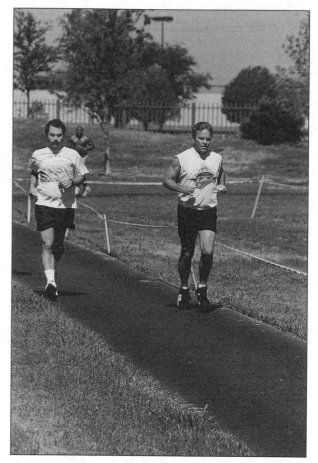

Courtesy of Dallas Texins Association

underactive or inactive but potentially amenable to lifestyle change. This 50 to 60 percent is the challenge for the future.

The marketing and programming focus for the future must be appealing to those on the cusp of initiating an exercise program, a healthy nutritional program, and other such healthy behaviors. The Exercise Lite program advanced by the American College of Sports Medicine and the American Heart Association encouraging moderate rather than vigorous exercise holds great promise in appealing to the underactive segment of our market. The trick will be how to best market the moderate exercise programs revolving around such activities as walking while not diminishing the commitments of those on vigorous exercise programs.

Consumer Awareness

The consumer is becoming more knowledgeable about health and fitness and is demanding more from health fitness programs in which they are actively participating. Many members subscribe to health and fitness magazines and are avid readers of such literature. Other media inundates the fitness enthusiast with information. The net effect of such exposure to health-related information is that the member is frequently as knowledgeable and, unfortunately, sometimes more knowledgeable than some staff working in health fitness programs. Member pressures on fitness center managers to hire individuals with specialized knowledge, skills, and abilities is increasing. Consequently, health fitness organizations are offering more broadly based programs to include nutrition, stress management, and other health topics that complement traditional fitness activities. Fitness and nutrition assessments, health risk appraisals, and other assessments of members as they enter, remain in, and exit from programs are now commonplace. Personal training programs developed in recent years are probable outgrowths of the increased demand of consumers for more sophisticated and comprehensive personalized health fitness programs.

Home-Based Fitness Programs

As discussed in chapter 1, the first half of the 1990s brought about a 82 percent increase in home-based exercisers. The continuing sales of home exercise equipment since then lends support that the trend is continuing. We can attribute this phenomenon to any number of factors. Convenience and time savings can account for some of the trend. The home exerciser can minimize the travel, clothes changing, and grooming time associated with exercising at a club. Improved home exercise equipment may also be a factor; equipment vendors have responded to the home exercise market by creating near-commercial grade equipment at more reasonable prices. Moreover, this equipment is user-friendly and frequently requires less caloric expenditure than most equipment found in the commercial environments. Also, there is no longer a stigma attached to cluttering up a spare bedroom with exercise equipment.

TECHNOLOGY

Certainly, new technology has hastened the maturation and development of the health fitness industry. New exercise equipment with programmable capabilities, software programs to access more heart healthy information, and other technology are rapidly becoming an accepted part of our lives.

Information

Welcome to the information age, where the most intimate details of your personal life are becoming so many bits and bytes sold by anyone who can ferret them out. Although the new technologies have much to offer consumers, they can also create dangerous new concentrations of power and invasions of privacy. The sweeping new telecommunications law is supposed to knock down the barriers that have kept local phone companies, long-distance carriers, and cable TV providers out of each other's markets. But if genuine competition doesn't lower costs, America could fracture into a nation of information haves and another of have-nots—people denied opportunities by lack of access to new technologies. This bifurcation of population groups inevitably impacts health fitness programs, which must appeal to both computer literate and illiterate users. User-friendliness is critical, especially as the membership ages and is less likely to remain abreast of the latest technologies. We need to consider technical and nontechnical alternatives when planning for innovative change in a program.

As technology advances and data become cheaper and quicker to gather, store, and exchange, a lucrative new industry is thriving by prying into—and selling—personal information about consumers' private transactions and even their intimate medical and fitness records. As we inevitably merge with the health care industry, greater safeguards must be in place to prevent unwarranted invasion of members' privacy. Membership data needs to become more difficult to access and manipulate. Yet, we must stay abreast of technological change.

> *We must view each technological challenge as a programming opportunity. It is conceivable that we can integrate the facility programs and home exercise activities with creative technology offered by innovative fitness professionals.*

It is conceivable that residential outreach programs might become a viable aspect of health fitness facilities. Personnel might travel to members' homes for personal training services. Distance learning programs might be broadcast into homes for fitness or nutrition activities. The Internet could easily be a platform for launching specialized health fitness services. The possibilities of such integration of club and home are limited only by one's imagination.

Computers

Computers have become an integral part of our professional and personal lives. The health fitness industry has embraced the computer in every aspect of program development and operation. We discussed the details of how we can use this computerization in operating and managing health fitness programs in chapter 19. However, the exercise equipment the programs are using is increasingly computer interfaced. Exercise equipment has evolved to third-generation levels. The first-generation equipment simply permitted workload settings. Second-generation equipment permitted programming of exercise loads. Third-generation exercise equipment now permits interaction between the user and the equipment during exercise. Target heart rates, for example, can be monitored and controlled during an exercise period by an interaction of the user and an accommodating workload on the equipment. Entertainment systems are now connected to exercise equipment to occupy members while they exercise. Programs are written to organize and orchestrate exercise classes. It is unlikely that we will avoid exponential computerization in the future of this industry.

HEALTH CARE AND HEALTH FITNESS

In the 1930s, when it was first advocated that all Americans be covered by national health insurance, millions of Americans lacked access to adequate medical treatment. Today, some 40 million people—a quarter of them children—lack health insurance. Health care costs, meanwhile, are climbing at a rate 60 percent higher than inflation. Both businesses and government are adding to the problem. As they try to rein in their own costs, employers are making employees carry more of the burden of paying for the medical treatment they and their families need. At the same time, succumbing to federal budget pressures, the government is proposing major rollbacks in projected increases in medicare funding for the elderly and in medicaid, the program that serves poor Americans and pays

for nursing home care for many people from the middle class. Also under the cost-cutting knife, health care providers are remaking the nation's medical delivery system in ways that are sometimes harmful to patients. Many new managed care networks reward doctors, hospitals, and clinics for keeping patient costs low—providing profit incentives for them to minimize treatment. Because the networks monopolize the delivery of care in many localities, patients often have little choice of either providers or available treatments.

The health fitness industry is both a problem and a partial solution to the health care difficulties we are facing. The health fitness industry is a problem to the extent that managers are increasing copay levels among employees and shifting more of the payroll to part-time and contract status. This means that the employer is saving on payroll expenses, but it also means that many employees who become contract labor for various employers may be unable to afford health insurance. There are many professionals in our industry going without health insurance; this will only exacerbate the problem. The uninsured's health care costs frequently go unpaid and ultimately result in providers and carriers exacting higher premiums to cover their costs. This creates a net increase in cost for employers providing health care benefits to their remaining staff.

However, our industry could become part of the solution to spiraling health care costs. We could become a major player in the health care system in this country by delivering preventive health care services as part of the managed care delivery system. The corporate health promotion programs have researched their cost benefit and cost effectiveness for decades and have concluded that health promotion is economically viable. Implementing health promotion programs has proven a wise investment in which the return on investment has averaged approximately three dollars for every dollar spent to keep employees well. In short, we know that prevention pays. Some programs, such as hypertension screening, have a quick return on investment. The screened employees with high blood pressure can be placed on medications and thereby be less likely to have a costly stroke. Other programs, such as exercise and nutrition, have a tremendous return on investment, but the payback requires years to see the yield. The net effect is that there is a demonstrated value in preventing disease and promoting health among our workforce. Then, what is the problem in getting the health care industry to implement more prevention and health promotion?

The first problem is that traditional fee-for-service medical care underwritten by insurance companies—currently accounting for well over half the health care in the country—does not generally reimburse patients' preventive and health promotion services. Insurance companies continue to focus reimbursement on the diagnosis and treatment of illness and disease. As long as this insurance reimbursement model for illness and disease exists there will be little opportunity for preventive services to flourish.

The second problem is that managed care, accounting for over one-third of the country's health care, is contracting with corporate clients for a fixed or *capitated annual rate* (about $4,500/year/person in 1997). The contract periods are usually for one year. Under this scenario, a managed care organization of, let's say, 100 hospitals agrees to provide for all health care needs of their contracted clients for the capitated rate identified in their contract. Companies, therefore, have a predictable and fixed rate for providing their employees with health care during the contract period. This creates a disincentive for companies—especially large companies who are self-insured—to continue budgeting their resources for in-house wellness programs in which their primary mission is the containment of health care costs.

Corporate health promotion programs, operating in environments with managed care contracts, must now justify their existence on such issues as increased morale, productivity, retention, and reduced absenteeism. These reasons alone are more than enough to justify a program's existence; however, many corporate health promotion programs are aligning themselves with managed care organizations, functioning as a preventive health care service to complement or joint venture with managed care.

Although managed care organizations recognize the benefits of prevention, they cannot afford to institute large-scale and costly prevention programs when their contract with company clients expires annually. In other words, they can't afford to expend their resources improving the health status of a client's employees when their contract is annual. It is conceivable that their competition could underbid them next year and reap the benefits of the healthy employees of their previous client. Therefore, annual contract periods do not give enough time for health promotion to be cost effective. Until there is the potential for contractual periods to extend to five years, health fitness will suffer in the health care system.

Paradigm Shift Toward Prevention

As our country moves toward more managed care (or some form of nationalized health care plan) to contain health care costs, we must make a *paradigm shift*. We can either emphasize more *demand management*, in which health care services are doled out to only a few in serious need of care, or we can emphasize prevention and health promotion, which reduces the burden of health care by minimizing illness and disease. Probably the best action would be to establish a reasonable demand management system while accentuating prevention and health promotion. We must accomplish this without diminishing the quality of care for patients. Yet, the major shift in focus will be from illness treatment toward health promotion. We must reduce the amount of illness treatment and increase the amount of health promotion. This shift toward health promotion might include more

- demand management (i.e., pretreatment screening, education, primary care),
- health education (i.e., smoking cessation, stress management),
- home health care (i.e., nursing, physical therapy taken to the home),
- community health screening (i.e., lipids, blood pressure, risk appraisal), and
- health fitness services (i.e., exercise, nutrition).

The health fitness industry is currently posturing itself for involvement with the health care industry. Many new programs and services being introduced into health fitness programs are health care related. Physical therapy, weight management, nutrition counseling, and aquatics classes for the obese and arthritic are just a few examples of the overlapping activities between health care providers and health fitness providers. There is a blurring of the differences between preventive managed care services, which are slowly developing, and ancillary medically oriented services currently being provided in the club industry.

Managed care systems are becoming monolithic structures through ongoing takeovers and mergers of smaller health care providers. As this process continues, there will be fewer systems available to provide health care. At some point, these major health care providers will make the commitment to provide comprehensive prevention and wellness, regardless of the length of contracts with major clients. At that time, a merger of the health care system and the health fitness industry could be affected. It is time to consider a model for such an alliance between health care providers and health fitness providers.

Comprehensive Health Care and the Health Fitness Model

Figure 21.1 illustrates a fictitious scenario that might serve as a model. In this illustration, the hospital, having a patient service area of approximately 30 to 40 miles, has established an alliance with commercial, corporate, and community agencies to complement the health fitness services provided by their on-site wellness center. This makes a lot of sense. The typical health fitness program can only market effectively within a 10- to 15-mile radius for its fitness services. In other words, people will travel farther to go to a hospital than they will to a fitness center for services. Because the hospital markets services in a much larger area for its traditional clinical services, it stands to reason that an alliance of a hospital and numerous health fitness facilities would be necessary to provide a market area coverage for wellness activities. It is conceivable that a hospital may joint venture with several different types of health fitness venues to establish their full market coverage of wellness services.

There is some research to support the contention that we need an alliance between health care providers and health fitness providers. According to a 1994 IHRSA survey, more than one-third of inactive Americans said they would switch to an HMO insurance plan that helped pay for health club membership; 73 percent of active Americans who were health club members would switch to such an HMO

insurance plan. Because the consumer sees the merits of such an alliance, it would seem that decision makers in the health care industry should follow with some alternative. The future may unfold to embrace an alliance of what we now consider the health care industry and the health fitness industry. It is conceivable that an amalgamation of the two may eventually yield total health care, which embraces promotion of health, prevention of disease, treatment of disease, and rehabilitation of patient populations. It may well be that the future health care industry in America will include what we now think of as fitness facilities, hospital facilities, and outpatient services combined to treat the entire spectrum of health. Although this sounds a bit outlandish at the moment, there is much to support such a contention as we move toward the 21st century.

IN CLOSING

In this chapter we presented factors that will have a long-term impact on the strategic planning process for health fitness professionals. The ongoing influences of aging Americans, the maturing of our industry, the role of technology, and the relationship of health care and health fitness will have a significant impact as we move into the 21st century. The adept health fitness professional needs to proactively respond to these changes, especially when the rate of change in our culture is becoming more compressed each year. Indeed, the future manager in our industry needs to respond not so much to change but to needs forecast if he or she hopes to be responsive in a meaningful way with our consumers.

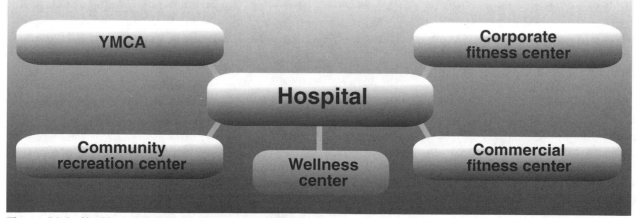

Figure 21.1 Health care and health fitness alliance model.

KEY TERMS

Baby boomers

Baby boomlets

Capitated annual rate

Certification

Demand management

Demographics

Licensure

Managed care

Paradigm shift

RECOMMENDED READINGS

American College of Sports Medicine. 1992. *ACSM's health fitness facility standards and guidelines*. Champaign, IL: Human Kinetics.

American College of Sports Medicine. 1995. *ACSM's guidelines for exercise testing and prescription*. Baltimore: Williams & Wilkins.

American Heart Association. 1992. Statement on exercise: Benefits and recommendations for physical activity programs for all Americans. *Circulation* 86: 340-344.

Association for Fitness in Business. 1992. *Guidelines for employee health promotion programs*. Champaign, IL: Human Kinetics.

Blair, S.N., E. Horton, A.S. Leon, I.-M. Lee, B.L. Drinkwater, R.K. Dishman, M. Mackey, and M.L. Kienholz. 1996. Physical activity, nutrition, and chronic disease. *Medicine and Science in Sport and Exercise* 28: 335-349.

Blair, S.N., H.W. Kohl, R.S. Paffenbarger, D.G. Clark, K.H. Cooper, and L.W. Gibbons. 1989. Physical fitness and all-cause mortality: A prospective study of healthy men and women. *Journal of the American Medical Association* 262: 2395-2401.

International Health, Racquet and Sportsclub Association. 1994. *Profiles of success. The 1994 IHRSA/Gallup industry data survey of the health and fitness club industry*. Boston: IHRSA.

International Health, Racquet and Sportsclub Association, 1997. *The 1997 IHRSA report on the state of the health club industry*. Boston: IHRSA.

Kaman, R.L., and R.W. Patton. 1994. Costs and benefits of an active versus an inactive society. In *Physical activity, fitness, and health*, ed. by C. Bouchard, R.J. Shephard, and T. Stephens, 134-144. Champaign, IL: Human Kinetics.

Markarian, M. 1993. How does your club compare to the typical club? *Club Industry* (February): 23-29.

Moffat, T. 1995. The home front. *Club Industry* (September): 25-31.

Pate, R.R., M. Pratt, S.N. Blair, W.L. Haskell, C.A. Macera, and C. Bouchard. 1995. Physical activity and public health: A recommendation from the Centers for Disease Control and Prevention and the American College of Sports Medicine. *Journal of the American Medical Association* 273: 402-407.

Patton, R.W., J.M. Corry, L.F. Gettman, and J.S. Graf. 1986. *Implementing health/fitness programs*. Champaign, IL: Human Kinetics.

Patton, R.W., W.C. Grantham, R.F. Gerson, and L.F. Gettman. 1989. *Developing and managing health/fitness facilities*. Champaign, IL: Human Kinetics.

U.S. Department of Health and Human Services. 1996. *Physical activity and health: A report of the Surgeon General*. Atlanta, Georgia: U.S. Department of Health and Human Services, Centers for Disease Control and Prevention, National Center for Chronic Disease Prevention and Health Promotion.

Wilson, B.R.A., and T.E. Glaros. 1994. *Managing health promotion programs*. Champaign, IL: Human Kinetics.

INDEX

ABOUT THE AUTHORS

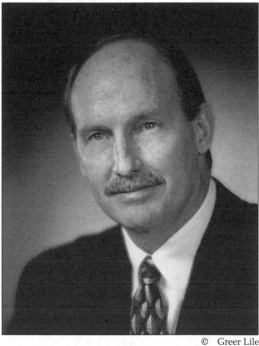

© Greer Lile

William C. Grantham is general manager of the Little Rock Athletic Club, which was named the best commercial fitness center in Arkansas in 1996 by both the Arkansas Governor's Council on Physical Fitness and the *Arkansas Times*. Selected in 1974 at the age of 25 to direct Dr. Kenneth Cooper's Aerobics Activity Center in Dallas, Texas, Grantham has since been involved in nearly every facet of health fitness facility management and operation. He has directed facility design and start-up, managed as many as 135 employees, and handled all areas of marketing, finance, member services, food and beverage, and pro shop management. In addition, he has served as a health fitness facility consultant and as a certified examiner for the American College of Sports Medicine (ACSM).

Grantham is the coauthor of *Developing and Managing Health/Fitness Facilities*. He is a member of the International Health and Racquet Sports Association and a graduate of the organization's Professional Management Institute. He is also a member of ACSM. Married to Jamie Grantham, William enjoys reading, cycling, and computers.

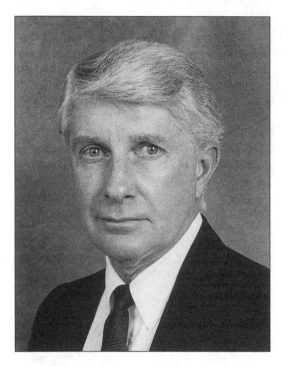

Dr. Robert W. Patton has been involved in the health and fitness field for the past thirty years. He is currently a regents professor of kinesiology at the University of North Texas in Denton, where he was instrumental in the development of the health fitness management and exercise physiology graduate programs. Patton is also president of Health Fitness Associates, a Texas-based company whose mission is planning, designing, equipping, staffing, programming, and evaluating health fitness facilities and programs around the world. His particular expertise is in the facility planning stages prior to construction and in the personnel and program development processes after construction. As a consultant and expert witness, Patton has served over fifty major clients, including corporations, hospitals, resorts, and hotels, as well as preventive medicine clinics and commercial fitness centers.

In addition to writing more than 80 journal articles and several encyclopedia chapters, Patton is the principal author of *Implementing Health/Fitness Programs* and *Developing and Managing Health/Fitness Facilities*. He is a fellow of the American College of Sports Medicine and a former chair of the organization's Health Fitness Director certification subcommittee. He is also a fellow of the Association for Worksite Health Promotion and the American Alliance of Health, Physical Education, Recreation and Dance's Research Consortium. Patton is married to Elisa Hardy Patton and has two grown children, Laura and Scott. He is an avid traveler and a fitness enthusiast who enjoys jogging and cycling as well as reading and gardening.

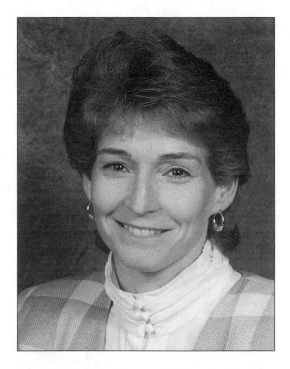

Tracy D. York serves as director of operations for the Lake Austin Spa Resort, a destination wellness spa located in Austin, Texas. Prior to accepting this position, she served as director of The Spa at the Crescent, a luxury spa, fitness, and wellness facility managed by Rosewood Hotels and Resorts, which oversees five-star hotels and resorts around the world. In this role, York was responsible for managing all aspects of the private fitness facility and public day spa. In addition to her management duties at The Spa, York served on the development team for Rosewood Hotels, designing spa and fitness facilities. She is a contributing author to *ACSM's Guidelines for Exercise Testing and Prescription (Fifth Edition)* and a section editor for the *ACSM's Resource Manual to the Guidelines (Third Edition)*. York is the recipient of a master's degree in health fitness management from North Texas State University. She is a lover of outdoor activities and enjoys jogging, cycling, weight training, yoga, and golf.

Mitchel L. Winick is a consultant, author, and speaker in the areas of professional service management, marketing, and communications. During the past 20 years, he has applied his expertise to two distinctly

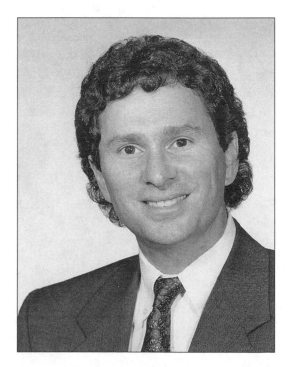

different industries. As a consultant in the health fitness industry, he provides management and marketing research, analysis, and advice to many of the United States' largest health fitness organizations, including the American College of Sports Medicine and the President's Council on Physical Fitness and Sports. As a licensed attorney, he serves as an adjunct professor of law, teaching law office management and technology, at Texas Tech School of Law and the University of Houston Law Center. He also serves as a faculty member and author for several professional organizations, including the Texas Center for Legal Ethics and Professionalism, the Center for Nonprofit Management, and the State Bar of Texas Professional Development Program. He is coauthor of *A Guide to the Basics of Law Practice* and *Law Office Management: Practice and Technology*. Winick received his JD from the University of Houston Law Center. He and his wife, Debbie, have two children, Tyler and Lezah.

You'll find other outstanding health and fitness at

www.HumanKinetics.com

In the U.S. call

1-800-747-4457

Australia	08 8277 1555
Canada	1-800-465-7301
Europe	+44 (0) 113 255 5665
New Zealand	0064 9 448 1207

HUMAN KINETICS
The Information Leader in Physical Activity
P.O. Box 5076 • Champaign, IL 61825-5076 USA